Pharmaceutical Technology
Fundamental Pharmaceutics

Pharmaceutical Technology

Fundamental Pharmaceutics

Eugene L. Parrott, Ph.D.
College of Pharmacy
University of Iowa
Iowa City, Iowa

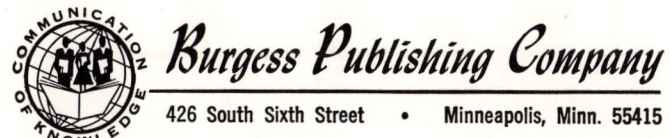

426 South Sixth Street • Minneapolis, Minn. 55415

Copyright ©1970 by Burgess Publishing Company
All rights reserved
Printed in the United States of America
Library of Congress Catalog Card Number 70-92313

Standard Book Number 8087-1628-X
Second Printing 1970

PREFACE

Pharmaceutical Technology is not an encyclopedic reference book; it is a textbook designed for the undergraduate student who has completed the required mathematics, organic chemistry, physics, and zoology. It contains the minimum pharmaceutical information and knowledge required as a prerequisite to the dispensing pharmacy course and to the proper practice of any occupational aspect of pharmacy.

Pharmaceutical Technology quantitatively correlates physicochemical theories with the characterization, development, evaluation, and preparation of dosage forms. The general objectives of courses in pharmaceutical technology are:

1. To impart a comprehension of chemical and physical principles pertinent to pharmaceutical phenomena, preparations, and problems, which can be used to understand and predict the behavior and efficacy of pharmaceuticals.

2. To develop skills and techniques upon which pharmaceutical processes are dependent through actual use of equipment, instruments, and laboratory manipulations.

3. To present professional and scientific terminology that will enable the pharmacist to express himself as an educated person as well as to read current literature.

4. To promote judgment based on critical, logical, and imaginative thought.

The discipline of pharmaceutical technology can be conveniently studied according to physical state: solids, solutions, and polyphasic and plastic systems. A schedule of three lectures and one laboratory weekly for a minimum of two semesters (preferably for three semesters) permits satisfactory coverage. For the interested teacher further discussions are found in *Proceedings Teachers' Seminar on Pharmacy 13,* 38 (1961); *American Journal of Pharmaceutical Education 27,* 198 (1963); and A. A. C. P., *Studies of a Core Curriculum,* 1968.

The objectives of a course in pharmaceutical technology cannot be achieved without a laboratory. The laboratory exercises should be designed to simultaneously correlate theory with pharmaceutical applications so that the student identifies the theory to be learned with a recognized need for it. The use of *Experimental Pharmaceutical Technology* in the laboratory facilitates the presentation of laboratory exercises concurrently with the discussion and theory presented in this book.

In the experience of the author the undergraduate student rarely reads references; thus, the traditional references are not provided. For those persons interested in additional reading, the references accompanying the figures and the references in the companion book, *Experimental Pharmaceutical Technology,* are helpful. The centimeter-gram-second system is used with few exceptions. All unspecified temperatures are expressed in the centigrade scale. More than 170 simple drawings are used to facilitate understanding of a relationship or the operation of equipment without the distraction of nonessential details. Seventy tables and 111 formulations are used to present specific examples to support the discussions. A concise review of mathematics is given in the Appendix.

It is intended that the student study this book with the concept that it contains core knowledge. The lecturer varies emphasis and presents facts in addition to this core knowledge according to his educational philosophy and experience and according to the curriculum of the individual college.

Eugene L. Parrott

CONTENTS

	Page
Preface	iii
Symbols and Physical Constants	vii

Part I. Solids

Chapter 1.	Characteristics of Particles and Powders	1
Chapter 2.	Comminution and Blending of Solids	37
Chapter 3.	Solid Pharmaceuticals	58
Chapter 4.	Properties of Solids	107

Part II. Solutions

Chapter 5.	Characteristics of Solutions	139
Chapter 6.	Dissolution Processes	158
Chapter 7.	Aqueous Pharmaceutical Solutions	170
Chapter 8.	Nonaqueous Pharmaceutical Solutions	238
Chapter 9.	Chemical Stability	250
Chapter 10.	Sterile Solutions	274

Part III. Polyphasic and Plastic Systems

Chapter 11.	Characteristics of Polyphasic Systems	295
Chapter 12.	Dispersion Processes	317
Chapter 13.	Fluid Pharmaceutical Suspensions and Emulsions	341
Chapter 14.	Plastic Pharmaceutical Suspensions and Emulsions	364
	Appendix	395
	Index	409

SYMBOLS AND PHYSICAL CONSTANTS

A	absorbance; area
Å	angstrom unit (10^{-8} cm)
C	capacitance; concentration; number of components
D	diffusion coefficient (cm^2 sec^{-1}); debye (10^{-18} esu cm)
E	energy; voltage
E_a	activation energy
F	number of degrees of freedom
G	free energy
ΔH	activation energy; heat of solution
J	joule
K	absolute temperature scale; equilibrium constant; partition coefficient
K_b	boiling-point constant (deg molal^{-1})
K_f	freezing-point constant (deg molal^{-1})
L	freezing-point constant ($L = iK_f$); specific conductance (ohm^{-1} cm^{-1})
M	molecular weight (g mole^{-1}); molarity
N	Avogadro number (6.024×10^{23} mole^{-1}); mole fraction; normality
P	number of phases; polarization; pressure
Q	flux (mass cm^{-2} sec^{-1})
R	gas constant (0.0821 liter atm mole^{-1} deg^{-1}; 1.987 cal mole^{-1} deg^{-1}; 8.315×10^7 ergs mole^{-1} deg^{-1})
S	area; solubility; specific surface
T	absolute temperature ($t + 273$)
ΔT_f	freezing-point depression
V	volume of 1 mole of a gas; volt
W	work
a	activity; radius of atom or ion
atm	atmosphere (14.7 lb in.$^{-2}$ = 760 mm of mercury)
c	concentration

cal	calorie = 4.184 absolute joules
cc	cubic centimeter (cm^3)
cm	centimeter
cp	centipoise
d	diameter
deg	degree
e	electron; electronic charge
f	force; fraction
g	acceleration of gravity (980 cm sec^{-2})
g	gram
h	height; thickness
hr	hour
i	van't Hoff factor
k	Boltzmann constant (R/N = 1.38 X 10^{-16} ergs deg^{-1} $molecule^{-1}$); reaction-rate constant
kcal	kilocalorie (1000 cal)
kg	kilogram (1000 g)
l	equivalent conductance of an ion; length
ln	2.303 log
m	mass; molality
min	minute
mμ	millimicron (10^{-7} cm)
n	number of moles; number of particles; transference number
o	as a subscript refers to variable in its pure state or its initial value
p	partial pressure
p	poise
pH	expression of hydrogen ion concentration; -log a_{H+}
pK	-log K
psi	lb $in.^{-2}$
q	flux (mass cm^{-2} sec^{-1})
r	radius
sec	second
t	centigrade temperature; time
$t_{1/2}$	half-life
v	volume
w	weight
z	valence of an ion

α (alpha)	degree of dissociation; polarizability
β (beta)	polymorphic form; beta particle; buffer capacity
γ (gamma)	activity coefficient; gamma ray; interfacial tension (dyn cm^{-1}); microgram (10^{-6} g)
Γ (capital gamma)	surface concentration
δ (delta)	inexact differential; small increment
Δ (capital delta)	a change given as final value minus initial value
ϵ (epsilon)	dielectric constant
ζ (zeta)	zeta potential
η (eta)	coefficient of viscosity (poise = dyn sec cm^{-2})
Λ (capital lambda)	equivalent conductance (cm^2 equiv^{-1} ohm^{-1})
μ (mu)	dipole moment; ionic strength; micron (10^{-4} cm)
π (pi)	osmotic pressure; surface pressure (dyn cm^{-1})
ρ (rho)	density (g cc^{-1})
σ (sigma)	standard deviation; surface energy (ergs cm^{-2})
Σ (capital sigma)	summation
ω (omega)	angular velocity (radians time^{-1})
Ω (capital omega)	ohm

Part I

Solids

1 | CHARACTERISTICS OF PARTICLES AND POWDERS

In the preparation of pharmaceuticals one is vitally concerned with the size of particles. The term "particle" is broad and encompasses a wide size range. The size inferred depends on the connotation and technology being used. The solute dissolved in a solution may be referred to as solute particles, which are molecular or ionic in size. In colloidal technology the particles under consideration consist of aggregates of molecules or ions and possess a size from 0.001 to 1 micron (1μ equals 10^{-4} cm). The solute particles in a solution follow certain behavioral patterns or laws of solutions, and the colloidal particles have their own characteristic behavior; however, certain terms and characteristics are common to both solute and colloidal particles. As particles from 1 to 10^3 μ are important in studying the characteristics of powdered drugs and dosage forms made from powdered drugs, this size of particle is used to introduce terminology common to all particulate systems.

STATISTICAL DIAMETERS OF IRREGULAR PARTICLES

Most particles in nature or as formed during grinding are irregular in shape. Since there is no known method of defining irregular particles in geometric terms, the expression of size of irregular particles becomes a matter of convention. The theory of dimensions only requires that the surface area be proportional to the square, and the volume be proportional to the cube, of a single dimension referred to as the diameter of the particle.

Various diameters have been defined in terms of spheres; to utilize these definitions with non-spherical particles a correction or shape factor is introduced. The mean surface area, S, per particle of a group of spherical particles with a mean diameter, d, is

$$S = \pi d^2$$

where π is the surface shape factor for spheres. A general equation may be written

$$S = \alpha_s d^2$$

where the surface shape factor, α_s, represents a proportionality factor for the ratio S/d^2.

Similarly, the general equation for the mean volume, V, per particle is

$$V = \alpha_v d^3$$

where the volume shape factor, α_v, represents a proportionality factor for the ratio V/d^3. For spherical particles the volume shape factor is $\pi/6$.

For a group of spherical particles the specific surface, S_v, per unit volume is equal to the total surface area of the particles divided by the total volume (see Appendix: Exponents):

$$S_v = \frac{\Sigma n \pi d^2}{\Sigma n \frac{\pi}{6} d^3} = \frac{6}{d}$$

where d is the mean diameter of the spherical particles, $\Sigma\, n$ * is the number of particles, and $\pi/(\pi/6)$ is the ratio α_s/α_v. The ratio α_s/α_v is an expression of the particle shape. Experiments have shown that this ratio is 6.1 for rounded particles and 6.4 for worn particles. It is 7.0 to 7.7 for sharp and angular particles, respectively.

The mean surface-volume diameter, d_{vs}, is used to express particle size in terms of surface area per unit volume. A unit volume of monosized particles with a diameter d_{vs} will have a total surface area identical with the surface of a unit volume of actual sample having a mean surface-volume diameter d_{vs}. The mean surface-volume diameter is used to express the size of particles in pharmaceutical phenomena, e.g., adsorption, coating, and surface degradation in suspensions, which are concerned with surface per unit weight or unit volume. The d_{vs} may be expressed in the form

$$d_{vs} = \frac{\Sigma\, nd^3}{\Sigma\, nd^2}$$

where n is the frequency or number of particles of diameter d. The value of this equation is that the shape factor does not have to be evaluated.

The specific surface, S_w, is defined as the surface area per unit weight. The relation between the two specific surfaces is

$$S_v = \rho S_w$$

where ρ is the density of the material. Substitution of the S_v term yields

$$S_w = \frac{\alpha_s}{\alpha_v} \frac{1}{\rho d_{vs}}$$

As the ratio α_s/α_v is 6 for spheres, the specific surfaces are inversely proportional to the diameter of spherical particles according to the equations

$$S_w = \frac{6}{\rho d_{vs}}$$

and

$$S_v = \frac{6}{d_{vs}}$$

---

*The symbol Σ indicates the addition or summation of all the individual values of a variable or measurement. The summation notation should include limits, and the summation of the total number of individual particles, n_i, from the first to the nth particle is correctly written

$$\sum_{i=1}^{i=n} n_i$$

In the text the subscript and limits have been omitted to simplify writing the equations. The student should use an interpretation of the simplified summation symbol to include all variables or measurements that would be reasonably and physically included in the particular discussion to which the equation is related. For example, the arithmetic mean diameter (see page 4) is defined by the equation

$$d_{av} = \frac{\sum_{i=1}^{i=n} n_i d_i}{\sum_{i=1}^{i=n} n_i}$$

and using the simplified summation symbol, the equation is written

$$d_{av} = \frac{\Sigma\, nd}{\Sigma\, n}$$

In the study of dissolution of solid particles in a solvent and in the flow of dry particulate materials, a specific shape factor may be used. If there are N particles of weight w and density ρ, based on the definition of density, the volume of an individual particle is

$$V = \frac{w}{\rho N}$$

As $V = \alpha_v d^3$, the diameter may be written

$$d = \left(\frac{1}{\alpha_v}\right)^{1/3} \left(\frac{w}{\rho N}\right)^{1/3}$$

The surface area of the individual particle is $\alpha_s d^2$; thus

$$S = \left[\alpha_s \left(\frac{1}{\alpha_v^2}\right)^{1/3}\right] \left(\frac{w}{\rho N}\right)^{2/3} = \alpha_{sv} \left(\frac{w}{\rho N}\right)^{2/3}$$

The term within the brackets is a measure of the particle shape and is known as the specific shape factor, α_{sv}. For spheres α_{sv} is 4.85 and for cubes it is 6. If the specific shape factor is greater than 6, the particles are irregular.

The particles of a powdered drug or granulation may appear uniform to the eye; however, there may be a wide variation in the size of the particles. Most of the particles will fall within a narrow range about the average particle size, but there will be some much larger and some much smaller in size.

The per cent frequencies of the various particles plotted against the mean of the size groups form a size frequency curve. The size frequency curve shown in Figure 1 is obtained by plotting the frequencies against the midgroup diameters for the 330 particles of Table I.

The frequency or percentage of total particles depends on the method of expression. For example, on a numerical or count basis as used in microscopy, 80 per cent of the particles in a sample of powder may have a diameter of 5 μ, but these particles may be only 20 per cent of the total weight as determined gravimetrically.

The size of a nonuniform powder is not completely defined by a single diameter. Any mean diameter is the diameter of a hypothetical particle that in some manner represents the total mass of the particles. Some of the statistical diameters used to express particle size will be discussed.

Some powders, such as the 330 particles given in Table I, have a distribution that produces a size frequency curve which follows a normal distribution that is symmetrical about the vertical axis. A Gaussian or normal distribution curve of this type is shown in Figure 2.

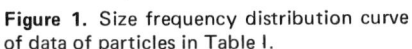

Figure 1. Size frequency distribution curve of data of particles in Table I.

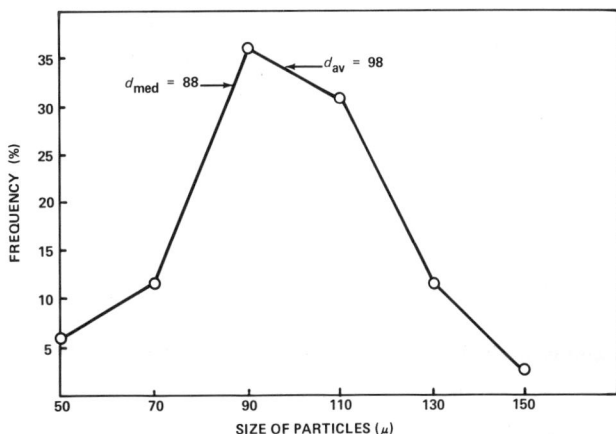

Table I Determination of the Average Diameter of 330 Particles Measured by an Optical Micrometer

Size Group (μ)	Midsize, d (μ)	Number of Particles in Each Size Group, n	nd
40-59.9	50	20	1,000
60-79.9	70	40	2,800
80-99.9	90	120	10,800
100-119.9	110	100	11,000
120-139.9	130	40	5,200
140-159.9	150	10	1,500
		$\Sigma n = 330$	$\Sigma nd = 32,300$

$$d_{av} = \frac{32,300}{330} = 98\ \mu$$

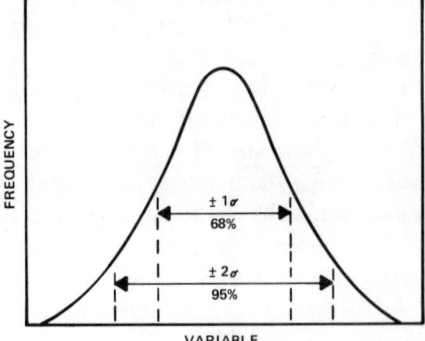

Figure 2. Normal distribution curve showing the percentage included within both ±1 and 2 standard deviations about the arithmetic mean.

In a normal probability distribution, where n is the frequency of particles of diameter d and Σn is the total number of particles, the position and shape of the size frequency curve is defined by the arithmetic mean diameter, d_{av}, and the standard deviation, σ. The d_{av} of the various particles is the sum of the diameters of the separate particles divided by the number of particles. If $n_1, n_2, \ldots, n_n$ are the number of particles having the diameters $d_1, d_2, \ldots, d_n$, then

$$d_{av} = \frac{n_1 d_1 + n_2 d_2 + \cdots + n_n d_n}{n_1 + n_2 + \cdots + n_n} = \frac{\Sigma nd}{\Sigma n} \qquad \textit{Arithmetic mean diameter}$$

The method of calculation can be illustrated by considering a group of 330 particles measured by a microscope. In Table I the size group is given in the first column, the midsize of the group is given in the second column, and the frequency or the number of particles in a size group is given in the third column.

An infinite variety of size frequency curves have a given average; therefore, an average size does not adequately characterize any sample of particles. In contrast, a size frequency distribution curve adequately describes a sample of particles because it expresses the per cent frequencies of the particles of a particular size group. The utilization in pharmacy of a size frequency curve can be illustrated by considering an injectible suspension. Excessively large particles would not flow readily through a hypodermic needle at the time of injection and would be mechanically irritating to the tissue after injection. The d_{av} of the suspended particles would not indicate if the solid were satisfactorily subdivided, because a wide size distribution with an equal number of very large and very small particles would provide an average diameter that would appear clinically acceptable. Furthermore, the flow properties of the suspension may depend on the ratios of the various size groups (see page 348). A size frequency curve would show the frequency of the size groups so that the material could be evaluated for unwanted large particles and for its flow properties.

The d_{av} may give undue weight to the smaller particles. A certain powder may contain a small weight per cent of extremely small particles but such a large numerical percentage that the calculated d_{av} is very small. Thus, the d_{av} has little physical significance; it indicates the size present in the greatest number.

The standard deviation is a special form of average deviation from the mean. The standard deviation, σ, is the root mean square of the deviation from the arithmetic mean*:

$$\sigma = \sqrt{\frac{\Sigma[n(d-d_{av})^2]}{\Sigma n}}$$

To illustrate the calculation of standard deviation, consider a sample of powder containing 151 particles that have been measured by an optical micrometer. The variable in this example is the diameter, and $(d - d_{av})$ represents the difference between the average diameter and the midsize of each size group. As shown in Table II, Σn is the total number of particles of 151.

In a normal distribution based on chance or probability, there is a 68.3 per cent probability that an item or variable chosen at random will be within $\pm 1\sigma$, and a 95.5 per cent probability that a variable picked will be within $\pm 2\sigma$ of the arithmetic mean. In powder technology, the standard deviation is a measure of the uniformity of sizes of the particles. According to statistical theory, approximately 95 per cent of the particles will have a size between $d_{av} \pm 2\sigma$.

The median is that diameter for which 50 per cent of the particles are less than the stated size. The median may be approximated by reference to the third column of Table I. It can be seen that 180 particles are smaller than 100 μ and that the median is between 80 and 100 μ. The exact value of the median can be found by plotting the percentage less (or greater) than the stated size against the particle size. The median, or 50 per cent value, as read from Figure 3 is 88 μ. The experimentally determined median and arithmetic mean for a sample are indicated in Figure 1. In a normal distribution the arithmetic mean divides the curve into two equal areas.

The mode is the value for the diameter for which the frequency curve is a maximum. If the distribution were symmetrical, the mode, mean, and median of the size frequency curve would have the same value.

If a size frequency distribution follows a normal distribution, a straight line is formed when the size frequency data are plotted on an arithmetic-probability grid. The abscissa consists of a probability

---

*For small samples the total number of items or measurements is replaced by $\Sigma n - 1$. When a single measurement is made on a sample, a rough estimate of the mean is obtained. This single measurement does not give an indication of the variability in the sample. With a second measurement there is a basis for estimating the population variability. Thus, two measurements provide one estimate of the variability of the sample. Consequently, all n values are not accessible for estimating the standard deviation, but one less than n. For small samples the standard deviation is

$$\sigma = \sqrt{\frac{\Sigma[n(d-d_{av})^2]}{\Sigma n - 1}}$$

When the number of items or measurements is large, the difference between $\Sigma n - 1$ and Σn is negligible and Σn is used in the equation.

Table II Calculation of the Standard Deviation of Particle Size Distribution of 151 Particles Measured by an Optical Micrometer

Size Group (μ)	Midsize, d (μ)	Number of Particles in Each Size Group, n	nd	$d - d_{av}$	$(d - d_{av})^2$	$n(d - d_{av})^2$
0-4.9	2.5	1	2.5	-24.24	587.5776	587.5776
5-9.9	7.5	12	90.0	-19.24	370.1776	4,442.1312
10-14.9	12.5	19	237.5	-14.24	202.7776	3,852.7744
15-19.9	17.5	24	420.0	-9.24	85.3776	2,049.0624
20-24.9	22.5	19	427.5	-4.24	17.9776	341.5744
25-29.9	27.5	19	522.5	0.76	0.5776	10.9774
30-34.9	32.5	16	520.0	5.76	33.1776	530.8416
35-39.9	37.5	15	562.5	10.76	115.7776	1,736.6640
40-44.9	42.5	12	510.0	15.76	248.3776	2,980.5312
45-49.9	47.5	8	380.0	20.76	430.9776	3,447.8208
50-54.9	52.5	2	105.0	25.76	663.5776	1,327.1552
55-59.9	57.5	0	0	30.76	946.1776	0
60-64.9	62.5	2	125.0	35.76	1,278.7776	2,557.5552
65-69.9	67.5	2	135.0	40.76	1,661.3776	3,322.7552
		$\Sigma n = 151$	$\Sigma nd = 4,037.5$			$\Sigma n(d - d_{av})^2 = 27,187.4176$

$$d_{av} = \frac{\Sigma nd}{\Sigma n} = \frac{4,037.5}{151} = 26.74 \ \mu$$

$$\sigma = \sqrt{\frac{\Sigma n(d - d_{av})^2}{\Sigma n}} = \sqrt{\frac{27,187}{151}} = 13.4 \ \mu$$

particles and powders • 7

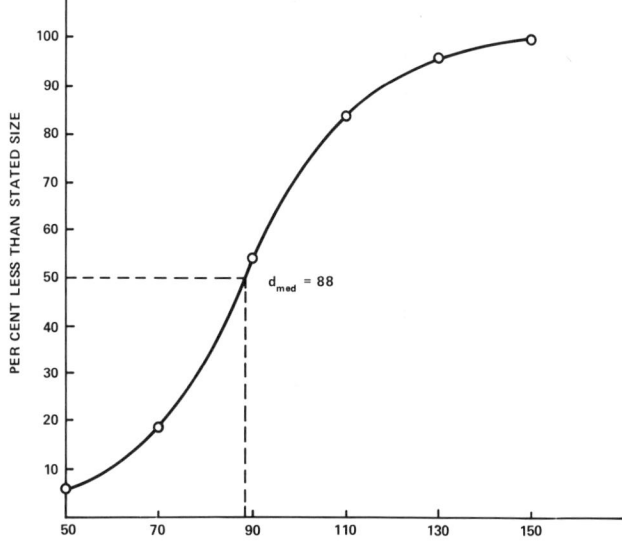

Figure 3. Determination of median size.

scale on which the cumulative percentage less (or greater) than a stated size is plotted. The ordinate consists of an arithmetic scale on which the sizes of the particles are plotted. When the data in Table I and Figure 1 are plotted on an arithmetic-probability grid as shown in Figure 4, a straight line is produced. The value of the 50 per cent size corresponds to the median. The standard deviation is

$$\sigma = 84.13 \text{ \% size} - 50 \text{ \% size}$$
$$= 50\% \text{ size} - 15.87\% \text{ size}$$

Most distributions of milled or chemically precipitated particles are asymmetrical or skewed. Many asymmetrical frequency curves have a logarithmic-probability distribution and can be made symmetrical if the logarithms of sizes are substituted for sizes. Then the geometric mean diameter, d_{geo}, and

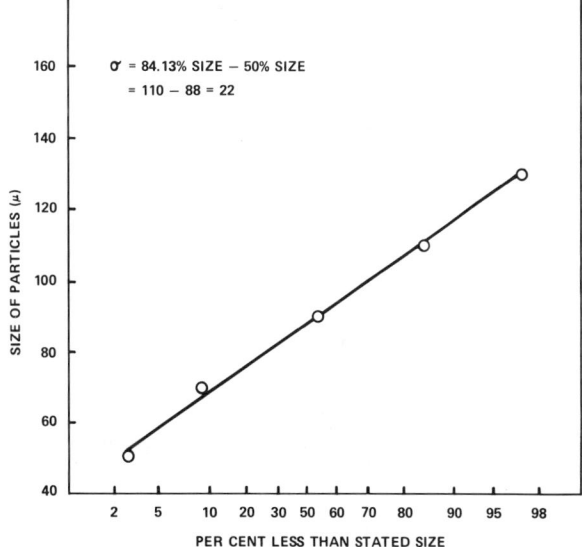

Figure 4. Arithmetic-probability plot of a normal distribution curve shown in Figure 1.

the geometric standard deviation, σ_{geo}, are determined from the logarithms (see Appendix: Logarithms) of sizes and are defined as

$$\log d_{geo} = \frac{\Sigma (n \log d)}{n}$$

and

$$\log \sigma_{geo} = \sqrt{\frac{\Sigma [n(\log d - \log d_{geo})^2]}{\Sigma n}}$$

The calculation of a geometric mean diameter is given in Table III for the same 330 particles.

Table III
Determination of the Geometric Diameter of
330 Particles Measured by an Optical Micrometer

Size Group (μ)	Midsize, d (μ)	Number of Particles in Each Size Group, n	Log d	$n \log d$
40 - 59.9	50	20	1.6990	33.980
60 - 79.9	70	40	1.8451	73.804
80 - 99.9	90	120	1.9542	234.504
100 - 119.9	110	100	2.0414	204.140
120 - 139.9	130	40	2.1139	84.556
140 - 159.9	150	10	2.1761	21.761
		$\Sigma n = 330$		$\Sigma n \log d = 652.745$

$$\log d_{geo} = \frac{652.745}{330} = 1.978 \qquad d_{geo} = 95 \, \mu$$

For a logarithmic-normal distribution d_{geo} is the diameter at which 50 per cent of the particles are smaller than a stated size. A graphic solution of these two parameters can be made by plotting the size frequency data on a special grid. The abscissa consists of a probability scale on which the cumulative percentage less (or greater) than a stated size is plotted. The ordinate consist of a logarithmic scale on which the sizes of the particles are plotted. If the size frequency curve is skewed, a straight line is formed when the data are plotted on a logarithm-probability grid. The d_{geo} is found by reading the size corresponding to a value of 50 per cent on the probability scale. Obviously, if the use of the logarithms of the diameters normalizes the distribution, the geometric mean diameter is also the median.

From the logarithm-probability plot the geometric standard deviation is

$$\sigma_{geo} = \frac{84.13\% \text{ size}}{50\% \text{ size}} = \frac{50\% \text{ size}}{15.87\% \text{ size}}$$

Based on size frequency distributions plotted on a logarithm-probability grid, the Hatch and Choate equations relate various types of diameters by the use of the geometric mean diameter and standard deviation. These statistical diameters are a function of the size and numerical frequency of the particles for a given size. The size is influenced by the shape of the size frequency curve, and therefore the particle size is expressed explicitly in terms of the mean diameter and the standard deviation. The

Hatch and Choate equations for expressing various diameters based on a numbers distribution, such as obtain by microscopy, are

$$\underline{\log d_{av}} = \log d_{geo} + 1.1513 \log^2 \sigma_{geo} \quad \text{\textit{Arithmetic mean diameter}}$$
$$\underline{\log d_s} = \log d_{geo} + 2.3026 \log^2 \sigma_{geo} \quad \text{\textit{mean surface diameter}}$$
$$\underline{\log d_v} = \log d_{geo} + 3.4539 \log^2 \sigma_{geo} \quad \text{\textit{mean volume diameter}}$$
$$\log d_{vs} = \log d_{geo} + 5.7565 \log^2 \sigma_{geo} \quad \text{\textit{mean-volume-surface diameter}}$$

In sieving and sedimentation analysis the particles are separated into weight fractions of various size; thus, a weight distribution is obtained. Fortunately, there is a set of Hatch and Choate equations that relate weight distribution data to statistical diameters:

$$\underline{\log d_{geo}} = \log d'_{geo} - 6.9078 \log^2 \sigma'_{geo} \quad \text{\textit{geometric mean diameter}}$$
$$\log d_{av} = \log d'_{geo} - 5.7565 \log^2 \sigma'_{geo}$$
$$\log d_s = \log d'_{geo} - 4.6052 \log^2 \sigma'_{geo}$$
$$\log d_v = \log d'_{geo} - 3.4539 \log^2 \sigma'_{geo}$$
$$\log d_{vs} = \log d'_{geo} - 1.1513 \log^2 \sigma'_{geo}$$

The prime on the geometric mean diameter and the standard deviation signifies a weight distribution. The geometric standard deviation for a weight and a numbers distribution are almost identical. When the geometric mean diameter and the standard deviation have been determined, the above equations permit the computation of various statistical diameters from a number or a weight distribution analysis.

Another statistical diameter is the harmonic mean diameter. The harmonic mean diameter, d_h, of a series of particles is the reciprocal of the arithmetic mean of the reciprocals of the diameters:

$$\frac{1}{d_h} = \frac{\frac{1}{d_1} + \frac{1}{d_2} + \cdots + \frac{1}{d_n}}{n_1 + n_2 + \cdots + n_n} = \frac{1}{\Sigma n} \Sigma \frac{n}{d}$$

The calculation of the harmonic mean diameter for 330 particles is given in Table IV. The harmonic mean diameter is sometimes used because of the inverse relationship between specific surface and diameter. A comparison of various statistical diameters for 330 particles is shown in Table V.

Table IV
Determination of the Harmonic Mean Diameter of
330 Particles Measured by an Optical Micrometer

Size Group (μ)	Midsize, d (μ)	Number of Particles in Each Size Group, n	$\frac{n}{d}$
40-59.9	50	20	0.4000
60-79.9	70	40	0.5714
80-99.9	90	120	1.3333
100-119.9	110	100	0.9091
120-139.9	130	40	0.3076
140-159.9	150	10	0.0667
		$\Sigma n = 330$	$\Sigma \frac{n}{d} = 3.5881$

$$\frac{1}{d_h} = \frac{1}{330} \times 3.5881 \qquad d_h = 92\ \mu$$

Table V Résumé of Statistical Diameters of a Distribution of 330 Particles Measured by an Optical Micrometer

Midsize, d (μ)	Number of Particles in Each Size Group, n	nd	nd^2	nd^3
50	20	1,000	50,000	2,500,000
70	40	2,800	196,000	13,720,000
90	120	10,800	972,000	87,480,000
110	100	11,000	1,210,000	133,100,000
130	40	5,200	676,000	87,880,000
150	10	1,500	275,000	33,750,000
	$\Sigma n = 330$	$\Sigma nd = 32{,}300$	$\Sigma nd^2 = 3{,}329{,}000$	$\Sigma nd^3 = 358{,}430{,}000$

$$d_{av} = \frac{\Sigma nd}{\Sigma n} = \frac{32{,}300}{330} = 98\ \mu \qquad d_v = \sqrt[3]{\frac{\Sigma nd^3}{\Sigma n}} = \sqrt[3]{\frac{358{,}430{,}000}{330}} = 102.8\ \mu$$

$$d_s = \sqrt{\frac{\Sigma nd^2}{\Sigma n}} = \sqrt{\frac{3{,}329{,}000}{330}} = 100\ \mu \qquad d_{vs} = \frac{\Sigma nd^3}{\Sigma nd^2} = \frac{358{,}430{,}000}{3{,}329{,}000} = 107.7\ \mu$$

The surface area and volume of irregular particles are related to the shapes of the size frequency curves. Small particles have a greater specific surface than larger particles. Thus, from a surface consideration the finer particles contribute more in proportion to their number than the coarser particles. A greater emphasis is placed on the effect of the smaller particles if a surface diameter is used instead of d_{av}. The surface area is proportional to the square of the size; thus, the surface area of the average particle in a sample of powder is

$$S = \alpha_s \frac{\Sigma nd^2}{\Sigma n} = \alpha_s d_s^2$$

The mean surface diameter, d_s, is

$$d_s = \left(\frac{\Sigma nd^2}{\Sigma n}\right)^{1/2}$$

Similarly, the volume of an irregular particle is proportional to the cube of its diameter; thus, the volume of the average particle in a sample of powder is

$$V = \alpha_v \frac{\Sigma nd^3}{\Sigma n} = \alpha_v d_v^3$$

and the mean volume diameter, d_v, is defined as

$$d_v = \left(\frac{\Sigma nd^3}{\Sigma n}\right)^{1/3}$$

Both d_s and d_v are functions of d_{geo} and σ_{geo}. It is possible for different distributions to have the same value of d_s and d_v; however, if the size is defined in terms of d_{geo} and σ_{geo}, only one size frequency curve is defined. If these two parameters are known, the percentage of particles below or above a stated size can be determined.

MEASUREMENT OF PARTICLE SIZE

Microscopic Method

In the microscopic method the average diameter of a particulate system is obtained by measuring the particles at random along a given fixed line. As these particles lie in a random manner, their diameters are measured with equal frequency in every direction; therefore, they may be considered as being replaceable by spherical particles of the same diameter d.

To provide statistically sound data a minimum of 200 particles should be measured. With pharmaceutical powders measurement is usually carried out by a microscope having a filar micrometer eyepiece or an image-splitting measuring eyepiece.

The eyepiece of the optical micrometer has a cross hair which is actuated by a calibrated micrometer drum. The cross hair is alined with one edge of the particle and the micrometer drum reading is taken. The cross hair is moved to the opposite edge of the particle and the micrometer drum reading is taken. The difference between the two readings is the measure of the particle length. The micrometer drum is calibrated with a stage micrometer so that the readings may be expressed in any units desired. A calibrated stage micrometer is necessary to calibrate the optical micrometer because the magnification is not equal to the product of the nominal magnification of the objective and the eyepiece.

The microscopic method is useful in the size range 0.5 to 100 μ. The diameter obtained by this technique is of statistical interest only, as it is two-dimensional, so the shape factor cannot be computed. More useful diameters for studying pharmaceutical systems are those related to weight, surface, or volume of the particles.

Method of Sieves

The simplest method of measuring the average size of particles is to use standard sieves. Sieves are made of wire mesh with openings of known size. The term "mesh" is used to denote the number of openings per linear inch.

Conventionally, sieves have square openings. With a square opening with a side l, a needle-shaped crystal may pass diagonally if its dimensions do not exceed $l\sqrt{2}$. The average size of a particle passing through one screen and retained on another can only be approximately determined from the size of the openings, because size separation depends on the shape of the particles and how they pass through the opening. For example, a needle-shaped crystal longer than $l\sqrt{2}$ will pass through a sieve if it is oriented with its long axis perpendicular to the sieve. Since a particle presenting its smallest dimension may pass through the sieve, the particles classified by sieves will have a somewhat broad distribution of sizes.

Standard sieves are those that have been calibrated so that they may be used for size determination. Although there are several sieve series, the most commonly used series in pharmacy is the U.S. Sieve Series shown in Table VI.

In determining particle size by the use of sieves, a nest of sieves with the coarsest on top is placed on a shaker and the powder sample is introduced onto the upper sieve. The material is classified as having passed through one sieve and being retained on the adjacent finer sieve. A diameter of the particles may be considered as the size of the opening in the larger or finer sieve, or as the size of the arithmetic or geometric mean of the openings of the two sieves. Whichever size is choosen, it should be stated and used throughout the study. The limit for the use of sieves in measuring particle size is 44 μ.

The diameter of particles that pass a 40-mesh sieve and are retained on a 60-mesh sieve (expressed 40/60) may be defined in terms of the larger sieve, i.e., 0.42 mm. The same particles might be expressed as the arithmetic mean of the openings of the two sieves, i.e., $(0.42 + 0.25)/2$ or 0.335 mm. The size of the particles could also be expressed as the geometric average of the two sieve openings, i.e., $(0.42 \times 0.25)^{1/2}$ or 0.324 mm.

Actually the material varies in size and none of the aforementioned expressions indicates the true mean size of the material. Particles of a given size might be found on several sieves. However, by using a uniform procedure and treatment of data a valid distribution curve may be obtained, as the particles are actually classified in subgroups with a limited range of size.

Table VI Nominal Dimensions, Permissible Variations, and Limits for Wire Diameter of U. S. Sieve Series

| Size | | Sieve Opening | Per Cent Allowable | Wire |
Microns	Number	(mm)	Variation in Average Opening	Diameter (mm)
5,660	3½	5.66	3	1.28-1.90
4,760	4	4.76	3	1.14-1.68
4,000	5	4.00	3	1.00-1.47
3,360	6	3.36	3	0.87-1.32
2,830	7	2.83	3	0.80-1.20
2,380	8	2.38	3	0.74-1.10
2,000	10	2.00	3	0.68-1.00
1,680	12	1.68	3	0.62-0.90
1,410	14	1.41	3	0.56-0.80
1,190	16	1.19	3	0.50-0.70
1,000	18	1.00	5	0.43-0.62
840	20	0.84	5	0.38-0.55
710	25	0.71	5	0.33-0.48
590	30	0.59	5	0.29-0.42
500	35	0.50	5	0.26-0.37
420	40	0.42	5	0.23-0.33
350	45	0.35	5	0.20-0.29
297	50	0.297	5	0.170-0.253
250	60	0.250	5	0.149-0.220
210	70	0.210	5	0.130-0.187
177	80	0.177	6	0.114-0.154
149	100	0.149	6	0.096-0.125
125	120	0.125	6	0.079-0.103
105	140	0.105	6	0.063-0.087
88	170	0.088	6	0.054-0.073
74	200	0.074	6	0.045-0.061
62	230	0.062	7	0.039-0.052
53	270	0.053	7	0.035-0.046
44	325	0.044	7	0.031-0.040
37	400	0.037	7	0.023-0.035

When a powder is passed through a series of standard sieves and the amount of material retained on each sieve is determined, a weight size distribution of material is obtained. Such a size analysis of boric acid granules is given in Table VII and the size distribution curve is plotted in Figure 5.

Table VII Size Weight Distribution of 96.0 g of Boric Acid Granules

Sieve Number (Passed/Retained)	Arithmetic Mean of Openings (mm)	Weight Retained (g)	Per Cent Retained	(Per Cent Retained) × (Mean of Opening)
10/20	1.420	0.81	0.84	1.1928
20/40	0.630	23.60	24.58	15.4854
40/60	0.335	52.30	54.49	18.2541
60/80	0.214	13.75	14.32	3.0645
80/100	0.163	4.72	4.92	0.8020
100/120	0.137	0.82	0.85	0.1164
		96.00	100.00	38.9152

$$d_{av} = \frac{\Sigma \text{(per cent retained)} \times \text{(average size)}}{100} = \frac{38.91}{100} = 0.389 \text{ mm}$$

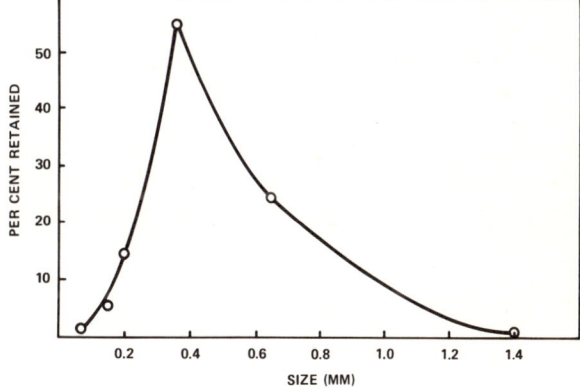

Figure 5. Size-weight distribution for 96.0 g of boric acid granules.

For distributions that follow the normal-probability or logarithm-probability law, Hatch extended the basic size distribution equations to apply to weight distribution curves in sieve analysis. If cumulative per cent by weight is plotted on the probability scale against the logarithm of the mean size opening of two adjacent sieves, the geometric mean diameter, d'_{geo}, and the geometric standard deviation can be graphically evaluated (see page 8). Knowing these values the relation between number and weight distributions can be calculated by the equations

$$\log d_{av} = \log d'_{geo} - 5.7565 \log^2 \sigma_{geo}$$
$$\log d_s = \log d'_{geo} - 4.6052 \log^2 \sigma_{geo}$$
$$\log d_v = \log d'_{geo} - 3.4535 \log^2 \sigma_{geo}$$
$$\log d_{vs} = \log d'_{geo} - 1.1513 \log^2 \sigma_{geo}$$

Sedimentation Method

For particles of subsieve size, such as one is often concerned with in pharmacy, the sedimentation method is based on the Stokes equation. The powder to be measured is suspended in a liquid in which the material is not soluble. The suspension is placed in a calibrated pipet from which samples may be drawn from a fixed depth at various times. These samples are evaporated to dryness and the residue weighed.

Each sample withdrawn has a smaller particle size than that corresponding to the settling velocity, because all particles of larger size will have fallen below the level of the tip of the pipet. The effective, or Stokes, diameter is calculated by the Stokes equation,

$$d = \sqrt{\frac{18h\eta}{(\rho_i - \rho_e)gt}}$$

where η is the viscosity of the suspending liquid in poises, h the distance between the liquid surface and the tip of the pipet when the sample is drawn, $(\rho_i - \rho_e)$ the difference in density between the particle and the suspending medium, g the gravitational constant, and t the time in seconds from the start of the measurements.

From the weight of the dried samples the percentages by weight of the original sample are calculated. The data are plotted with the calculated particle size as the abscissa and the percentage by weight as the ordinate. From this smooth curve, the percentage by weight of any particle size in the sample may be found.

In utilizing the sedimentation method to measure the size of irregular particles, one should realize that the diameter obtained is a relative size equivalent to that of a sphere having the same settling rate. The shape factor will affect the rate of settling; in general, the greater the irregularity and the deviation from a spherical shape, the slower the rate of settling will be.

The mathematical characterization of sedimentation may be complex. In utilizing the Stokes equation, it is assumed that the particles to be measured are initially uniformly distributed and that they fall independently of each other. These assumptions are valid for dilute suspensions; however, if the concentration exceeds 5 per cent, the particles begin to interact with possible coagulation. It is common practice not to exceed a 2 per cent concentration to ensure that there is no interaction among the particles.

Elutriation Method

The elutriation method of particle size measurement is the reverse of the sedimentation method. Air is introduced into the lower end of a column containing the sample to be measured. At the upper end of the column there is a filter to collect the material. Air enters the column at a known velocity and carries upward with it particles, smaller than a certain size, which are collected on the filter and weighed. The method is based on the fact that an air column moving at a certain velocity is capable of supporting only particles smaller than a certain size, and as the velocity is increased, larger particles are airborne to the filter.

The size frequency curve is drawn by plotting the weight of particles less than a stated size against the particle size.

Centrifugal Method

Centrifuging is used only for the determination of size of very fine particles or high-molecular-weight polymers. Essentially, the diameter may be calculated by the Stokes equation, with the gravitational constant replaced by the centrifugal acceleration, $\omega^2 x$, where ω is the angular velocity in radians per unit time and x the distance of the particle from the center of rotation.

Using the symbols as previously defined, the diameter is given by

$$d = \frac{6}{\omega}\sqrt{\frac{\eta \log(R_2/R_1)}{2t(\rho_i - \rho_e)}}$$

where R_2 is the distance from the axis of rotation to the bottom of the centrifuge tube and R_1 the distance from the axis of rotation to the meniscus of the suspension.

PACKING AND FLOW OF POWDERS

The size of container required to hold a given weight of granular or powdered drug depends on the way in which the particulate material will pack. In production of compressed tablets, the manner in which the granulation flows through the tablet machine will determine the uniformity of the finished tablets. The efficiency of automatic filling apparatus in packaging powders and granules is dependent on the flow and packing properties of the material being packaged. An understanding of packing arrangement and the flow of particles is important in many other pharmaceutical processes.

Systematic Packing of Spheres

Closest Packing. Packing systems are defined for spheres of uniform size. In Figure 6 the rhombohedral arrangement is formed when the spheres are piled in a triangular pyramid in which the top sphere rests in the hollow formed by the three immediately below it. The three spheres in the second row rest on six spheres in the third row, and so on.

This arrangement is known as closest packing because the greatest number of uniform-sized spheres can be packed into a given volume by the rhombohedral arrangement. The resulting pore or void arrangement can be seen by studying Figures 6 and 7, which have identical symbols. The relative frequency of the various types of pores are

3 rhombus : 3 square : 2 triangle

and, as shown in Figure 7, the angles between the particles are 120, 90, and 60° for the rhombus, square, and triangle, respectively.

A unit cell is the smallest portion of any packing which provides a complete picture of the packing arrangement. With closest packing, if d is the diameter of the spherical particle, the volume of the unit cell is $0.71d^3$ and the volume of the void is $0.18d^3$. There is a continuous, tortuous pore within the space bounded by lines P and P' of Figure 6.

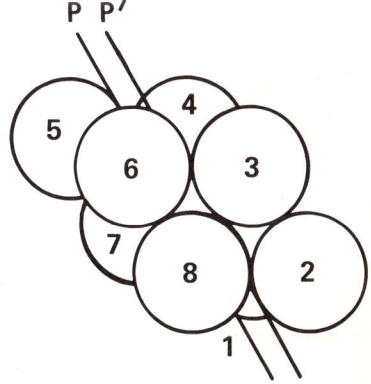

Figure 6. Closest packing or rhombohedral arrangement of uniform spherical particles.

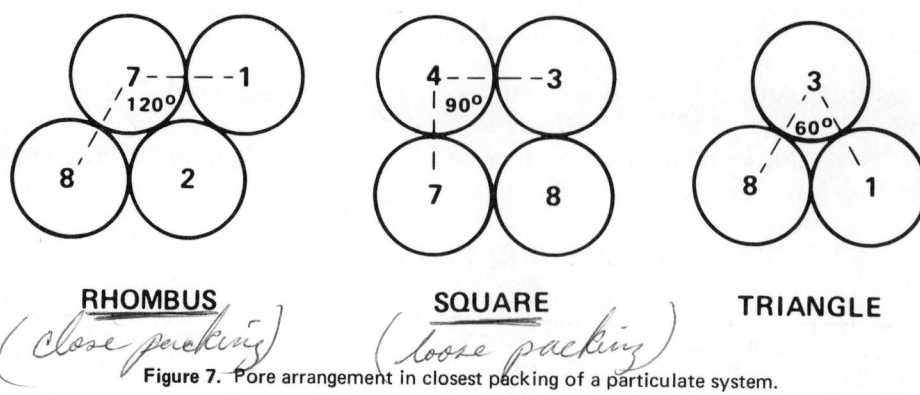

RHOMBUS (close packing)   **SQUARE** (loose packing)   **TRIANGLE**

Figure 7. Pore arrangement in closest packing of a particulate system.

Figure 8 shows how this continuous pore arises in closest packing. The solid-line spheres represent the first layer and the dashed-line spheres represent spheres lying in the depressions formed by the first layer. Each depression into which a sphere fits is marked D. Each cell so formed is a closed tetrahedral cell.

There is a second set of tetrahedral cells, T, formed by spheres in the first layer, fitting into three spheres immediately above in the second layer. The cells R are formed by six spheres; they are rhombohedral. Thus, the depressions formed by R cells are not occupied and form a continuous, twisted pore or channel through the closest packing arrangement.

Cubical Packing. The cubical (most open) packing of uniform spheres occurs when they are piled so that each lies immediately above the other on a rectangular base arrangement. In cubical packing the volume of the unit cell is d^3, and the volume of the void is $0.48d^3$.

In cubical packing each sphere is surrounded by six other spheres, and the porosity is 47.64 per cent. In closest packing each sphere is surrounded by 12 other spheres and the porosity is 25.95 per cent. Between these two theoretical extremes there are possible intermediate arrangements of packing of uniform spheres that produce any porosity from 25.95 to 47.64 per cent. In real particulate systems there are also particles of various sizes which will slip between the larger particles and further decrease the void space, so that almost any degree of porosity of less than 26 per cent is possible.

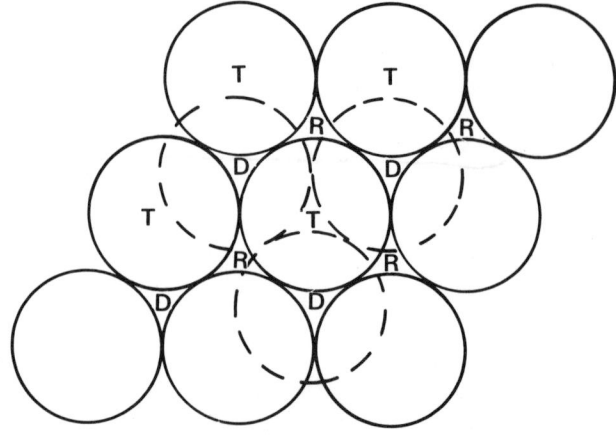

Figure 8. Closest packing system, illustrating the tetrahedral cells formed by spheres designated as D and T and rhombohedral cells designated as R. The depressions R form a continuous pore.

Terminology

Porosity and Density. In real particulate systems, void or porosity cannot be calculated, but they must be experimentally determined. Porosity is the per cent of void space; it is the void multiplied by 100. Void may be calculated in terms of measurement of true volume, V, and bulk volume, V_{bulk}, of the material:

$$\text{void} = \frac{V_{bulk} - V}{V_{bulk}} = \frac{\text{void volume}}{\text{bulk volume}}$$

True volume refers to the volume occupied by the solid substances exclusive of space larger than the spacing between molecules, ions, or atoms in the crystal lattice of the solid. Bulk volume is the total volume occupied by a powder or by particles when placed in a container; it includes the true volume plus the volume of the internal pores and the volume of the spaces between the particles.

Although the bulk volume may vary with the treatment of a powder, satisfactory measurements may be made by means of a standardized procedure. A 50-ml sample of the powder is passed through a 20-mesh sieve and placed into a 100-ml graduated cylinder. The cylinder is dropped onto a wood surface three times from a height of 1 in. at 2-second intervals. The volume in milliliters is the bulk volume.

Apparent density, ρ_a, is obtained by dividing the weight of the sample by the bulk volume; it is the weight of a unit volume of packing. True density, ρ, refers to the density of the substance, excluding the entire pore volume larger than the spacings of molecular or atomic dimensions that exist in the crystal lattice of the solid.

The true density of magnesium carbonate is 3.0 g cc^{-1}. By the technique described above it is found that 3.5 g of light magnesium carbonate occupies 50 ml. The true volume of the sample is 1.1667 ml. The void space is

$$\text{void} = \frac{V_{bulk} - V}{V_{bulk}} = \frac{50 - 1.1667}{50} = 0.977$$

The porosity of this batch of light magnesium carbonate is 97 per cent.

The void space may be calculated by the use of densities. The previous equation may be written in the form

$$\text{void} = \frac{V_{bulk}}{V_{bulk}} - \frac{V}{V_{bulk}} = 1 - \frac{V}{V_{bulk}}$$

and as $\rho = w/V$, w/ρ may be substituted for V:

$$\text{void} = 1 - \frac{w/\rho}{w/\rho_a} = 1 - \frac{\rho_a}{\rho}$$

Porosity is a characteristic of powders, and in real powders extreme values range from 90 to 10 per cent porosity, although no single material has so great a range. Theoretically, the void for a system of spherical particles is independent of the size; in real powders the void is generally increased as the particle size is decreased. These deviations from ideal packing arise in a real powder because the particles are not of a single size and are not spherical. In addition to these geometric considerations of size and shape, there may be electrostatic interaction between the particles that further affects the porosity.

In pharmacy the terms "light" and "heavy" are applied to powders to indicate the fineness of subdivision. A light powder is one that has a very fine particle size with a resulting low apparent density and a large bulk volume. A heavy powder, relative to a light powder, indicates that another form of the substance has a greater apparent density and a smaller bulk volume than the light form. If a sample of heavy magnesium carbonate had an apparent density of 0.39 g cc^{-1}, the porosity would be

$$\text{porosity} = 100 \left(1 - \frac{\rho_a}{\rho}\right) = 100 \left(1 - \frac{0.39}{3.0}\right) = 87\%$$

Bulkiness. Bulkiness is defined as the reciprocal of apparent density. Usually bulkiness increases with decreasing particle size. Mixtures of different-sized particles decrease bulkiness by making more efficient use of the void space.

Reduction of bulk is advisable for ease of packaging and for economy of shipment. In the preparation of some chemicals and drugs, the control of temperature, concentration, and rate of crystallization may yield a more dense mass. High-speed milling may entrap air and increase the bulk of the ground powder. Entrained air may at times be removed by placing the powder under a vacuum or by moistening the powder with a limited volume of solvent and drying in warm air. Occasionally a bulky powder is compressed by rollers or a tablet machine and then ground to reduce bulk.

In the preparation of capsules, a size must be used that can be conveniently swallowed by the patient. If the dose or weight of medicinal ingredients is too bulky to be placed in a capsule that can easily be swallowed and it cannot be decreased in bulk by one of the above methods, the medication may be administered in a liquid form as a suspension or solution. In the manufacture of compressed tablets the granulation is compressed with high forces to markedly decrease the void or bulk. Most compressed tablets have a void of less than 0.1.

Angle of Repose. If a powder is poured freely onto a plane surface it forms a cone that has a constant angle between the surface of the pile and the horizontal plane. This angle is known as the angle of repose, and for most pharmaceutical powders it ranges from 34 to 48°. The angle depends on the mutual friction between the particles. With an increase in friction, there is an increase in angle of repose. As the irregularity of the particles becomes greater, the friction and the resistance to flow is increased.

In preparing compressed tablets, the granulation to be compressed must flow easily and uniformly through the tablet machine to produce tablets of uniform weight. The angle of repose permits evaluation of the granulation before compression is attempted; a small value for the angle of repose indicates that the granulation will flow readily. As spherical particles flow most easily, it is desirable to have tablet granules approach a spherical shape.

The angle of repose of tablet granules increases with a decrease in particle size, as illustrated in Figure 9. In order that the tablet granules flow properly, an excessive amount of fines or very small particles is generally avoided in tablet production.

Rate of Flow. A rotary tablet machine may compress 5000 tablets per minutes; a capsule filler may fill and cap 650 hard gelatin capsules per minute; an auger filler may deliver powder or granules into a hundred containers per minute. With the use of such high-speed machines, which require a high rate of flow, it seems that a measurement of flow rate is more meaningful in evaluation of the mobility of a formulation than the repose angle, which is a static characteristic of a particulate system. The movement of a powder or granulation is more appropriately expressed in a dynamic term, the rate of flow from a flowometer. As shown in Figure 9 there is poor, if any, correlation of repose angle and rate of flow. The uniformity of movement may be determined by plotting the weight flowing from the flowometer against time. If the plot produces a straight line, the flow and movement is uniform. If the plot produces a wavy line, the flow is not uniform and the movement through the equipment may not be satisfactory.

The rate of flow may be used to evaluate the effectiveness of a lubricant. For example, the flow rate and the repose angle of a batch of aspirin crystals are 11.2 g sec^{-1} and 40.3°, respectively. When 1 per cent talc is added, the flow rate and repose angle are 10.51 g sec^{-1} and 41.3°. When ¼ per cent magnesium stearate is added, the flow rate and repose angle are 12.6 g sec^{-1} and 36.8°. The increase in rate of flow and the decrease in angle of repose indicate that magnesium stearate is a good lubricant.

particles and powders • 19

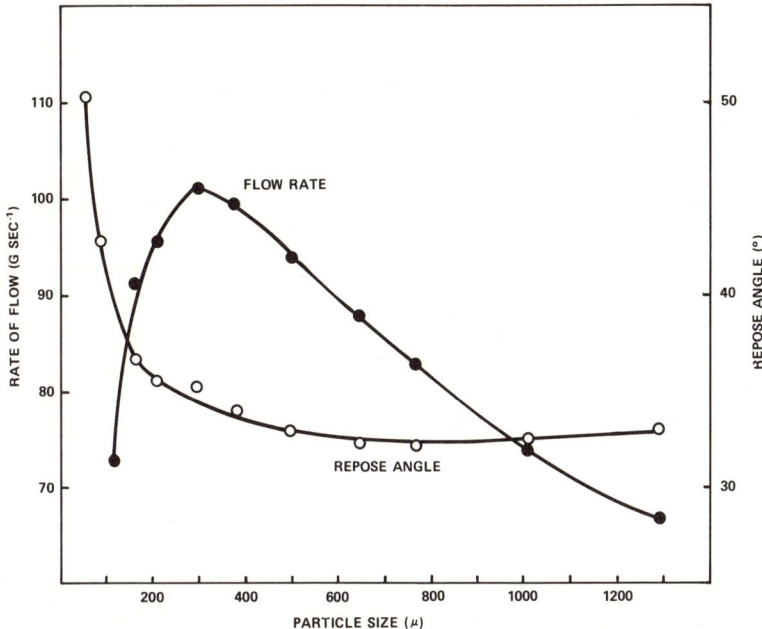

Figure 9. Flow rate and repose angle of granules for a sodium chloride tablet as a function of particle size.

PHENOMENA INFLUENCED BY PARTICLE SIZE
Chemical and Electrical Activity

The time required for a reaction to occur is influenced by the particle size of the reactants. In the solid state, a chemical change is not as rapid as in the gaseous or liquid state. If the time required for a reaction is to be shortened, the solids are ground or triturated to a small particle size. The small particles present a greater specific surface, which increases the number of reaction sites between the reacting molecules.

Fine particles suspended in the air may be explosive if the concentration of particles and the temperature are optimum. After ignition the flame is propagated through adjacent particles, resulting in an explosion. The chemical nature of the dust, the concentration of dust and air, the ignition temperature, and the particle size affect the flammability.

With a decrease in particle size and the accompanying increase in surface area, the flammability will increase. Such commonly milled pharmaceutical adjuvants as starch and sugar are not generally thought to be dangerous, yet without proper dust removal the airborne dust may be ignited by a spark.

On occasion a large-sized particle is preferred in pharmaceuticals. Vitamin A readily undergoes atmospheric oxidation. A highly stable preparation of vitamin A acetate is available in the granular form. The vitamin is enveloped in a matrix of gelatin plasticized by syrup. The use of a granule serves a dual purpose. The spherical granule is free flowing and the granule presents less surface and fewer reaction sites to the atmosphere than a powdered preparation.

When a solid is milled to a very small particle size, the particles frequently acquire an electrostatic charge. The electrification of the particles may be produced by friction or contact of dissimilar materials. The electrification of particles may also be produced by interparticulate friction. The charge developed in the latter case results from the difference in size and mass of the particles.

It is assumed that all particles carry a rather loosely bound layer of negatively charged particles of the nature of "free" electrons. If two particles of equal mass collide, there will be an equal exchange of negative charge. If a large particle collides with a small particle, the smaller particle is accelerated so fast that it loses its attached charge, and the amount of charge is gained by the larger particle.

This localized electron deficiency and excess exerts a profound influence on the behavior of small particles. The electrostatic force is so small that it has not been measured, but it is observed and expressed in terms of the behavior of the particles.

For example, powdered plastic that will flow freely in an uncharged state can acquire a charge by agitation. This mechanical work upsets the neutral balance of electron state on the surface of the particles. Immediately the mass ceases to flow freely. The particles adhere and agglomerate. With time, the attracting forces holding the agglomerate together tend to relax somewhat. Any factor that promotes electron flow will speed relaxation.

The electrostatic attraction for these particles may cause them to adhere to the walls of containers and to equipment. This nuisance may often be avoided by increasing the relative humidity. The beneficial effect of high humidity is mainly the result of a film adsorbed on the surface of the solid material. The moisture reduces the tendency to separate the charges and aids in the dissipation of the electrical charges.

Adsorption

The properties of the surface layer of a substance are different than those of the bulk phase. As the degree of subdivision of a material is increased, the specific surface area is increased and the surface phenomena become more pronounced in their effect. The traditional illustration of the large increase in surface accompanying subdivision is the consideration of a cube of material 1 cm on edge and with a total surface of 6 cm^2. If the cube is cut into cubes 1 μ on edge, the total surface area is 60,000 cm^2. The large surface of the small cubes presents many more reaction sites and makes the surface properties highly significant.

Adsorption occurs in pharmaceuticals. Granules, powders, and compressed tablets adsorb atmospheric moisture. The flow properties of powders and granules are affected by moisture; usually as the amount of moisture adsorbed is increased the flow is slowed. The adsorbed moisture may react chemically with the drug, causing degradation. The adsorption of a layer of molecules from the atmosphere may prevent contact between the surface of the solid and a solvent, so that dissolution does not occur readily. Recently, it has been realized that in mixing the finely divided ingredients in preparing solid formulations, the medicinal compound may be adsorbed upon a therapeutically inert diluent or adjuvant with an alteration in the clinical availability of the drug.

Surface Tension and Surface Energy. An interface is a boundary between two phases; a surface is an interface between a liquid and a gas or a solid and a gas. At the surface of a liquid the molecules are subjected to an unbalanced force of molecular attraction, as the molecules of the liquid tend to pull those at the surface inward. Owing to this unbalanced force, a liquid tends to maintain a minimum surface area. This unbalanced force is known as surface tension. If sulfur is sprinkled on the surface of water, even though the density of sulfur is greater than water, surface tension will support the powdered sulfur on the surface of the water.

Surface tension is the force acting perpendicular to a unit length of a line in the surface. As shown in Figure 10, surface tension may be visualized by considering a movable bar on a wire frame against which a liquid film is stretched. When a force, f, in dynes is exerted on the length of the bar, l, in centimeters, the surface tension, γ, is

$$\gamma = \frac{f}{2l}$$

The factor 2 arises because there are two liquid surfaces on any film. Surface tension is expressed in dyn cm^{-1}.

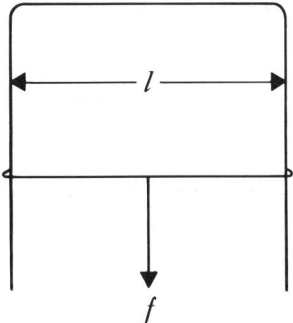

Figure 10. Dupré frame used to define surface tension.

If the length l is 10 cm and the mass required to break a film of liquid on the frame is 0.75 g, the surface tension is

$$\gamma = \frac{0.75 \text{ g} \times 980 \text{ cm sec}^{-2}}{2 \times 10 \text{ cm}} = 36.75 \text{ dyn cm}^{-1}$$

If the wire is pulled 10 cm, the work done in increasing the area 100 cm² is equal to the surface tension multiplied by the increase in surface area, ΔA,

$$W = \gamma \, \Delta A = 36.75 \text{ dyn cm}^{-1} \times 100 \text{ cm}^2 = 3675 \text{ ergs}$$

Thus, the energy expended in increasing the surface by 1 cm² or the energy per unit area is 3675/100 or 36.75 ergs cm⁻². Since 1 dyn cm⁻¹ is equal to 1 erg cm⁻², the surface tension in dyn cm⁻¹ is numerically equal to the energy in ergs cm⁻².

Neither the surface tension nor the surface energy of a solid has been directly measured; however, both are important factors in the adsorption or accumulation of molecules of a vapor at a gas-solid interface.

Vapor-Solid Adsorption. When a molecule of a vapor phase approaches the surface of a solid, it is attracted by the unbalanced force of the surface molecules. If the interaction force is sufficiently great, the vapor is adsorbed or held on the surface. The substance that is adsorbed is known as the adsorbate. The extent of adsorption of a vapor by a solid depends on the surface area and the chemical nature of the adsorbent, i.e., the substance used to adsorb the vapor. Charcoal is a good adsorbent because the cellular nature of the vegetable or animal material from which it is prepared provides a large surface. Silica gel is widely used in chromatography because the many pores and crevices in its fine particles provide a large surface and a large capacity for adsorption.

Adsorption depends on the temperature and the pressure of the vapor phase. The relation between the amount of vapor physically adsorbed on a gram of solid and the equilibrium pressure or concentration at a constant temperature is known as an adsorption isotherm. In general there are five types of adsorption isotherms. The type I adsorption isotherm as shown in Figure 11 is for a monomolecular layer of adsorbed vapor and is described by the Freundlich and Langmuir equations. Other isotherms shown in Figure 12 represent the adsorption of multimolecular layers.

Adsorption may be a physical or a chemical process. In chemical adsorption (chemisorption) the adsorbate is strongly held to the surface of the solid by a chemical reaction, and for practical consideration chemisorption is irreversible. The energy involved in chemisorption is considerably greater than in physical adsorption. In chemisorption a surface compound is formed and no more than a monomolecular layer is adsorbed. Chemisorption may be a stepwise process in which the vapor molecules undergo physical adsorption and then diffuse over the surface of the solid to reaction or chemisorption sites.

Physical adsorption, or van der Waals, adsorption, involves weak interaction between a solid and a vapor. Since the interaction is weak, the process is reversible; most of the vapor can be removed

22 • particles and powders

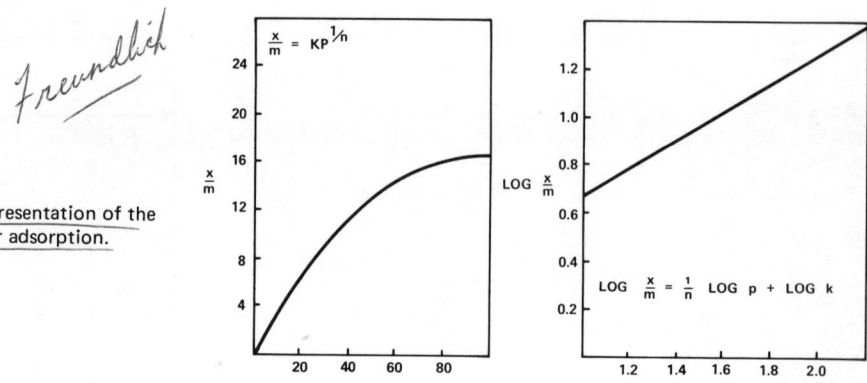

Freundlich

Figure 11. Graphic representation of the Freundlich isotherm for adsorption.

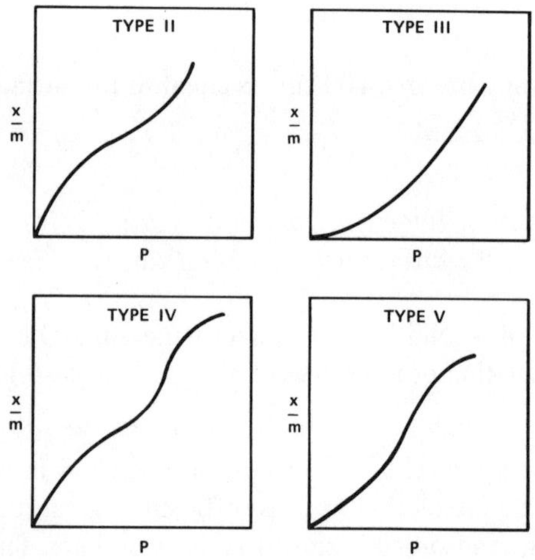

Figure 12. Types of isotherms for multilayer adsorption.

or desorbed from the solid by evacuation at the same temperature at which adsorption occurred. With elevated temperature and lowered pressure, adsorption is decreased and the adsorbate is released.

The type I physical adsorption isotherm is shown in Figure 11; its curve is satisfied by the empirical Freundlich equation

$$y = \frac{x}{m} = kp^{1/n}$$

where y is the mass of vapor, x, adsorbed per unit mass, m, of the adsorbent; p is the pressure; and k and n are constants. For convenience of evaluating the constants, a plot of the equation

$$\log \frac{x}{m} = \frac{1}{n} \log p + \log k$$

is made, and from the straight line formed the constants can be evaluated, as $\log k$ is the y intercept and $1/n$ is the slope of the line (see Appendix: Analytic Geometry).

According to the Freundlich equation, the amount adsorbed increases indefinitely with increasing pressure or concentration. At high pressures this is not a fact and the Freundlich equation does not apply.

Assuming that adsorption occurs only to the extent of a monomolecular layer, Langmuir derived an equation based on the kinetic consideration that adsorption is dependent on the rate of evaporation, r_e, and the rate of adsorption, r_a, of the adsorbate. If f represents the fraction of sites occupied by the vapor molecules at pressure p, then $(1-f)$ represents the fraction of sites not occupied by the vapor.

At a constant temperature the rate of adsorption is proportional to the unoccupied sites and the pressure,

$$r_a = k_1 (1-f) p$$

The rate of evaporation of molecules from the surface is proportional to the fraction of the surface occupied,

$$r_e = k_2 f$$

At equilibrium, the rate of adsorption equals the rate of evaporation, so that

$$r_a = r_e = k_1 (1-f) p = k_2 f$$

By multiplying and rearranging,

$$k_1 p = k_2 f + k_1 f p = f(k_2 + k_1 p)$$

and, by dividing by $k_2 + k_1 p$,

$$f = \frac{k_1 p}{k_2 + k_1 p} = \frac{\frac{k_1}{k_2} p}{1 + \frac{k_1}{k_2} p}$$

If, for convenience, k_1/k_2 is replaced by b and f is replaced by y/y_{max}, where y is the mass of vapor adsorbed per gram of adsorbent at pressure p and y_{max} the mass of vapor that 1 g of adsorbent can adsorb when a monolayer is complete, the equation may be written

$$y = \frac{y_{max} b p}{1 + bp}$$

This may be inverted and multiplied by p to obtain

$$\frac{p}{y} = \frac{p}{y_{max}} + \frac{1}{b y_{max}}$$

so that a plot of p/y against p is a straight line from which y_{max} and b can be evaluated from the slope and the y intercept. Such a plot, using concentration, C, instead of pressure, is shown in Figure 13.

Langmuir assumed that (1) the adsorbed gas behaves ideally in the vapor phase, (2) the adsorbed gas is restricted to a monomolecular layer, (3) the affinity of each adsorbing site on the surface for the vapor molecule is the same, (4) there is no lateral interaction between the adsorbate molecules, and (5) the adsorbed molecules do not move on the surface. In reality these assumptions are valid only under certain conditions. The first two assumptions are valid only at low pressures. As the pressure is increased the behavior of the vapor molecules departs from ideality; and as the pressure is increased more than a single layer of vapor molecules are adsorbed. Thus, the Langmuir equation does not apply at low temperatures and high pressures. Real surfaces are not homogenous and the affinity for the adsorbate is different at various regions on the surface. The initially adsorbed molecules are held at the more active adsorption sites, and the lack of homogeneity leads to a decrease in interaction force as the surface coverage is increased, with the less-active sites holding the adsorbate at higher pressures. There is some lateral attraction of adsorbed molecules caused by the nonhomogeneity of the surface, and an adsorbed molecule still has a certain amount of two-dimensional mobility at the surface.

24 • particles and powders

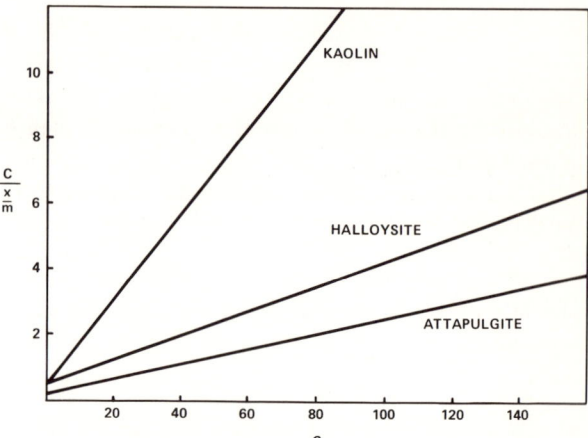

Figure 13. Adsorption isotherms at 24° for strychnine by gastric juice-washed clays. [N. Barr and E. Arnista, *J. Am. Pharm. Assoc.* **46**, 489 (1957).]

If the pressure term is replaced by concentration, the Langmuir isotherm applies to the adsorption of a solute from solution by such solids as charcoal, alumina, and clay. This has been demonstrated for such drugs as quinine, strychnine, and atropine, which have been adsorbed from aqueous solution by kaolin and other clays. Figure 13 compares the effectiveness of various clays in adsorbing strychnine from solution. It has been suggested that this phenomenon be utilized for the adsorption of toxins from the gastrointestinal tract.

Adsorption is not always a desired process. Aluminum hydroxide particles when administered orally with oxytetracycline will adsorb the antibiotic on their surface so that the antibiotic is not as readily available for systemic absorption from the gastrointestinal tract. Quaternary ammonium compounds, e.g., cetylpyridinium chloride, have been used as oral antiseptics in the form of troches. In troches using talc as a lubricant, the cetylpyridinium chloride is adsorbed on the talc and its antiseptic activity is lost.

The BET theory was developed by Brunauer, Emmett, and Teller for multimolecular-layer adsorption; it is expressed by the equation

$$\frac{p}{V(p^0 - p)} = \frac{1}{V_{max}b} + \frac{(b-1)p}{V_{max}bp^0}$$

where V is the volume of vapor adsorbed per gram of powder at pressure p at a temperature at which the vapor pressure of the liquefied vapor is p^0; V_{max} is the volume of vapor in cubic centimeters, converted to standard temperature and pressure, required to form a monolayer on a gram of the powder; and b is a constant, which is related exponentially to the difference between the heat of liquefaction and the heat of adsorption of the adsorbate. For type II adsorption isotherms a plot of $p/V(p^0 - p)$ against p/p^0 is a straight line with a slope of $(b-1)/bV_{max}$ and an intercept of $1/bV_{max}$. Figure 14 illustrates this plot for some pharmaceutical powders. At low pressures at which multimolecular layers are not formed, the BET equation reduces to the Langmuir equation. Extensions of the BET equation include all five types of isotherms.

Similar to the Langmuir theory, the BET theory assumes that (1) the surface is homogenous, (2) the adsorbate molecules do not move at the adsorption site, and (3) there is no lateral interaction between the adsorbed molecules. It assumes that molecules can be adsorbed in multimolecular layers and that the area available for a layer is equal to the coverage of the preceding layer. It assumes that the energy of adsorption of the first layer is constant and that the energy of adsorption in succeeding layers is equal to the energy of liquefaction of the vapor. A failing of the BET theory is the last assumption — that one molecule may be adsorbed on top of an isolated adsorbed molecule and that the energy involved is the same as if the vapor were condensed to a liquid in which each molecule is surrounded by 12

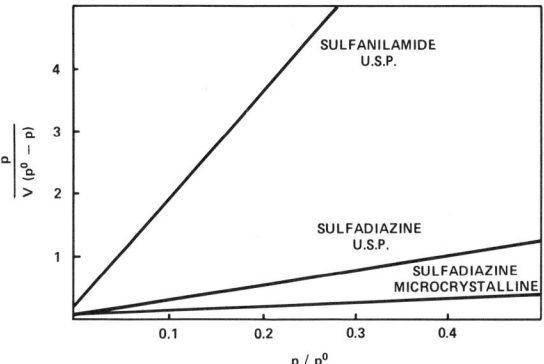

Figure 14. Adsorption data for nitrogen on sulfanilamide and sulfadiazine plotted according to the BET equation. [J. Swintosky, S. Riegelman, T. Higuchi and L.W. Busse, *J. Am. Pharm. Assoc., 38,* 312 (1949).]

adjacent molecules, i.e., closest packing. In all the adsorption theories presented, it is the lack of surface homogeneity that makes an exact mathematical representation of adsorption difficult.

The BET equation has found application in the measurement of the surface area of a powder. The measurement of surface area is important in pharmacy, as the bulk, chemical activity, adsorption, and therapeutic availability of drugs may depend on the surface.

The experimental determination of the surface of pharmaceutical powders is best accomplished by measuring the volume of adsorbed vapor forming a monomolecular layer on the surface of the particles. The apparatus shown in Figure 15 is used to measure the van der Waals adsorption isotherm of nitrogen near its boiling point. The sample is placed in the BET apparatus and evacuated at a low pressure to remove any adsorbed substances. Nitrogen is then admitted, and the volume adsorbed is determined at various pressures.

The result of the measurement of the volume of nitrogen adsorbed by a sample of microcrystalline sulfdiazine at various relative pressures is shown in Figure 16. The point V_{max} at the lower extreme of the linear portion of the isotherm represents the volume of adsorbed nitrogen required to form a monomolecular layer. For this sample V_{max} is equal to 3.47 cc. V_{max} is best evaluated from the slope and intercept values obtained from the plot of the BET equation as shown in Figure 14.

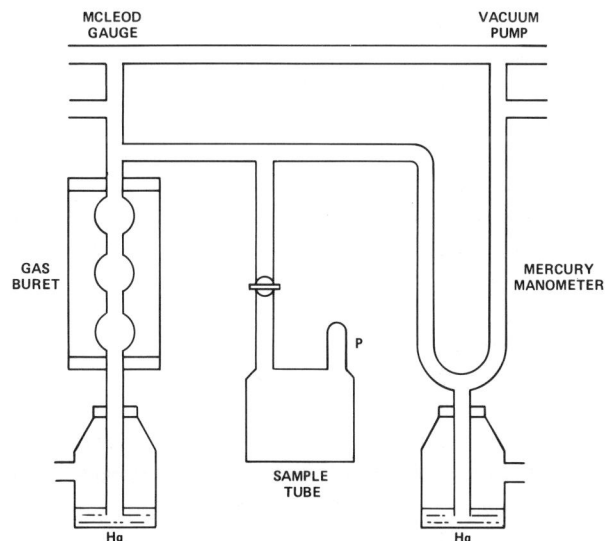

Figure 15. Schematical arrangement of BET apparatus.

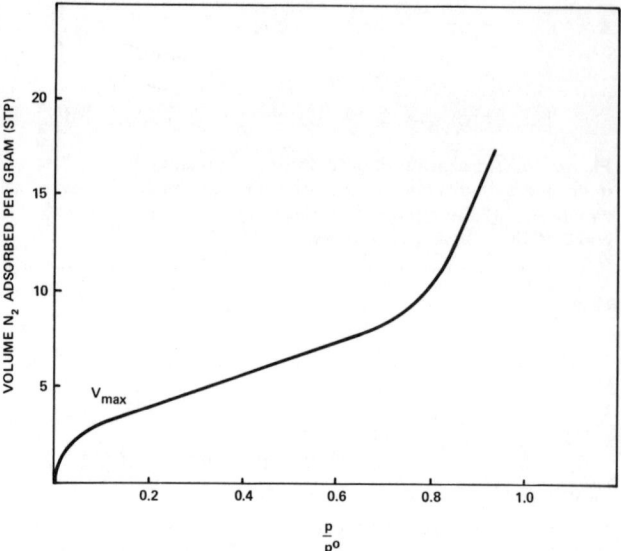

Figure 16. Isotherm showing the volume of nitrogen adsorbed on sulfadiazine powder at varying pressure ratios. Point V_{max} is the volume of the adsorbed nitrogen corresponding to completion of a monomolecular film. [J. Swintosky, S. Riegelman, T. Higuchi and L.W. Busse, *J. Am. Pharm. Assoc. 38*, 311 (1949).]

The area, s_m, occupied by a molecule of a vapor in a closest packed surface is

$$s_m = 3.464 \left(\frac{M}{4\rho\sqrt{2}\,N} \right)^{3/2}$$

where M is the molecular weight of the vapor, N Avogadro number, and ρ the density. The area occupied by a single molecule of nitrogen is 16.24×10^{-16} cm^2 and by a single molecule of water vapor is 10×10^{-16} cm^2.

For the monomolecular-layer type of adsorption, if s_m and V_{max} are known the specific surface, S_w, may be calculated:

$$S_w = \frac{s_m N}{\dfrac{M}{\rho}} V_{max}$$

where M/ρ, the molar volume of gas at standard temperature and pressure, is 22,400 cc and N is the Avogadro number. For nitrogen adsorption the equation becomes

$$S_w = \frac{16.24 \times 10^{-16} \times 6 \times 10^{23}}{22,400 \times 10^4} V_{max} = 4.35\, V_{max}$$

where the 10^4 in the denominator converts square centimeters to square meters so that the specific surface is expressed in square meters per gram of powder. The specific surface of the sample of microcrystalline sulfadiazine is

$$S_w = 4.35 \times 3.47 = 15.1 \text{ m}^2 \text{ g}^{-1}$$

Assuming that the particles of the sulfadiazine are spherical, the particle size may be expressed as

$$d = \frac{6}{\rho S_w} = \frac{6}{1.5 \times 15.1 \times 10^4} = 0.26 \times 10^{-4} \text{ cm } (0.26\,\mu)$$

The specific surface and diameter of some pharmaceutical powders are given in Table VIII. Some chemicals, such as zinc oxide and bismuth subcarbonate, are very fine as obtained from the manufacturer; they may be incorporated directly into ointments and suspensions without further subdivision. Other drugs, such as sulfathiazole and bismuth subnitrate, are relatively coarse and must be reduced in size if pharmaceutically elegant suspensions and ointments are to be made. Although the tabulation gives the approximate size of these medicinal chemicals, the size and surface show appreciable variation among manufacturers and among batches from one manufacturer.

Table VIII Specific Surface Area and Average Particle Size of Some Drugs as Determined by The BET Method *

Drug	S_w (m² g⁻¹)	Diameter (μ)	Density (g cc⁻¹)
Ammoniated mercury U.S.P.	0.96	1.19	5.2
Ammoniated mercury, spray dried	4.06	0.28	5.2
Barium sulfate	2.42	0.551	4.5
Bismuth subcarbonate U.S.P.	5.56	0.157	6.86
Bismuth subnitrate U.S.P.	0.63	1.93	4.93
Mercuric sulfide	0.33	2.24	8.1
Sulfadiazine U.S.P.	1.57	2.55	1.5
Sulfadiazine, microcrystalline	15.1	0.265	1.5
Sulfanilamide	0.28	14.4	1.4
Sulfathiazole, microcrystalline	4.12	0.971	1.5
Sulfathiazole, micronized	2.10	1.90	1.5
Sulfur U.S.P.	0.26	11.1	2.07
Sulfur, colloidal	3.96	0.732	2.07
Sulfur, spray dried	1.73	1.68	2.07
Titanium dioxide	13.7	0.114	3.84
Zinc oxide	3.56	0.308	5.47

* J. V. Swintosky, S. Riegelman, T. Higuchi and L. W. Busse, *J. Am. Pharm. Assoc.* **38**, 210, 308 (1949).

Solubility

Theoretical derivation based on surface energy of particles indicates that by reducing particle size, the solubility may be increased. If d_2 is the diameter of a small particle and d_1 is the diameter of a large particle, the relative solubility of the two particles may be expressed as

$$(1 - \alpha - n\alpha)\frac{RT}{M} \ln \frac{S_2}{S_1} = \frac{4\sigma}{\rho}\left(\frac{1}{d_2} - \frac{1}{d_1}\right)$$

where α is the degree of dissociation, n the number of ions from the compound of molecular weight M, R the gas constant (8.31 X 10⁷ ergs mole⁻¹ deg⁻¹), T the absolute temperature, ρ the density, and σ the surface energy.

If a nondissociating compound with a molecular weight of 150 g mole⁻¹ and a density of 2.3 g cc⁻¹ has a diameter of 10⁻⁴ cm and a surface energy of 50 ergs cm⁻², one may calculate the reduction in particle size necessary to increase the solubility 10 per cent. As no dissociation occurs upon substituting the values, one has

$$\frac{2.303 \times 8.31 \times 10^7 \times 298}{150} \log \frac{1.1}{1} = \frac{4 \times 50}{2.3}\left(\frac{1}{d_2} - \frac{1}{10^{-4}}\right)$$

$$d_2 = 5.3 \times 10^{-6} \text{ cm}$$

A particle of 10^{-4} cm has a small surface energy. To have appreciable surface energy a particle must be of the magnitude of 10^{-6} cm or smaller. The reality of this phenomenon of increased solubility is evident only in the colloidal range less than $0.1\ \mu$. For practical purposes, the solubility remains unchanged with a change in particle size.

In parenteral suspensions the particle size of the suspended particles injected is an important factor. The absorption of the drug from the particles often increases with an increase in specific surface, i.e., a reduction of particle size. The size of the particles in a parenteral suspension should be sufficiently small so they do not cause mechanical irritation to the tissue at the site of injection. To be properly administered a parenteral suspension must flow readily from the syringe through the hypodermic needle into the injection site. This flow is affected by the size and shape of the suspended particles.

Although the size range is carefully controlled, the size frequency distribution will have a small fraction of very fine particles near the colloidal size. The dispersing medium of the suspension will become saturated with the sparingly soluble drug. Saturation is an equilibrium phenomenon in which some of the molecules in solution are returning to the crystal face and condensing, while other molecules are dissolving or leaving the crystal face and going into solution (see page 141).

The colloidal particles have a greater solubility than the larger particles and dissolve. To maintain the dynamic equilibrium of saturation, some of the dissolved drug crystallizes on the surface of the larger particles. The net result is the growth of particle size of the suspension with the loss of the very small particles.

On long storage pharmaceutical suspensions may have an increase in particle size, which is often accompanied by caking of the sediment. A molecule returning to the solid phase may condense in such a manner that it joins or bridges two particles. When a large number of such bridgings occur between the closely packed particles of the sediment, aggregation or caking into a nondispersible mass occurs. In the formulation of a suspension the pharmacist attempts to retard this process by adding a surface-active agent to lower the surface energy of the particles.

Rate of Dissolution. If one wishes to dissolve a solid, most persons will intuitively subdivide the solid into smaller pieces to hasten the dissolution process. A single lump of alum will dissolve quite rapidly when agitated in water; however, if the same lump of alum were pulverized, it would dissolve in less time under the same agitation. The reduction of particle size increases the total surface of the solid in contact with the solvent, and solution occurs in a briefer time.

The dissolution process is complex, and the rate of dissolution depends on many factors. The free surface energy and the shape of the particles affect the rate of dissolution. The temperature, type of agitation, amount of material already in solution, and viscosity and volume of the solvent influence the rate of dissolution. The exposure of new surfaces and the condition of the surface modifies the rate; if gas pockets or an insoluble coat form on the surface, the rate of dissolution will be decreased. It will be noted that the specific surface is of major importance and that it is a factor related to the effect of most variables.

Under standard agitation and temperature Noyes and Whitney proposed the relationship

$$\frac{dw}{dt} = -K'S(C_S - C)$$

where the loss of weight of a particle per unit time, dw/dt, is at any instant proportional to the surface, S, and the difference in concentration between a saturated solution and the concentration existing in solution at that instant, $(C_S - C)$. The constant, K', is a function of all other variables and applies for a given set of conditions.

The rate of dissolution, $\frac{dw}{dt}\frac{1}{S}$, is the amount of substance dissolved per unit area per unit time (see Appendix: Differentiation). For most solids this is expressed in terms of g cm^{-2} min^{-1}. The rate of dissolution is expressed

$$\frac{dw/dt}{S} = K'(C_s - C)$$

As the solid dissolves the surface area S is changing with time. This variable may be related to the weight of the particles by use of the specific shape factor

$$S = \frac{\alpha_{sv}}{\rho^{2/3}} w^{2/3} = aw^{2/3}$$

where a is a convenient means of expressing the ratio $\alpha_{sv}/\rho^{2/3}$.

Although the general case for expressing the rate of dissolution is mathematically complex, some special cases are simply expressed. For the condition in which the initial weight of the particles is the weight required to saturate the solvent, the following relation applies:

$$V\frac{dw}{dt} = K'Sw = K'aw^{5/3}$$

where V is the volume of the solvent and w the weight of the particles. The integrated form of this equation is

$$\frac{K'at}{V} = w^{-2/3} - w_0^{-2/3}$$

where w_0 is the initial weight of the particles and w the weight of the undissolved particles at time t.

More useful to pharmaceutical science is the special case in which the concentration of the solution does not change significantly, i.e., $C_s \gg C$. Under this condition

$$-\frac{dw}{dt} = 3kS = 3kaw^{2/3}$$

where the constant, k, is a function of all other variables in the dissolution system in which the concentration does not change, and the rate of dissolution, $\frac{dw}{dt}\frac{1}{S}$, is equivalent to $3k$. The integrated form of the above equation is useful in numerically evaluating the rate of dissolution,

$$kat = w_0^{1/3} - w^{1/3} \quad \text{Cube root law or Hixson-Cromwell Eq.}$$

where w is the weight of the undissolved particles at any time t.

Figure 17 shows the curve used to calculate the rate of dissolution of a spherical particle of benzoic acid in water at room temperature under a given set of conditions. Experimentally, the weight of the particle is measured at various time intervals and the difference between the cube root of the initial weight and the cube root of the weight at time t is plotted against time on the abscissa. For this particular sphere with a density of 1.124 g cc^{-1}, the slope ka is equal to 0.0627. Substituting the density and the specific shape factor, which for a sphere is 4 85, the constant a is

$$a = \frac{\alpha_{sv}}{\rho^{2/3}} = \frac{4.85}{1.124^{2/3}} = 4.49$$

k is equal to 0.0140, and the rate of dissolution is $3k$ or 0.042 g cm^{-2} hr^{-1}.

In the gastrointestinal tract the rate of dissolution of a solid drug or dosage form may be slower than the process of absorption through the walls of the gastrointestinal tract. Then the dissolved drug is absorbed as rapidly as it dissolves, and for all practical purposes the drug concentration in the lumen is unchanged. This equation then applies to *in vivo* rates of dissolution.

particles and powders

Galenical Extraction. Galenical extraction is the process of dissolving or leaching out of the soluble constituents of crude drugs. With intact cells of crude drug, the solvent does not come into immediate contact with the solute to be extracted, and extraction is impractical. To facilitate extraction the crude vegetable or animal drugs are comminuted or ground. This ruptures the cell wall or membrane and allows the solvent to come into direct contact with the solute. The solute dissolves; its solution may be separated from the extraneous crude material.

The extent of subdivision of a crude drug depends on its physical structure. Cascara sagrada and sarsaparilla are soft tissues, which are readily extracted, so a very coarse powder is used. Ipecac is more difficult to extract, so a fine powder is used. The descriptive terms used to express the fineness of powdered crude drugs are defined in Table IX.

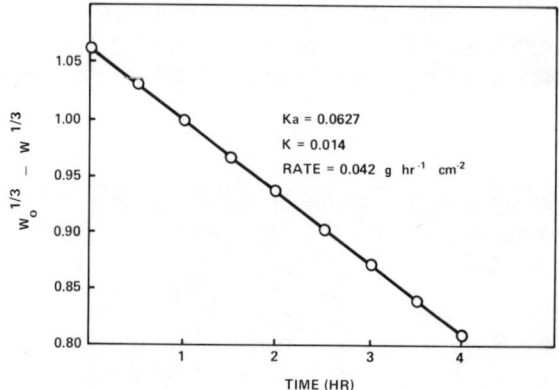

Figure 17. Determination of the rate of dissolution of a spherical benzoic acid pellet in water when the concentration of the solution is unchanged.

Table IX Classification of Powders by Fineness *

Classification of Powder	Vegetable and Animal Drugs			Chemicals		
	Nominal Designation No.† of Powder	Fineness Limit‡		Nominal Designation No.† of Powder	Fineness Limit‡	
		%	Sieve No.		%	Sieve No.
Very coarse	8	20	60			
Coarse	20	40	60	20	60	40
Moderately coarse	40	40	80	40	60	60
Fine	60	40	100	80	100	80
Very fine	80	100	80	120	100	120

* *National Formulary,* Mack, Easton, Pa., 12th ed., 1965, p. 487.
† All particles of the powder pass through a sieve of the nominal designation.
‡ Limit of the percentage that passes through a sieve of the size designated.

Physiological Activity

Absorption of Drugs. The therapeutic efficacy of a dosage form may be affected by the particle size. As the particles of the drug are reduced in size, there is an increase in specific surface area. Since the solution of a given weight of a drug is proportional to the exposed surface, with an increased surface area, there is more rapid solution and greater amounts of the drug are absorbed from the site of administration.

The effect of particle size on absorption has been admirably demonstrated by the administration of a single 3-g dose of a suspension of sulfadiazine in humans. Serum concentrations of the sulfadiazine were determined at various time intervals after giving the oral suspension. Figure 18 compares the serum levels obtained from U.S.P. and microcrystalline sulfadiazine. The microcrystalline powder appears more rapidly and in higher concentrations in the serum because, with its greater specific surface area, as indicated in Figure 14 and shown in Table VIII, the microcrystalline sulfadiazine dissolves and is absorbed faster into the blood stream.

Novobiocin also shows the effect of particle size on solution and absorption. When the crystalline, acid form of novobiocin is given orally, practically no absorption occurs, as indicated by serum levels. If the antibiotic is micronized or precipitated in a finely divided amorphous form, it becomes an effective oral drug. The more effective absorption of finer particles has been experimentally demonstrated with other drugs, such as arsenic trioxide, calomel, chloramphenicol, estrone, griseofulvin, and sulfethylthiadiazole.

The more effective absorption of finer particles is a general effect with sparingly soluble drugs; however, with rapidly dissolving drugs the solution of the solid drugs is no longer the rate-limiting step in gastrointestinal absorption. This is manifested with tetracycline and its salt.

Tetracycline base is soluble 1:2500 in water and it has a slow rate of dissolution. If a 200-mg dose is given orally as a pellet with a surface of 2.8 cm^2 and as a capsule containing a powder with a surface of 85 cm^2, the absorption of the slowly dissolving tetracycline is increased by a greater specific surface area. A comparison of the excretion rates shows that the powder was absorbed and excreted faster and in greater amounts, as shown in Figure 19.

When the experiment was repeated with the more rapidly dissolving tetracycline hydrochloride, no significant difference was found between the orally administered pellet or powder, as shown in Figure 20. With a drug that intrinsically dissolves rapidly, a reduction of particle size will have little, if any, effect on the speed with which absorption occurs.

Although the therapeutic level of a drug in the body depends on the solubility and the size of particles of the solid drug administered, many other factors must be considered in designing a proper dosage form. The region of the gastrointestinal tract in which the drug is to act influences the design of a preparation. Phenothiazine is used as a veterinary anthelmintic in sheep. The activity of the slowly dissolving phenothiazine is increased in the small intestines by increasing the specific surface area; however, the activity is increased in the large intestine if larger particles are used. Apparently the smaller particles dissolve and are absorbed before reaching the large intestine, so no anthelmintic effect is exhibited in the large intestine. The drug, in larger particles, dissolves more slowly and is able to reach the large intestine, providing activity.

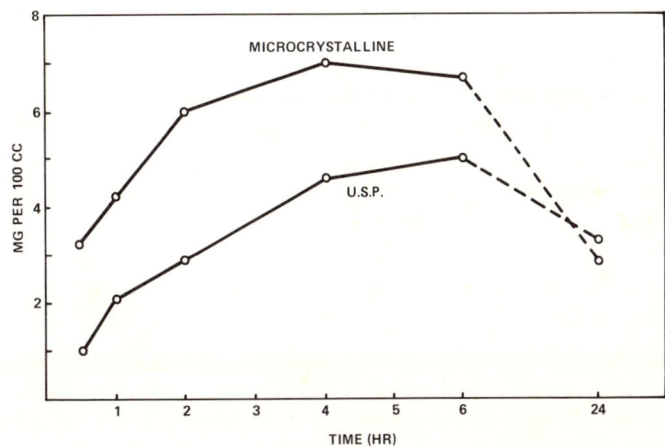

Figure 18. Serum levels in humans after one 3-g dose of sulfadiazine. Microcrystalline sulfadiazine with the smaller particle size produces a higher serum level. [J.G. Reinhold, F.J. Phillips, M.F. Flippin, and L. Pollack, *Am. J. Med. Sci.* **210,** 141 (1945).]

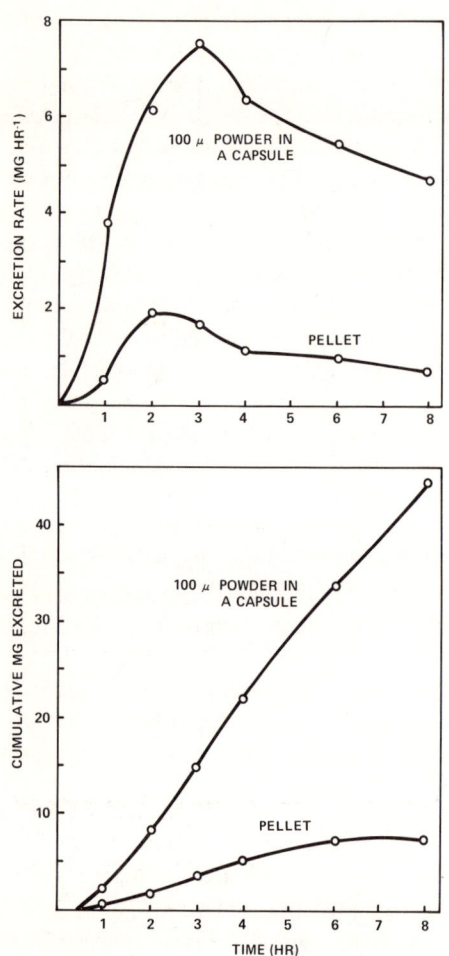

Figure 19. Comparison of cumulative amount excreted and excretion rate curves for 200 mg of tetracycline administered orally as a pellet and as a powder in a capsule. [E. Nelson, *J. Am. Pharm. Assoc. 48,* 96 (1959).]

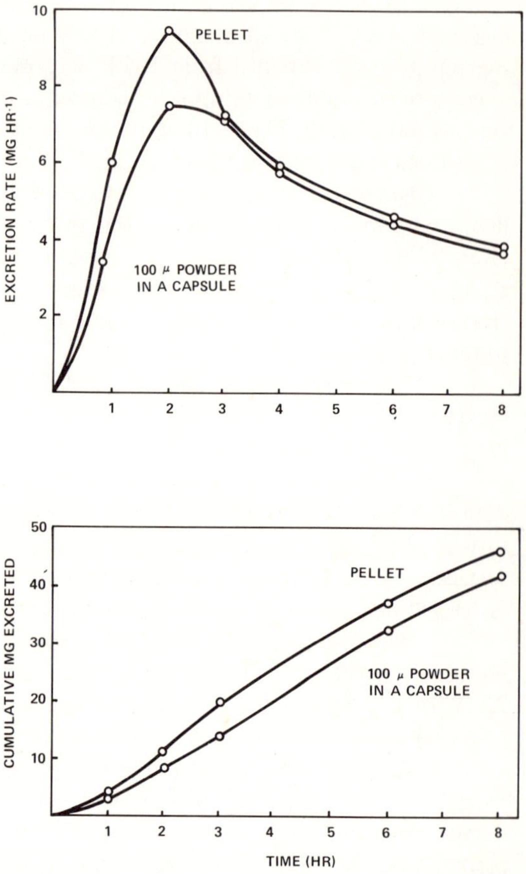

Figure 20. Comparison of cumulative amount excreted and excretion rate curves for 200 mg of tetracycline administered orally as the hydrochloride as a pellet and as a powder within a capsule. [E. Nelson, *J. Am. Pharm. Assoc. 48,* 96 (1959).]

Many types of insulin are available for subcutaneous injection in the treatment of diabetes mellitus. In one type, insulin is combined with zinc in the presence of acetate buffer to form an insoluble complex. The size of the particles formed is controlled by the pH at which complexation occurs. The amorphous form is known as Semilente Iletin®; the larger-sized form is known as Ultralente Iletin®. Chemically they are identical, but the physical difference of size results in a different onset of activity and length of activity. With Semilente Iletin® there is a greater specific surface, so the insulin dissolves rapidly in the tissue fluid and circulates through the body to give a rapid effect with maximum activity from 2 to 6 hours after injection. As the particles dissolve and exert their effect more rapidly than Ultralente Iletin®, the duration of activity is shorter, varying from 12 to 16 hours. With the larger particles of Ultralente Iletin® the onset is slower, but the duration of activity is longer lasting, up to 36 hours. A comparison of the two forms is given in Figure 21. By mixing these two forms, intermediate ranges of activity may be obtained. A mixture of 70 per cent Ultralente and 30 per cent Semilente is called Lente Iletin®.

particles and powders • 33

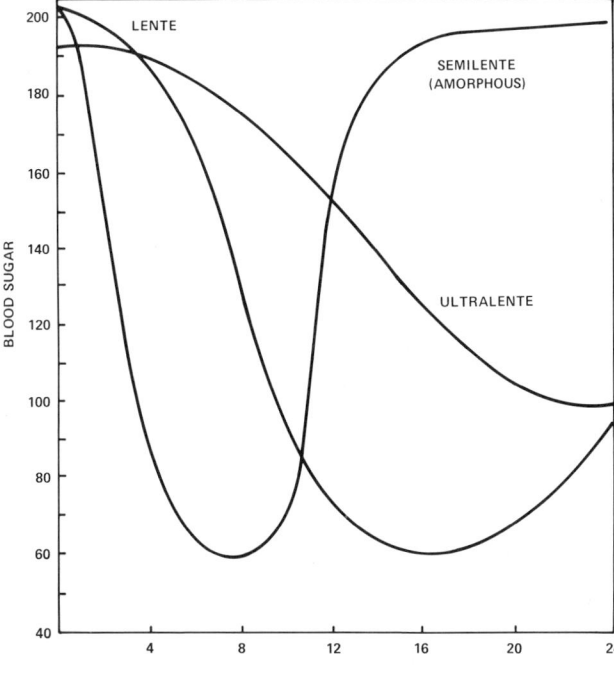

Figure 21. Graphic drawing of duration and intensity of action of insulin as function of particle size.

As most patients are adverse to the use of the hypodermic needle, the research pharmacist strives to develop parenteral products so that fewer injections are required daily. The early aqueous solutions of penicillin required six to eight intramuscular injections daily to maintain therapeutic blood levels. Pharmaceutical research since then has developed numerous "insoluble" penicillins, which dissolve slowly, releasing the drug in amounts so that only a single injection is required every 1 or 2 days. Procaine benzyl penicillin was the first therapeutically successful "insoluble" penicillin. It has been found that aqueous procaine benzyl penicillin suspensions containing from 40 to 70 per cent solids would provide prolonged activity and would still flow easily from the syringe through the hypodermic needle if the specific surface exceeded 10,000 cm^2 g^{-1} and there was a broad size frequency distribution of particles.

With a narrow size distribution there is less friction and a lower angle of repose, and the injection fans out at the site of injection. With a broader size distribution the depot in the muscle assumes a spherical shape, which presents less surface for leaching out of the penicillin. With a broad distribution the depot is more compact and with the high solid-to-water ratio the depot is more viscous; thus, absorption is delayed to the extent that only a single injection is required every 48 hours.

The experimental data presented in Table X illustrate the effect of particle size on the absorption of procaine benzyl penicillin from aqueous suspension when administered to rabbits. The large particles of procaine benzyl penicillin delay absorption from the aqueous system, whereas the small particles accelerate absorption.

A parenteral suspension of procaine benzyl penicillin in sesame oil may be used for repository effect. Upon injection the oily suspension, which is insoluble in the aqueous tissue fluid, forms a depot in the muscle. The penicillin is dissolved or leached from the interface of the oily depot and the tissue by the aqueous body fluid. As the interfacial area is limited and the movement of the penicillin particles in the oil toward the interface is slow, the oily suspension provides a slow release and prolonged action of penicillin. If micronized procaine benzyl penicillin (95 per cent less than 5 μ) and the milled antibiotic

Table X Effect of Particle Size of Procaine Penicillin G in Aqueous Suspensions (300,000 units cc^{-1}) on Serum Concentrations in Rabbits *

Mesh Size	Particle Size (μ)	Average Blood Levels (units ml^{-1}), hr					
		1	4	24	28	48	72
60/100	150-250	1.37	1.29	0.82	0.86	0.31	0.12
100/140	105-150	1.24	1.50	0.76	0.28	0.16	0.01
140/250	58-105	1.54	1.44	0.47	0.25	0.12	0.04
250/400	35-58	1.64	1.51	0.62	0.33	0.15	-
400	35	2.40	2.36	0.33	0.16	0.07	-
Micronized	1-2	2.14	2.22	0.06	0.02	-	-

* From F. H. Buckwalter and H. L. Dickison, *J. Am. Pharm. Assoc., Sci. Ed.* 47, 661 (1958).

(150 to 175 μ) are used to prepare identical oily suspensions except for particle size, the larger particles are absorbed more slowly and provide a more prolonged effect.

A single deep muscular injection of 300,000 units of procaine benzyl penicillin in 1 ml of oil is detectable in the blood for up to 24 hours, and the addition of 2 per cent aluminum monostearate maintains a therapeutically effective level of 0.03 unit ml^{-1} for 2 to 4 days. In the presence of aluminum monostearate the particles micronized to 5 μ give more prolonged effect than the larger particles, as shown in Figure 22. Apparently the gel structure formed with the aluminum monostearate holds the smaller particles within the intersticial spaces of the hydrophobic aluminum monostearate, reducing the diffusion or movement of the penicillin particles. With less movement the penicillin is not leached out of the depot as readily, because less body fluid is brought in contact with the surface of the particle. The larger particles are bigger than the intersticial spaces of the gel structure; thus, they are not retarded by the gel.

Medicinal aerosols are suspensions or solutions of drugs in a propellant under pressure (see page 323). The low-boiling propellant has a vapor pressure of approximately 35 lb. in.$^{-2}$. When the valve is opened, the pressure forces out the ingredients, which strike the orifice of the valve, causing a fine spray to be formed. The size of the aerosol particles can be regulated by the pressure, nature of the propellant, and design of the valve. The size of the particles controls the effect of the drug in inhalation therapy.

In inhalation therapy, as used with drugs such as epinephrine, ergotamine, isoproterenol, octyl nitrate, and penicillin, particles larger than 30 μ are carried to the trachea, and particles from 10 to 30 μ reach the terminal bronchioles. In these regions local effects may be evident, but there is no significant systemic effect.

If systemic absorption of the drug is desired, the particles must be deposited in the alveolar region. Aerosol particles from 1 to 3 μ reach the alveolar sacs, from which they are absorbed into the body. It is possible that the particles can be too small. Particles less than 0.5 μ reach the alveolar sacs but remain dispersed by Brownian movement and are exhaled back into the external environment.

Pellets or implantation tablets have been developed for subcutaneous implantation of hormones. The sterile pellets are generally placed by incision in the thigh, where they serve as a depot, slowly releasing the hormone. Effects have been observed for several months after implantation.

The rate of dissolution and absorption are proportional to the surface area of the implant at a given time. The surface area decreases with time, and the relationship between the decrease in release of drug is described by the change in area as a function of time. Figure 23 illustrates that as a spherical implant dissolves and the surface area decreases, the amount of drug dissolved and absorbed per unit time progressively decreases.

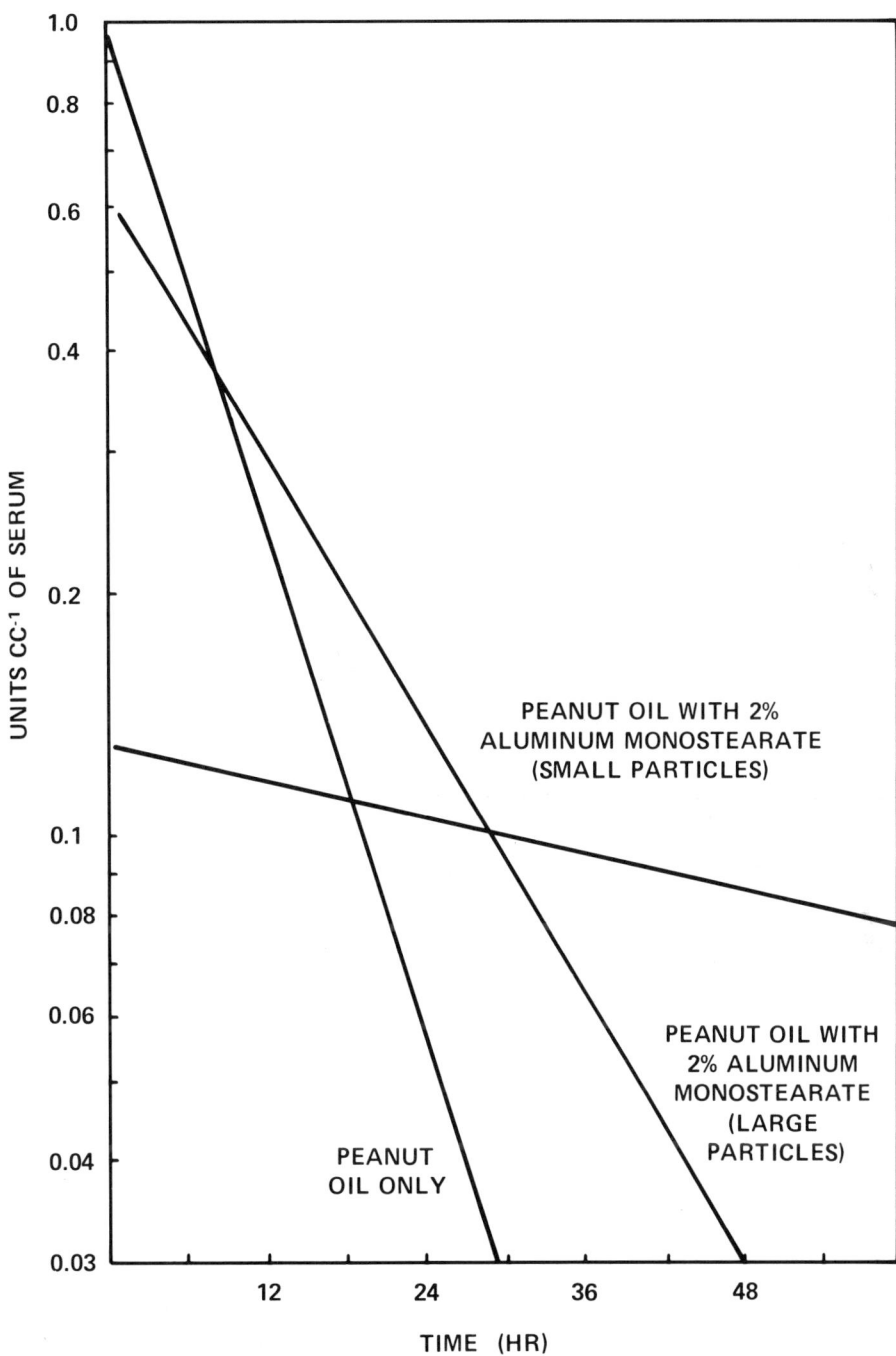

Figure 22. Average penicillin blood concentrations in humans produced by a single injection of 300,000 units of procaine penicillin in various peanut oil vehicles. [F.H. Buckwalter and H.L. Dickinson, *J. Am. Pharm. Assoc. 47,* 661 (1958).]

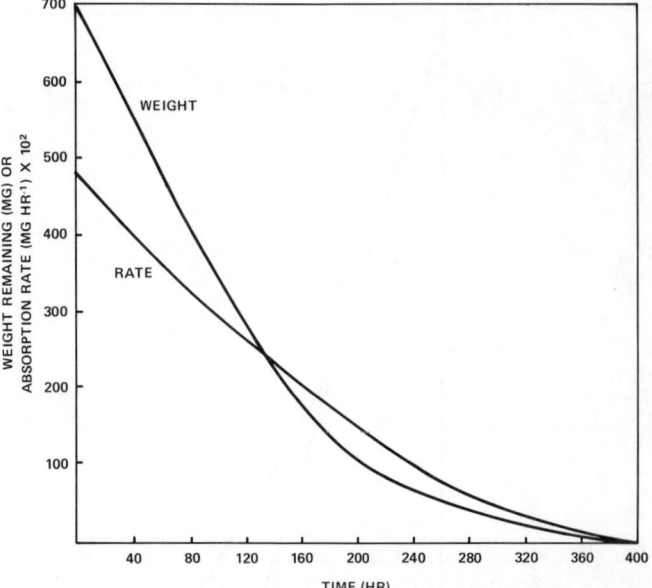

Figure 23. Decrease in weight and rate of change of weight of a spherical implant as a function of time. [B.E. Ballard and E. Nelson, *J. Pharm. Sci. 51*, 915 (1962).]

Mechanical Irritation. When applied, large irregular particles incorporated into various dosage forms may irritate the tissue by abrasion. The talc used in baby powder and the abrasives used in dentifrices must pass a 325-mesh sieve (44 μ) to be acceptable. It would appear that similar specification should be applied to pharmaceutical powders. Dusting powders are applied to irritated, diseased, or denuded skin, and smaller particles are less likely to cause further irritation. In other dermatological products containing insoluble particles, such as lotions and ointments, very fine size is meritorious to avoid irritation.

Intraarticular injection of adrenocortical suspensions for rheumatoid arthritis should be finely subdivided or further damage to the synovial membrane may result. Ophthalmic suspensions are rather restricted in usage; however, some of the adrenocortical drugs are administered in this fashion. Ophthalmologic studies have reported that most individuals experience a gritty sensation and irritation from the instillation of suspended particles possessing a diameter of 50 μ. Although a particle-size limit for such products is arbitrary, 5 μ might be accepted as the maximum allowable size.

2 | COMMINUTION AND BLENDING OF SOLIDS

The reduction of particle size of drugs is of paramount importance in pharmacy. In Chapter 1 it was shown that particle size affects the physiological availability and efficacy of solid drugs. It is well recognized that reducing the particle size of the reactants will accelerate a chemical reaction. Dissolution and extraction processes are influenced by size. The effect of particle size on the blending of drugs will be discussed in another section.

To ensure that a uniform dose of medication is given to the patient with each administration, all dosage forms must be uniformly mixed. If the initial drugs are markedly different in size, they should be reduced to approximately the same size before mixing. It is time consuming and inefficient to attempt to mix particles of considerable difference of size. If fine particles are mixed with large particles, the fine particles tend to migrate through the void space formed by the larger particles and accumulate in the bottom of the container.

SMALL-SCALE COMMINUTION AND MIXING

Comminution is a mechanical process of reducing a solid to a smaller state of subdivision. Small-scale comminution is accomplished in the community pharmacy by the use of the mortar and pestle or by a spatula and tile.

Trituration is the process of rubbing a solid in a mortar with a pestle. Trituration serves a dual purpose. It reduces particle size and intimately mixes the powder until it is uniform. The pestle is held firmly in the palm with the fingers and thumb wrapped about the handle, allowing moderate downward pressure. The pestle is given a circular motion beginning on the solid in the mortar and extending in larger circles until the side of the mortar is touched. During trituration the sides of the mortar should occasionally be scraped. In compounding a prescription adequate trituration must be used to mix the powdered ingredients.

A glass mortar is used with drugs that stain and in preparing solutions, as it provides a visual means of determining if all the solid has dissolved. The rough surface of a porcelain mortar makes it more effective in reducing particle size than the smooth surface of a glass mortar.

The pestle used should be of proper size for the mortar. There should be maximum contact between the surface of the mortar and pestle. The efficiency of trituration depends on the area of grinding surface and the pressure applied. The energy needed to comminute is proportional to the increase in surface area.

After a solid has been reduced by trituration, it may be passed through a sieve to further reduce the particle size or to make certain that the proper degree of subdivision has been obtained.

Levigation is used in the extemporaneous compounding of ointments. Levigation is the process of reducing the size of solid particles, made into a paste by the addition of a small amount of a liquid or ointment base, by rubbing with a spatula on a tile. This liquid or ointment base is known as a levigating agent. For example, ammoniated mercury is levigated with mineral oil before it is incorporated into petrolatum, which is the base for ammoniated mercury ointment.

In compounding a prescription order for solid ingredients, all solid material is reduced to a fine powder. In mixing the pulverized ingredients, the drug present in the smallest amount is placed in the mortar with an equal bulk of the next most abundant or potent drug. The two drugs are triturated until intimately mixed. An equal bulk of the remaining ingredients is added and the mixture is triturated until intimately mixed. This procedure is repeated until all the material has been added and thoroughly mixed. This process is known as mixing by geometric dilution, because each portion added is equal in bulk to the material already in the mortar.

INDUSTRIAL MILLING

The terms comminution and grinding are synonymously used for the process of size reduction. Milling is the mechanical operation of reducing the particle size of solids. There is no individual all-purpose mill that will satisfactorily handle all products. In general, the amount of work required in milling is proportional to the surface produced. Milling is inefficient, however, as much of the energy is wasted as heat.

Size reduction of glandular and plant materials is accomplished by cutting edges such as are found in knives and graters. The Wiley mill is widely used for contusion or cutting of fibrous crude drugs such as roots, leaves, and dried plant tissues. In the Wiley mill the rotor is fitted with four knives, which rotate against six stationary knives set in the frame. The clearance between the blades may be adjusted. Below the grinding chamber there is a removable screen through which the material is delivered after it has been ground. The Wiley mill may be used for coarse grinding, but it is not a fine grinder.

As many drugs and pharmaceutical necessities are of synthetic origin, the cutting processes are much less important today than they were in the nineteenth century. Milling of blends or crystals by grinding, attrition, and impact to the small particle sizes required in pharmaceutical products will be considered. Crushers and grinders such as those used in the coal and flour industries will not be discussed; only the fine-grinding equipment used in pharmacy will be mentioned.

Factors in Milling

Abrasion. When sufficient force is applied to a solid, the stress causes cracks. The continued application of force provides transverse stress at the initial crack and causes fragmentation. Abrasion or the wearing away by friction is probably the most important factor in milling. For example, the surface of a certain chemical may wear away the hammer and screens of a hammer mill so readily that it is not economical to use; however, a roller mill, which is less sensitive to abrasion, may be used to provide suitable size reduction.

Abrasion is a nebulous term; it has been suggested that it be expressed as abrasion index, which is determined by the following method. A small micropulverizer operating at 14,000 rpm with a Stellited forged swing-hammer rotor is used with a screen having freshly drilled 0.027-in. perforations. A 5-lb sample of the material to be assigned an abrasion index is passed through the mill. An abrasive material will gouge out the sides of the perforations farthest from the entrance point. The amount of gouging in microns as determined by a microscope is the abrasive index. If the abrasive index is zero, the hammer has an indefinite life. If the abrasive index is $100\,\mu$, the solid is too hard to be milled in this manner. An abrasive index of $20\,\mu$ is acceptable for practical, economical milling.

It has been suggested that the term "grindability" be applied to the work necessary to produce a given amount of new surface. "Grindability" has been used in the coal industry, where it means the number of revolutions of a ball mill required to reduce the coal so that 80 per cent will pass a 200-mesh sieve.

Friability is the tendency of a particle to break into smaller sizes in the normal course of handling. In pharmacy the Roche friabilator has been suggested as an apparatus for expressing the friability of compressed tablets. The tablets are weighed and placed in a drum, which rotates for 4 minutes (100 rotations). The tablets are then removed and weighed. The loss of weight, as per cent of initial weight, is the friability; a maximum loss limit of 0.8 per cent is usually acceptable.

With hard, crystalline material a high-speed hammer mill provides an effective abrasive action for particle-size reduction. Fibrous material tends to mat and compress in a hammer mill and it is best reduced in size by a cutting action. Elastic material will tend to deform under stress and does not mill readily. Usually elastic material is cooled by the use of "dry ice" or liquid nitrogen until it becomes brittle and will fragment.

Size. An ideal milling process would be a single operation in which the material could be fed into an easily cleaned machine from which the desired finished particle size would be obtained. The size of the material fed into the mill may present a problem if the mill capacity is low and the ultimate particle size is to be very small. In such cases, a small feed opening should be used and milling should be in stages. It has been found that a uniform rate of feed produces a more uniform shape and size distribution of milled particles.

In pulverizing sugar using a high-speed hammer mill, a coarse crystal will yield a finer milled sugar than a less coarse crystal. As a crude approximation, a soft material may be fed in a 2- to 5-mesh size, and a hard material may be fed in a 4- to 14-mesh size for a product size of 100 mesh.

Moisture. Wet grinding and dry grinding both have advantages. Inks, paints, and cellulose pulps can only be wet ground. Many gels if thoroughly dried become hard and abrasive. Gels may appear dry when filtered but may contain as much as 50 per cent moisture. These are fine ground and then dried. Upon drying the particle size is further reduced, as the gel shrinks.

The concentration of moisture affects grindability. Cellulose and clays with 1 per cent water are not grindable; however, with 2 to 5 per cent moisture they may break up easily.

Water of crystallization may be driven off by the heat generated during milling. It is impractical to mill highly hydrated substances, e.g., aluminum sulfate, potassium, and ammonium alum, so that all the milled material will be of the desired size. The moisture driven off tends to wet portions of the material and clog the mill. In practice the materials containing water of crystallization are milled so that approximately 50 per cent will pass a 100-mesh sieve. The material is then classified or separated according to size, and the larger particles are milled again.

Mills may be water jacketed to cool the material. Generally this is not effective, but it may be effective if the mill surface is large with respect to the amount of product in the mill.

Flammability. Many common compounds used in pharmaceuticals are combustible; starch, sugar, and sulfur dusts may burn with explosive violence. Oxidizers such as nitrates and chlorates require care in milling.

The explosive hazard of drugs depends mainly on the moisture content, particle size, and dispersibility of the particles. Acacia with 11 per cent moisture is not explosive; however, acacia with 5.5 per cent moisture can be made to explode. Anhydrous acacia powder is approximately four times as explosive as acacia containing 5.5 per cent moisture.

As a means of comparison, it has been suggested that the explosive hazard be expressed as EW_{50}, i.e., the concentration of powder dust cloud that will have a 50 per cent probability of exploding under test conditions. Table XI shows the effect of particle size on EW_{50} for salicylamide. Another expression of explosive tendency is the average rate of pressure rise, i.e., the ratio of the maximum pressure to the time interval from the initiation of explosion until maximum pressure is reached. The effect of particle size of dextromethorphan on average rate of pressure rise is shown in Figure 24.

In general, there seems to be a greater probability of an explosion with smaller particles. Agglomeration of fine particles tends to decrease flammability. For example, crystalline saccharin with $d_{vs} = 16\ \mu$ has an $EW_{50} = 92.1$ mg liter^{-1}, while spray-dried saccharin with $d_{vs} = 5.6\ \mu$ has an $EW_{50} = 145.7$ mg liter^{-1} because of agglomeration.

Table XI Effect of Particle Size on EW_{50} for Salicylamide

d_{av} (μ)	d_{vs} (μ)	EW_{50} (mg liter^{-1})
46.1	58.9	35.4
54.6	72.7	39.4
68.4	89.9	83.7
79.9	106.0	110.0

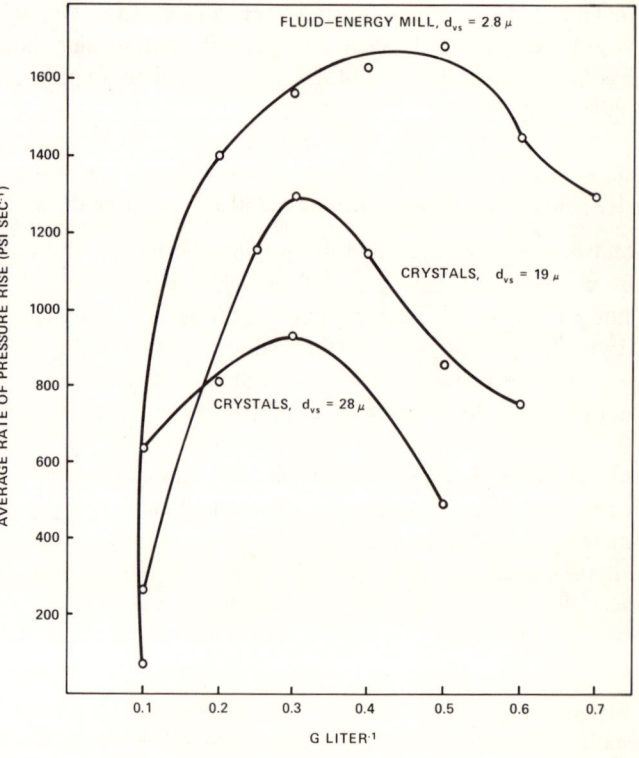

Figure 24. Relation between the particle size of a dextromethorphan salt and its explosive hazard. (W.E. Smith and J. Buehler, Midwestern Industrial Pharmacy Meeting at Chicago, 1964.)

Sparking from the discharge of static electricity must be prevented. All equipment should be grounded. Fortunately, stainless steel, which is used almost universally in pharmacy, sparks less readily than ordinary steels. In extreme circumstances a silicone lubricant should be used instead of combustible oils and an inert atmosphere may be employed.

Temperature. Many materials tend to bond and agglomerate at higher temperatures. Some compounds tend to soften and to present viscous liquid surfaces as the temperature rises. Materials containing a high oil or fat content require cooling to prevent clogging the mill. With cocoa or nut materials air conditioning is often adequate cooling.

At low temperatures elastic materials tend to become brittle and susceptible to abrasion. Proteins, methylcellulose, and methyl methacrylate are cooled by "dry ice" or liquid nitrogen to facilitate fracture.

Whenever work is done, heat is produced. The heat produced by the milling procedure may be sufficient to cause degradation of thermolabile drugs or the heat may interfere with the grinding operation. The thermal effect may be represented as

$$2546.4P = T(wk_m - 60VK_a) - L$$

where P is the motor input in horsepower, T the temperature rise of material and air in degrees Fahrenheit, w the weight of material milled in lb hr^{-1}, V the volume of air passing through the mill in ft^3 min^{-1}, L the loss due to radiation in the machinery in Btu, K_m the specific heat of the material in Btu lb^{-1} deg^{-1}, and K_a the specific heat of air (0.0183 Btu ft^{-3} deg^{-1}).

The high ratio of the mill surface to the amount of material being milled in a ball mill permits reduction of temperature by use of a water jacket. At times cooling may condense moisture and hinder milling operations; fortunately, an air-conditioned laboratory will normally keep the humidity low enough so the dew point is not reached if the jacket is water-cooled.

Jet and fluid-energy mills use a gas, either steam or air, at 120 to 150 psi (see page 45). With thermolabile drugs steam cannot be used, but compressed air or nitrogen may be used, as they cool upon expanding and permit fluid-energy mills to be used in fine grinding of costly, heat-sensitive drugs.

Toxicity. With all milling operations it is advisable for the workers to wear dust respirators. With drugs that are irritating and toxic, safety promotion is vital. Workers must be periodically examined and impressed with the safety precaution of respirators and goggles. Wet grinding will eliminate dust and reduce hazards. Sealed units such as the ball mill will confine obnoxious materials.

Chemical Composition. Chemicals may react with the mill. Crystalline copper sulfate as the pentahydrate sets up an electrolytic effect and corrodes iron parts. Bromides and iodides will corrode iron surfaces. Fortunately, stainless steel, which is standard material for pharmaceutical equipment, is resistant to corrosion.

Equipment

Ball Mills. The ball mill is one of the most common and versatile grinding units. As shown in Figure 25, the ball mill is a horizontally rotating cylinder, with the material to be reduced and balls sealed within the cylinder. Ball mills may be used for pulverizing and/or blending of both wet and dry mixtures. In wet grinding the charge should be above the level of the grinding medium, but it should not occupy more than 60 per cent of the total jar volume.

In dry grinding the jar is half filled with the grinding medium or balls, and enough material to be ground is added to fill the voids between the balls up to the level of the balls. Usually the material will not exceed 25 per cent of the jar volume.

Round balls are used to obtain as many points of contact as possible between the balls and the material. For a given weight of a grinding medium, smaller balls are more numerous and provide more points of contact than larger balls. The balls may be too small and tend to ride with the mass of material to be pulverized. As a guide, 20-mesh charge uses balls from ¾ to 1 in., and a 100-mesh charge uses balls from ½ to ¾ in.

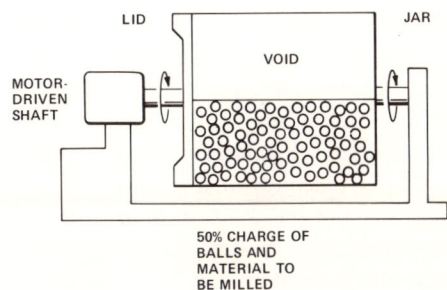

Figure 25. Diagrammatic cross section of a ball mill.

Balls of high-density materials are more effective in grinding than balls of low-density materials. Ball mills are used to fine grind to a size less than 100 mesh. As grinding with a ball mill is rather a slow process, coarse material should be milled to less than 10-mesh size prior to introduction into the jar. Although the process is slow, it is an economical one because labor costs are low.

The ball mill is sealed so that dust, evaporation, and contamination are controlled. It is easily cleaned. In parenteral suspensions and in ophthalmic ointments, where a very small particle size is required, the ball mill is often used in pharmacy. The ball mill has the advantage that the unit may be charged and sterilized; as the unit is sealed, it will remain sterile during all processes until packaged aseptically. The impact and erosion action of the ball mill produces particles with rounded edges and easy flowing characteristics.

Roller Mills. A roller mill, as shown in Figure 26, consists of rollers having a finely cut corrugation in a slight spiral pattern on their surface and operating at different speeds. The size and shape of the milled particles depend on the relation of the corrugations on the rollers. Particles that are reduced to the desired size are constantly removed. Roller mills have largely replaced Buhrstone mills. For some operations up to five rollers are used in a single machine. Pharmaceutically these mills have their greatest use in the preparation of ointments.

Hammer Mills. As illustrated in Figure 27, a hammer mill utilizes rigid or swing hammers on a rotating shaft in a housing incorporating a screen about the rotor. High-speed hammer mills use peripheral speeds up to 21,000 ft min^{-1} with a controlled feed rate. The material is discharged through a screen during operation.

Particles from 200 to 325 mesh are readily made by hammer mills. The particles are sharp and have irregular edges. If the hammers are across the entire width of the rotor, a maximum of fines is produced. If knife-like hammers or blades are used on a fraction of the width, fines are minimized.

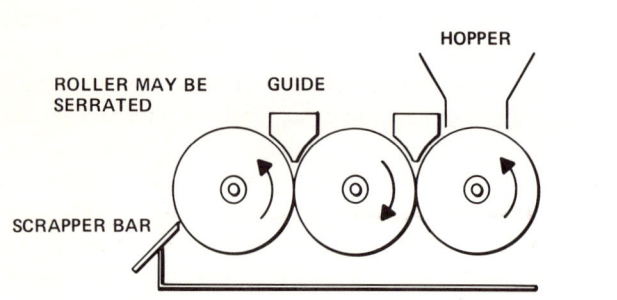

Figure 26. Diagrammatic cross section of a three-roller mill.

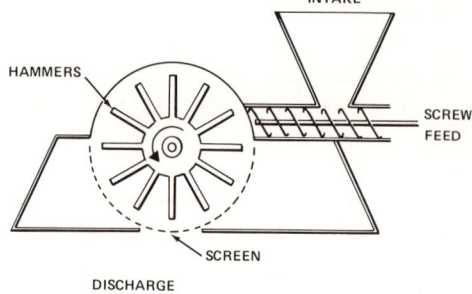

Figure 27. Diagrammatic cross section of a hammer mill.

Although the screens are interchangeable, the openings in the screen have less effect on particle size than the speed of the hammers. Material does not pass radially through the screen but follows a tangential path, as shown in Figure 28. The milled particle is smaller than the screen opening. At high speeds, the approach angle of the particle to the screen hole will approach a tangent, thus making a round hole appear as an ellipse, and finally decreasing to a slit at highest speed. Accordingly, with the same size screen but with a higher speed, a smaller particle is obtained.

The thickness of the screen affects the particle size, as shown in Figure 28. When the screen opening and the speed are constant, the use of a thicker screen will produce a smaller particle. If a heavier screen must be used for strength, but no decrease in particle size is desired, it is necessary to use a screen with larger openings.

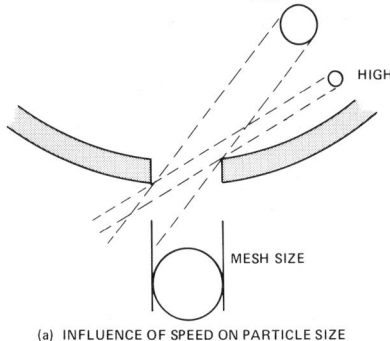
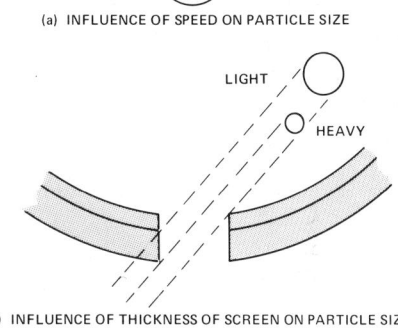

Figure 28. In a hammer mill particle size is a function of speed (a) and thickness of screen (b). (a) Influence of speed on particle size; (b) influence of thickness of screen on particle size.

The capacity increases in a direct ratio to the screen opening. As heat is generated in the milling process, low-melting substances require cooling by passing a coolant through a jacketed mill or by milling "dry ice" with the material if clogging of the screen is to be avoided.

The speed and type of hammers affect the particle size. In general, as the speed of the hammers is increased, the particle size is decreased. A higher speed does not invariably produce a finer powder. At very high speed there may not be sufficient time between hammers for the product to fall for impacting, so a slower speed or a smaller hammer or blade should be used.

Flat-edge blades or impact edges are used to pulverize and emulsify. The knife-like edges are used for chopping and granulating when fines are undesirable or fibers and tissues are to be milled. In the Fitzpatrick comminuting machine there is an impact edge on one side of the hammer and a knife edge on the other side. By reversing the rotor with its hammers, the most advantageous edge is made available. The hammer mill is one of the most versatile comminutors and is used in pharmacy for milling ointments, comminuting and blending wet masses, granulating tablet granulations, and pulverizing dry solids.

Obviously, the particles of a milled product are not all the same size, but they possess a size frequency distribution. To an extent the width of the size frequency distribution may be controlled.

Figure 29 illustrates the effect of speed on size frequency distribution. The product and the screen are constant, but the speed is varied. The maximum and minimum size limits are the same for all speeds, but three distributions exist. It should be recognized that such a size frequency variation in pharmaceuticals will cause batch-to-batch variation in color, taste, flowability, density, and reconstitution.

An air-swept closed grinding system produces a narrower size frequency distribution, because the particles are removed as soon as formed and no further attrition occurs to form fines. Tangential feed submits all of the product to the same actions and forces which results in a narrower size frequency distribution than with axial feed.

44 • comminution and blending

The location of the feed inlet can affect the amount of fines. A horizontal inlet produces the finest grinding, as it provides the maximum metal surface for rebound. For friable material the forward, vertical inlet is best when fines are unwanted, because the product is immediately exposed to the screen, and thereby the amount of solid surface for impact is minimized. This tends to give a narrower size frequency distribution.

Lack of uniform feeding produces a wide size frequency distribution because the packed material passes radially and the loose, open material passes tangentially. With a heavy feed there are more fines, owing to attrition between particles. Variation in the original size produces the same effect; thus, particles of grossly dissimilar sizes should be coarse ground prior to passing through the mill if a narrower size frequency distribution is desired.

Colloid Mills. The use of the colloid mill shown in Figure 30 is limited to pastes and liquids. A colloid mill consists of two parallel disks, one a rotor and the other a stator. The clearance between the two disks is adjustable and regulates the particle size. The material is fed into a central point and the discharge is at the periphery. Colloid mills are widely used in preparing pharmaceutical dispersions and emulsions.

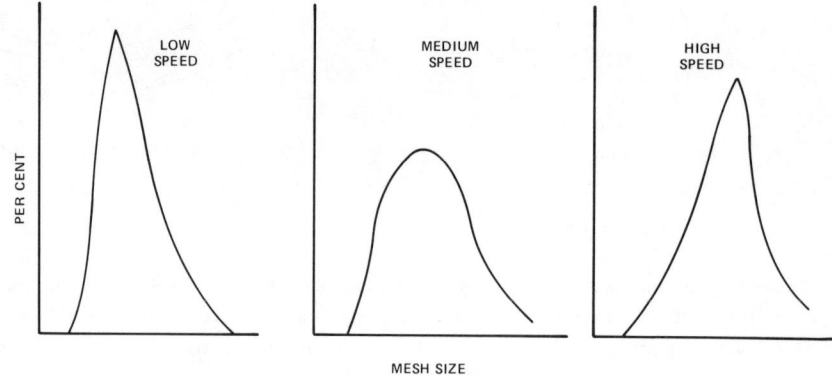

Figure 29. With a constant product and screen, the speed will affect the size frequency distribution.

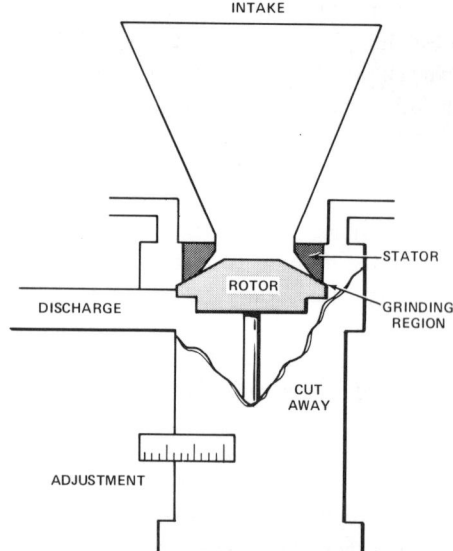

Figure 30. Diagrammatic cross section of a colloid mill.

Fluid-Energy Mills. Micronizers, or fluid-energy mills, produce particle sizes at or below the limit of most mechanical mills, i.e., below 250 mesh. This is the degree of size reduction desired for injectable and ophthalmic suspensions of drugs such as procaine penicillin, cortisone, and the sulfa drugs. Some data on micronized drugs are given in Table XII.

As shown in Figure 31, a fluid-energy mill consists of a shallow, vertical, cylindrical milling chamber in which a circulating charge of the material to be milled is acted upon by a series of impinging jets of gas introduced through orfices around the periphery. The particles are impelled at high speed in the turbulent gas flow and are reduced in size upon impact with other particles. A sequential series of impacts and size reductions occurs until particles of the desired size are formed. These are carried toward the center by the inward movement of gas, which overcomes centrifugal force. Centrifugal force keeps the larger particles in the impact zone. The pressure of the milling fluid controls the particle size obtained. A built-in cyclone removes the particles of desired size. A cyclone consists of a vertical cylinder with a conical bottom, a tangential inlet near the top, and an outlet for dust. The incoming air stream from the mill receives a rotating motion on entering the cyclone. The vortex formed provides centrifugal force, which propels the particles radially toward the wall of the cyclone. The air stream follows a downward spiral adjacent to the wall and reaches to the bottom; the air then moves upward in

Table XII Particle Size of Some Micronized Drugs

Drug	Grinding Fluid	Average Particle Size (μ)
DDT	Air	5 - 6
Procaine penicillin	Air	5; max. 20
Sodium benzoate	Air	2
Sulfur	Air	3 - 4
Talc	Steam	2
Titanium dioxide	Steam	0.2 - 0.5

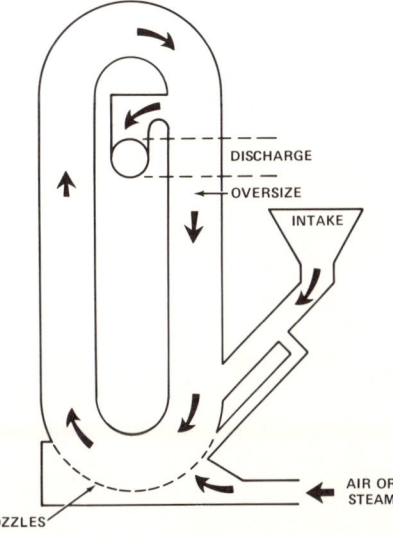

Figure 31. Diagrammatic cross section of a fluid-energy mill or micronizer.

46 • comminution and blending

a smaller spiral concentric with the first spiral and leaves through the outlet. The airborne particles attain velocities corresponding to their size. The finer particles are retained in the air and may be collected in a filter at the outlet; the larger particles settle rapidly and are collected at the periphery or bottom of the cyclone.

The milling fluid is steam at 100 to 250 psi or air at 45 to 115 psi. Steam is not used in pharmacy because of the thermolability and low melting point of many drugs. Compressed air expands on entering the milling chamber and exerts a cooling effect, so air may be used as a milling fluid for most pharmaceuticals. If the drugs are susceptible to atmospheric oxidation, an inert gas may be used as a milling fluid.

The micronizer has the advantage that grinding and classification occur in one unit. As the larger particles are held in the milling chamber by centrifugal force until reduced in size, the size frequency distribution of these ultrafine particles is narrow.

In addition to pulverizing, fluid-energy mills may be used to blend, to dry wet slurries or filter cakes, and to remove water of hydration.

A summary of the use of various mills for grinding is given in Table XIII.

Table XIII Mills Used for Intermediate and Fine Grinding of Some Drugs *

Key to types of mills:

a fluid-energy mill *(micronizer)*
b ball mill
c colloid mill
d roller mill
e hammer mill

Drug	Intermediate (8 to 40 mesh)	Fine (less than 40 mesh)
Acetanilid	be	be
Alum	be	be
Aluminum chloride	e	a
Aluminum sulfate	e	a
Ammonium bromide	e	e
Ammonium chloride	e	ae
Ammonium nitrate	e	ae
Ammonium sulfate	e	abe
Antibiotics	be	abce
Ascorbic acid	be	ab
Barium sulfate	e	ace
Barks	be	abe
Bentonite	be	abe
Benzoic acid	e	ae
Betanaphthol	e	ae
Borax	be	abe
Boric acid	be	b
Botanicals	be	abe
Caffeine	e	e
Calcium bromide	e	abe

Calcium carbonate	be	abe
Calcium chloride	e	ae
Calcium gluconate	e	ae
Calcium lactate	e	ae
Calcium phosphate	e	abde
Calcium sulfate	e	abe
Carbon, activated	b	abe
Carboxymethylcellulose	be	abce
Citric acid	e	ae
Color pastes	ai	ae
DDT	be	abe
Detergents	e	ae
Diatomaceous earth	be	abe
Dry colors	be	abe
Ferrous sulfate	e	abe
Gelatin	e	ae
Glutamic acid	e	ae
Gums	e	ace
Hexamethylenetetramine	e	abe
Iodine	e	ae
Kaolin	be	abe
Kieselguhr	be	abe
Lake colors	e	e
Magnesium carbonate	be	abe
Magnesium oxide	be	abe
Magnesium stearate	e	ae
Mercuric oxide	e	ab
Methylcellulose	be	be
Paraffin	e	be
Paraformaldehyde resin	e	abe
Penicillin	e	abce
Polyvinyl alcohol	e	ae
Potassium bromide	e	ae
Potassium carbonate	be	ae
Potassium chlorate	e	ae
Potassium chloride	e	ae
Potassium permanganate	e	ae
Resins	e	abe
Rochelle salt	e	ae
Shellac	be	abe
Sodium acid phosphate	e	ae
Sodium benzoate	e	ae
Sodium bicarbonate	e	abe
Sodium chloride	e	abe
Sodium citrate	de	ade
Sodium metaphosphate	e	ae
Sodium phosphate	e	ae
Sodium salicylate	e	ae
Sodium sulfate	ae	ae

48 • comminution and blending

Starch	e	ce
Stearic acid	e	ae
Sugar	be	abe
Titanium dioxide	be	abce
Zinc stearate	e	ae

* Modified from A. L. Stern, *Chem. Eng.* **69**, 134 (1962).

Lyophilization. Size reduction is most economically achieved by comminution or milling of larger particles into smaller particles; however, particles in a fine state of subdivision may be obtained by condensation of molecules from solution. One such technique is lyophilization, or freeze drying.

Freeze drying is a process for drying substances using a low temperature and a high vacuum. It is used for dehydrating biologicals, antibiotics, and other thermolabile products that cannot be dried by the application of heat. In freeze drying the water is sublimed, i.e., passes directly from the solid to the vapor phase without liquefying, at a temperature less than $-40°$ and at a fraction of a millimeter of mercury of pressure, as shown in Figure 32.

In the laboratory model, the liquid to be dried is placed in a flask and quickly frozen in a thin shell about the inner surface of the flask. The freezing bath consists of "dry ice" with low-freezing solvents such as acetone or alcohol. The frozen layer should not be more than 1 cm thick, as water vapor diffuses slowly through ice. Freezing should occur at a temperature less than $-40°C$ to avoid separation. If freezing takes place too slowly, some materials tend to concentrate near the top of the tray or at the inside of the flask. In drying there is the tendency for these fractions to thaw out upon the application of heat; this might impair the therapeutic potency.

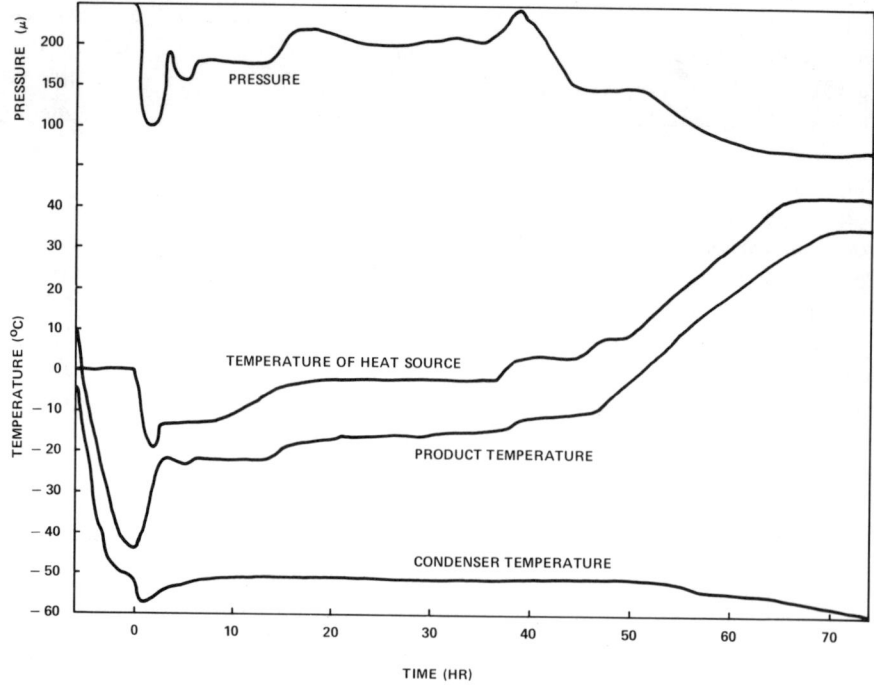

Figure 32. Typical bulk lyophilization curve for 20 per cent w/v solution with a 30-mm depth.

The flask is next connected, as shown in Figure 33, to a vacuum chamber or condenser, which is chilled by a freezing mixture. The water sublimes and collects as ice in the condenser. As the water vaporizes and heat is removed, the temperature drops. When an equilibrium temperature is reached, it becomes necessary to carefully introduce heat to complete the drying cycle. When the water content reaches 10 per cent, the material shrinks and breaks away from the side of the flask. Heat is applied by use of infrared lamps, as very little of the material touches the sides of the flask and heat transfer by conduction is very limited.

When the moisture content is reduced to 1 per cent, there is no longer any cooling from evaporation and the material assumes the temperature of the heating medium. Care must be taken that the infrared lamp is discontinued or degradation may occur. The dried material is sealed in the flask ready for use. Freeze drying requires from 6 hours to several days, depending upon the material and the size of the batch.

Production models consist of cast-iron vacuum chambers with gasketed doors and shelves. The shelves may be hollow so that cooling or heating may be accomplished by circulating fluid through the shelves. The material to be dried is placed in trays and frozen if it is to be handled as bulk material. Ampuls, vials, and bottles are filled with the correct amount of liquid and are placed in a refrigerated bath so that the product freezes in a shell on the inner surface of the vial. They are then placed in trays and lyophilized.

From the stability point of view, products prepared by freeze drying retain their original potency throughout the drying process and may be stored in sealed containers for extended periods.

Lyophilization has been suggested as a method for producing particles of less than 1 μ diameter for parenteral suspensions of slightly soluble drugs. For example, pregnenolone has been lyophilized from frozen organic solution in an attempt to produce massive nucleation from a supersaturated solution but with only slight growth of nuclei, resulting in particles of submicron size.

Many dry medicinal suspensions or solutions for reconstitution contain gums and dispersing agents that dissolve slowly. Long periods of shaking and stirring by the community pharmacist are eliminated when the pharmaceutical manufacturer lyophilizes the product. The lyophilized material is very porous, with a large specific surface, so that, upon the addition of water, reconstitution is extremely rapid because of the large surface in contact with the solvent. Some of the dispersing agents with which this technique has been successfully used are acacia, agar, algin, carboxymethylcellulose, methylcellulose, pectin, and tragacanth.

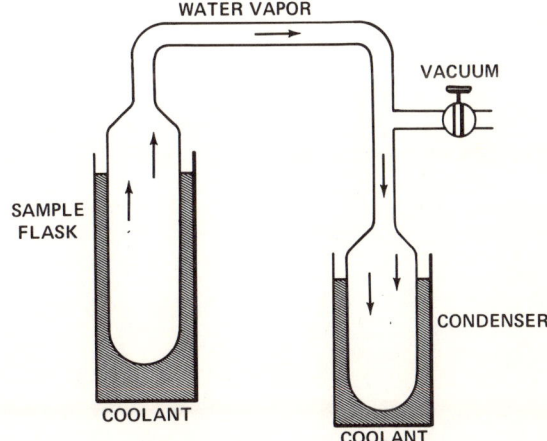

Figure 33. Diagrammatic lyophilization apparatus.

comminution and blending

Spray Drier. As shown in Figure 34, a spray drier consists of a conical drying chamber, a source of hot gases, an atomizer for the liquid feed, and a method of separating the dry powder from the exhaust gases. In operation the liquid or slurry is sprayed by a centrifugal atomizer under pressure into the drying chamber where warm air almost instantaneously removes the water, which is carried out with the exhaust air. The dry solid falls as a fine powder or is separated by a cyclone collector.

The atomizer produces a highly dispersed liquid state in the warm-air zone. The large surface of contact between the droplets and the air makes possible very rapid heat transfer and quick removal of water, so the material is only briefly in contact with warm air. The evaporation of the water keeps the intimate surface of the particle at a lower temperature than the surrounding air. Thus, under proper conditions spray drying may be used with thermolabile substances.

Spray drying has been used in pharmacy to dry hygroscopic and readily oxidizable materials and to prepare granules. Spray drying, e.g., of boric acid and methylcellulose, produces very small particle size, as shown by the increased bulkiness and decreased time required for solution. When they are suspended, spray-dried mercuric sulfide, sulfadiazine, and sulfur settle more slowly with less aggregation, indicating a small particle size. Table VIII (page 27) permits a comparison of the diameter of ammoniated mercury and sulfur powder to the diameter of spray-dried ammoniated mercury and spray-dried sulfur.

Spray-dried particles approach a spherical shape. When a liquid is atomized, the droplet assumes a spherical shape. If a hardened outer shell forms on the droplet in its initial drying stage, the liquid from the interior of the particle is prevented from reaching the surface. As heat transfer is very rapid, the liquid at the center of the particle vaporizes, causing the outer shell to expand and form a hollow sphere. If a hole is blown through the wall, the surface is greatly increased and solution occurs more rapidly.

A spherical shape makes a spray-dried powder free flowing. This method may be used to form free-flowing powders of highly irregular particles that have high interparticular friction and a high angle of repose. Spray-dried lactose is used as a diluent in the direct compression of tablets because it flows readily through the tablet machine. Tablet granulations may be prepared by spray drying a slurry of the excipient, disintegrant, binder, and color. With production units the particle size is from 100 to 250 μ. These are mixed with the active medicinal ingredient and compressed. In addition to being free flowing the granulations are uniformly colored, as they are almost instantly dried and there is little chance of migration of the colorant.

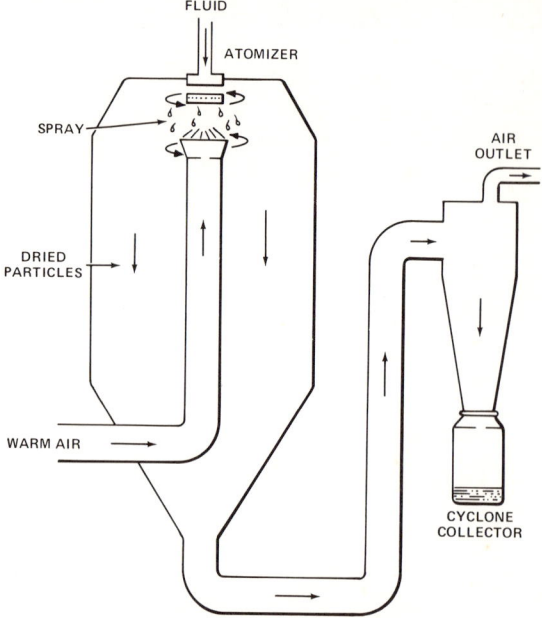

Figure 34. Diagrammatic spray-dry apparatus.

INDUSTRIAL SOLID-SOLID BLENDING

While he is compounding a prescription for solid dosage forms, the community pharmacist is concerned with the proper, uniform mixing of diluents with active drugs which in their pure form are too potent for safe and convenient use. The magnitude of the blending problem is increased for the industrial pharmacist. In addition to the diluent and the drugs, buffers, colors, flavors, preservatives, and other adjuvants must be added, often in amounts smaller than the drugs. This mixture must then be precision blended.

In industrial pharmacy blending is involved in situations other than dosage-form preparation. Plant processes, no matter how carefully controlled, sometimes produce a substandard material. This variation between batches may be compensated for by blending the substandard batch with other batches to achieve a satisfactory material. For example, after growth and extraction, the fermentation process for antibiotic production may produce a particular batch of low potency. At times this batch may be blended with a high-potency batch to obtain a mixture that is of acceptable potency.

Factors in Blending

Shape. The shape of particles is related to their structure and the way in which they were formed. Crystals assume the characteristic shapes of their ordered molecular structure. In blending one is apt to consider a solid as having a definite shape and size; however, blending at times may alter the shape and size by erosion or fragmentation.

Mechanical force can shatter a particle into smaller particles. The fragmentation products may resemble crystals or have a random shape and size. Mechanical force can exert an abrasive or erosive action in which small portions of the particle are worn from its surface. An eroded particle more or less maintains its original shape, and the fines are flakes, chips, or filaments. If and to what extent this occurs depends on the shape of the particle, its resiliency, its brittleness, and the force exerted on it. Certain industrial processes, such as the Wurster process and spray drying, produce nearly spherical particles.

The significance of the shape lies in its effect on flow characteristics. Spherical or oval particles flow readily. Rough, fractured particles are less mobile. Needle-shaped particles interlock in the manner of a miniature logjam and flow with difficulty.

Irregular-shaped particles have more surface area than an equivalent sphere. This affects adsorptivity, and sometimes mechanical forces will bring the surfaces close enough to bring molecular adhesive forces into effect, and small particles may join together into larger ones or agglomerates. With more surface the irregular-shaped particles are more likely to form an aerated suspension or dust during blending.

Size. In pharmaceutical operations the particles being blended range from $1\ \mu$ to the size of a granule, and their size distribution affects the blending process. A random motion is modified by agglomeration, coating, particle breakdown, and segregation so that a random distribution is not necessarily achieved. Large and small particles tend to segregate when blended with random motion. As the larger particles gain their mobility by rolling and flowing over one another, and the smaller particles achieve their mobility more by aerated suspension, the fines tend to dust out as the larger particles settle. This segregation of dust may be minimized by slowing the random motion.

Contrarily, in some mixtures of fines with larger, irregular particles, the fines support the coarser particles during agitation. If charcoal is placed in a thin layer on the surface of tablet granulations in a glass column attached to the hopper of a tablet machine, the vibration of the tablet machine will cause the charcoal to pass through the void between the granulations and to eventually collect on the bottom of the column. This segregation occurs with a tablet granulation that has excessive fines.

Certain pigments adhere to one another so that the dry particles behave similar to a paste. In rare cases their angle of repose approaches 90°. This is due to the extreme fineness of the particles. The fineness enhances the electrostatic effect, and it permits close packing, which emphasizes the electrostatic interaction force. Grinding and impingement of other materials may break up these agglomerations. If this fails, a surface-active agent may aid; however, the indiscriminate use of surface-active agents is not permissible in pharmacy.

Small particles tend to coat larger ones. The coated ingredient should be of uniform size or the fines with their greater specific surface will adsorb a greater portion of the coating material, and the blend would not be uniform.

Surface coating usually promotes agglomeration, but at times it lubricates each particle so that the particles will not adhere. Powders to be encapsulated and granules to flow through a tablet machine usually have a fraction of 1 per cent of a solid lubricant added. The lubricant has very small particle size and coats the powder or granule so that it does not agglomerate and will flow freely.

Density. Radical density differences of particles of the same size tend to promote separation. The heavy ones settle and the light ones rise. This is aggravated if the heavy particles are coarse and the light particles are fine. On the other hand, size differences and density differences may balance out if the fines happen to be more dense than the coarse particles.

The density of most substances used in pharmaceuticals is not extremely different, and generally this effect has little significance.

Electrostatic Force. It has been said that the control of electrostatic charge is the most important consideration in blending solids. If the particles of two different materials have acquired mutually repellent charges, this can produce a situation in which segregation forces are remarkably powerful. It may be impossible to mix these particles by mechanical means. Materials being blended must have an attraction for one another.

Surface conductivity is the ability of a particle to hold a static charge or to dissipate electron imbalances readily. Organic compounds tend to accumulate static electricity. It is not uncommon for micronized organic drugs to adhere in an oriented pattern to containers and machinery. This makes blending or any other manipulative operation a questionable one. In general, metals and inorganic salts dissipate a static charge more readily than organic compounds.

It is surface conductivity that makes the technology of solid-solid and liquid-solid blending different. In a liquid-solid system the electrical conductivity is relatively high, but in a solid-solid system it is low. Thus, the random motion of the blender serves to make unblending possible. The surface electron states are unbalanced by the frictional effects of the particles as they rub against one another, and as the surface conductivity is low, the electrostatic charge is built up. Generally, the particles will adhere to one another and they form agglomerates. Under other conditions the particles will be mutually repelled and will adhere to their container.

Limits of Blend. It is generally agreed that a homogeneous dispersion is required for all mixtures of pharmaceuticals; however, this statement requires some qualification. For a pharmaceutical product a blend of active and inert ingredients that assures a uniformly safe, effective amount of the drug in each patient dose will be a satisfactory blend.

In a blend of two or more solids, the active ingredient is the one constituent whose uniform dispersion throughout the blend is most important. Critical quantity is the smallest amount of a blended material in which the accuracy of mixing will be significant during use. In pharmacy, the critical quantity is the smallest dose of a blend that will be administered, e.g., a capsule or a tablet.

In a pharmaceutical blend the concentration of the active ingredient is controlled by careful weighing when the batch is placed in the blender. The active ingredient is often only a few per cent of the blend. Obviously, the product of the percentage of active ingredient in the blend and the critical quantity is the amount of active ingredient desired in the critical quantity of the blend. For example, if a blend contains 2.0 per cent of a medicinal compound to be blended into 250 mg of powder to be filled into a capsule, the amount of active ingredient desired in the critical quantity is 250 x 0.02 or 5 mg.

With a knowledge of the particle size of the active ingredient, the number of particles of the active ingredient desired in the critical quantity of the blend can be computed. Any mixture that would require less than 100 active particles in a critical quantity is impractical. Figure 35 shows in a random distribution the relationship between probable error and the number of active particles in the critical quantity. Obviously, the active ingredient should be broken down into the smallest, most uniform particles that are practical.

In a 50:50 binary mixture, there may be thousands of active particles in the critical quantity. In a 1:99 blend of the same materials, there are 1/50 as many active particles present in the same critical quantity. In a 0.1:99.9 blend only 1/500 as many active particles are present in the same critical quantity.

Refer to the capsule that is to contain 5.0 mg of active ingredient. The formula must be blended to the extent that every 250 mg of the mixture will contain 5.0 mg of active ingredient; however, this does not theoretically require that the 5.0 mg of active ingredient be completely randomized throughout the 250-mg critical quantity.

Blending Equipment

The most effective solid-particle blenders apply a motive force to the entire batch of material simultaneously. The ideal blender for solid particles should have efficient mixing action so that blending will be accomplished rapidly. The mixing action should be gentle, with a minimum scraping friction and maximum mobility. Mechanically the blender should be easily cleanable, dusttight, and provide complete discharge.

Blending equipment may be divided into two types: In one, the tumbler uses gravity to impel flow, and in the other the tumbler pushes the material with blades or paddles. A tumble-type blender is better than a blender with blades or impellers. In tumbling the gravity action is sustained throughout the mass.

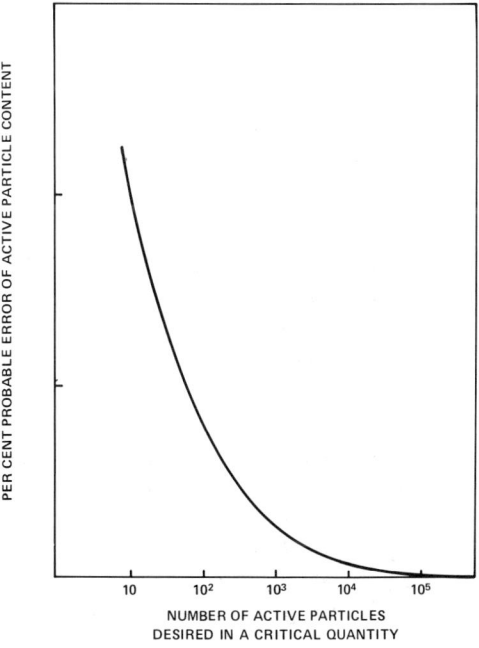

Figure 35. Qualitative representation of the relationship between probable error in random distribution and number of active particles in a critical quantity.

54 • comminution and blending

Tumble Blenders. Drum-type blenders with the axis of rotation horizontal to the center of the drum lack good cross flow along the axis. Baffles may be added to improve the cross flow. Discharge is through an adjustable chute. Drum-type blenders are not recommended for pharmaceutical operations because of the poor cross flow and the difficulty of cleaning.

Cubical and polyhedron-shaped blenders are available with rotating axis disposed at various angles. The flat surfaces of the vessel produce a sliding flow that is not conducive to mixing. When particles slide, they move in a fixed relative position to one another; mixing occurs from flat surfaces when the particles are dropped or bounced. The sliding action also causes abrasion of the particles. The many corners make sanitary cleaning of the vessel difficult.

In the double-cone blender shown in Figure 36, two cones are joined to a relatively short cylindrical section and the axis of rotation is centrally located on the cylindrical portion. Usually the cones have a 90° included angle or a 45° discharge angle. This type of blender provides a constantly changing cross-sectional flow as the vessel rotates. There are no flat spots, so all motion is rolling. Its maximum charge is 50 per cent of its total capacity; this assures complete displacement from cone to cone as the vessel rotates. As it is free of baffles and corners, it is easily cleaned.

As illustrated in Figure 36, a twin-shelled blender is formed from a cylinder cut at an angle and joined together to form a V shape. It provides a nonsymmetrical shape about the axis of rotation, which is located at a point that provides equal torque loading throughout a full rotation. The twin-shell blender combines the efficient blending action of the inclined cylinder with the intermeshing action that occurs when two inclined cylinders combine their flows. The charge of all tumble blenders should not exceed 50 per cent of their capacity. The twin-shelled blender is the fastest of the precision blenders. For tumble blenders the scale-up from laboratory size is precise; in fact, larger tumble blenders may have a higher blending efficiency than smaller units. The twin-shelled blender is completely discharged from a central valve. It is accessible from both ends and is easily cleaned.

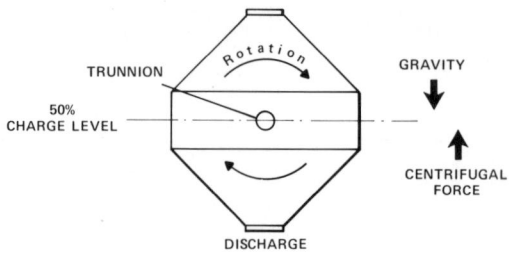

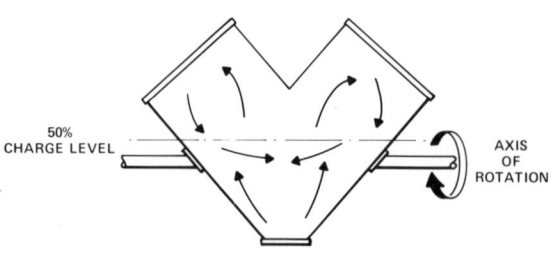

Figure 36. Precision tumbler blenders: (a) double-cone blender; (b) twin-shell V blender.

Blade and Paddle Blenders. The ribbon blender shown in Figure 37 is a stationary-trough type of shell approximately three times as long as it is wide, with a semicircular bottom fitted with a longitudinal shaft on which are mounted arms that support slender spiral ribbons. Usually there is an outer spiral ribbon to move material in one direction and an inner spiral ribbon to move material in the opposite direction. This opposing of ribbon helices provides for axial flow and prevents pile up of material in one direction. The amount of material moved by the ribbons is relatively small, so blending cycles are quite long. The outer ribbon must have a fairly close clearance with the semicircular cross section of the shell bottom so that no undisturbed material remains on the bottom surface. With fine powders this is hard to accomplish. The ribbon blender is not a precision blender. The ribbon blender imposes a grinding action and should not be used when blending fragile particles. Its power requirement is many times that required by tumbler blenders.

Sigma blade mixers and planetary paddle mixers are primarily for liquid-solid blending. The sigma blade mixer is widely used in the pharmaceutical industry to incorporate liquids into solids, such as a granulating solution into a tablet formula, but it is not a precision blender for solid-solid systems.

INDUSTRIAL LIQUID-SOLID BLENDING

Liquid-solid blending in pharmacy refers to precision blending in which the liquid comprises only a relatively small portion of the total blend. The individual particles retain their identity and the blend appears to be dry. The liquid may be adsorbed in a thin surface layer or the liquid may be trapped in the interstices of the particles. The liquid is probably held to the particles by a combination of adsorption, absorption, and entrapment in fissures.

When properly blended a liquid may be added to small particles and the resulting powder will be apparently dry and free flowing, with a high degree of uniformity. In general, it is best to first blend the solids precisely before the liquid is introduced. Any liquid present tends to maintain segregation, and any solid-solid blending problems should be corrected before the liquid is added.

Factors in Blending

Electrostatic Force. In a liquid-solid system the electrical conductivity is relatively high, and no appreciable electrostatic charge accumulates on the particles. As a result the liquid-solid system has less adherence and agglomeration. This is the only blending problem that is improved by the addition of a liquid to a powder.

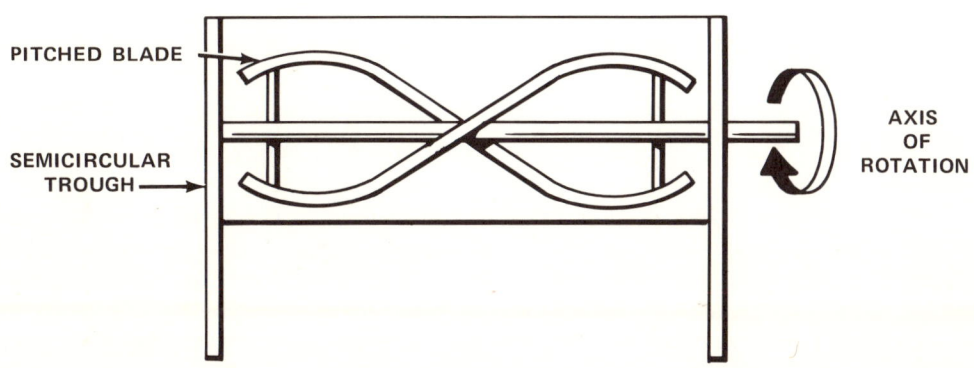

Figure 37. Ribbon blender.

56 • comminution and blending

Size. Particle size must be uniform if a desired weight-to-weight uniform distribution is to be attained. The smaller particles with a greater specific surface will hold more of the liquid on their surface than the larger particles, preventing the desired uniform weight-to-weight distribution.

Consider the blending of a liquid with a substance having particles with diameters d_l and d_s equal to 400 and 40 μ, respectively. If the subscripts l and s refer to the larger and the smaller particles, respectively, the ratio of the weights W to the volumes V is

$$\frac{W_l}{W_s} = \frac{\rho V_l}{\rho V_s} = \frac{(\pi/6)d_l^3}{(\pi/6)d_s^3} = \frac{400^3}{40^3} = 1000$$

The ratio of the surface area, S_l, of the larger particles to the surface area, S_s, of the smaller particles is

$$\frac{S_l}{S_s} = \frac{\pi d_l^2}{\pi d_s^2} = \frac{400^2}{40^2} = 100$$

In practical blending one is generally concerned with the distribution of a certain weight of liquid on a given weight of solid. On the basis of surface per unit weight, the larger particle above will have

$$\frac{S_l/W_l}{S_s/W_s} = \frac{\pi d_l^2/(\pi/6)d_l^3}{\pi d_s^2/(\pi/6)d_s^3} = \frac{1}{10}$$

as much surface on which a liquid may be adsorbed. Consequently, with a mixture of 40- and 400-μ particles, the liquid would probably be distributed to a greater extent on the smaller particle than on the larger and the desired weight-to-weight distribution would not be achieved.

Mobility is affected by the ratio of the surface to the weight of a particle. Fines with a high specific surface tend to float or dust, and their mobility depends on aeration. Excessive dusting or selective aeration can be eliminated by blending in a vacuum. Large particles with smaller surface-to-weight ratios tend to move by rolling or sliding. Although a liquid tends to inhibit both types of movement, it is best to reduce the size of the particles to the same magnitude before blending and the addition of the liquid.

Moisture. Depending on the ability of a substance to hold moisture, an apparently dry powder is seldom completely moisture free and may contain various amounts of moisture. Certain substances, if completely dry, have so strong an affinity for the liquid added that all is sorbed immediately by the first few particles it contacts. The sorbed liquid is not available for coating other portions of the powder. Uniform distribution in such conditions may be helped by wetting the solids with another volatile liquid before adding the active liquid ingredient. A simple increase in humidity may have the same effect.

If the liquid is not attracted by the solid, a slight excess of a volatile, penetrating liquid may be added to aid in dispersing the active liquid, and the volatile dispersing agent may then be removed by mild heat. The excess liquid dispersing agent may also be removed by tumbling and drying under a vacuum.

Viscosity and Surface Tension. Liquids with low surface tension are more readily distributed than those with high surface tension.

With an increase in viscosity it becomes more difficult to break a liquid into colloidal droplets. A viscid liquid tends to remain in larger particles, which require high shearing force to reduce to colloidal size. Liquid contact with the vessel should be avoided, as the liquid adheres to the walls and lumps are created.

To blend liquids with high viscosity and surface tension high shearing force is required. An increase in temperature will decrease viscosity and surface tension; thus, an increase in temperature may facilitate blending.

Liquid-Solid Ration. Colloidal clays may sorb up to 20 per cent water and remain apparently dry and particulate, however, beyond this further addition of water produces a dough or slurry. Volatile oils may be added to talc without a change in appearance; the oil will progressively be rubbed from one particle and spread in thin coats on others until almost slurry-producing proportions are reached.

In preparing a uniform liquid-solid blend, there should be sufficient surface to hold all the liquid. If there is more solid surface than there is liquid to provide a monomolecular coating of the dry surface, all the solid cannot be covered; thus, this blend cannot be homogeneous, although it may be uniform.

Blending Equipment

The basic requirements to have satisfactory liquid-solid blending are that (1) both the liquid and the solid be finely divided, (2) both must be suspended in space, and (3) the liquid and solid must be kept in motion, so that fresh materials are constantly exposed.

A spray nozzle is used to spray colloidal droplets of the liquid into a tumbler or blender. A whirling agitator in a V blender as shown in Figure 38 may be used. The agitator rotates at a high speed, e.g., 4000 ft min^{-1}, forming an interior void about the agitator. The liquid is sprayed through the hollow shaft of the agitator through high-pressure nozzles with blades. The blades are pitched so that a colloidal mist is formed. The colloidal droplets and the solid particles mix under conditions of high mobility, and new solid particles are continuously brought into contact with the spray.

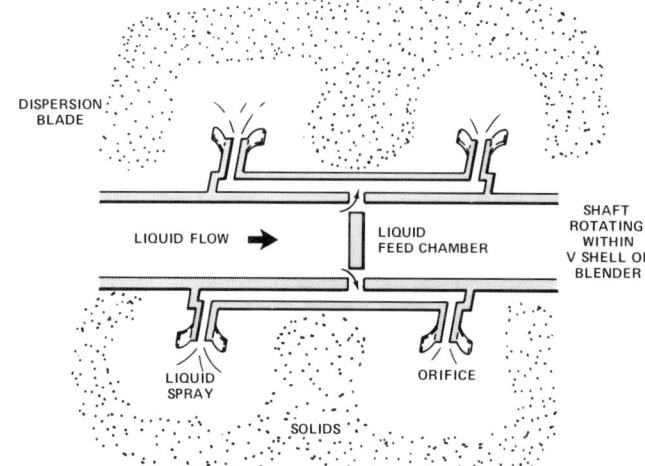

Figure 38. Diagram of whirling dispersion blades used in a V blender for liquid-solid blending.

3 | SOLID PHARMACEUTICALS

POWDERS

Powders are mixtures of drugs and medicinal chemicals in a dry, fine state of subdivision. Powders are used internally and externally. Their versatility is shown by the many types of powders used today: bulk powders, dental powders, dusting powders, divided powders, douche powders, and insufflations. The greater specific surface area of the powders provides more rapid dispersion or solution of the ingredients than compacted dosage forms such as a tablet.

Some very soluble drugs, in the form of a capsule or tablet, cause nausea and irritation. This may be caused by the high localized concentration of drug in contact with a small portion of the gastric mucosa. The administration of a rapidly diffusing powder diminishes this type of irritation.

From the medical viewpoint, powders provide a flexible dosage form that may be extemporaneously compounded by the community pharmacist. The physician may prescribe any drugs, dose or bulk, most favorable for a certain patient without being restricted by prefabricated dosage forms.

For children and some adults who experience difficulty in swallowing a tablet or capsule, powders may be used. The powder is stirred in part of a glass of water or fruit juice and is immediately swallowed. Some adults prefer to place the powder on their tongue and then swallow it with a drink of water. Some drugs are so bulky that the size of the encapsulated or compressed dose would be prohibitive. These large, bulky doses may be administered in the form of a powder.

Drugs possessing an unpleasant taste should not be prime candidates for an oral powder. Readily oxidizable and moisture-attracting drugs should not be dispensed as powders with their large surface area exposed to the atmosphere but in a dosage form protected from the air. For example, ferrous sulfate is easily oxidized and should be dispensed as a coated tablet.

As discussed in Chapter 2, all drugs to be used in a solid dosage form should be comminuted to powders of approximately the same size to avoid stratification during blending. The pulverized ingredients are then mixed by geometric dilution. In the pharmacy, the mortar and pestle is the best means for comminution and blending. Gentle trituration produces a light, bulky powder; heavy and prolonged trituration reduces granules and crystals to a fine powder. Heavy trituration of resinous drugs causes unwanted caking of the powder. Routine sifting ensures proper mixing and reduction of particle size.

Whether compounding a prescription for 25 capsules or manufacturing a batch of 1 million tablets, qualitative and quantitative accuracy are vital. The industrial pharmacist has an elaborate system for controlling the accuracy of a product during its manufacture and after its production is completed; this system is known as quality control.

To ensure qualitative accuracy in a compounded prescription, the pharmacist should read the labels on the bottles of drugs at least three times. The label is first read when the drugs and chemicals are assembled at the prescription counter and are placed on the left side of the balance. The label is read again at the time the ingredients are weighed and the bottle placed on the right side of the balance to indicate that the substance has been weighed. The label is read for the third time when the drugs are returned to the shelves.

All drugs are carefully handled to avoid waste and loss during transfer and compounding. An error of ±5 per cent is generally permissible and can be achieved with standard equipment in the pharmacy. As the prescription balance is used many times to weigh life-giving medicinals, it is essential that the pharmacist completely understand its operation, correct usage, and limitations. For this reason a review of weighing with a prescription balance is presented.

The National Bureau of Standards sets standards for balances. The Class A prescription balance is required at every prescription counter. A Class A prescription balance has a sensitivity requirement of 6 mg with no load and with a load of 10 g on each pan. The prescription balance usually is used to weigh quantities up to 120 g.

Prior to weighing, the balance is leveled by means of the thumbscrew and is adjusted to obtain equal swings of the pointer to the right and left (or up and down, depending on the type of indicator) or to obtain rest with exact alignment of the double pointers. The rider on the graduated beam must be at its zero position during this operation.

Medicinal substances are weighed on powder papers. The paper protects the pans from chemical corrosion and eliminates the need for repeated washing of the pans. A new paper for each item prevents contamination. Another advantage to the use of a paper is that it serves as a transfer funnel.

Weighing papers should have a smooth surface so that no appreciable amount of drug will adhere to the paper. This is especially important when small amounts are to be weighed. A paper should be chosen so it is of reasonable size, giving a maximum weighing area without touching any part of the balance except the pan. The papers should be creased diagonally from each corner to the opposite corner and then flattened before being placed on the pans. If desired, tared watch glass or special stainless steel pans may be used.

To weigh, the pharmacist places the creased papers on the balance pans and adjusts the balance by means of the leveling screws so the index pointer is at zero. Powder papers from the same container can vary in weight by as much as 65 mg. If equilibrium is not established after the papers are placed on the pans, an error as great as 30 per cent can result in the weighing of 200 mg of material.

With the balance arrested, the pharmacist opens the balance lid and places the desired weights on the right pan and/or the weighbeam. The material to be weighed is placed on the left pan, and then the balance is unlocked to observe if the correct weight of material was deposited. A spatula is used to remove or add material until the correct amount is deposited; the balance is arrested each time a transfer is made. When equilibrium is established, the balance is arrested, the lid is closed, and the arrest is released to check the equilibrium. The arresting knob is most conveniently operated by the left hand.

The amount that can be weighed on a balance depends on its sensitivity requirement. The sensitivity requirement is the weight that must be added to one pan to produce a change of one index plate division in the rest point of the indicator. A balance that requires a smaller weight to move the indicator one division is more sensitive than a balance that requires a greater weight.

When it is stated that a substance has a certain weight, the figure includes not only the true weight but also the possible excessive or deficient weight resulting from the error introduced by virtue of the sensitivity of the balance. The sensitivity requirement is used to determine the per cent of possible error for a given amount of material being weighed.

If 200 mg of drug is to be weighed on a balance with a sensitivity requirement of 5 mg, the actual weight could be between 195 and 205 mg. The percentage of possible error is

$$\frac{5}{200} = \frac{x}{100}$$

$$x = 2.5\%$$

solid pharmaceuticals

In general, the inherent percentage of error for any given weighing may be expressed

$$\text{per cent error} = \frac{\text{sensitivity requirement} \times 100}{\text{amount desired}}$$

The same relationship is used to calculate the smallest amount that can be weighed within a particular permissible percentage of error. If the permissible error is 5 per cent and the sensitivity requirement of the balance is 5 mg, the smallest amount that can be weighed within this limit of error may be calculated:

$$5 = \frac{5 \times 100}{W}$$

$$W = 100 \text{ mg}$$

To achieve 99 per cent accuracy, i.e., to permit a 1 per cent error, the amount weighed must be at least 100 times as great as the sensitivity requirement of the balance. To ensure an error no greater than 5 per cent, an amount at least 20 times the sensitivity requirement must be weighed.

Most ingredients may be weighed on a Class A balance; however, when the amount of the drug is too small to be weighed with the desired accuracy, an aliquot method of weighing may be employed. The aliquot method consists of weighing an excess of the drug equal to a multiple of the quantity needed and diluting this to a convenient weight. Then the aliquot, or part of the dilution which represents the desired amount of the drug, is used.

Using a balance with a sensitivity requirement of 5 mg, consider weighing 15 mg of atropine sulfate with 95 per cent accuracy. A multiple quantity is first selected. The smallest amount that can be weighed to ensure an error no greater than 5 per cent is at least 20 times the sensitivity requirement,

$$5 \times 20 = 100 \text{ mg}$$

Thus, an amount of drug 21 times the sensitivity requirement of the balance, or 105 mg, is weighed. The size of this multiple quantity is determined by the degree of accuracy desired, the convenience of the multiple, the availability of weights, and the cost of the drug.

The amount of inert diluent to be added must be a quantity large enough to be weighed within the desired limit of error. The weight of aliquot must be at least as much as the multiple quantity, and to reduce the error its weight should usually be somewhat greater. In this example, the multiple quantity weighs 105 mg, so the aliquot must weigh at least 105 mg or more.

If 125 mg is chosen as the aliquot to contain 15 mg of the drug and 105 mg of atropine sulfate is weighed, the weight of the total dilution is

$$\frac{15}{125} = \frac{105}{W}$$

$$W = 875 \text{ mg}$$

Thus, the total dilution of 875 mg will contain 105 mg of atropine sulfate and 770 mg of diluent.

Industrially, triturates of potent drugs may be used if the amount cannot be weighed directly. These are usually 1 or 10 per cent triturations with inert diluents such as lactose.

Whether a fraction of a gram or several hundred kilograms is being weighed, the same procedure and limitations apply to the size and type of balance being utilized.

Bulk Powders

Only powders that are nonpotent and can be measured in a spoon may be safely dispensed as a bulk powder for oral administration. In modern therapy this almost limits internal bulk powders to antacids, dietary supplements, laxative, and a few analgesics.

Bulk powders are dispensed in screw-capped glass jars with a wide mouth. The opening should be large enough to admit a spoon. A glass container protects the product from moisture and retards the loss of volatile components.

1. Phenobarbital   0.45 g
   Belladonna extract   0.30 g
   Calcium carbonate   45.00 g
   Magnesium oxide   18.00 g
   Magnesium trisilicate   30.00 g
   Dried aluminum hydroxide gel   18.00 g
   Peppermint oil   0.50 ml

   Sig.: ʒ i in water every 4 hours

The belladonna extract, the phenobarbital, and the peppermint oil are triturated in a porcelain mortar until homogeneously mixed. Approximate quantities of 1, 2, 4, and 11 g of magnesium oxide are added in sequence with trituration after each addition. The dried aluminum hydroxide gel is added, and the mixture is triturated. The magnesium trisilicate is added, and the mixture is triturated. Finally, the calcium carbonate is added and blended until the bulk powder is uniform.

2. Hard soap, 100 mesh   50 g
   Calcium carbonate, 325 mesh   935 g
   Sodium saccharin   2 g
   Peppermint oil   4 ml
   Cinnamon oil   2 ml
   Methyl salicylate   8 ml

   Sig.: N.F. Dentifrice

The sodium saccharin, the oils, and the methyl salicylate are gradually blended with approximately one-half of the calcium carbonate. The soap is passed through a 100-mesh sieve and gradually blended with the remainder of the calcium carbonate. The two powders are mixed thoroughly and pass through a 325-mesh sieve or bolting cloth.

Dusting powders are fine medicinal powders intended to be dusted on the skin by means of sifter-top containers. A single medicinal agent may be used as a dusting powder; however, a base is frequently used to apply a medicinal agent and to protect the skin from irritation and friction. Bentonite, kaolin, kieselguhr, magnesium carbonate, starch, and talc are used as bases for dusting powders. Power bases absorb secretions, exerting a drying effect, which relieves congestion and imparts a cooling sensation. Cooling results, as the moisture is sorbed on a large surface and increased evaporation from this large surface facilitates the removal of heat.

Dusting powders are prepared in the same manner as other powders. All extemporaneous dusting powders should be passed through a 100-mesh sieve to ensure that they are grit free and will not further mechanically irritate traumatized areas. Commercial dusting powders pass through a 200-mesh sieve. In general, powders that are to be packaged as powder aerosols must not contain particles greater than 50 μ if they are to be sprayed successfully.

3. Menthol   10 g
   Salicylic acid   30 g
   Tannic acid   100 g
   Alum   100 g
   Boric acid   760 g

   Sig.: Astringent foot powder

62 • solid pharmaceuticals

The crystals of menthol and salicylic acid are pulverized in a mortar. Powdered tannic acid is added and blended; then the powdered alum is added and blended. After the powdered boric acid is added to the mixture and it is thoroughly blended, the foot powder is passed through a 100-mesh sieve.

4. Clove oil   2 ml
   Cinnamon oil   2 ml
   Undecylenic acid   20 g
   Zinc undecylenate   200 g
   Boric acid   776 g

   Sig.: Dust on affected area t.i.d.

Douche powders are prescribed as a matter of convenience for the patient, as a powder is more portable than a bulky solution. The formula is developed so that a teaspoonful of powder dissolved in a specified volume of water provides the desired concentration. The pH usually ranges from 3.5 to 5 when the solution is prepared. Feminine bulb syringes or fountain syringes are used for vaginal irrigation.

Since many of the ingredients are volatile, e.g., menthol, thymol, and volatile oils, douche powders should be packaged in glass jars with a wide mouth. Some commercial douche powders are available in metal-foil packets, which contain the proper amount of powder for a single douche.

5. Boric acid   72.00 g
   Alum   23.00 g
   Phenol   2.00 g
   Eucalyptus oil   1.25 ml
   Methyl salicylate   1.00 ml
   Thymol   0.25 g
   Menthol   0.50 g

   Sig.: ʒ ii in qt warm water

The phenol, the eucalyptus oil, the methyl salicylate, the thymol, and the menthol are triturated in a mortar. To this liquid, boric acid powder is added in divided portions with trituration after each addition until the liquid is adsorbed. The remainder of the boric acid and powdered alum are added, and the mixture is triturated until homogeneous.

6. Sodium lauryl sulfate   0.375 g
   Papain   1.500 g
   Citric acid   24.000 g
   Lactose   123.000 g
   Methyl salicylate   0.375 ml
   Menthol   0.375 g

   Sig.: ʒ ii in qt warm water

Insufflations are extremely fine powders to be introduced into body cavities. To administer an insufflation the powder is placed in an insufflator, and when the bulb is squeezed, the air current carries the fine particles through the nozzle to the region for which the medication is intended. All extemporaneously compounded insufflations must be passed through a 100-mesh sieve.

7. Iodochlorhydroxyquin   250 g
   Boric acid   100 g
   Lactic acid   25 ml
   Zinc stearate   200 g
   Lactose   425 g

   Sig.: Insufflate 2 g intravaginally

solid pharmaceuticals • 63

Lactic acid is a syrupy liquid; it is mixed with the boric acid. The lactose is then uniformly incorporated. The iodochlorhydroxyquin and zinc stearate are then added and the powder is mixed.

For inhalation, isoproterenol is an example of an insufflation administered by the oral route. A cartridge, containing 10 per cent isoproterenol diluted with lactose, is inserted in the inhaler. The apparatus is placed in the mouth and a deep breath is taken. The incoming air drives a ball against the cartridge, releasing a small quantity of powder that is immediately drawn into the respiratory tract. It is the opinion of some authorities that the powder is more irritating to the mucous membrane and causes more side effects than when the solution is inhaled.

Divided Powders (Chartulae)

Divided powders are single doses of powdered medicinals individually wrapped in cellophane, metallic foil, or paper. The divided powder is an accurate dosage form because the patient is not involved in measurement of the dose. Cellophane and foil-enclosed powders are better protected from the external environment until the time of administration than paper-enclosed powders.

The technique of mixing the ingredients in divided powders is the same as previously discussed for the pulverizing and blending of solids. Briefly, all drugs are reduced to a powder before weighing. The weighed drugs are then blended by geometric dilution or by mixing in ascending order of quantity. As powder papers vary in weight, a pair of counter balanced weighing papers are used, and each weighed portion of the powder is transferred to the paper in which it will be wrapped. If the therapeutically active ingredients are less than 300 mg, it is advisable to add an inert diluent to increase the bulk. It is then easier for both the pharmacist and patient to handle the powders without appreciable percentage loss.

In the community pharmacy, divided powders are folded in a traditional manner as shown in Figure 39.

1. The long edge of the paper is folded over approximately ½ in. This fold will be the top of the finished powder paper. To save time and to get a uniform fold, several papers may be folded at once.

2. With the fold away from the pharmacist, the powder papers are laid side by side with a slight overlap.

3. The correct weight of powder is placed in the center of each paper.

4. The lower edge of the paper is brought up and fitted under the top fold.

5. The top fold is pulled toward the pharmacist until it divides the remainder of the paper approximately in half.

6. The folded paper is picked up with the thumb and index finger of each hand, and the ends are folded over a powder box so that the finished paper will just fit into the box. All folds should appear uniform.

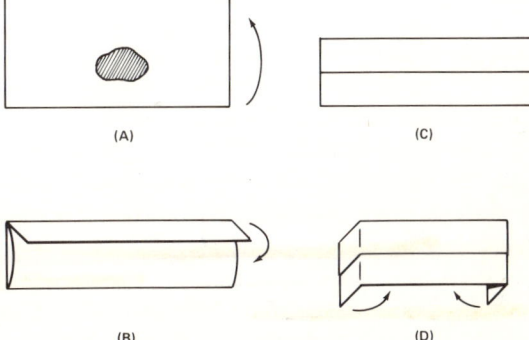

Figure 39. Stages in the folding of a divided powder (see the text for explanation).

64 • solid pharmaceuticals

The divided powders are placed in a hinged-cover cardboard box with the label affixed inside the cover. Normally, the powder papers face in the same direction, with the top fold uppermost. A shouldered box is made so that the folded powders project slightly above the edge of the base without being crushed when the cover is closed. This permits the patient to more readily remove a powder from the box.

The traditionally folded paper may be replaced by cellophane envelopes, which protect the medication from atmospheric moisture and are prepared more rapidly. Seamed cellophane tubing with a closed and an open end is available in several sizes. To use a cellophane envelope, the correct weight of medication is placed into the envelope, taking care not to spill powder on the open end. The open end is folded over approximately ½ in. and is sharply creased. It is laid on a tile and is sealed by passing a heated spatula over the creased end. The cellophane envelopes are dispensed by stacking one on top of another in a box.

8. Sodium bicarbonate, 60 mesh   30 g
   Potassium sodium tartrate, 40 mesh   90 g
   Tartaric acid, 40 mesh   26 g

Sig.: One dozen Seidlitz powders

In preparing the classical Seidlitz powders, dry drugs must be used. The sodium bicarbonate and potassium sodium tartrate are intimately mixed, and 10 g of the blend is wrapped in each blue powder paper. The tartaric acid is divided into 12 equal parts and wrapped in a white paper. The contents of one white and one blue paper are placed in half a glass of water and are drunk just after effervescence begins to subside.

9. Sodium nitrite   0.1 g
   Potassium nitrate   0.3 g
   Sodium bicarbonate   1.0 g

Sig.: One powder in water for visceral crisis

GRANULES

Medicinal granules are particles ranging from 4 to 10 mesh in size. Granules are not used with potent drugs because of the inherent error when a patient measures the dose with a teaspoon. Examples of dietary supplements marketed as granules are Calcigranules® and Somagen®. Some bulk laxatives administered as granules are Bassoran®, Gentlax®, Mucara®, and Mucilose®.

Certain drugs are unstable in water and are prefabricated as granules, which are dissolved or suspended in water by the pharmacist before the prescription is dispensed. Compocillin-VK®, Granules for Oral Suspension, and Sulfa-Sugracillin® Flavored Granules are granules for reconstitution by the pharmacist.

Granules are formed by moistening the blended powders and by passing this mass through a screen or granulator. The moist granules are then air or oven dried.

As discussed in Chapter 1, granules may be prepared by spray drying a slurry or solution of the drugs. Somagen® is commercially prepared by this technique. Spray-dried flavor granules are widely used in pharmaceuticals. An emulsion of the flavor oils with a gum, e.g., acacia, is spray dried. Up to 16 per cent oil is entrapped within the porous granule formed without any oil appearing on the surface. The granules are free flowing and the oils are more stable to the atmosphere.

Effervescent granules contain mixtures of citric acid, tartaric acid, or sodium biphosphate with a bicarbonate and a medicinal agent. When the granules are placed in water, effervescence occurs and the solution is carbonated. Since the evolution of carbon dioxide is very rapid, a powdered formulation might effervesce violently enough to spill the solution from the glass. With granulation there is less surface and effervescence is less violent. It is recommended that the patient use cold water, as the reaction occurs less readily and carbonation is more complete.

The carbonated solution is a pleasant vehicle and lessens the bitter and saline taste of salts, e.g., magnesium sulfate. Viewing the effervescence may have some psychological benefit to the patient. Speciality products, which are effervescent granules, are Citrocarbonate® and Bromo Seltzer®. These are packaged in wide-mouth jars that permit the entrance of a spoon or in jars that have a cap that will hold a dose of the granule. Moisture must be excluded to avoid a reaction.

The two methods for the preparation of effervescent granules are the fusion and the wet method. The formulation is the same regardless of the method of manufacture. Although the weight of 1 teaspoonful of material depends on the density of the material and the size of the granules, 1 heaping teaspoonful of an effervescent granule is considered in practical therapy to weigh 5 g.

A pharmacist is requested to develop a formula for an effervescent bromisovalum granule containing 600 mg of bromisovalum per teaspoonful to be packaged in a 120-g unit. As each teaspoonful weighs 5 g, there are 24 doses per bottle; the effervescent granule will consist of 14.4 g of bromisovalum and 105.6 g of granulation base.

A mixture of acids will be used because tartaric acid produces a chalky, friable granule, and citric acid is too sticky to manipulate. It is desired that citric acid and tartaric acid be used in the ratio 1:2. The amount of sodium bicarbonate required to react with this ratio of acids is calculated from the equations of the reaction

$$3 NaHCO_3 + HO-C(CH_2COOH)_2-COOH \cdot H_2O \rightarrow 4H_2O + 3CO_2 + HO-C(CH_2COONa)_2-COONa$$

3 X 84   210 (citric acid)

The amount of sodium bicarbonate to react with 1 g of citric acid is

$$\frac{1}{210} = \frac{x}{3 \times 84}$$

$$x = 1.2 \text{ g}$$

$$2 NaHCO_3 + \begin{matrix} COOH \\ CH-OH \\ CH-OH \\ COOH \end{matrix} \rightarrow 2H_2O + 2CO_2 + \begin{matrix} COONa \\ CH-OH \\ CH-OH \\ COONa \end{matrix}$$

2 X 84   150 (tartaric acid)

The amount of sodium bicarbonate to react with 2 g of tartaric acid is

$$\frac{2}{150} = \frac{x}{2 \times 84}$$

$$x = 2.24 \text{ g}$$

Thus, with the acids in the ratio 1:2, it has been calculated that 3.44 g of sodium bicarbonate is required to neutralize 3 g of the combined acids. To enhance the flavor a small amount of acid is left unreacted so the sodium bicarbonate may be reduced to 3.4 g. The 105.6 g of effervescent base is prepared in the ratio

citric acid	1
tartaric acid	2
sodium bicarbonate	3.4
	6.4

The amount of citric acid to be used is

$$\frac{1}{6.4} = \frac{x}{105.6}$$

$$x = 16.5 \text{ g}$$

After similar calculations for the other ingredients, the final formula is

10. Bromisovalum 14.4 g
    Sodium bicarbonate 56.1 g
    Tartaric acid 33.0 g
    Citric acid 16.5 g
    ─────────
    120.0 g

To prepare the granule by the fusion method all ingredients except the citric acid are passed through a 60-mesh sieve and dried at 100°. The citric acid should be uneffloresced, as its water of crystallization is the source of moisture for granulation. All ingredients are blended and the mixture is placed in a fusion pan or in a large evaporating dish in an oven preheated to 100°. In a few moments the heat releases the water of crystallization from the citric acid. As the mass is stirred, it becomes coherent. Working rapidly, the cohesive mass is granulated through a 6-mesh sieve and dried.

In the wet method, heat is not employed. A small amount of liquid with limited solvent capacity, e.g., alcohol, is mixed with the powders until a cohesive mass is formed. This is then passed through an appropriate sieve and dried.

The control of humidity and temperature is important in the commercial preparation of effervescent granules. Pharmaceutical elegance is achieved by the addition of sweetening agents and color. A steam-jacketed fusion pan is used to heat the mixture, a mechanical granulator is used to granulate the mass, and a vacuum drier is used to dry the granules.

A high degree of automation has been achieved in a few plants that continually make large-volume, over-the-counter granules. The mixture is conveyed by belt through a heated chamber, with automatic temperature and time regulation to ensure proper release of moisture. The mass is passed through sieves and is received on a belt moving through a drying chamber and is finally delivered to the packaging machine.

11. Exsiccated sodium phosphate 200 g
    Sodium bicarbonate 477 g
    Tartaric acid 252 g
    Citric acid, uneffloresced 162 g

    Sig.: Effervescent sodium phosphate granules

CAPSULES

Capsules are gelatin shells filled with the powdered and blended ingredients that make up an individual dose. Dry powders, semisolids, and liquids that do not dissolve gelatin may be encapsulated.

To the physician, the capsule is a flexible-unit dose form that may be used to administer almost any combination of drugs. The bulk of certain remedies prohibits placement in a single capsule; this problem is solved by dispensing the dose in several smaller capsules that can be easily swallowed.

Generally, the capsule is placed on the tongue and swallowed with a drink of water. Although few persons have difficulty swallowing a capsule, it is best not to administer capsules to small children. On rare occasions the physician may direct that capsules be given rectally or vaginally; these capsules should be dipped in warm water to facilitate insertion. At times a capsule is used as a convenience in preparing a solution; its contents are dissolved in a specified volume of water to make a solution of desired concentration.

solid pharmaceuticals • 67

To the patient the capsule affords an almost tasteless mode of administering unpleasant drugs. A thin gelatin shell encloses the drugs so they do not come in contact with the taste buds. Rapid release of the drug occurs from the capsule, as the gelatin shell usually dissolves and releases the content of the capsule within 5 minutes after the capsule is swallowed.

Hard Gelatin Capsules

The hard gelatin capsule consists of a base or body and a shorter cap, which fits firmly over the base of the capsule. For human use, eight sizes of capsules are available. The capacity of each size varies according to the combination of drugs and their apparent densities. To aid in the selection of the appropriate size, a table, with the capacity of five common drugs for that particular size of capsule, is printed on the box of the capsules. As a guide for the novice, the capacities of capsules in terms of aspirin are as follows:

Capsule Size	mg	
000	1000	17 gr
00	600	10 gr.
0	500	9 gr.
1	300	5 gr.
2	250	4 gr.
3	200	3 gr.
4	125	2 gr.
5	60	1 gr

Trial and error soon develops the judgment of the beginning pharmacist. Veterinary capsules are available in Nos. 10, 11, and 12. Their approximate capacities are 30, 15, and 7.5 g, respectively.

The commercially marketed capsules appear in all colors; however, the community pharmacist uses colorless and pink capsules. A pink capsule for one prescription may be used to distinguish two capsule prescriptions for the same person. A pink capsule may also be used to encapsulate ingredients that would appear unattractive in a colorless capsule.

To hand fill capsules at the prescription counter, the ingredients are triturated to the same particle size and then mixed by geometric dilution. The powder is placed on a powder paper and smoothed with a spatula to a height approximately half the length of the capsule body. The base of the capsule is held vertically and the open end is repeatedly pushed into the powder until the capsule is filled; the cap is then replaced to close the capsule. Each filled capsule is weighed using an empty capsule as a counterpoise. Powder is added or removed until the correct weight has been placed in the capsule. The filled capsule is tapped so that no air spaces are visible within the contents.

To remove traces of drug from the outside of the filled capsules, they are rolled between the folds of clean towel or shaken in a towel that has been gathered into the form of a bag. The attraction of gelatin for moisture forces the pharmacist to observe care in compounding capsules. Moisture from the hands leaves fingerprints and a dull finish on the capsule. The most sure method of protecting the capsule is to wear finger cots or rubber gloves.

The simplest method by which a capsule may be kept free of moisture during compounding is to wash the hands well, dry them, and keep the fingers dry by stripping a towel through the cleansed fingers until warmth is felt.

An alternative method is to use the base of one capsule as a holder for other bases during the filling operation. The capsules do not come in contact with the fingers.

Infrequently, semisolid substances, liquids, or a combination of a dry and a liquid substance are to be placed in a capsule. If possible a plastic mass is formed and rolled into a cylinder, which is cut into

(massed capsule)

the proper number of segments. These segments should be slightly longer than the capsule so that the ends of the capsule are filled.

Liquids, e.g., alcohol and fixed oils, that do not dissolve in gelatin may be dispensed in capsules. By calibrated dropper or pipet the correct volume of liquid is delivered into the empty capsule base supported by a box with holes that fit the capsule base. To ensure proper sealing none of the liquid should touch the edge of the capsule and the size of the capsules should be chosen so that the liquid does not completely fill the base. The capsule is sealed by moistening the lower portion of the inside of the cap with warm water using a camel's hair brush. The moistened cap is placed on the base and given a half turn. The capsules should be placed on a paper and inspected for leakage.

Capsules absorb moisture and soften in high humidity; in a dry atmosphere they become brittle and crack. To protect capsules from the extremes of humidity, they are dispensed in plastic or glass vials. A pledget of cotton may be added to keep the capsules from rattling.

12. Ephedrine sulfate   0.025 g
    Phenobarbital   0.015 g

    Make 24 capsules

    Sig.: One cap. q.i.d. (DTD)

To make 24 capsules 0.6 g of ephedrine sulfate and 0.36 g of phenobarbital are required. These amounts of the powdered drugs may be weighed directly on a prescription balance. To increase the bulk, 3.84 g of lactose is added as an excipient to make the content of each capsule weigh 200 mg. The lactose is added with trituration in divided portions. The uniform powder is filled into No. 3 capsules.

13. Codeine phosphate   0.06 g
    Aspirin   0.25 g
    Acetophenetidine   0.12 g
    Caffeine   0.03 g

    Make 18 capsules

    Sig.: 1-2 p.r.n. to relieve pain

Several small, manually operated capsule-filling machines were once available for filling from 20 to 36 capsules. It is unfortunate for the community pharmacist that most of these machines are no longer available.

For the small-scale filling of capsules the industry uses a semiautomatic machine, which consists of a perforated ring or disk that may be separated into two portions. Empty hard gelating capsules are pulled from the hopper and positioned in the perforations by a vacuum. The operator pulls the ring apart so that the caps are in the upper portion of the ring and the bases are left in the lower portion. The lower portion of the ring is placed under a hopper and the bases are filled. The two portions of the ring are put together and closed by a blast of air. The capsules are removed by placing the ring on a series of pegs corresponding to the openings in the ring containing the filled capsules. To facilitate flow and fill in an automatic capsule-filling machine, a fraction of 1 per cent of a lubricant may be added to aid the flow of the ingredients being encapsulated.

In one type of automatic capsule-filling machine a vane rises intermittently in the hopper containing empty capsules and allows a capsule to slide down a delivery tube to the rectifier, which positions the capsule with the base upward. A vacuum pulls the capsule body down an intake tube to the indexing turntable, where the cap is retained and the body is drawn up to cam-actuated plungers. The caps are held in the turntable, which rotates simultaneously with the bodies of the capsules held in the plungers overhead. By means of a cam, the plunger pushes the capsule body down eight or nine times into the powder. The body and cap are jointed and the filled capsule is ejected. This method cannot be used with materials that will not remain in the inverted capsule body during the cycle.

One model of the Zanasi automatic capsule-filling machine consists of a turntable with 48 stationary dies which receive and hold the bodies of the capsules during the filling process. Twelve groups of four movable dies are positioned slightly above the turntable. These groups move in a horizontal plane and the dies in these groups move in a vertical plane. The movable dies receive and hold the caps of the capsule during the filling process. Filling is by means of two groups of four filling tubes. When four filling tubes are discharging material into the capsule bodies, the other four filling tubes are obtaining powder from the hopper. The filling unit consists of a tube that is open at one end and contains an adjustable piston. The weight of the powder to be encapsulated is controlled by adjustment of the piston. The powder is compacted as the tube is filled. The degree of compaction is adjusted by varying the length of stoke of the piston and the compacting arm. The compacted powder is ejected into the capsule body. The upper dies are positioned over the lower dies and are pushed down so that the caps are joined to the bodies of the capsules. Then the capsules are pushed up by ejection pins into cleaning dies, where they are held by rubber rings. The rubber rings form a chamber in which a vacuum is drawn to ensure final closure and cleaning of the capsules. The capsules are ejected. This Zanasi machine will encapsulate from 250 to 290 capsules per minute.

Elastic Capsules

Elastic capsules are industrially prepared soft gelatin capsules filled with a liquid, suspension, or powder. The soft gelatin capsules are prepared from gelatin, glycerin, and water.

Elastic capsules may be produced automatically and continuously by a rotary die process. A molten gelatin formulation is delivered through a spreader onto a metal drum, where continuous gelatin ribbons are formed. The ribbons converge between a pair of rotary cylinders with dies cut into the cylinders and an injection apparatus as shown in Figure 40. A vacuum pulls the gelatin ribbon into the dies. As an accurate volume of liquid is metered under pressure, the rotary dies simultaneously seal and cut the finished capsule from the gelatin ribbons. Production is increased by the use of several adjacent units.

Ointments and pastes may be filled into capsules; solids are often milled with a liquid and the resulting slurry is encapsulated. Very stable, elastic capsules can be produced. Special ingredients may be incorporated in the gelatin formulation to absorb wavelengths of light that decompose photosensitive drugs. Oxidizable drugs are processed under an inert atmosphere and are hermetically sealed in the capsule.

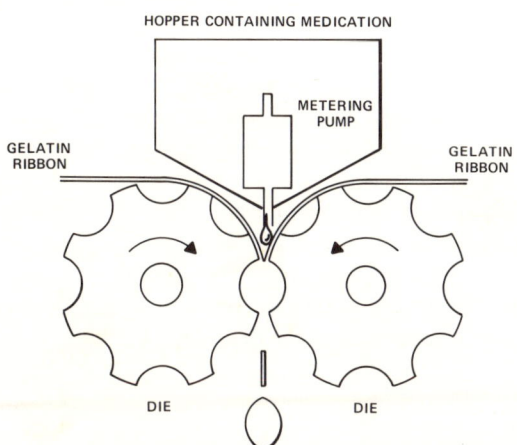

Figure 40. Diagram of rotary elastic capsule machine.

MOLDED DOSAGE FORMS

Tablet Triturates (T.T.)

Tablet triturates are tablets approximately 5 mm in diameter with opposing flat surfaces. Tablet triturates are friable, as they are made by forcing moistened ingredients into a mold by manual or low pressure. Rapid solution, the advantage of a tablet triturate, results from the very soluble lactose or lactose and sugar used as the diluent. Only potent drugs can be formulated into tablet triuartes, because of their small size.

The simplest hand mold consists of a hard rubber plate perforated with 50 holes and a lower plate with the corresponding number of pegs, which fit into these holes and eject the molded tablets. To prepare tablet triturates in such a mold, the drug and lactose are pulverized and mixed by geometric dilution. Fifty per cent alcohol is carefully added until the powder is moist enough to adhere but is not pasty; as an approximation, 0.8 ml of alcohol is sufficient to moisten 4 g of lactose.

With a spatula the mass is forced into the cavities of the upper plate placed on a tile. Firm pressure is exerted while the spatula is moved in a circular motion on the upper plate so that the tablets will be smooth and flat. Both sides of the plate should be examined to ensure complete filling of the cavities. After a moment the filled upper plate is placed bevel downward on the matching pegs of the lower plate and is gently pressed downward, forcing the tablet triturates from the mold. The tablet triturates are removed from the pegs and allowed to dry before packaging.

Although tablet triturate molds are assigned a capacity by the manufacturer, the variation of apparent density and porosity of each formulation requires that the mold be calibrated. A simple method of calibration is outlined below.

1. The active ingredient is blended with an amount of diluent known to be insufficient to fill the required number of cavities of the mold.
2. The powders are dampened with 50 per cent alcohol.
3. The moist powders are filled into the holes of the upper plate.
4. An additional portion of the diluent is moistened and the cavities are completely filled.
5. The tablet triturates are punched, crushed, mixed intimately, moistened if necessary, and filled into the cavities again.

Conceivably, lactose might be called the universal pharmaceutical excipient. Its wide use stems from its white color, physiological inertness, and high solubility. With lactose a solution of alcohol and water is used as a moistening agent. By its solvent action water provides a binding effect, and the alcohol hastens drying. Hardness may be varied slightly by the percentage of water used. As the percentage of water increases, the tablet becomes slightly harder. A high percentage of alcohol makes a soft, crumbly tablet.

With an extremely water soluble drug, the concentration of water should be reduced in the moistening agent. For example, in a tablet triturate containing 30 mg of sodium nitrite, the water content of the moistening liquid should be reduced to 20 per cent or the tablet triturates will be too sodden to mold.

In excessively moistened tablet triturates the capillary action and evaporation of the solvent may carry one of the ingredients to, and concentrate it, at the surface of the tablet. This is especially noticeable with colored materials.

The small size of a tablet triturate precludes the incorporation of much liquid. It is often expedient to replace a liquid with an equivalent amount of a solid form of the drug.

14. Belladonna tincture   0.5 ml

    Make 50 T.T.

    Sig.: One p.c.

One-half milliliter of belladonna tincture is too great a volume to be incorporated into a single tablet triturate. The tincture can be replaced by an equivalent weight of belladonna extract which contains 1.2 g of total alkaloids per 100 g as compared to the 0.03 g of total alkaloids per 100 ml of the tincture.

Hypodermic tablets are sterile tablet triturates intended to be dissolved under aseptic conditions to prepare solutions for injection. They are approximately 4 mm in diameter so that they may be dropped into the barrel of a syringe. A hypodermic tablet must dissolve rapidly and completely. As they are fragile, they are usually packaged in tubes of 20 tablets to prevent breakage and to restrict contamination. Tablet triturates are packaged in bottles with cotton to reduce breakage.

A few tablet triturates are made commercially by compression, but they tend to be harder and dissolve more slowly than molded tablet triturates; thus, most are produced manually, although automatic tablet triturate machines exist. As the cost of labor does not make tablet-triturate production economically profitable, the production of tablet triturates now marketed can almost be considered a service to fulfill a limited medical need.

Pills

Pills are an oval or spherical medicinal containing masses weighing from 100 to 300 mg. Although a few over-the-counter remedies are sold in pill form, pills are an archaic dosage form; yet the technique and knowledge used in preparing pills is a part of pharmaceutical technology that can be applied to other pharmaceutical operations.

In preparing extemporaneous pills, the powdered drug or liquid medicament is triturated with approximately an equal bulk of a mixture of the less potent powdered ingredients. To this mixture, the remainder of the mixed powders is added in divided portions with mixing after each addition. Usually a liquid excipient is required to form a cohesive mass. The liquid excipient should be added gradually with adequate heavy trituration after each addition until the mass is plastic enough to be molded. Excessive excipient will make the mass too soft to be molded.

The mass is taken from the mortar and kneaded with the hands until it is soft and pliable. It is then placed on a tile and rolled into a cylinder. A small flat board will aid in forming a uniform cylinder. Using the scale on the tile, the cylinder is cut into the required number of segments of equal lengths.

Each segment is shaped into a pill by rolling it in the palm of one hand with a finger of the other hand. The pill may be dusted with a dusting powder to prevent sticking of the packaged pills. Licorice, starch, and talc have been used as dusting powders. After a light dusting, the pills are set aside to dry.

The medicinal ingredients of a pill may not adhere when moistened, and an excipient must be added so that a mass may be formed. The excipient chosen must disintegrate rapidly in the gastrointestinal tract, produce a mass easily without a great increase in bulk, and be harmless. Alcohol, liquid glucose, syrup, and water are liquid excipients that are used. Solid excipients include acacia, althea, calcium phosphate, licorice, and magnesium oxide.

The choice of the excipient depends on the properties of the drugs. The mucilaginous carbohydrate material in powdered vegetable drugs absorbs water, forming a satisfactory mass. Crystalline chemicals are commonly massed with liquid glucose or syrup. Resinous medicinals are hydrophobic and are massed with alcohol or soap and water, which facilitates admixture of the hydrophobic and hydrophilic constituents. Oils and balsams cannot be evaporated to dryness, but they may be adsorbed on an inert solid with a great specific surface area, such as magnesium oxide. For those who are interested, the earlier texts on dispensing pharmacy abound with specific suggestions and detailed formulations.

15. Cascara sagrada extract   1.6 g
    Aloin   1.6 g
    Podophyllum resin   1.0 g
    Belladonna extract   0.8 g
    Ginger oleoresin   0.4 g
    Glycyrrhiza   1.0 g
    Liquid glucose   q.s.

Make 100 pills

Sig.: Hinkle's pills

Triturate the belladonna extract, the ginger oleoresin, and the podophyllum resin until uniform. Add the cascara sagrada extract, the aloin, and the glycyrrhiza and triturate to a uniform mixture. Add the liquid glucose to form a mass with kneading. Divide and form 100 pills.

To prevent sticking and flattening, pills should be dry before they are packaged. With extemporaneous pills there may be insufficient time to dry the pills before they are dispensed. If these are dispensed in a cardboard box, air drying will continue after the patient has received his medication.

Lozenges

Lozenges or troches are medicated disks intended to be held in the mouth, where they dissolve slowly. The slow dissolution and the viscosity of the resulting solution maintain the drug in contact with the oral mucosa for an extended time. Troches are used for the local effect of antiseptics, astringents, and local anesthetics.

Lozenges may be prepared by several methods. An older method is to mold a mass consisting of the medicinal agent, sugar, a gum, and flavors. The operative procedure is similar to that used to manufacture pills, but the final shape is different.

16. Tannic acid   3.0 g
    Sucrose   100.0 g
    Acacia   7.0 g
    Tolu tincture   2.0 ml
    Purified water, q.s.

Make 100 troches

Sig.: Dissolve slowly in mouth

The tannic acid is dissolved in 2 ml of water and mixed with the sugar and the acacia. The tolu tincture is added, and with the gradual addition of water the mass is kneaded to the proper consistency. The mass is rolled to form a sheet of uniform thickness and is cut by a knife or cutter to the correct size.

Many of the industrially prepared troches are manufactured by compression. Compressed troches are formulated with more binder and no disintegrating agent and are compressed harder than compressed tablets so that they will dissolve slowly and not disintegrate in the mouth.

Other troches are prepared from a hot mass which gels upon cooling. Pastilles are soft, translucent lozenges consisting of gelatin or a glycerogelatin base. Some of the over-the-counter pastilles contain no medication, but they are pleasantly flavored and have aesthetic appeal.

17.
Terpin hydrate	6.0 g
Thymol	0.2 g
Menthol	1.5 g
Gelatin	15.3 g
Glycerin	38.5 ml
Purified water	38.5 ml

Make 100 pastilles

Sig.: Let dissolve in mouth

The gelatin is added to the water and the mixture is heated until the gelatin dissolves. The glycerin, thymol, menthol, and terpin hydrate are added. The molten mass is allowed to cool almost to the congealing temperature and is poured into molds.

Candy or confectionary troches are prepared by heating a solution of sugar corn syrup under a vacuum to withdraw the water. The drug, flavor, and color are added to the molten mass, which is mechanically kneaded and drawn into a thin rope. The rope is cut and shaped by a die-compressing machine. Jets of air cool and congeal the troches as they pass on a conveyer belt.

Troches are wrapped in foil or cellophane to minimize the absorption of moisture if they contain hygroscopic ingredients.

COMPRESSED TABLETS

A compressed tablet is a unit dosage form prepared by compressing granulated medicinal substances under several hundred kilograms of force per square centimeter into a discoid or other shape by means of punches and dies. Although the conventional tablet is discoid with a thickness somewhat less than half its diameter, there are tablets of many distinct shapes, sizes, and colors. In 1962 the American Medical Association published the *Identification Guide for Solid Dosage Forms*, which permits tentative identification of a tablet from its physical dimensions and color. Confirmation of the identity is then made by chemical assay.

The fact that approximately half of the prescriptions written are for compressed tablets verifies that the tablet is the most popular dosage form today. The oral tablet is probably the easiest dosage form for self-medication; it is swallowed whole with a drink of water. The size of the tablet is determined by the bulk of the dose; the diameter should not exceed 7/16 in. When the dose exceeds 500 mg, the therapeutic dose is often divided between two tablets, and two tablets become the prescribed therapeutic dose.

For children and for persons who find it psychologically impossible to swallow a tablet, the tablet may be crushed and moistened with water prior to administration. Deaths have resulted from tablets becoming fixed in the larynx of children. The chewable tablet is made of a soluble-flavored base such as mannitol or glycine, which can be swallowed, chewed, or allowed to dissolve in the mouth. Many pediatric tablets are of the chewable type.

A dosage form should be appealing to the patient so that he will be cooperative in maintaining the dosage regimen recommended by his physician. Tablets may be coated to conceal an unpleasant taste. The coating, coloring, flavoring, design, and appealing packaging make tablets attractive to children. Tablets and all medication must be kept out of the reach of children, who may mistake them for candy. This does not imply that medication should not be elegant, but it does mean that people should be aware of the safe storage of medicinals.

Tablets are compact and are easy to package, transport, and store. The patient finds they are easy to carry on his person, and he does not need a bothersome teaspoon for measurement and administration. Although the tablet is a unit dosage form with one tablet representing a single dose, on occasion a tablet may be scored into halves or quarters so that the patient may break it into smaller doses.

Elegant tablets are marketed at a reasonable price because mass-production methods are used to increase production and reduce the cost of labor. A pharmaceutical marketed by a reliable firm implies that problems of stability, availability, incompatibility, and formulation were solved before its release for general use. Thus, the community pharmacist, acting on faith and the reputation of a firm, accepts the label claims and dispenses medication to a patient with an implied warranty that the purity and dosage is correct.

Usually a compressed tablet is considered an oral medication; the tablet is swallowed and passes into the gastrointestinal tract, where it disintegrates or dissolves, and the dissolved drug is absorbed and so produces its therapeutic effect. Generally, rapid release of the drug is desired so that the therapeutic effect will occur rapidly; however, for convenience a tablet may be prepared so it will release the drug over an 8- to 12-hour interval, producing a prolonged therapeutic effect with only a single administration. These sustained-release tablets have become popular.

Other tablets are formulated and shaped for special purposes. Troches made by compression contain more binder and no disintegrant and are compressed harder than oral tablets. Troches dissolve slowly and retain the dissolved medication in the oral cavity.

Inserts are specially shaped tablets for insertion into the vagina. Lactose or sodium bicarbonate are often used as the base.

Buccal tablets and sublingual tablets are small, flat or kidney-shaped tablets that are placed between the cheeks and the gums and under the tongue, respectively. Absorption of the drug occurs through the buccal mucosa into the systemic circulation. This is an advantageous route for drugs that are destroyed by the enzymatic action of the gastrointestinal tract. Unfortunately, all drugs are not readily absorbed by this route. Buccal tablets are compressed with moderate force so they dissolve in approximately 30 minutes. Flavors and sweetening agents are not added as they would stimulate salivation, which would cause unnecessary swallowing and loss of the drug.

Pellets or implants are sterile tablets compressed from the pure, crystalline drug under aseptic conditions. These 3.2 by 8 mm pellets are implanted subcutaneously by Kearns or Perloff injectors or by incision, and they serve as a repository from which the drug is slowly released over a period of from 1 to several months. Implants are available for hospital and clinical use and are limited to hormones, e.g., estradiol and testosterone.

Some tablet triturates and hypodermic tablets are made by compression; they are still considered to be such because of their appearance and properties. Hypodermic tablets are compressed with small force. The need for complete solubility restricts the diluents used to β-lactose, dextrose, and sodium sulfate.

A few tablets are used to make solutions for local use when dissolved in a specified volume of water. Potassium permanganate and Mercurochrome tablets are available to prepare cleansing and disinfecting solutions. One mercury bichloride large poison tablet dissolved in 1 pint of water yields a 1:1000 solution which is used for chemical sterilization of instruments.

Tablets for diagnostic aids are routinely used for self-diagnosis and testing for ketonuria, urinary bilirubin, and other pathological signs.

Manufacture of Compressed Tablets

Only a few substances can be compressed directly into a tablet without additional treatment. Some chemicals that may be compressed directly are ammonium chloride, benzoic acid, citrated caffeine, methenamine, potassium bromide, potassium chloride, potassium iodide, potassium permanganate, sodium chloride, and sodium citrate.

It has been suggested that crystalline structure may be a factor in determining if a substance can be directly compressed. The cubic crystalline structure (see page 113) appears to lend itself best to direct compression. During the compression of a material, the particles are fractured and forced close to one another. Since the cubic structure is the same along all axes, there is no orientation required for ionic or van der Waals bonding between the particles. If the system were not cubical, some orientation would be necessary and bonding between the particles would be less probable.

Most materials require pretreatment to ensure tablet formation and free flow in the tablet machine. This pretreatment is known as granulation. Granulation is the process by which fine powders are converted to granules with the above properties to assure a uniform fill of the die cavity, formation of a tablet, and easy ejection of the finished tablet.

The wet granulation method and precompression are the two major methods of manufacturing compressed tablets.

Wet Granulation Method. In the wet granulation method a granulating solution is used to impart adhesiveness to the ingredients so they will form granules and a firm tablet when compressed. Generally, a granulating solution is used because a solution of a binder is more effective than the same amount of dry, powder binder. Some of the more frequently used granulating agents are tabulated in Table XIV.

Table XIV Granulating Agents Used in the Wet Granulation Method

Substance	Percentage of Granulating Fluid
Acacia	10-20
Alcohol	-
Cellulose derivatives	5-10
Gelatin	10-20
Glucose	25-50
Polyvinylpyrrolidone	3-15
Starch	5-10
Sugar	70-85
Water	

With the potent, synthetic medicinal chemicals used today, the active ingredient often constitutes only a small part of the total tablet. A diluent is then used to increase the bulk of the tablet to a convenient size. Common pharmaceutical diluents are calcium carbonate, calcium sulfate dihydrate, dicalcium phosphate, glycine, mannitol, and lactose.

In industrial pharmacy, a batch ticket or photocopy is made of a master formula to avoid errors in transposition. By appropriate use of the batch ticket the ingredients are ordered and delivered to the production area. Each ingredient is checked and weighed by at least two persons. All ingredients are reduced to a powder and mechanically blended by standard mixing techniques (see Chapter 2).

Granulation is important, as it is this step in the process that determines the operation of the tablet machine and the properties of the tablet. By choosing a suitable granulating solution in the correct amount, the fine powder is converted into a granular form that will flow freely and uniformly from the hopper to the die cavity while possessing adhesive properties.

In small developmental batches the granulating solution is added gradually with kneading. The mass should not feel sticky, but it should form a ball when squeezed in the hand. Excessive granulating solution will cause the mass to become sticky so that it will be difficult to pass through a screen during the granulation process and will require a longer drying time. Excessive granulating solution may also make a hard tablet with a long disintegrating time. Insufficient binder leads to poor adhesion with capped tablets, i.e., tablets with the tops split.

The granulating solution is blended thoroughly into the mass by use of a ribbon or other suitable blender. The wet mass is passed through a screen, e.g., 6 to 8 mesh, by an oscillating granulator or a hammer mill, and the wet granules are collected on a paper-lined tray.

The granules are spread on a tray in a layer not exceeding ½ in. and are placed in a drying oven with circulating air at 40 to 60°. The granules must be dry before compression or they will stick to the punches and die. A drying cycle varies from 6 to 18 hours. Very rapid oven drying is avoided, as the outsides of the granules will lose their moisture first and bake to a hard shell, which will prevent the moisture from escaping from the interior. Upon compression the granule is broken and the liberated moisture will cause the punches to stick.

The oven-dried granules are reduced in size depending on the dimensions of the finished tablet. For small tablets, e.g., ¼ in., a 30-mesh granule is prepared; for large tablets, e.g., 7/16 in., a 12-mesh granule is prepared. With a colored tablet or an imprinted tablet, a granulation as small as 40 mesh may be used to avoid a mottled coloring or imperfect lettering. An oscillating granulator or a hammer mill is used to reduce particle size, because as soon as a particle is reduced to the desired size, it falls through the screen away from the grinding action and is not further reduced in size. Grinding-type granulators and comminutors tend to fracture the granules and produce an excess of fines.

A tablet machine measures the amount of granulation to be compressed into a single tablet by volume, i.e., the fill of the die cavity above the lower punch. The size frequency distribution of the granulation should be moderately narrow, with some small particles to fill the interparticular spaces so that each delivery of granulation to the die will have the same weight and uniform tablets will be produced. Ideally, the granules should approach a spherical shape so that they will flow readily. The angle of repose gives some indication of how well these goals have been attained.

A lubricant is a substance that is added to the granulation to aid in the flow of the granulation, to reduce die wall friction, to prevent sticking to the surface of the punches and die, and to aid in ejection of the finished tablet. A lubricant has a high specific surface, which enables it to coat a large number of granules. Lubricants are usually passed through a 200-mesh sieve to ensure their small particle size. The amount of the lubricant employed should not exceed 1 per cent. Common lubricants are calcium stearate, glycine, magnesium stearate, stearic acid, Sterotex®, and talc.

A disintegrating agent is added to the granulation to cause the tablet to rupture into small particles in the gastrointestinal tract. The large number of small particles present a greater surface to the dissolving fluid than an intact tablet does; therefore, the drug dissolves more rapidly and is absorbed faster. The common disintegrating agent, e.g., starch or algins, absorbs moisture and swells, causing the tablet to disintegrate. Dried starch is the most used disintegrating agent; it should be dried at 100° to remove the water that has been absorbed from the atmosphere.

The lubricant and the disintegrating agent are added to the granulation and gently mixed so the granules are not broken. The formulation is now ready for compression.

A single-punch tablet machine consists fundamentally of a die fitted with an upper and lower punch as shown in Figure 41. By means of cams the machine is engineered so that when the upper punch is out of the die, the lower punch is at its lowest position and the feed shoe connected to the hopper is filling the die cavity with granulation. The height of the lower punch may be adjusted to control the size of the die cavity and hence the weight of the tablet.

As the feed shoe withdraws, the upper punch descends compressing the granulation in the die cavity. The upper punch forms the upper surface of the tablet, and the lower punch forms the lower surface of the tablet.

The upper punch now begins to rise, and after a brief lag the lower punch begins to rise. As the lower punch rises it pushes the tablet from the die. The lower punch rises until it is flush with the upper surface of the die. The feed shoe ejects the tablet and then fills the die cavity as the lower punch descends. The height to which the lower punch rises is adjustable. If it were too low, the feed shoe would split or cap the tablet during ejection. If it were too high, the feed shoe would strike the lower punch with mutual damage.

solid pharmaceuticals • 77

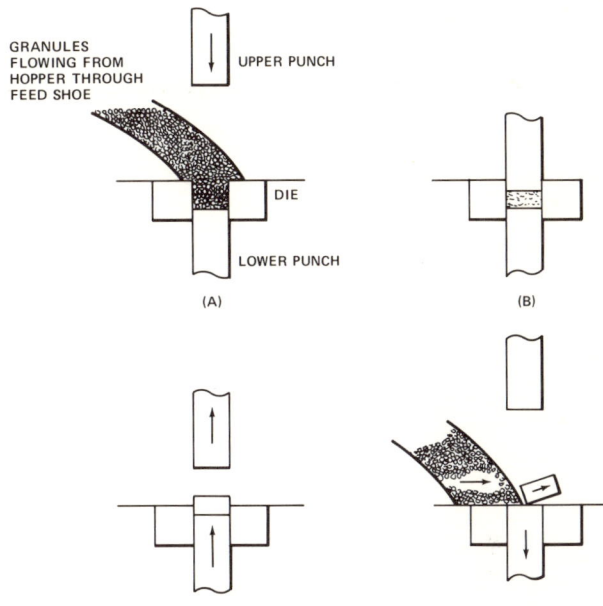

Figure 41. Compression cycle for a single-punch tablet machine: (a) granulation filling die cavity; (b) granules are compressed into a tablet; (c) tablet is pushed from die cavity by lower punch; (d) tablet is ejected by feed shoe.

The upper punch is adjusted to control the thickness and hardness of the tablet. A harder and thinner tablet is formed by lowering the position of the upper punch.

The ejected tablets move down a vibrating wire tray or under an exhaust system to remove any loose powder. The tablets are kept in quarantine until they have been assayed and released for packaging.

The wet granulation method may be summarized in the following stages:

1. The granulating solution is prepared.
2. The powdered ingredients are weighed and blended.
3. The blended ingredients are moistened by adding a proper amount of a granulating solution and kneading to the correct consistency.
4. The wet mass is passed through a sieve to form granules.
5. The granules are dried in an oven.
6. The dried granules are ground to a size appropriate for compression.
7. A lubricant and disintegrating agent are added.
8. The blended formulation is compressed into a tablet.

For the developmental pharmacist, a simple lactose granulation may be a starting formulation in which to incorporate a drug with a small dose.

18. | | |
|---|---|
| Lactose | 350.00 g |
| Starch | 26.00 g |
| Color | 0.25 g |
| Magnesium stearate | 5.00 g |
| Starch paste, 10% | 140.00 ml |

Using the geometric dilution technique, the color, starch, and lactose are uniformly mixed. The starch paste is prepared by making a slurry of the starch in a small amount of water and then adding boiling water to final volume. The starch paste should be a translucent gel. The starch paste is added to the mixture and uniformly incorporated. The wet mass is passed through a 6-mesh sieve. The wet granulation is dried in the oven at 60°. The dried granulation is reduced to a 20- mesh to 40-mesh size,

78 • solid pharmaceuticals

depending on the desired size of the finished tablet. The granulation is mixed with the magnesium stearate and compressed into tablets.

		mg/tablet
19.	Calcium carbonate	135
	Magnesium carbonate	100
	Sodium chloride	50
	Starch paste, 10%	80
	Magnesium stearate	5
	Dried Starch	15

Sig.: Antacid tablet

The sodium chloride, the magnesium carbonate, and the calcium carbonate are mixed until homogeneous. The starch paste is added, and the wet mass is passed through a 6-mesh sieve. The wet granules are dried in an oven at 55° for several hours. The dried granules are passed through a 14-mesh sieve. The magnesium stearate and the dried starch are added, and the mixture is tumbled until uniformly mixed. The tablets are compressed using a 13/32 in. standard concave punch and die set. Figure 42 shows the shape of some punches.

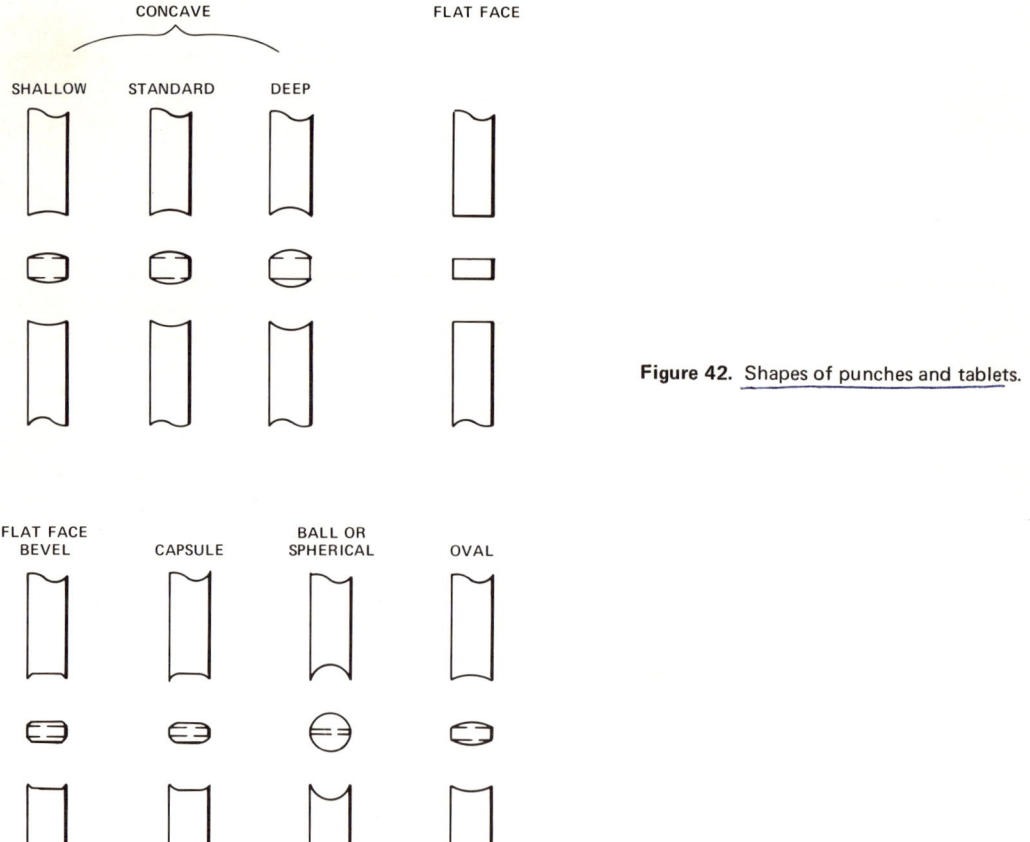

Figure 42. Shapes of punches and tablets.

20.
Vitamin A, as Crystalets®	5000 U.S.P. units
Vitamin D	1000 U.S.P. units
Ascorbic acid	50.0 mg
Thiamine mononitrate	1.0 mg
Riboflavin	1.5 mg
Pyridoxine hydrochloride	1.0 mg
Cobalamin concentrate, as Stablets®	2 mcg
Calcium panthothenate	2.0 mg
Niacinamide	10.0 mg
Saccharin, soluble	0.3 mg
Orange flavor, dry	7.0 mg
Mannitol	234.8 mg
Acacia	6.5 mg
Magnesium stearate	6.5 mg
Talc	7.0 mg

Sig.: Chewable multivitamin tablets

All vitamins except vitamins A and D, ascorbic acid, and 10 per cent of the riboflavin are blended with the mannitol and acacia. The soluble saccharin is dissolved in water to make a 0.9 per cent solution, which is used to granulate the dry blended ingredients. The wet mass is passed through a 8-mesh sieve and dried at 50°. The dried granulation is passed through a 16-mesh sieve. The flavor, ascorbic acid, magnesium stearate, vitamins A and D, and remainder of the riboflavin are blended with the talc and then mixed well with the initial blend. The tablets are compressed to a hardness (see page 82) of 3 to 4 kg using a 3/8 in. standard concave punch and die set.

Precompression Method. ("Dry" process) In the precompression method of manufacturing compressed tablets, the dry formulation is compressed into an oversized tablet or slug which is ground to a uniform size for recompression into the finished tablet. A heavy-duty tablet machine is used to make slugs 1 in. or greater in diameter. As they are to be ground, it is not necessary that the slugs be perfectly shaped. Since considerable dust may be formed, it is desirable to have the working parts of the machine housed.

The precompression method is used with drugs that are decomposed by moisture and heat. In addition to circumventing the deleterious effect of moisture and heat, the precompression method saves time and labor, as it eliminates the operations of wet mixing, drying, and granulating. By eliminating water, mixtures of drugs that react in the presence of moisture may be compressed into a single tablet, e.g., the bicarbonate and acids in an effervescent tablet.

All tablets cannot be made by this process. To be successful a formula must possess a reasonable adhesiveness, be moderately dense, and flow easily. Recently, spray-dried lactose has been suggested, with drugs having a small dose, as a diluent that lends itself to precompression.

21.
	mg/tablet
Reserpine, 1% triturate	25.0
Lactose	123.8
Sucrose	123.8
Starch	27.5
Magnesium stearate	3.0

Sig.: Reserpine tablet, 0.25 mg

Properties of Tablets

The patient, the pharmacist, and the physician expect a tablet to be elegant. A speckled or unevenly colored tablet visually indicates improper and incomplete blending. In scored tablets the drug must be uniformly distributed so that the patient will receive the desired portion of the total drug in a tablet when it is divided.

Any change in appearance may cause a loss of confidence in the product. Certain deterioration in tablets may be organoleptically detected. Aspirin tablets that are improperly formulated or stored produce acetic acid, which is quickly discernible. The eye is very perceptive to a change in color, whether due to a change of the drug or the fading of a colorant. In extreme cases, one of the drugs or a degradation product of the drug may volatilize and condense as crystals in the neck of the container.

The above changes are easily detected, but more subtle evaluations are made before a tablet is marketed. At all times and in all products the chemical identity and purity of all ingredients in pharmaceuticals are determined by chemical analysis. The methods of analysis and control are more appropriately discussed in a text on pharmaceutical chemistry; this discussion will be concerned with the physical aspects of tablets.

Dimensions. During the production of tablets frequent inspection maintains the thickness and weight within specifications. Twenty uncoated tablets are weighed individually and their average weight is calculated. To be acceptable by U.S.P. standards, the weights of not more than two of the tablets may differ from the average weight by no more than the percentage tabulated in Table XV, and no tablet may differ by more than double the percentage.

Influence of Compressional Force. As the granules in a tablet machine are compressed there is an increase in specific surface area as the force of compression increases. This increase in specific surface area indicates that the granules are fractured into smaller particles. In the sulfathiazole table shown in Figure 43, the initial specific surface area (0.18 m^2 g^{-1}) is increased roughly five times when compressed at 1600 kg cm^{-2}.

Bonding of the granules in the plane parallel to the direction of compression seems to be stronger than bonding in the plane normal to the direction of compression. In measuring the hardness of a tablet it is found that the tablet is harder in the parallel plane, owing to the flattening or distortion of the granules. This is obvious in the manner in which poorly formulated tablets cap or split during attempted compression.

The true density of a tablet is not affected by the force of compression. The apparent density, i.e., the quotient of the weight of the tablet and its geometric volume, is a sensitive function of the force of compression. As illustrated in Figure 44, the apparent density of a tablet is proportional to the logarithm of the force.

As the force of compression increases, the porosity, i.e., per cent void space, decreases. The relationship of logarithm of force to porosity is linear and has a negative slope. Porosity and apparent

Table XV Weight-Variation Tolerances for Uncoated Tablets

Average Weight of Tablet (mg)	Percentage Difference
130 or less	10
130-324	7.5
More than 324	5

density are inversely proportional. As shown in Figure 45, tablets seem to exhibit a maximum specific surface area at a porosity of 10 per cent, even though the forces at which the maxima are obtained vary from formulation to formulation.

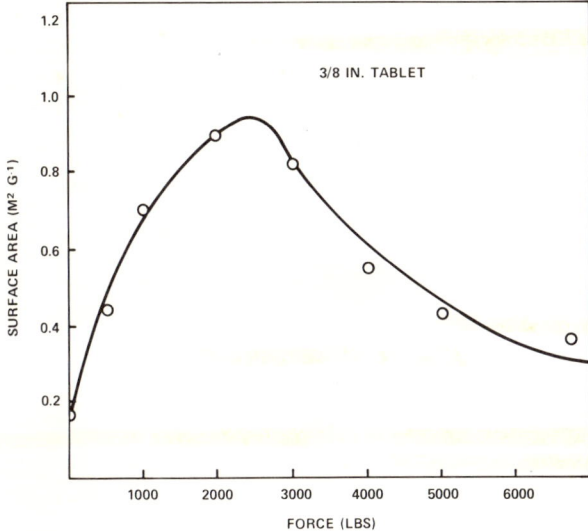

Figure 43. Effect of compressional force on the specific surface area of flat-faced sulfathiazole tablets. [T. Higuchi, A.N. Rao, L.W. Busse, and J.V. Swintosky, *J. Am. Pharm. Assoc. 42,* 196 (1953).]

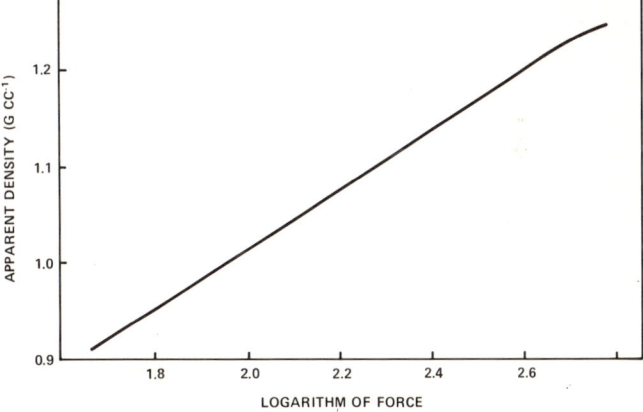

Figure 44. Apparent density of a spherical benzoic acid tablet is proportional to the logarithm of compressional force.

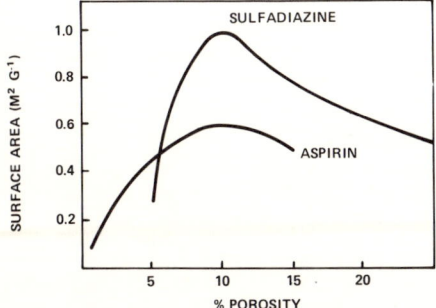

Figure 45. Porosity as a function of specific surface area of sulfadiazine and aspirin tablets. [T. Higuchi, L.N. Elowe, and L.W. Busse, *J. Am. Pharm. Assoc. 43,* 686 (1954).]

Hardness. Hardness is a term used to describe the resistance of tablets to mechanical wear as shown in breakage and abrasion during high-speed packaging and transportation. The resistance of a tablet to mechanical wear is dependent on its modulus, i.e., ratio of stress to strain, and tensile strength, i.e., breaking stress per unit cross section; however, suitable methods of measuring the modulus of a tablet have not been developed and hardness is used as a measure of compressive tensile strength. Hardness is conveniently measured by the Pfizer, Stokes, or Strong Cobb hardness tester. The hardness is supposedly expressed in kilograms of force required to crush the tablet held in the jaws of the instrument used. It has been reported that a constant ratio of hardness results with the Strong Cobb tester, giving results 1.6 times those of the Stokes tester.

As shown in Figure 46, hardness is proportional to the logarithm of compressional force. In making tablets, the hardness and apparent density increase and the porosity decreases as the force of compression increases. An increase in hardness may produce a shiny and less friable tablet, but the reduction in porosity will lessen penetration of the pores of the tablet by gastrointestinal fluids, and the disintegration of the tablet will be slowed or prevented.

Tablets have a hardness of 4 to 8 kg. Troches and certain sustained-release tablets are compressed to a hardness of at least 10 kg and as great as 20 kg. Chewable tablets have a hardness of approximately 3 kg.

Disintegration. The U.S.P. disintegration apparatus consists of a basket-rack assembly containing six open-ended glass tubes with a 10-mesh screen on the bottom. The basket-rack assembly is immersed in an appropriate fluid at 37° in a 1-liter beaker. The basket rack is raised and lowered through a distance of 5 to 6 cm at a rate of 30 strokes per minute. The volume of the fluid is adjusted so that the basket rack is never less than 2.5 cm below the surface of the fluid or above the bottom of the beaker.

To determine disintegration time, a tablet is placed in each glass tube and a disk may be added. The disks are perforated and grooved, intended to simulate the movement of the gastrointestinal tract. The disintegration time is the time required for a tablet to rupture and the particles to fall through the screen or until a soft mass having no palpably firm core remains on the screen.

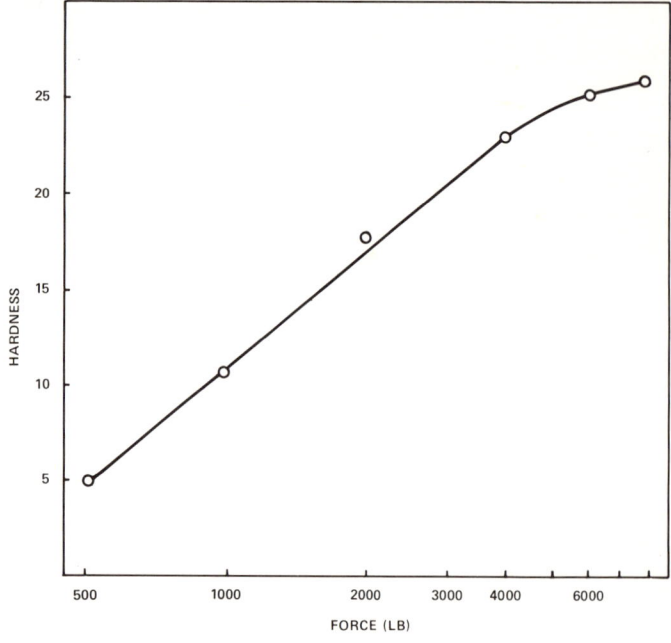

Figure 46. Relation of compressional force to the hardness of sulfadiazine tablets. [T. Higuchi, L.N. Elowe, and L.W. Busse, *J. Am. Pharm. Assoc.* **43**, 687 (1954).]

The disintegration of a tablet depends on the physical and chemical properties of a granulation and the hardness and porosity of a tablet.

If one or two tablets do not disintegrate within the time specified, the test is repeated with 12 additional tablets. Not less than 16 of the 18 tablets must disintegrate within the specified time limit to meet U.S.P. specifications.

Coated tablets are placed in the disintegration apparatus and immersed in water at room temperature for 5 minutes to wash off the soluble external coat. A disk is added to each glass tube. The apparatus is operated for 30 minutes using artificial gastric fluid at $37°$. If the tablets have not completely disintegrated, they are immersed in simulated intestinal fluid and should disintegrate within specifications.

22. Sodium chloride   2.0 g
    Pepsin   3.2 g
    Hydrochloric acid   7.0 ml
    Purified water, q.s.   1000 ml

    Sig.: Simulated gastric fluid, pH 1.2

23. Monobasic potassium phosphate   6.8 g
    Sodium hydroxide solution, 0.2 N 190.0 ml
    Pancreatin   10.0 g
    Adjust to pH 7.5 with 0.2 N NaOH
    Purified water, q.s.   1000 ml

    Sig.: Simulated intestinal fluid

Enteric coated tablets are tested by placing a tablet in each glass tube and immersing the basket rack in warm water at room temperature to wash off any soluble external coat. The disintegration apparatus is operated for 1 hour in simulated gastric fluid at $37°$. At the end of 1 hour the basket rack is withdrawn and the tablets are observed. No dissolution or disintegration should be seen. A disk is added to each glass tube and the apparatus is operated in simulated intestinal fluid according to specifications. At the specified time all the tablets should have disintegrated.

Buccal tablets are tested in the same manner as tablets but without disks. The basket rack is operated in water for 4 hours. At the end of this time all the buccal tablets should have disintegrated. Sublingual tablets are testing in the same manner as buccal tablets; however, the disintegration time is specified in the individual U.S.P. monograph.

The logarithm of disintegration time is proportional to the force of compression, as shown in Figure 47. As the hardness increases, the disintegration time becomes longer because the tablet is less porous and the fluid does not penetrate as readily. A granulating agent may prolong disintegration if it is slow to hydrate or absorb moisture. Lubricants, i.e., calcium stearate, stearic acid, and talc, have a pronounced effect on disintegration time. As shown in Figure 48, a small increase in concentration of a lubricant may greatly increase the disintegration time. Most lubricants are hydrophobic and excessive amounts tend to make a tablet waterproof.

A disintegrating agent is incorporated into a tablet to hasten rupture of the tablet into granules, which will dissolve or release the drug faster than the intact tablet. A disintegrating agent should not become sticky or gel, as this viscous layer would retard disintegration and dissolution. Dried starch is probably the most frequently used disintegrating agent.

An interesting observation on the effect of compressional force on the disintegration time of a tablet containing starch as a disintegrating agent is shown in Figure 49. With low compressional forces the tablet has a large void space and the water readily penetrates the tablet. It has been postulated that the wetted grains of starch swell and there is a lag period until they have swollen sufficiently to fill the void and to touch the structure of the tablet on which stress is then exerted. At high compressional

84 • solid pharmaceuticals

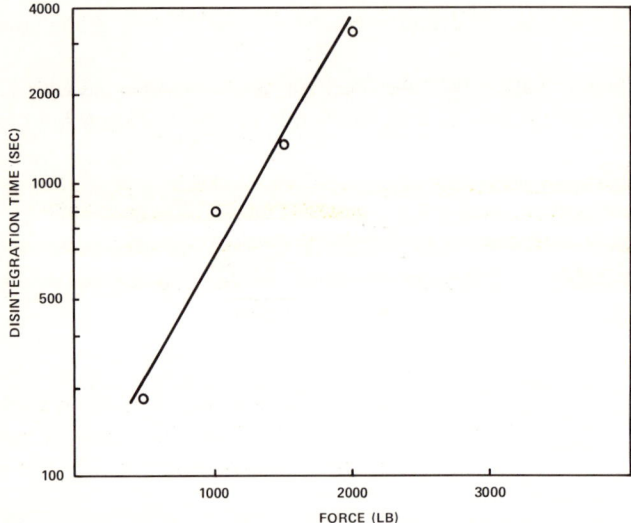

Figure 47. Effect of compressional force on the disintegration time of 3/8-in. flat-faced sulfadiazine tablets. [T. Higuchi, A.N. Rao, L.W. Busse, and J.V. Swintosky, *J. Am. Pharm. Assoc. 42*, 196 (1953).]

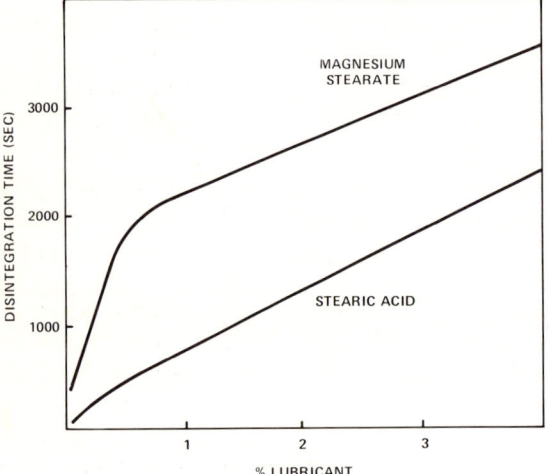

Figure 48. Effect of the concentration of lubricant in a sodium bicarbonate granulation compressed at 900-kg force upon disintegration time. [W.A. Strickland, E. Nelson, L.W. Busse, and T. Higuchi, *J. Am. Pharm. Assoc. 45*, 51 (1956).]

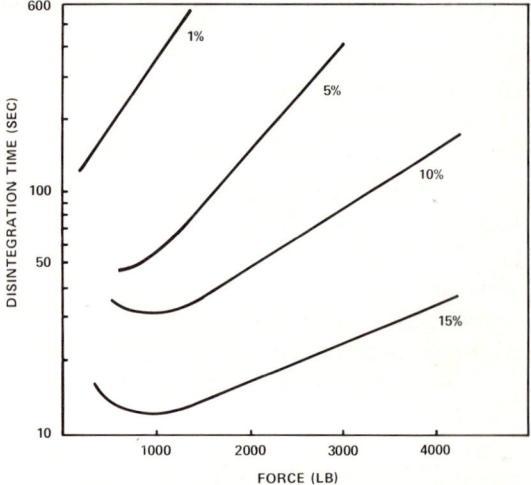

Figure 49. Effect of compressional force on the disintegration time of sulfadiazine tablets with various percentages of dried corn starch. [T. Higuchi, L.N. Elowe, and L.W. Busse, *J. Am. Pharm. Assoc. 43*, 688 (1954).]

forces the porosity is low and the pore size is small. Disintegration time is increased, as it is a slow process for water to penetrate into the tablet and the starch does not function as a disintegrating agent until it is wetted. At a critical compressional force, there is a minimum in the curve. At this force the grains of starch must fill the void spaces and the pores are large enough to be rapidly penetrated by water. If the starch swells, stress is immediately applied to the tablet structure, resulting in the most optimum disintegration time.

A representation of the steps involved in the release of a drug from a compressed tablet is given in Figure 50.

Dissolution. Any *in vitro* attempt to simulate *in vivo* conditions cannot be entirely successful because it is not possible to completely reproduce all physiological conditions. The disintegration method is an

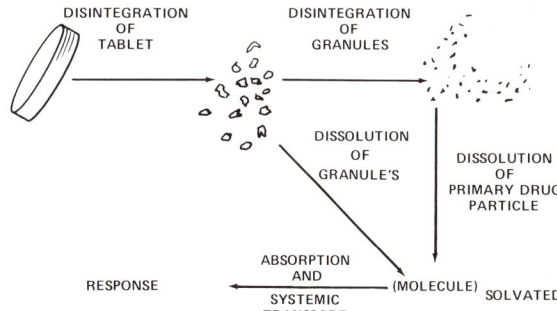

Figure 50. Steps involved before a drug administered in a compressed tablet will elicit a response.

arbitrary one which is valuable for batch-to-batch control in production. For instance, the disintegration time of multivitamin tablets has been correlated with the availability of riboflavin. In humans it was demonstrated that if the tablet did not disintegrate in 60 minutes, the riboflavin was not completely available to the body.

It is possible that a very soluble drug might be leached out of a tablet before the tablet disintegrated and that the tablet would be rejected because it did not meet disintegration standards. Conversely, a tablet may disintegrate rapidly but the drug may be unavailable to the patient; this tablet would be acceptable according to the disintegration test but it would be therapeutically unacceptable and potentially dangerous. The availability of a drug from a tablet must be proved on a clinical basis for a given formulation. Then arbitrary mechanical tests may be designed and correlated with clinical data for purpose of production control.

Usually the dissolution rate of a drug in the gastrointestinal tract is the rate-limiting step in drug transport. If the pharmacist were certain that the drug would be in solution shortly after administration, one of his major problems would be solved. A dissolution time would be more indicative of the availability of a drug from a tablet than the disintegration test.

By use of a standardized apparatus and technique, the amount of drug in solution at various time intervals can be found. The release of the drug from the tablet might be expressed as the rate of dissolution, or more simply as the time required for a certain quantity of the drug to be dissolved. Dissolution time in a few cases has been related to the rate of excretion of the drug. This is probably a happy coincidence, as there is no reason to assume that an arbitrarily developed dissolution apparatus should be related to dissolution in the gastrointestinal tract or to the complex processes of absorption and excretion.

The dissolution of a tablet or a capsule may be determined in a modified U.S.P. disintegration apparatus (see page 82). In the dissolution apparatus the basket rack has a 40-mesh stainless-steel screen and is positioned so that it descends to 1.0 cm from the bottom of the vessel on the downward stroke. Disks are not used in the dissolution procedure. This apparatus is used where the solubility is less than one dosage unit per 100 ml.

Another apparatus for determining the dissolution of a tablet or a capsule consists of a rotating basket in which the tablet or capsule is placed. The rotating basket is a cylinder 3.6 cm in height and 2.5 cm in diameter. The sides and bottom of the rotating basket are of 40-mesh stainless-steel cloth. The rotating basket is attached by three clips to a 30-cm rod with a diameter of 6 mm. The rotating basket and rod are attached to a stirring motor with a speed-regulating device that may vary the speed from 25 to 200 rpm. In a dissolution test 900 ml of dissolution fluid at 37° is placed in a 1000-ml resin flask fitted with a four-hole cover. A thermometer is placed in one of the holes of the cover. After a tablet or a capsule is placed in the rotating basket, the stirring rod is passed through the center hole in the flask cover and attached to the stirring motor. The apparatus is assembled so that the basket is immersed to 2.0 cm from the bottom of the flask. Stirring is then initiated at the specified speed. At appropriate time intervals samples for analysis are withdrawn through the two holes in the cover of the flask. This apparatus is used where the solubility is less than one dosage unit per 100 ml.

The solvents for dissolution tests, in order of preference, are: purified water, simulated gastric fluid without pepsin, and buffers of pH 4, 5, 6 or 7. A solvent should be selected so that the concentration of the drug during the test does not exceed 50 per cent of saturation in the volume selected.

COATING OF SOLIDS

Capsules, granules, and pills may be coated; however, for the sake of simplicity this discussion will most often refer to tablets. The original purpose of coating of pills was to cover the unpleasant taste of drugs. Today the glossy, colored, and more palatable tablets appeal to the patient. A distinctive coating and lettering on tablets serve to associate the product with its manufacturer. A coating protects drugs from atmospheric moisture and oxidation. The loss of volatile ingredients is reduced by coating. The release of a drug may be controlled by a coating. An enteric coating prevents the release of a drug in the stomach, but it releases the drug in the intestine, where the therapeutic action is wanted. Special coatings will provide a repeat action or sustained release from a single dosage form for 8 to 12 hours.

Pan Coating

The equipment used for pan coating is a motor-driven coating and polishing pan to which an exhaust and hot-air system with a blower is attached, as shown in Figure 51. Steam kettles are used to keep the coating solutions in a pourable state. The stainless-steel pans are available from 6 to 72 in. in diameter. A 36 in. pan will hold approximately 180,000 3/8 in. tablets. In selecting the proper size of pan, it should be realized that the sugar-coated tablet will be approximately twice the weight of the uncoated tablet. The polishing pan may be a coating pan lined with canvas or a canvas drum supported in a metal frame.

Sugar Coating. The majority of the coated dosage forms are covered by a sugar coating. Tablets that are to be coated are compressed with a deep concave punch and die. This shape permits the tablet to be more uniformly covered in a shorter time. The tablets are compressed slightly harder than uncoated

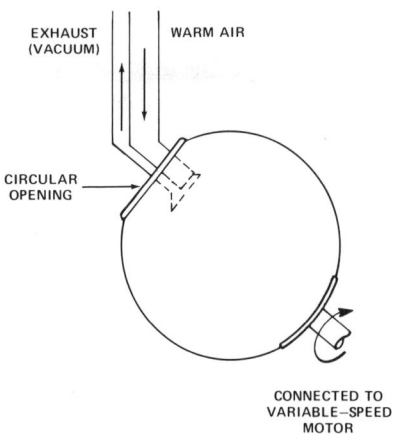

Figure 51. Apparatus for pan coating of tablets.

tablets so that they can withstand the additional processing. Dust is removed before coating so that irregularities will not form.

If the drug in a tablet is hygroscopic, a sealing coat may be applied to the tablet to prevent the absorption of moisture from the subcoating solution. Unwanted moisture may cause discoloration and deterioration of the tablet. A 40 per cent solution of pharmaceutical glaze or shellac in alcohol may be used as a sealing coat. A small volume of shellac solution is added to the tablets rolling in a rotating pan. The operator ensures even distribution by mixing the rolling tablets with his hand. After rolling for 5 minutes, the cool air is turned on to dry the tablets. The exhaust system will remove vapors. In approximately 10 minutes the tablets are dry and a second quantity of shellac solution equal to one-half the volume of the first coat is applied and dried. Two coats are adequate for sealing. Care must be taken that excessive shellac is not applied or the tablet will not disintegrate properly.

The thickness of the coating varies from 0.4 to 0.5 mm and results from the application of more than 100 applications or coats. The entire coat consists of deposits of subcoating powder and sugar.

24.
Acacia	2.25%
Gelatin	2.25%
Sucrose	57.25%
Purified water	38.25%

Sig.: Medium subcoating syrup

25.
Calcium carbonate	35%
Kaolin	16%
Talc	25%
Sucrose	20%
Acacia	4%

Sig.: Subcoating powder

The application of the subcoating is the first step in the sugar-coating process. Subcoating is the alternate wetting of the tablet with a subcoating solution and the application of a subcoating powder when the tablets are partially dry. The subcoat rounds out the edges and builds the tablet to the desired shape. Modified syrup and gelatin solutions are generally used as subcoating solutions.

In process the gelatin syrup at 60° is added to the tablets in a preheated rotating pan. The tablets are stirred by hand immediately to distribute the solution. When the gelatin syrup is partially dry, the tablets begin to form a ball. Then the subcoating powder is immediately dusted onto the tablets until no wet tablets show and the tablets again tumble freely. When the subcoating powder has been taken up by the tablets, the warm air is turned on until the tablets are dry. The excess subcoating powder is removed by the exhaust system. When the tablets are dry, the warm air is shut off and the coating procedure is repeated from 5 to 15 times until the tablets have been correctly shaped.

Smoothing is the alternate wetting with a smoothing syrup and drying until the tablets are properly rounded and smoothed. A 60 per cent sucrose solution may be used as a smoothing syrup.

In process the smoothing syrup at 60° is added to the subcoated tablets in a rotating pan. After 5 to 10 minutes the tablets appear dull and tumble freely. The warm air is turned on and the tablets are dried. From 5 to 25 coats may be necessary to smooth the tablets.

Coloring is the gradual buildup of color by repeated applications of a color syrup. A stock coloring syrup may contain from 0.1 to 0.6 per cent of a F.D.A.-approved colorant. The initial color syrup is prepared by dilution of the stock coloring syrup to as low as 0.005 per cent colorant. As the color deepens, the concentration of the colorant in the color syrup is increased until the desired hue is obtained.

Finishing is the slow, controlled drying of the last application of syrup. The pan is covered and is manually rotated through one-half revolution every 10 to 15 minutes during a 2-hour period. Finishing imparts a luster to the coating.

The sugar-coated tablet is completed by applying a thin layer of polish to produce a gloss. A solution of beeswax and carnauba wax in carbon tetrachloride or petroleum benzin is added to the tablets, which are allowed to roll in a polishing pan until the solvent has evaporated and a high gloss has been given to the coating. Sometimes the powdered wax mixture is sprinkled on the rolling tablets in a polishing drum.

A suggested modification of the sugar-coating method utilizing pigments and titanium dioxide reduces the time involved and yields a coating approximately one-half as thick. First a shellac sealing coat is applied. The tablets are given two coats of an acacia-gelatin syrup containing a dye. Powdered acacia is used as the subcoating powder. A pigment and titanium dioxide are suspended in a coating syrup by means of a wetting agent. Approximately 25 coats of the suspension are applied to the tablet. They are then polished.

Enteric Coating. An enteric coating is one that does not disintegrate in the stomach but rapidly disintegrates or dissolves in the intestine. An enteric coating is used when a drug, e.g., erythromycin, is inactivated by the gastric fluid; when a drug, e.g., aminophyllin, is irritating to the gastric mucosa; and when a drug, e.g., gentian violet, is to be placed in the specific region of the intestine.

Obviously, the release of the medication depends on the emptying time of the stomach, which varies from a few minutes to as much as 12 hours, depending on physiological and psychological factors. The developmental pharmacist uses an average stomach-emptying time of 6 hours for designing an enteric coating. As solids stay for a shorter time in an empty stomach than a full stomach, enteric-coated products are administered 2 hours before meals in the hope of a more uniform emptying time.

Enteric coatings usually are prepared with ingredients that have acidic groups. At the low pH, i.e., 1.5 to 2.5, of the stomach the ionization of the acidic substance is suppressed and the enteric substance exists in an undissociated, insoluble form. As the pH increases along the gastrointestinal tract, more of the acidic substance is ionized to a more soluble form. The coating then dissolves and releases the medication. The pH of the intestinal tract varies from pH 3.6 to 7.9. An alkaline pH is not required for dissolution of these acidic substances. Cellulose acetate phthalate begins to dissolve at pH 5.7; ammoniated shellac dissolves at pH 6.4.

The disintegration of an enteric coating may depend on either the hydrolysis of the enteric ingredients by enzymes of the intestines or the emulsification and dispersion by the bile salts or both. Ethylcellulose, hydroxypropylene methylcellulose, fats, and fatty-derivative coatings are removed by this mechanism. The ester butyl stearate is hydrolyzed by esterases to butanol and stearic acid. As the butanol dissolves the stearic acid flakes off and the enteric coating is removed.

A third mechanism for the removal of an enteric coating depends on the length of time it is in contact with moisture. One such enteric coating consists of powdered carnauba wax and stearic acid with vegetable fibers of agar and elm bark. After administration the vegetable fibers absorb moisture and swell, causing the coat to rupture. The time required for disintegration depends on the thickness of the coating and the ratio of the vegetable fibers to the wax.

Cellulose acetate phthalate is widely used in commercial enteric coated products. The cellulose acetate phthalate coating dissolves at pH 5.7. The coating is made more pliable and resistant to cracking by the addition of a plasticizer, e.g., diethyl phthalate, triacetin, dibutyl tartrate.

26. Cellulose acetate phthalate 12.0 g
    Diethyl phthalate 3.0 ml
    Ethyl acetate 67.5 ml
    Isopropanol 67.5 ml

Sig.: Enteric coating solution

The tablets are made with a deep concave punch and die. About 8 ml of the enteric coating solution is added to 1000 preheated tablets. The tablets are stirred by hand and dried with warm air. Usually 10 to 30 coats are required, as determined by tests after applying various coats during the coating process.

The community pharmacist may extemporaneously prepare enteric coated capsules and tablets by dipping them in a 10 per cent solution of cellulose acetate phthalate. Four or five coats will render them enteric coated.

Film Coating. Film coating is a rapid process by which a thin film of water-permeable coating material is applied or sprayed onto tablets. The film is so thin that there is no significant increase in the size of the tablet and imprinted designs are clearly seen. The film coating masks the unpleasant tastes and protects the tablet from the atmosphere, yet the film coating disintegrates rapidly in the gastrointestinal tract. A film coating may be applied faster and more economically than a sugar coating.

The film coating consists of cellulosic derivatives, which are film-forming substances, and water-dispersible waxy materials. Cellulose acetate phthalate, sodium carboxymethylcellulose, and hydroxyethylcellulose are film-forming compounds. Polyethylene glycols and glyceryl monostearate are water-dispersible, waxy materials that are responsible for the rapid disintegration of the coating in the gastrointestinal tract. Propylene glycol and vegetable oils may be added as plasticizers.

27. Cellulose acetate phthalate   30.0 g
    Propylene glycol   9.0 ml
    Span® 80   3.0 ml
    Alcohol   120.0 ml
    Polyethylene glycol 6000   70.0 g
    Colorant   0.5 g
    Castor oil   1.3 ml
    Stearic acid   5.0 g
    Acetone, q.s.   500 ml

Sig.: Film-coating solution

Dissolve the cellulose acetate phthalate, propylene glycol, Span® 80, and alcohol in approximately 200 ml of acetone. The remainder of the acetone is warmed and the polyethylene glycol, stearic acid, castor oil, and colorant are added. The two solutions are mixed and sprayed or poured onto the tablets tumbling in a coating pan. Roughly 5 ml of film-coating solution is needed to coat 1000 tablets. After the coating has dried, additional applications are made until the coating is complete.

Press Coating

Press coating or compression coating is the process by which a fine, dry granulation is compressed about a core tablet, forming what has been called a "tablet within a tablet." There are two basic types of press-coating machines. The Kilian Prescoter, the Stokes Press-Coater, and the Colton Compression Coater coat cores that have been compressed on other tablet machines. These cores are placed in a vibrating hopper, which feeds the cores to a transfer system that places the cores on a bed of coating granulation. As the turret rotates, the die is completely filled with granules. The granules are then compressed about the core.

The Manesty DryCota® consists of two rotary tablet machines connected by a transfer system. The cores are compressed on the first turret and transferred to the turret of the second machine. As they are transferred, the cores pass over a vacuum which removes the dust and any granulation. The core is deposited in the coating die, coated, and compressed.

The particle size of the coating granulation influences the centering of the core. The granulation of the outer layer should have a narrow size frequency distribution to aid the flow of the coating granulation about the core without displacing it from its center position. If the coating granules are excessively hard, the coating layer in the die offers little resistance to the centrifugal force applied to the core by the rotation of the turret and the core will be compressed off center. With a good granulation the speed of the machine does not affect the centering of the core.

The core granulation should be larger, i.e., 14 to 16 mesh, than the coating granulation, i.e., 30 to 40 mesh, so that the core will be porous. The finer outer granulation is compressed with more force so that the finer granules will penetrate the core and bond to it more firmly. The core has a hardness from 4 to 9 kg. At times the coating may not bond to the core; this might be remedied by the addition of a waxy material.

28. Polyethylene glycol 6000   2.5%
    Ammonium calcium alginate   2.0%
    Starch   5.0%
    Stearic acid   2.0%
    Alcohol, q.s.
    Purified water, q.s.
    Lactose   88.5%

    Sig.: Typical core granulation

29. Tragacanth   2.0%
    Sucrose   15.0%
    Colorant   0.5%
    Talc   5.0%
    Magnesium stearate   1.0%
    Lactose   76.5%
    Alcohol, q.s.
    Purified water, q.s.

    Sig.: Typical coating granulation

Press coating has the advantage of being an anhydrous process, so moisture-sensitive drugs, e.g., aspirin and penicillin, can be coated by this process. Incompatible ingredients may be combined in a press-coated tablet by placing one of the ingredients in the core and the other in the coating. Press coating has found wide usage in repeat-action tablets. In a repeat-action tablet the initial dose is in the coating, which dissolves immediately, while the core has been treated so that the second dose will not be released for from 4 to 6 hours. Press coating may be applied to any shape of tablet, whereas sugar coating is limited to rounded tablets.

A multiple compressed tablet is a modification of a press-coated tablet. The first layer of a conventional granulation is compressed into a tablet; then a second granulation is delivered and compressed onto the initial tablet, forming a two-layered tablet. Two- and three-layered multiple compressed tablets are marketed. Incompatibilities have been circumvented and prolonged release has been achieved by the use of layered tablets or press-coated tablets.

Air-Suspension Coating

The Wurster air-suspension coating process for the coating of particles and tablets consists of supporting the particles in a column of heated air while the particles pass an atomizing nozzle that applies the coating material in the form of a spray. Enteric and film coating of tablets by this process requires approximately 30 minutes. Coating materials that have been successfully used include cellulose acetate phthalate, ethylcellulose, hydroxypropyl methylcellulose, polyethylene glycol, and zein.

The Wurster apparatus for coating tablets, as shown schematically in Figure 52, consists of a vertical column in which the tablets to be coated are suspended and are given a controlled cyclic

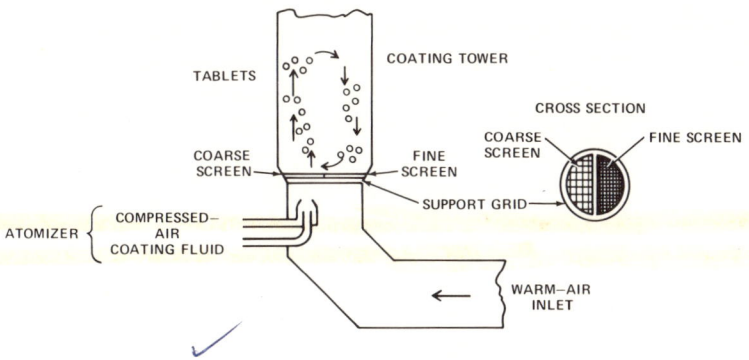

Figure 52. Diagram of the Wurster air-suspension coating apparatus.

movement by a rising stream of warm air. An air-supply system that controls the humidity and temperature of the air is connected to the vertical column. The velocity of the air is regulated by a damper.

An air-suspended or fluidized bed of particles has a random movement. If tablets move in and out of a coating zone in a random manner, the coating can be applied only at a slow rate. The Wurster apparatus, by imparting a controlled cyclic movement without randomness, provides better drying and eventually a more uniform coating. A support grid at the bottom of the vertical column holds a coarse screen, e.g., 10 mesh, and a fine screen, e.g., 200 mesh. The fine screen offers considerably more resistance to the air flow than the coarse screen; thus, the greater amount of air flows through the coarse screen. The air flowing through coarse screen lifts the tablets upward in the column. As the velocity of the air stream is reduced because of diffusion of the stream and resistance of the tablets, the upward movement of the tablets ceases. Then the tablets enter the region of a still lower velocity air stream above the fine screen, where they dry and gently settle. As the dried and partially coated tablets approach the grid, they are again introduced into the higher-velocity air stream above the coarse screen and enter into another cycle.

Below the grid support for the coarse screen, the coating fluid is dispersed by atomization under pressure. A compressed-air inlet is connected to the atomizer to aid in atomizing the solution or slurry of the coating material. The tablets, which are suspended above the coarse screen, have little contact with each other, so the coating fluid is readily distributed onto the surface of the tablets in the moving bed. As the cyclic movement of the tablets continues, the tablets are presented many times in many different positions to the atomized spray; therefore, a uniform coating is built about the tablets. Coating is controlled by the weight of the coated tablets, formulation of the coating, temperature, time, and air velocity.

Modifications of this equipment may be used for granulation and for coating granules. The dry, blended ingredients are injected into the column and the granulating solution is atomized into the column. The air pressure and flow pattern are controlled, so the particles never touch the lower part of the column. Dust is no problem, as the system is enclosed. The turbulent air flow prevents sticking to the sides of the column. The granulations are spherical and free flowing.

EVALUATION OF A COATING

A coating cannot be adequately tested or evaluated by a single test method. A sugar coat, a film coat, and a press coat should disintegrate or dissolve and permit contact of the dosage form with the gastrointestinal fluids in not more than 15 minutes. An *in vitro* disintegration test may be used to evaluate a coating during the product-development stage. Disintegration specifications may be a useful part of quality control during production.

The water-vapor permeability of a coating is determined by exposing the coated dosage form to 90 per cent relative humidity at 45°. The water-vapor permeability may be expressed in terms of an increase in weight, a softening of the coat, or an altered surface appearance.

The durability of a coating is tested in a mechanical shaker or in actual shipment to evaluate the extent of attrition and chipping of the coat. The effect of aging on the properties of the coating should be studied at several temperatures and under exposure to light.

An enteric coating should be intact after 1 hour of exposure to simulated gastric fluid in a disintegration apparatus with disks, and it should disintegrate in simulated intestinal fluid within 2 hours. After the product-development pharmacist has formulated a promising coating, the coated product should be submitted to *in vivo* testing. A correlation of *in vitro* and *in vivo* testing provides a more adequate picture of the release of the medicament.

Roentgenography has been used to follow the progress of enteric coated dosage forms through the gastrointestinal tract. Usually barium sulfate tablets coated with the film to be evaluated are given alone or with coated tablets of the drug. This method provides a simple means of determining the emptying time of the stomach and gives a good indication of the location in the gastrointestinal tract of the dosage form when it disintegrates.

Another technique is to attach a string to the coated dosage form so that it may be withdrawn at a given time after swallowing and visually examined. It has been reported that 20 in. of string is required to reach the stomach and 30 in. of string is required to reach the intestine.

Radioactive materials, e.g., ^{24}NaCl and ^{131}I, have been used in small amounts to study disintegration. As the enteric coated dosage form containing the radioactive material traverses the gastrointestinal tract, it is followed by a movable Geiger counter. A second, stationary counter within a lead shield measures the radioactivity in the hand of the subject. While the coating is intact, the radioactivity of the hand is only the background activity, but when the coating ruptures, there is a rapid increase in radioactivity. This method detects an imperfect or permeable coating, but it does not define the site of disintegration.

Although *in vitro* and *in vivo* disintegration tests show that the drug has been released, this does not assure the availability or absorption of the drug. Certain drugs are absorbed by a selective portion of the intestine; if the dosage form has passed this portion before disintegration of the coating occurs the drug is totally unavailable to the body. At times a comparison of the percentage of administered dose available from the coated dosage form and from a control form, e.g., a solution, is the best method of evaluating the success of a coating in clinical use. For example, approximately 30 per cent of salicylates administered orally are recovered in a 48-hour urine collection. A comparison of the untreated dosage form with the coated dosage form will show a 30 per cent recovery of salicylates if the drug is available from each form.

SUSTAINED RELEASE

For many drugs there is a satisfactory correlation between therapeutic response and blood level or concentration of the drug. In such a case, knowledge of the concentration obtained in the blood after the administration of a chemotherapeutic agent provides a time-dose relationship that is helpful in the design of standard and sustained-release dosage forms and dosage regimen.

If one predominant mechanism for drug elimination exists, the characterization of elimination rate may be expressed by a simple rate expression. Although the data of the absorption phase may be useful, this discussion will primarily consider the postabsorptive phase. A first-order elimination of a drug from the blood is expressed by the equation (see Appendix: Analytic Geometry)

$$\log C = -\frac{kt}{2.3} + \log C_0$$

where C is the concentration of the drug in the blood at any time t, k the biological velocity of elimination constant, and C_0 the theoretical maximum blood level, which is found by extrapolation of the straight line obtained when the logarithm of concentration is plotted against time to the concentration axis at zero time. The velocity constant is expressed in reciprocal time units; when k has a value of 0.17 hr^{-1}, the drug is eliminated at the rate of 17 per cent per hour. For a considerable number of drugs, e.g., aminophylline, aprobarbital, barbital, caffeine, digitoxin, penicillin, phenobarbital, sulfapyridine, sulfathiazole, streptomycin, and tetracycline, the net absorption and elimination in the range of therapeutic usefulness has been found experimentally to be described by a first-order expression. In practice this first-order elimination is most frequently seen after completion of the absorption phase.

The rates of elimination of a drug from the blood may be described by giving a numerical value to k, or by giving a biological half-life $t_{1/2}$, which is the time necessary for half of a given amount of drug to be eliminated from the blood. For a first-order elimination

$$t_{1/2} = \frac{0.693}{k}$$

Like other biological parameters, k and $t_{1/2}$ values for a drug are subject to physiological variations; however, they represent a mean scalar value, which permits comparison and tabulation. In most subjects receiving a single dose, the half-life of sulfaethidole may vary from 7 to 10 hours, with the greatest number of persons having a value of 8 hours. This biological variation still affords a quantitative comparison of the elimination of sulfaethidole with sulfamethylthiadiazole and sulfmethyoxypyridazine, which have half-lives of 2 and 34 hours, respectively. The utilization of k and $t_{1/2}$ permits better design and evaluation of dosage forms and regimens of the sulfa drugs.

Since many drugs undergo loss from the body by several routes, a biological constant of elimination from the blood, which is measured in an exponential plot of data, is the sum of the coefficients of the routes by which the drug activity disappears. As the elimination is by several routes, the order of such an exponential elimination is more properly known as a pseudo-first-order elimination.

Sulfaethylthiadiazole is a thoroughly studied drug and is an example of a drug that is eliminated by a first-order process. As shown in Figure 53, a plot of blood level against time on semilogarithmic paper produces a straight line after the absorptive phase. The blood levels at the first hour show that absorption of the orally administered sulfaethylthiadiazole is not complete; however, 2 hours after administration the drug has been absorbed and diffusion equilibrium has been attained. The velocity constant, k, may be evaluated by multiplying the slope of the line by 2.3. The biological velocity constant for sulfaethylthiadiazole is 0.085 hr^{-1}. Within the therapeutic dose range the velocity constant is not affected by the size of the dose. The biological half-life may be read directly from the graph or calculated from the relation

$$t_{1/2} = \frac{0.693}{k} = \frac{0.693}{0.085} = 8 \text{ hr}$$

Thus, within a practical dose range, k and $t_{1/2}$ can serve as a useful guide in product development and evaluation. The value of C_0 is dependent upon the size of the dose. Extrapolation of the straight line until it intercepts with the concentration axis permits numerical evaluation of C_0. It should be noted in Figure 53 that an administration of twice a dose of sulfaethylthiadiazole does not give a twofold increase in C_0.

Orally administered salicylates are absorbed over a long period of time and have a long half-life, 19 hours.* For such drugs a relatively large dose is required to yield a therapeutic blood level, but once

---

*Salicylates are rapidly hydrolyzed in the blood to salicylic acid, which is conjugated chiefly with glycine to form salicyluric acid. If the dose of salicylate is small, so that elimination is mostly as salicyluric acid, the half-life of salicylate elimination from the blood is from 2 to 4 hours. With large doses of salicylate the formation of salicyluric acid reaches a maximum rate, and the amount of salicyluric acid eliminated is negligible compared to the amount of drug eliminated as unconjugated salicylate. With large doses of salicylate, the half-life of salicylate elimination from the blood varies from 15 to 30 hours.

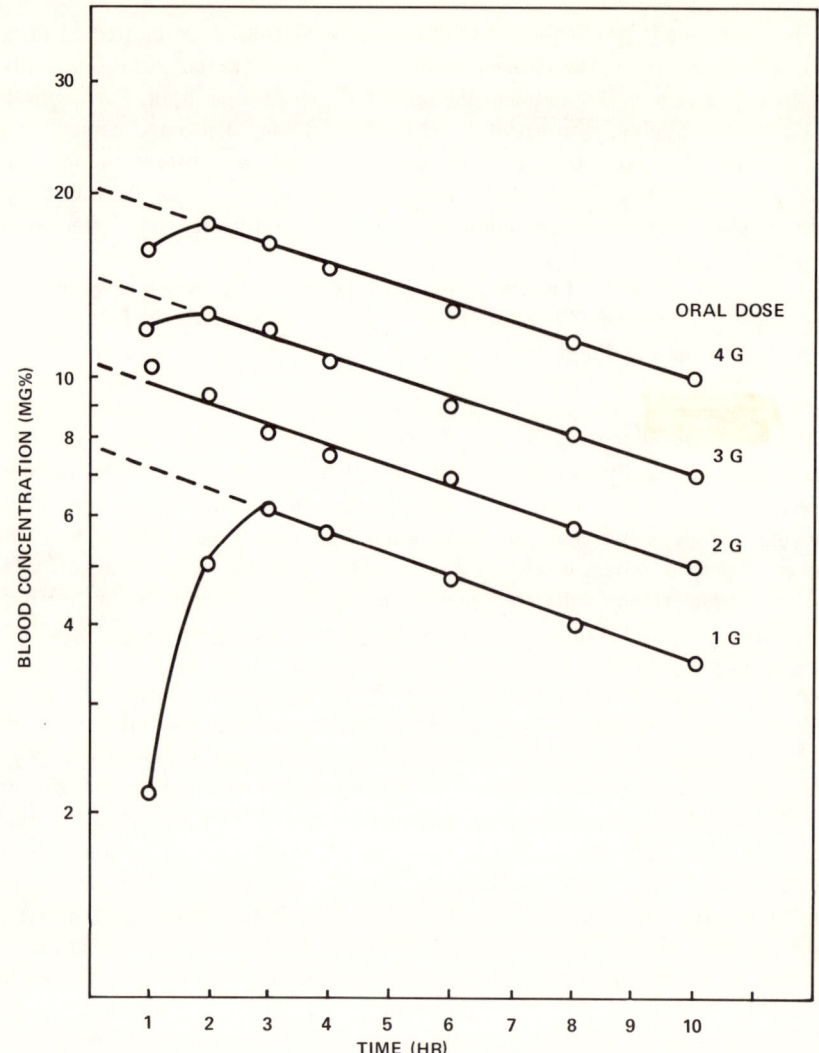

Figure 53. Sulfaethylthiadiazole concentrations in the blood for a subject following oral doses of 1.0, 2.0, 3.0, and 4.0 g. [J.V. Swintosky, M.J. Robinson, E.L. Foltz, and S.M. Free, *J. Am. Pharm. Assoc. 46*, 400 (1957).]

the therapeutic level has been established, only small and infrequent doses are necessary to maintain the therapeutic level. Too frequently administration of salicylates without regard to their long half-life may result in salicylism.

Conversely, penicillin has a half-life of less than 1 hour and requires frequent administration to maintain adequate blood levels. With a knowledge of the blood level needed for therapeutic efficacy, $t_{1/2}$ and k enable one to give a rational size and frequency of doses.

A hypothetical drug administered in a capsule provided blood levels shown in Table XVI. The blood level required to produce the desired therapeutic effect in the majority of patients, i.e., the minimum effective dose (M.E.D.), was 20 γ ml^{-1}. The data are plotted in Figure 54, and $k = 0.17$ hr^{-1} and $t_{1/2} = 4$ hr. Knowing these constants the concentration of the drug may be calculated for any time by the equation

$$C = C_0 10^{-kt/2.3}$$

Table XVI Blood Levels of a Hypothetical Drug at Various Times after Administration

Time (hr)	Blood Level (γ ml^{-1})
1	85
4	50
8	26
12	13

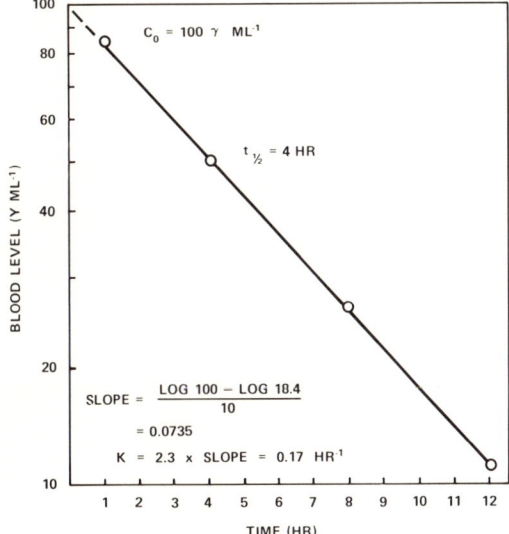

Figure 54. Semilogarithmic plot of the blood level of a hypothetical drug against time, illustrating first-order elimination of a drug.

or its logarithmic form,

$$\log C = -\frac{kt}{2.3} + \log C_0$$

For example, the concentration in the blood 6 hours after administration is

$$\log C = -\frac{0.17 \times 6}{2.3} + 2.00 = 1.557$$

$$C = 36 \; \gamma \; \text{ml}^{-1}$$

If the exponential form of the equation is used, substituting the data and solving,

$$C = 100 \times 10^{-0.17 \times 6/2.3} = 36 \; \gamma \; \text{ml}^{-1}$$

Realizing that the blood level should not fall below the M.E.D., the research pharmacist may wish to know the duration of efficacy of a single dose. The above logarithmic equation rearranges to

$$t = \frac{2.3}{k} \log \frac{C_0}{C}$$

For a single dose of the hypothetical drug with a M.E.D. of 20 γ ml^{-1} and $C_0 \doteq 100 \; \gamma$ ml^{-1}, the length of time this single dose will provide a blood level exceeding the M.E.D. is

$$t = \frac{2.3}{0.17} \log \frac{100}{20} = 9.4 \text{ hr}$$

Frequently a conventional tablet or capsule is administered three or four times a day to evoke and to maintain a therapeutic response. With the older drugs the medical profession has empirically determined the dose and frequency of administration required to produce the desired therapeutic effect. The frequency of dose depends on the half-life of the drug. Digitoxin is generally given as a 1.2-mg initial dose followed by a daily maintenance dose of 0.1 to 0.2 mg. This single daily dose provides satisfactory therapeutic response because the clinical half-life of digitoxin is 5.3 days. If the half-life for a first-order elimination is known, the blood level can be calculated for repeated doses of the drug at fixed time intervals.

For parenteral administration or if the time delay in absorption and the attainment of diffusion equilibrium is disregarded, the concentration of drug at any time t is expressed as

$$C = C_0 \, 10^{-kt/2.3}$$

If the same dose is administered at fixed time intervals of t, the total drug present will be the residue from the initial dose, $C_0 \, 10^{-kt/2.3}$, plus the C_0 of the second dose, or

$$C_0 + C_0 \, 10^{-kt/2.3}$$

After the third dose the total drug is

$$C_0 + C_0 \, 10^{-kt/2.3} + C_0 (10^{-kt/2.3})^2$$

and after n doses the total drug is

$$C_0 \, [1 + 10^{-kt/2.3} + (10^{-kt/2.3})^2 + \ldots + (10^{-kt/2.3})^{n-1}]$$

Since $10^{-kt/2.3}$ is less than 1, C_n approaches an upper limit as n increases. By letting $n \to \infty$, the sum of the geometric progression within this limit is

$$C_{max} = \frac{C_0}{1 - 10^{-kt/2.3}}$$

The minimum steady-state concentration of the drug is expressed by

$$C_{min} = \frac{C_0 \, 10^{-kt/2.3}}{1 - 10^{-kt/2.3}}$$

With a given dose repeated at uniform time intervals after an infinite number of administrations, the blood level will reach a maximum or steady level. If the hypothetical drug discussed were given in a dose that yielded $C_0 = 100 \, \gamma \, \text{ml}^{-1}$ and this dose was given every 6 hours, the blood level would rise to a maximum value of

$$C_{max} = \frac{100}{1 - 10^{-0.17 \times 6/2.3}} = 155 \, \gamma \, \text{ml}^{-1}$$

The minimum steady-state blood level would be

$$C_{min} = \frac{100(10^{-0.17 \times 6/2.3})}{1 - 10^{-0.17 \times 6/2.3}} = 56 \, \gamma \, \text{ml}^{-1}$$

It is interesting to note that if the drug has a relatively long half-life, the steady state is attained with relatively few doses. In the example cited, the maximum blood level for the dose repeated at 6-hour intervals is obtained with the fourth dose administered,

$$C_{4\,th} = 100[1 + 10^{-0.17 \times 6/2.3} + (10^{-0.443})^2 + (10^{-0.443})^3] = 155 \, \gamma \, \text{ml}^{-1}$$

When a drug is given orally, there is a time lag before a peak blood level is obtained. The time lag is due to the time required for dissolution and absorption of the drug. This time lag, t', corresponds to the time that has elapsed from the administration of the dosage form to the beginning of the first-order elimination of the drug from the blood after each dose. If one wishes to consider the delay caused by absorption of an oral dosage form, the maximum and minimum blood levels, resulting when the drug is administered in consecutive, fixed doses and at fixed time intervals, are given by

$$C_{max} = \frac{C_0 10^{-kt'/2.3}}{1 - 10^{-kt/2.3}}$$

and

$$C_{min} = \frac{C_0 10^{-kt/2.3}}{1 - 10^{-kt/2.3}}$$

In using these equations it should be realized that for equal doses, C_0 does not have the same value by parenteral and oral administration.

Sustained-release products have been formulated for some drugs that have a relatively short half-life and are readily eliminated from the body. A sustained-release product is one in which the drug is initially made available to the body in an amount sufficient to cause a rapid onset of desired therapeutic response, after which the level of the therapeutic response is maintained at the optimum level for a desired time. In theory, a sustained-release product rapidly releases the amount of drug required by the average person to produce the desired therapeutic effect and then releases the drug at a rate equivalent to that at which the drug is eliminated by being excreted, degradated, and/or biotransformed. During its action a sustained-release product maintains the concentration of the drug in the body at a constant or steady level.

In general, an orally administered sustained-release solid dosage form exerts its effect for approximately 12 hours. A single massive dose may provide a prolonged effect; however, the high initial concentration of the drug may cause toxic and unwanted side effects. As shown in Figure 55, the administration of twice a dose results in prolonging the serum level for an additional 1.4 hours, but the higher initial serum level approaches the toxic concentration and may elicit side effects. As the desired therapeutic response is achieved at the M.E.D., the excess of drug from a massive single dose is wasted as well as being potentially dangerous.

An advantage of sustained-release medication is the avoidance of high maxima and low minima in drug concentration or blood level. The blood level provided from a single conventional dosage form frequently decreases below the M.E.D. and then elicits no therapeutic benefit until another dose is administered to raise the blood level. In theory, with a sustained-release product a smaller initial dose produces a drug concentration approximating the M.E.D., and this drug concentration is maintained by the sustained-release process. In essence, the total drug given is less than by multidose administration, and the side effects may be diminished.

An un-ionized, water-soluble drug exhibits a first-order elimination from the blood and has a M.E.D. of 0.4 mg 100 ml^{-1}. The biological half-life of this drug is 3 hours; the biological elimination velocity constant is 0.23 hr^{-1}. The administration of 250 mg of drug in a capsule produces a maximum blood level of 0.9 mg 100 ml^{-1} and a blood level which exceeds the M.E.D. for 3.5 hours. As the dissolution of the capsule shell and the drug and the absorption of the drug are rapid processes, the time involved in these processes is small and for simplicity is ignored.

If a capsule containing 250 mg of the un-ionized, water-soluble drug is administered every 6 hours, i.e., three times a day, during the 18 awakened hours, the blood level as shown in Figure 56 would be adequate approximately 70 per cent of this time, with the blood level falling below the M.E.D. for 5.4 hours. The blood level at any time is the sum of the residue concentration of drug contributed by each capsule administered during this time interval. For example, immediately prior to the administration of the second capsule at 6 hours, there is a residue from the initial capsule of

$$C = C_0 10^{-kt/2.3} = 0.9 \times 10^{-0.23 \times 6/2.3} = 0.225 \text{ mg } 100 \text{ ml}^{-1}$$

98 • solid pharmaceuticals

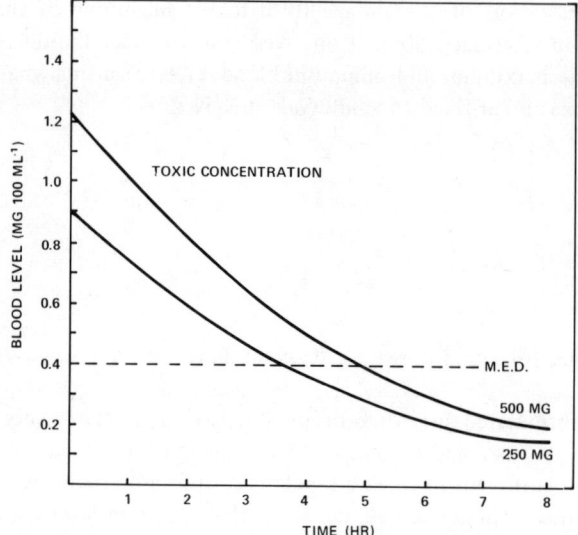

Figure 55. Large dose provides a longer period of activity, but the initial blood level may rise to toxic concentration.

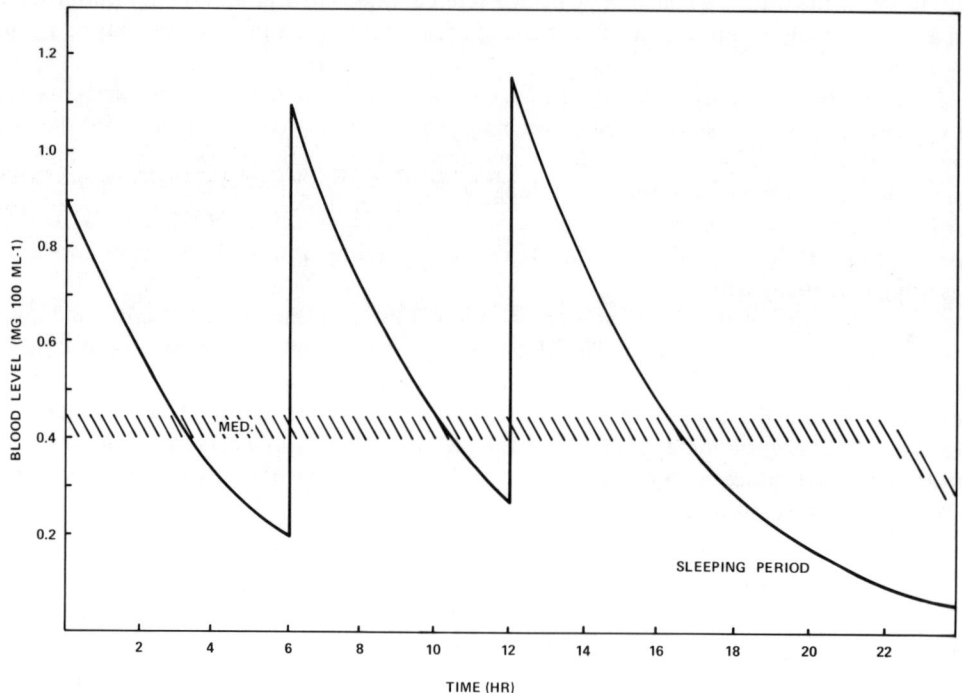

Figure 56. Blood level obtained by the administration of 1 capsule three times a day (q. 6 hr) compared with the blood level from an ideal sustained-release product represented by the diagonal-line curve.

Thus, with the administration of the second capsule at 6 hours, the blood level is the sum of drug concentration contributed by the second capsule (0.9 mg 100 ml^{-1}), and the residue from the initial capsule (0.225 mg 100 ml^{-1}), or 1.125 mg 100 ml^{-1}. As no medication is given during the sleeping hours, the blood level during a 24-hour period falls below the M.E.D. for a total of 11.6 hours. Thus, a dosage regimen of three tablets given at 6-hour intervals will provide the patient with an adequate therapeutic blood level for 12.4 hours of a 24-hour period.

An ideal sustained-release dosage form of this drug would release an initial concentration of drug corresponding to a blood level of 0.4 mg 100 ml^{-1} and would continue to release the drug so a uniform and sustained blood level at the M.E.D. would exist, as shown in Figure 55. As the maxima of multidose administration are eliminated, no drug would be wasted and the side effects would be lessened.

The total amount of a drug in a sustained-release product is the sum of the initial dose and the sustaining dose. For most drugs the initial dose is determined early in its clinical testing. The sustaining dose is released over a 10- to 12-hour period at a rate equal to the rate of elimination. The rate of elimination, $\frac{dE}{dt}$, is expressed by (see Appendix: Differentiation)

$$\frac{dE}{dt} = kb$$

where b is the amount of the drug present in the body to provide the M.E.D. and k is the biological elimination velocity constant. For convenience this may be expressed in terms of half-life, i.e., $t_{1/2} = \frac{0.693}{k}$, and since the rate of release, $\frac{dR}{dt}$, from the sustaining dose must equal the rate of elimination, the above equation upon substitution becomes

$$\frac{dR}{dt} = \frac{0.693b}{t_{1/2}}$$

The amount, A, of drug required to maintain the M.E.D. for the number of hours of sustained action, h, is

$$A = \frac{0.693bh}{t_{1/2}}$$

If the drug undergoes simultaneous degradation in the body, the equation is modified to

$$A = 0.693 \left(\frac{1}{t_{1/2}} + \frac{1}{t_{1/2}^d} \right) bh$$

where $t_{1/2}^d$ is the half-life of the degradation reaction and $t_{1/2}$ is the half-life of elimination of drug that has not degraded.

As a lesser advantage, sustained-release medication is a convenience to the ambulatory patient and for the nursing staff of a hospital in that considerable time is saved by administering a single dose in the morning and evening instead of multiple doses. A more important therapeutic advantage of sustained-release medication is that the required medication is continued during the sleeping hours without interruption of sleep or medication.

The release of the drug from a sustained-release product is a continuous or an incremental type of release. Continuous release provides a steady, uninterrupted release or solution of the drug from the initial to the final amount of the drug released. The sustained-release products functioning on an erosion, ion-exchange resin and a leaching mechanism give a continuous release.

In incremental release the drug is released or dissolved in a discontinuous manner with intervals during which no drug is released. The controlled-disintegration type of sustained-release medication provides incremental release.

Techniques of Obtaining Sustained Release

Attempts have been made to achieve sustained release by biological, chemical, and pharmaceutical means. One medical technique prolongs the effect of a drug by the administration of a second drug, which blocks the excretory mechanism for the therapeutic agent and consequently prolongs its effect. Penicillin, which has a half-life of less than 1 hour, is rapidly excreted by the kidney. Historically, penicillin was the first major drug that stressed the need for a prolonged-acting dosage form. The simultaneous administration of probenecid blocks renal excretion, and the penicillin remains in the body and exerts its action for a longer time. Unfortunately, it is not possible to control the excretion of all drugs by this method.

Certain drugs, e.g., chlortrianisene and dibenamine, are very lipid-soluble and are partitioned and deposited in the adipose tissue after administration. This drug depot in the fatty tissue establishes an equilibrium with other tissues, and it gradually releases the drug to provide a prolonged effect. Other drugs, e.g., mepacrine, phenylbutazone, and suramin, are reversibly bound to blood and/or tissue protein. This protein binding protects the drug from degradation and permits slow release of the free drug according to equilibrium conditions.

Drugs may be inactivated by an enzymatic system of the body. If a secondary drug is administered which inactivates or modifies the enzymatic system, the activity of the primary drug is prolonged. The inactivation of acetylcholine is due to hydrolysis by the enzyme cholinesterase. Neostigmine inhibits the action of cholinesterase, thus promoting the accumulation and prolonging the action of acetylcholine in the tissue.

Medical techniques are restricted to the use of the physician and at present have limited application. Often a massive dose of the secondary drug is necessary to prolong activity; with a large dose of the secondary drug, side effects may occur and the risk involved in prolonging duration exceeds the advantage over a standard dose regimen.

A chemotherapeutic agent may be chemically modified to form an inactive derivative that liberates the parent compound in a manner giving a prolonged effect. Originally, the palmitate ester of chloramphenicol was synthesized to reduce the bitter taste of the antibiotic. The insoluble, tasteless chloramphenicol palmitate has little antibiotic activity. As the chloramphenicol palmitate passes along the gastrointestinal tract, it is continuously hydrolyzed to the active alcohol, which is absorbed to give a longer duration of activity; e.g., an oral suspension equivalent to 500 mg of chloramphenicol provides a detectable blood level for 12 hours. Similarly, the benzoate, cyclopentylpropionate, and dipropionate esters of estradiol are absorbed and slowly hydrolyzed to the parent compound, resulting in an increased duration of action.

Some drugs, e.g., digitoxin, isopropamide, and sulfamethoxypyridazine, are inherently long in action when administered orally, owing to their physical and chemical properties, which confer a long half-life to the molecule. Obviously, such drugs need no further treatment to make them long acting.

The duration of drug activity may be lengthened by reducing the rate of absorption, delaying biotransformation and retarding excretion. The pharmaceutical technique used to formulate sustained-release products is based on the reduction of the rate of drug release or availability as the rate-limiting step for controlling the rate of absorption.

Controlled Disintegration. Enteric coating has been known for almost a century as a method for controlling the release of an orally administered drug. The disintegration of the enteric coating has been said to depend on the pH or enzymatic action of the gastrointestinal tract, or the water permeability of the coating. Currently, it is believed that the variation in pH of the gastrointestinal tract renders the dependence on pH the least predictable method. The most reliable release is based on the water permeability of the enteric coating. An enteric coated solid, which releases the medication in the intestine or 6 hours after ingestion, is a controlled, but not a sustained-release, dosage form.

A repeat-action tablet consists of a tablet within a tablet from which the outer shell rapidly disintegrates, releasing the initial dose of the drug for immediate effect. Repeat-action tablets are also known as delayed-action and timed-release tablets. They may also take the form of a layered tablet. Usually the core is enteric coated with shellac or some resistant coating which protects the core from fluids for approximately 4 hours, after which the coating and the core disintegrate, releasing a second dose of medication. The outer shell may be applied to the core by pan coating or press coating. The repeat-action product is not a sustained-released dosage form because the amount of drug released from the shell exceeds the immediate need and the drug level may drop in a conventional manner below the M.E.D. before the core disintegrates. With the disintegration of the core, the drug level is the same as from the initial dose supplied by the shell. Unless these two releases overlap, no therapeutic advantage is gained with a repeat-action tablet. The advantage of a repeat-action tablet is for those persons who require a second dose of medication during the hours of sleep.

If coatings of various thickness are applied to small particles, the particles with the thinner coating release their medication sooner than particles with a thicker coating. The concept of sustained release based on different thicknesses of coatings on several hundred pellets was commercially introduced in this country as the Spansule.® The Spansule® is a hard gelatin capsule containing a large number of coated pellets to provide a sustaining release and uncoated pellets to provide an initial drug concentraiton. The coated pellets do not release at any set interval. All coated pellets are essentially the same, with two or three groups representing levels of coating. Sustained release is obtained by statistical distributions within the groups of coating of thin spots, imperfections, and pores. In a typical product four groups of 100 pellets each are employed. Each group contains approximately an equal amount of the drug, and the total amount of the drug is from two to four times the average adult dose given in a standard dosage form.

Although any desired release theoretically can be obtained by a multiplicity of coatings, in most products the coated pellets seem to fall into three groups of thicknesses. The thickness of the coating in any coated group ranges from 30 to 40 per cent of the average value. Since within a coated group some pellets disintegrate sooner and some later than the average, the net release from a group is a steadier and a more nearly ideal sustained release than from a group with an absolutely uniform thickness of coating.

In production each pellet begins as a 12- to 40-mesh nonpareil, e.g., sphere of sugar, or a granule of the drug and sucrose. Using syrup the nonpareils are coated with the drug by a standard pan-coating technique. Numerous coats are applied to the nonpareils until chemical analysis indicates that the proper weight of the drug has been placed on the pellet. One-fourth of these uncoated pellets will provide the drug for immediate effect; the other uncoated pellets are pan coated by spraying a warm solution of glyceryl monostearate and beeswax in carbon tetrachloride onto the rotating pellets. Variations in the formulation of the coating are possible by using other water-insoluble, indigestible lipids, e.g., bayberry wax, carnauba wax, cholesterol, and paraffin, in combination with other water-dispersible, digestible substances, e.g., diglycol stearate, high-molecular-weight fatty alcohols, stearic acid, and esters of fatty acids of high molecular weight.

In a similar manner, two-thirds of the first group of coated pellets are further coated, forming a second group of coated pellets with a coating of intermediate thickness and having an intermediate disintegration time. One-half of the pellets of the second coated group are coated to yield a third group of coated pellets that disintegrate at 9 hours. The four groups of pellets, each containing the same weight of drug, are blended and placed in capsules.

The disintegration of Spansule® granules depends on the moisture permeability of the coating, and it is controlled by the composition and the thickness of the coating. The many pellets in a Spansule® provide a more uniform distribution of the drug in the gastrointestinal tract. If a single coated tablet fails to disintegrate, the entire dose is lost. If a few pellets of a Spansule® fail to disintegrate, only a small amount of the total drug is lost and the gross therapeutic effect is only slightly affected.

Medules® consist of a capsule containing a large number of pellets of uniform size. They are coated with a styrene-maleic acid copolymer that is pH sensitive and does not disintegrate in the stomach. The composition and thickness of the coating determines the release of the drug from the pellet.

This concept has been applied to compressed tablets. Coatings that delay disintegration, e.g., ethylcellulose and shellac, are applied to particles that have been coated with an active ingredient. These coated pellets are blended with a conventional granulation and compressed into a tablet. For the most part, the coatings appear to be sufficiently elastic so they are not ruptured during compression.

Similarly, a sustained-release tablet may be formed by compressing a mixture of a conventional granulation and a sustained-release granulation. A sustained-release granulation is prepared by the use of a slowly dispersible, hydrophobic granulating agent, e.g., cellulose acetate, ethylcellulose, zein, and glyceryl esters with fatty acids and alcohols.

Erosion. In the erosion technique of obtaining sustained release the tablet does not disintegrate but maintains its geometric shape as it passes through the gastrointestinal tract. The release of the drug is independent of pH and depends on the attrition of small particles from the surface of the tablet and dissolution of the drug from these particles. As erosion occurs continuously from the surface, the release of the drug is continuous, but the amount released is decreased as the surface area progressively becomes less. This effect may be lessened by compressing a cylindrical tablet with a large diameter relative to the thickness of the tablet. The eroding surface then remains essentially constant and the drug is released and dissolves at a nearly constant rate.

In production the powdered drug is dispersed in molten fats and waxes. The molten suspension is congealed by spreading it on cooling drums. The solid blend is ground at low temperature, granulated, and compressed into tablets. A sustained-release tablet based on the erosion mechanism may be modified by a press-coated or a pan-coated shell. This shell disintegrates rapidly to provide the initial concentration of drug, after which the eroding core provides a sustained release.

Leaching. In the leaching technique of obtaining sustained release, there is a steady dissolution of the drug from an insoluble, intact matrix. The matrix consists of a water-insoluble polymer, e.g., methyl acrylate and methyl methacrylate, polyethylene, polystyrene, and cellulosic polymers, which passes unaltered through the gastrointestinal tract and is eliminated in the feces. When the compressed tablet reaches the gastrointestinal tract, the drug is rapidly leached from the superficial channels and pores to provide an immediate effect. As the tablet passes further along the gastrointestinal tract, the drug is leached from the deeper pores. Release of the drug is controlled by varying the porosity and the ratio between the exposed surface of the dissolving drug and the insoluble matrix. Enzymatic concentration and pH do not affect the rate of release of the drug.

Ion-Exchange Resin. Ionic drugs may be complexed with resins to form insoluble drug resinates from which the drug is released by mass action as its ions are displaced by those of the gastrointestinal tract. The rapidity with which this type of equilibrium is usually attained suggests that only lack of water or slowed diffusion from the resinate bead would provide a sustained release. In most products of this type, an amine or basic drug, e.g., amphetamine, ephedrine, and phenyltoloxamine, is absorbed on a cation-exchange resin, e.g., sulfonated polystrene. It is claimed that the formation or dissociation of the resinate proceeds at a finite rate. The insoluble drug resinate releases the drug by double decomposition, in which the drug is replaced by hydrogen ion in the stomach,

$$\underset{\cdots\text{-CH-CH}_2\text{-}\cdots}{\underset{}{\text{C}_6\text{H}_4}}\text{-SO}_2\text{O(drug)} + \text{HCl} \rightarrow \underset{\cdots\text{-CH-CH}_2\text{-}\cdots}{\underset{}{\text{C}_6\text{H}_4}}\text{-SO}_2\text{OH} + (\text{drug})^+ + \text{Cl}^-$$

and by a cation in the intestine,

$$\underset{\cdots\cdot\text{-CH-CH}_2\cdots}{\underset{|}{\bigcirc}}\text{SO}_2\text{O (drug)} + \text{NaCl} \rightarrow \underset{\cdots\text{-CH-CH}_2}{\underset{|}{\bigcirc}}\text{SO}_2\text{ONa} + (\text{drug})^+ + \text{Cl}^-$$

The rate of release depends on the proper selection of resin and on the concentration of ions in the gastrointestinal tract. If the rate of release depends only on the concentration of ions, which is nearly constant in the gastrointestinal tract, the release from a given resinate should be predictable, continuous, and controlled.

If the bead size of the resin is small, the drug is released more rapidly than from a large bead. The greater specific surface area of the smaller bead gives faster elution or ion exchange; thus, the smaller bead does not give as prolonged a duration as the larger bead. In preparation of the resinate the amount of drug removed during elution and the degree of cross-linkage of the resin affects the rate of release.

An insoluble tannate complex may be prepared by reacting an alcoholic solution of a therapeutically active amine with a 20 per cent excess of tannic acid. At low pH and in the presence of electrolytes the drug is released from the insoluble tannate. The release may be further retarded by the addition of polygalacturonic acid to the product. As the release is influenced by pH, the release may vary considerably, as pH fluctuates because of biological variation. Obviously, this method is restricted to those drugs that form insoluble tannates.

Evaluation of Sustained-Release Pharmaceuticals

By definition the rate of drug release from a sustained-release product should be equal to the rate of elimination. In fact, commercial sustained-release products do not make the drug available at a constant rate. Although they provide a release of the drug which appreciably increases the duration of activity, the rate of release of the drug becomes progressively less than the rate of elimination. Many drugs are absorbed in the upper intestine to a greater extent than in the lower intestine; consequentially, the drug released after 6 to 8 hours should be greater than the drug released at 4 to 5 hours, to compensate for decreased absorption.

For many sustained-released products the release of the drug is approximated by a first-order equation; i.e., the rate of release of the drug from the sustaining dose is proportional to the amount of drug remaining,

$$-\frac{da}{dt} = ka$$

and upon integration,

$$\log \frac{a}{a_0} = -\frac{kt}{2.3}$$

where a_0 is the total dose of the drug in the dosage form; a the fraction of the total dose left in the sustained-release preparation at time t, if a_0 is 1; and k the apparent specific release constant. Figure 57 shows the amount of drug that has been released by a first-order process from the sustaining dose as a function of time; the intercept on the ordinate is the total amount of drug that was in a sustained-release form. If the sustained-release dosage form immediately releases a fraction of the total dose, f_i, and another fraction, f_s, exponentially from the sustained portion, the amount of drug released at any time is

$$a_r = a_0 f_i + a_0 f_s (1 - e^{-kt}) = a_0 f_i + a_0 f_s (1 - 10^{-kt/2.3})$$

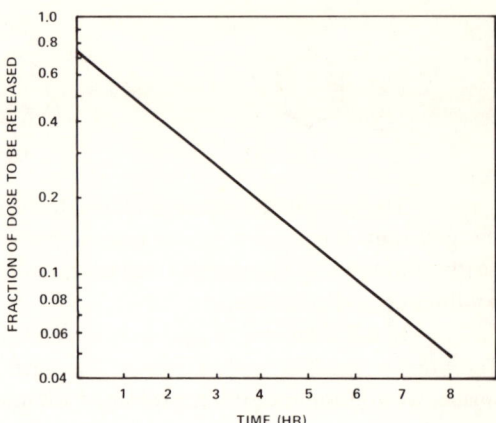

Figure 57. Logarithm of the fraction of hexocyclium methylsulfate remaining in a Gradumet® sustained—release tablet is a linear function of time. [R.G. Wiegand and J.D. Taylor, *Drug Std. 27,* 165 (1959).]

When all the drug has been released, $f_i + f_s = 1$. If this sum is less than 1, all the drug has not been released. With the ion-exchange technique, this sum is at times less than 1, indicating that the drug is not completely released from the resinate.

With different techniques of sustained-release preparation, the release of the drug may deviate somewhat from a first-order release; however, the leaching, ion-exchange, and erosion types release the drug according to the above equation. A multiple-pellet sustained-release product can be made to have a variety of release patterns by varying the composition and the thicknesses of the coatings.

Solid dosage forms to be given occasionally should have an f_i value sufficient to produce a rapid effect. If the product is to be given repeatedly, f_i should be small, because the drug level is not at zero after the first dose.

Sustained-release medication has certain restrictions. It should not be used for drugs that have a very critical dose because biological variance may alter the normal release pattern and not provide the precise dose required. This is especially important with persons known to have impaired or erratic gastrointestinal absorption. As there are three to four times as much drug in a sustained-release dosage form as in a conventional dosage form, only drugs with a substantial margin of safety should be in a sustained-release product. An erosion type of tablet is intended to be swallowed whole; if it were chewed, an overdose of the drug would be immediately available.

From the viewpoint of product development, it is not feasible to produce a sustained-release dosage form for a drug that has a large dose. The bulk of the drug and the pharmaceutical necessities for producing sustained release make a tablet or capsule too large to be easily swallowed. Drugs that are absorbed from a restricted site of absorption in the gastrointestinal tract should not be administered in sustained-release form because most of the drug is released in nonabsorbing regions and the total amount of drug absorbed will be grossly insufficient.

There appears to be no general *in vitro* method for testing the availability of a drug from a sustained-release product. Each technique for producing sustained release requires a specific testing method. During the product-development stage, *in vitro* testing serves as a tool in estimating the rate of release and reduces the number of formulations to be submitted for *in vivo* testing. All *in vitro* methods are valid only after being correlated with *in vivo* release patterns. The *in vitro* method then serves as a quality-control tool for production batches.

The following *in vitro* method for determining the amount of drug released from sustained-release capsules and tablets is useful in establishing test criteria to assure product uniformity. It may generally be used as a routine control test; however, through actual experience it may be found unsuitable for some products. The apparatus consists of a horizontal rotating shaft fitted with clamps for holding round, screw-capped bottles which are approximately 150 mm long and 30 mm in diameter. The bottles are clamped at right angles to the axis of the shaft and are immersed in a constant-temperature water bath. The speed of the shaft can be varied from 6 to 50 rpm.

The following five extraction fluids are prepared from simulated gastric fluid and simulated intestinal fluid: (1) pH 1.2 consists of simulated gastric fluid, (2) pH 2.5 consists of 46 ml of simulated gastric fluid and 54 ml of simulated intestinal fluid, (3) pH 4.5 consists of 39 ml of simulated gastric fluid and 61 ml of simulated intestinal fluid, (4) pH 7 consists of 17.5 ml of simulated gastric fluid and 82.5 ml of simulated intestinal fluid, and (5) pH 7.5 consists of simulated intestinal fluid.

The sustained-release capsules or tablets are placed in each of five bottles containing 60 ml of pH 1.2 extracting fluid at 37°. The bottles are capped and rotated in the apparatus at 40 rpm at 37° for 1 hour. Then the pH 1.2 extracting fluid from each bottle is decanted through a separate 40-mesh screen and as much residue is retained in four of the bottles as is conveniently possible. Any decanted residue on each of the four screens is quantitatively returned to its respective original bottle by washing the screen with 60 ml of pH 2.5 extracting fluid at 37°. The four bottles are then replaced in the apparatus and rotated for an additional hour. The content of the fifth bottle is quantitatively transferred onto the 40-mesh screen using 30 ml of water. The residue is assayed for content of drug.

After a total rotational time of 2 hours, the four bottles are removed from the apparatus. The residue from one bottle is collected on a screen as previously described and retained for assay. The pH 2.5 extracting fluid from each of the other three bottles is decanted through a separate screen and any residue is returned to its original bottle by using 60 ml of pH 4.5 extracting fluid at 37°.

At the end of 3.5 hours of total rotation time all the bottles are removed from the apparatus. The residue from one bottle is quantitatively collected and assayed. The pH 4.5 extracting fluid is decanted from each of the other two bottles through a separate screen and any residue is returned to its original bottle using 60 ml of pH 7 extracting fluid at 37°. The two bottles are replaced in the apparatus.

At the end of 5 hours of total rotation time both bottles are removed. The residue from one is quantitatively collected on a screen and assayed. The pH 7 extracting fluid is decanted through a screen and any residue is quantitatively returned to the bottle using 60 ml of pH 7.5 extracting fluid at 37°. The remaining bottle is replaced in the apparatus.

At the end of 7 hours of total rotation time the remaining bottle is removed from the apparatus. The residue is quantitatively collected on a screen and assayed.

Roentgenographic methods (see page 92) have been used to evaluate sustained-release products containing barium sulfate. This method has been questioned on the basis that a soluble drug may be leached from the sustaining coat or barrier, whereas the barium sulfate is insoluble. In radiopaque studies it has been shown that the contents of a capsule administered on an empty stomach are scattered throughout the initial segment of the small intestine within 1 hour. Possible tissue damage due to radiation exposure and the rare availability of radioactive drugs severely limits the use of these methods of evaluation.

Toxicity tests in animals may be used in the development of a sustained-release dosage, if the drug has a relatively high toxicity. In evaluating ion-exchange resinates the dose producing death in 50 per cent of the test animals, i.e., LD_{50}, of the untreated drug is compared to that of the resinate. If the LD_{50} is greater and the time until death is longer, the release is more prolonged. After initial developmental research the toxicity tests are of little value, as they give no indication of the overall pattern of release and cannot be applied to humans.

The therapeutic effect elicited by a drug is a function of its concentration at the site of action in the body. Methods for measuring the concentration of drug at the receptor sites are still unknown, but since the tissues of the body are in equilibrium, any changes in drug concentration of the blood should reflect concentration changes at the receptor sites and in other tissues of the body. It is convenient to evaluate the physiological availability of a drug by measuring blood levels. If the minimum blood level or M.E.D. required to produce a therapeutic activity is known, blood-level studies will demonstrate the onset and duration of action of a dosage form. Two disadvantages of blood-level determinations are the lack of a satisfactory analytical method and at times the necessity of giving a dose larger than the therapeutic dose to facilitate chemical assay.

For certain drugs there is a relationship between urinary excretion rate and the concentration of the drug in the blood. As there is a relation between therapeutic response and blood levels, a relation exists logically between the therapeutic activity and the rate of excretion in the urine. Urinary drug levels have been useful in preliminary evaluation of sustained-release products as a means of comparison between conventional and sustained-release dosage forms in regard to the rate of excretion and the total excreted drug.

Ultimately all dosage forms must be evaluated by properly designed clinical studies with humans. Subjective impressions of the physician and subjective values based on the opinion of the patient are unreliable and should be avoided if possible. In properly designed experiments quantitative analysis of the drug concentration in the body fluids and tissues provides unbiased data. Likewise, clinical studies should be objective. The efficacy of a mydriatic may be evaluated by measuring the diameter of the pupil and the length of time dilation exists. Peripheral vasodilators may be evaluated by a capacigraph which measures the blood volume change produced by the pulse wave in a finger.

4 | PROPERTIES OF SOLIDS

BONDING FORCES PRESENT IN SOLIDS

Intramolecular attractive forces between atoms are responsible for the existence of molecules; intermolecular attractive forces between molecules are responsible for the condensed state of a substance. Intramolecular forces are large. For example, approximately 220 kcal are required to break all the O-H bonds in 1 mole of water. The force between molecules is considerably less than the intramolecular force. Approximately 12 kcal is sufficient to disrupt the intermolecular forces in 1 mole of ice so that it can be dispersed in the gaseous phase as individual molecules.

Although the intermolecular force may appear weak, it is a significant force that maintains substances in a liquid or solid state. The attractive force between two similar molecules is usually the sum of two types of force: dipole-dipole force and van der Waals force. The contribution of each in maintaining a condensed state depends on the electronic configuration of the molecules. It is the intermolecular force that determines the physical properties of a substance and is important to the pharmacist.

Dipole-Dipole Interaction

In many molecules the electrons are arranged so that the centers of positive and negative electricity do not coincide, although the molecules as a whole are not charged. In a molecule of cetyl alcohol, the electron pair responsible for the O-H bond is not equally shared by the two atoms as in a purely covalent bond. The kernel, i.e., the nucleus and all except the valence electrons, of the oxygen atom has a higher central charge and a greater affinity for the bonding electrons than the hydrogen atom. Consequently, the electrons are somewhat displaced toward the oxygen atom, producing an asymmetrical distribution of electrons with a deficiency in the region of the hydrogen atom. This may be considered as a partial transfer of the bonding electrons to the oxygen, making it more electronegative than the hydrogen. Polarization of a bond resulting from electronic shifts produced by differences in the electrostatic affinity of the bonded kernels for the bonding electrons is known as the inductive effect (or I effect).

The inductive effect results in the separation of electrical centers of a cetyl alcohol molecule with the negative center residing with the oxygen atom and the positive center with the hydrogen atom. Molecules having a noncoincident negative and positive center are known as dipolar molecules or dipoles. Conventionally, a dipole such as cetyl alcohol is represented as

$$\text{CH}_3\text{-(CH}_2)_{14}\text{-CH}_2\overset{\delta-\;\;\delta+}{\diagup \text{O: H}}$$

The dissymmetry in the electrical charge distribution makes these dipoles responsive to electrical fields. The dipoles tend to orient themselves parallel to the field with the negative portion toward the positive side of the field and the positive portion toward the negative side of the field. The

properties of solids

extent of this orientation in an electrical field depends on the dipole moment of the molecule. Dipole moment, μ, is defined as the product of the charge and the distance between the two average centers of positive and negative electricity. The values in debye units, D, of some dipole moments are given in Table XVII.

Table XVII Dipole Moments

Compound	Debye *
H_2O_2	2.13
H_2O	1.87
H_2S	1.1
CH_4	0
CH_3Cl	1.86
CH_2Cl_2	1.59
$CHCl_3$	1.01
CCl_4	0
C_2H_6	0
$(CH_3)_2 \cdot C = O$	2.88
C_2H_5OH	1.7
C_6H_6	0
C_6H_5OH	1.45
$C_6H_5NH_2$	1.53
C_6H_5Cl	1.73
$C_6H_5NO_2$	4.23
$C_6H_5OCH_3$	1.38
$C_2H_5OOCCH_3$	1.78
$CH_3CO \cdot NH_2$	3.6
$(NH_2)_2C = O$	4.56
HCl	1.08
HBr	0.78
HI	0.38
N_2	0
Cl_2	0

*1 Debye = 10^{-18} esu cm

The attraction of the oppositely charged fields causes the positive end of a polar molecule to be attracted to the negative portion of an adjacent dipole, forming an intermolecular bond. The negative end of the same molecule is attracted to the positive portion of other polar molecules. This interaction is called dipole-dipole interaction. The dipole-dipole interaction that maintains cetyl alcohol and boric acid in a solid state may be diagrammatically represented as

Cetyl alcohol   Boric acid

Dipole-dipole interaction becomes a stronger force if the positive center is located in a hydrogen atom. The small size of the hydrogen atom permits the negative ends of adjacent dipoles to approach much closer to the electropositive hydrogen atom than is possible with any other atom in a similar position. Further, if the negative center resides in a strong proton acceptor, e.g., fluorine, nitrogen, or oxygen atom, the interaction between the two oppositely charged electrical centers forms a strong intermolecular bond. This type of bonding, frequently encountered in the biological sciences and pharmacy, is a special case of dipole-dipole interaction known as hydrogen bonding. Hydrogen bonding has an energy of approximately 2 to 10 kcal mole^{-1}.

A dipole may also exist as a consequence of resonance. According to valence-bond theory, the actual structure of a resonance hybrid is intermediate between written configurations. The electronic structure of benzoic acid is probably a hybrid structure between the following electronic configurations:

(A)   (B)

Resonance form (B), which requires higher energy content, contributes only slightly to the overall resonance structure; however, this slight contribution is sufficient to withdraw some of the electrons from the hydroxyl group. Polarization of this type is known as the electromeric effect (or E effect). The electromeric effect exists to some extent in nearly all unsaturated compounds, i.e., acids, aldehydes, ketones, and amides. Traditionally, a curved arrow is used in writing a formula to indicate the direction of flow of electrons.

Benzoic acid is a dipole by virtue of the electromeric effect. The negative center residing with the oxygen atom is attracted to the positive electrical center of an adjacent benzoic acid molecule. This hydrogen bonding that holds benzoic acid in a solid state may be diagrammatically shown as

Nearly all solid organic compounds other than salts and hydrocarbons are held in the condensed state by dipole-dipole interaction. The dipole arises due to either the inductive shift or the electromeric shift. Some pharmaceutical examples of molecular solids having permanent dipole interactions are given in Table XVIII.

Table XVIII Organic Functional Groups Common to Pharmaceuticals and Their Primary Bonding Interaction

Functional Group	Crystalline Example	Major Type of Bonding
Acid	Citric acid, nicotinic acid, stearic acid, tartaric acid, aspirin	Hydrogen bonding
Alcohol	Inositol, stearyl alcohol, sorbitol	Hydrogen bonding
Phenol	Phenol, resorcinol, thymol	Hydrogen bonding
Amide	Acetamide, nicotinamide, phenacetin, urea	Hydrogen bonding or dipole - dipole
Amine	Codeine, glycine, morphine	Hydrogen bonding or dipole - dipole
Aldehyde	Chloral hydrate, paraldehyde	Dipole - dipole
Ketone	Acetophenone, camphor, diphenadione	Dipole - dipole
Ester	Methylparaben, salol, wax	Van der Waals
Ether	Benzophenone, chlorotrianisene	Van der Waals
Halogen	Benzene hexachloride, iodoform	Van der Waals
Hydrocarbon	Paraffin, petrolatum	Van der Waals

Van der Waals Interaction

Nonpolar molecules that have a zero dipole moment are known to exist as liquids, e.g., benzene and carbon tetrachloride, and solids, e.g., hexachloroethane and naphthalene. The intermolecular force maintaining an electrically neutral and symmetrical molecule in a solid state arises from a transient, internal electronic polarization of the molecules.

Any molecule at a given instance may have a temporary dipole arising from electronic oscillations within the molecule. Such internal oscillations induce further vibrations in adjacent molecules, and as these would tend to be in phase, there is intermolecular attraction. This is known as induced dipole-induced dipole attraction because the attraction arises from the induced polarization of the interacting molecules. The induced dipole-induced dipole force is also known as van der Waals force and London force. As the molecular weight increases, the molecules have a greater number of electrons per molecule and van der Waals force is stronger. Thus, as the molecular weights of nonpolar compounds increase, the melting points increase.

As van der Waals force is weak, solids held together by an induced dipole-induced dipole interaction have a low melting point and are relatively volatile. Docosane and codeine have approximately the same molecular weight, but the melting point of the hydrocarbon is only 44°, reflecting the weak interaction of van der Waals force as compared to the stronger dipole-dipole interactions in codeine, as reflected by a melting point of 155°.

Van der Waals force exists in all compounds, and it contributes somewhat to compounds also held together by dipole-dipole interaction. The contribution of each type of intermolecular force depends on the relative proportion of polar and nonpolar groups in the molecule.

Ionic Interaction

According to valence-bond theory, the atom may be considered as a positively charged nucleus surrounded by a sufficient number of electrons, moving in well-defined orbits, to make the whole atom neutral. The number and configuration of the outer or valence electrons determines the chemical properties of the element. The inner electrons that do not take part in forming chemical bonds and the nucleus are collectively known as the kernel of the atom. The charge of the kernel is always opposite and equal to the total charge of the valence electrons. The kernel of an oxygen atom has a charge of +6.

Atoms tend to take up electrons, so the configuration of the valence electrons and any acquired electrons resemble that in the outer shells of the rare gas elements. For many common elements, this results in eight electrons outside the kernel. The electrons necessary to achieve this octet may be acquired by a transfer or sharing of electrons with other atoms, i.e., covalent bonding.

If the electron transfer is from one atom to another, an ion is formed; e.g., sodium atom gives up its outermost electron, becoming a cation, while the chlorine atom acquires a single electron, forming an anion. The oppositely charged ions are attracted by an electrostatic or coulombic force, binding them together as a sodium chloride crystal:

$$:\ddot{\underset{..}{Cl}}\cdot + Na\cdot \rightarrow :\ddot{\underset{..}{Cl}}\bar{:}\ Na^+$$

The sodium chloride crystal is made up of positively charged sodium ions and negatively charged chloride ions as shown in Figure 61. Each sodium ion is surrounded by six chloride ions; each chloride ion is surrounded by six sodium ions. As each of the ions is equidistant from an oppositely charged ion, no particular pair of ions has a greater affinity than any others; therefore, the term "molecule" is not applicable to this structure. For this reason the structure of the solid is known as an ionic lattice.

The ionic interaction energy is much greater than molecular interaction energies. About 184 kcal mole^{-1} is required to separate crystalline sodium chloride into individual gaseous ions. This strong interaction in sodium chloride is reflected in its high melting point, 801°. Dipole-dipole interactions involving less energy than ion-ion interactions produce lower melting points; e.g., benzoic acid melts at 122°. Solids held together by the weaker van der Waals force have still lower melting points for compounds of equivalent molecular weight. Naphthalene melts at 80°.

The molecules of a solid held together by van der Waals force have a tendency to escape from the solid into the vapor state. Sublimation is the process by which a solid passes directly into the vapor state without an intermediate passage through the liquid state. Naphthalene and paradichlorobenzene readily sublime at room temperature because only a weak van der Waals force is operative in these solids.

Covalent Interaction

With crystals of some nonmetals each atom is joined to adjacent atoms by covalent bonds, allowing each atom to complete its electron octet. These crystals are hard and have a high melting point.

The effect of a crystal lattice may be illustrated by comparing graphite and diamond in Figure 58. Graphite has a hexagonal network in sheets with 1.34 Å between the atoms in this plane. The distance between these atomic layers is 3.41 Å; this is too great a distance to correspond to a chemical bond, so each carbon atom is attached to three other carbon atoms. In two directions graphite is as strongly bonded as in diamond; however, in the third direction the force of attraction is less and one layer can slip over another. Graphite crystals are flaky and the planar structures slip readily over one another, providing a lubricating action. In a diamond each carbon atom is covalently bonded to four other atoms in a tetrahedral arrangement, which provides a more rigid lattice and results in a very hard crystal.

Other examples of covalent solids are fused aluminum oxide, iodine, quartz, silicon carbide, and zinc sulfide.

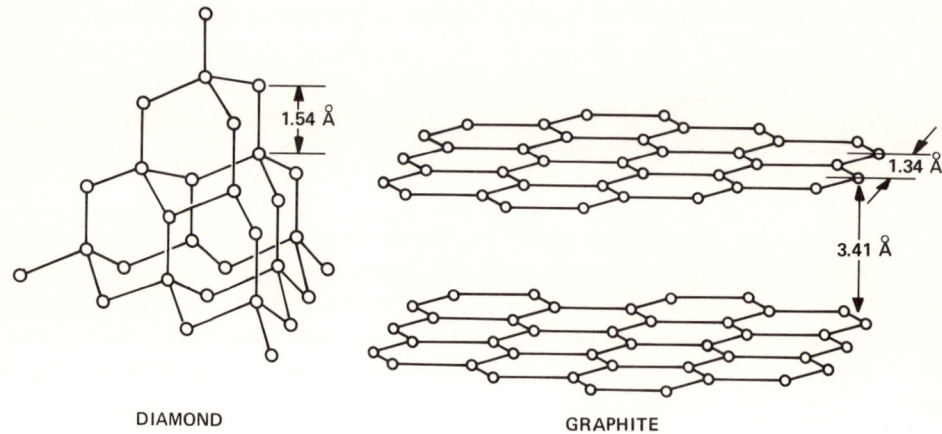

DIAMOND   GRAPHITE

Figure 58. Diagrammatical comparison of the space lattices of diamond and graphite.

Metallic Interaction

In a metal the atoms lose some of their electrons, becoming positive ions. The metallic crystal is held together by the electrostatic force between the free or cloud electrons and the lattice-held positively charged metallic ions. The bonding does not have a strong directional nature and the arrangement of the atoms frequently corresponds to a closest packing of spheres. The ductility and malleability of metals is associated with the close packing of the atoms. Under stress a metal distorts along the planes most densely occupied by atoms. In these planes the atoms are closest and the interaction forces is greatest, so the metal can yield and be less brittle. The high electrical conductance of metals is due to the mobile free electrons.

Substances bonded by covalent or metallic interaction are of limited consequence in medicine and pharmacy and will not be further discussed. For a summary of the various types of solids see Table XIX.

Table XIX Comparison of Types of Solids

	Molecular	**Ionic**	**Covalent**	**Metallic**
Units in crystal lattice	Molecules	Anion and cations	Atoms	Positive ions in electron cloud
Bonding force	Van der Waals, dipole - dipole	Electrostatic	Shared electrons	Attraction between cation and electrons
Hardness	Soft	Hard, brittle	Very hard	Hard to soft
Melting point	Low	High	Very high	Moderate to high
Volatility	High	Low	Low	Low
Example	Cetyl alcohol, resorcinol, paraffin, aspirin	Potassium citrate, sodium bromide, potassium iodide	Iodine	Copper, iron

THE STRUCTURE OF SOLIDS

A solid has a rigid form and a definite shape. The shape or habit of a crystal of a given substance may vary, but the angles between the faces are always constant. This interfacial angle is of value in characterizing crystals.

A crystal is made up of atoms, ions, or molecules in a regular geometric arrangment or lattice constantly repeated in three dimensions. The constantly repeated pattern of this lattice is known as the unit cell. If a crystal has the same appearance n times per 360° rotation about an axis, it is said to possess an n-fold rotation axis.

For convenience crystal lattices have been classified, as illustrated in Figure 59, into six major crystal systems, which are further divided into 32 classes. In the cubic system there are three axes of equal length intersecting at right angles. Cubic crystals are isotropic, i.e., have identical properties in all directions. All crystals in the cubic system may be typed as a simple cubic, face-centered cubic, or body-centered cubic lattice. As shown in Figure 60, the simple cubic crystal has units only at the corner of each unit cell. Each unit cell of the simple cubic lattice has a coordination number of 6. The number of equidistant adjacent ions surrounding a given ion is the coordination number. The face-centered lattice in addition has units at the center of each face. The body-centered lattice has a unit in the center of each cube as well as at the corners; its coordination number is 8.

114 • properties of solids

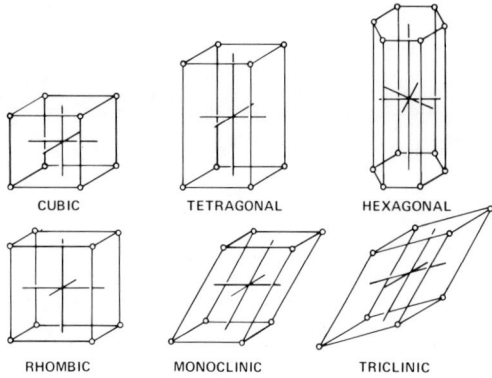

Figure 59. Unit cells of the major classes of crystal systems.

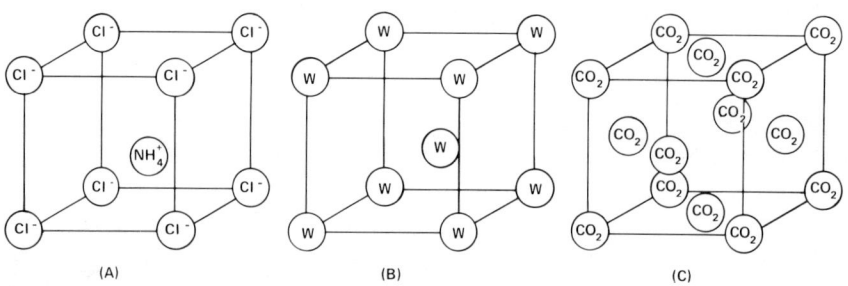

Figure 60. Unit cells in the cubic crystal system: (a) simple; (b) body-centered; (c) face-centered.

The solids in Figure 60 have been selected to illustrate that within a particular crystal system the units of a crystal may be atomic, ionic, or molecular. The simple cubic lattice is demonstrated by an ionic crystal of ammonium chloride in which there is a chloride ion at the corner of the unit cell with an ammonium ion at the center of the cell. This is not body centered, as it does not have the same type of ion at each lattice point. The body-centered cubic crystal is illustrated by an atomic crystal in which a metallic atom of tungsten is represented by each circle. The face-centered cubic crystal is represented by a molecular crystal of "dry ice," in which a molecule of carbon dioxide is represented by each circle.

To study a crystal structure, sodium chloride is considered in detail. The sodium chloride crystal is a face-centered cubic lattice; it is composed of two interpenetrating lattices of ions: one of sodium ions and one of chloride ions. In Figure 61 the square connecting the sodium ions contains a face-centered sodium ion. Likewise, the chloride ions may be connected, forming a square with a face-centered chloride ion. These interpenetrating face-centered lattices overlap by half the length of the face; thus, a corner of an interpenetrating sodium cube is halfway between the corners of a chloride cube. In diagonal planes through the sodium chloride cubes only sodium or chloride ions appear in a single plane; thus, diagonally there are alternating planes of sodium and chloride ions.

The radius of the sodium ion is 0.95 Å and that of the chloride ion in 1.81 Å. Although diagrammatic representations of the crystal often show atoms or ions as points or circles separated by some distance, the atoms or ions in a crystal practically touch one another. The distance of closest approach of sodium and chloride ions in the crystal would be the sum of the ionic radii, or 2.76 Å. The ions cannot approach closer to each other because of the repulsive electrostatic forces between the electron shells of their kernels. Experimentally the length of the unit cell of sodium chloride has been evaluated at 5.64 Å. This value is in good agreement with the length of the unit cell based only on the consideration of ionic radii, as shown in Figure 62.

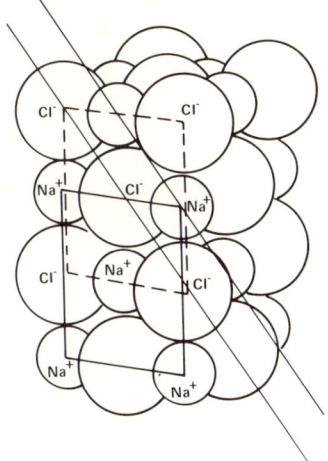

Figure 61. Interpenetrating face-centered lattice of sodium chloride; square connects face-centered lattice of sodium ions; dashed line connects face-centered lattice of chloride ions.

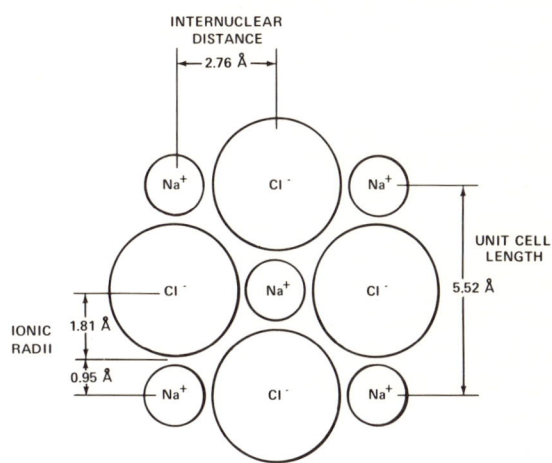

Figure 62. Distances in the sodium chloride crystal lattice.

Other examples of cubic crystals encountered in pharmacy are ammonium bromide, ammonium chloride, "dry ice," methenamine, potassium bromide, potassium chloride, potassium iodide, sodium bromide, and zinc sulfide.

The tetragonal system contains three axes intersecting at right angles, but two axes are equal in length and the third is longer or shorter. Mercurous chloride, pentaerythritol tetranitrate, titanium dioxide, and urea exist in the tetragonal form.

The hexagonal system has three axes of unit length in the same plane and intersecting at 60°, and a fourth axis longer or shorter and perpendicular to the plane of the others. Barbital, iodoform, silver iodide, and thymol are hexagonal crystals.

The rhombic system has three axes of unequal length and all intersect at right angles. Some crystals in this system are acetanilid, iodine, magnesium sulfate, potassium nitrate, potassium permanganate, sodium biphosphate, sulfacetamide, terpine hydrate, and zinc sulfate.

The monoclinic system has three axes of unequal length, two of which intersect at right angles while the third axis is perpendicular to one and not the other. Pharmaceutical substances existing in the monoclinic system are aluminum sulfate, benzoic acid, betanaphthol, chloral hydrate, ferrous sulfate, naphthalene, phenacetin, salicylic acid, sodium acetate, and sucrose.

The triclinic system has three axes of unequal length, no two of which intersect at right angles. Aminopyrine, boric acid, copper sulfate, naphazoline hydrochloride, and phenolphthalein are triclinic crystals.

The structure of a crystal depends on the type of binding force, the unit grouping, and the relative size of the units. In ionic crystals the structure is determined by how many ions can be packed about an oppositely charged ion while maintaining electrical neutrality. Although most alkali halides have face-centered cubic lattices, cesium chloride has a body-centered cubic lattice because of the size of the ions. The relatively large cesium ion is approximately the same size as the chloride ion, and eight chloride ions can pack about it in a body-centered cubic structure with a coordination number of 8. As the size of the positive ion decreases to that of sodium, i.e., 0.95 Å, only six chloride ions fit about the cation to form a face-centered cubic lattice. Although the radius of the chloride ion would allow more than six sodium ions, the electrical neutrality of the crystal permits only six sodium ions to be associated with a chloride ion. The ions then assume the stable lattice previously discussed.

The ratio of the radius of the positive ion to the negative ion has been used to suggest the type of lattice to be formed by the ions. If this ratio is greater than 0.73, eight anions at the corners of a cube may be in contact with one cation, i.e., coordination number of 8. With this ratio the body-centered cubic lattice predominates. If this ratio lies between 0.73 and 0.41, the coordination number is 6 and the face-centered cubic lattice is common. If the ratio is from 0.22 to 0.41, the coordination number is 4; i.e., four anions are packed at the corners of a tetrahedral about one cation. If the ratio is from 0.15 to 0.22, three cations surround one anion.

In molecular crystals the structure depends on the configuration of the molecules. The molecules in a linear hydrocarbon, e.g., paraffin, are aligned parallel to the length of the chain and packed so that each molecule is surrounded by six other molecules in an arrangement analogous to the closest packed system. This results in a structure that falls into the hexagonal system. In solid carboxylic acids, e.g., adipic, benzoic, and cinnamic acid, the hydrogen bonds are parallel to the long axes of the needle-shaped crystals.

PHYSICAL PHENOMENA AFFECTING SOLID PHARMACEUTICALS
Melting Point

The melting point and the freezing point of a pure crystalline solid is that temperature at which the pure liquid and solid are in equilibrium. Although pressure affects the melting point, for most practical purposes the melting point is usually determined and reported at atmospheric pressure.

The heat absorbed when 1 g of a solid melts is known as the latent heat of fusion. The molar heat of fusion, ΔH_f, is the amount of heat absorbed when 1 mole of a solid melts; e.g., the molar heat of fusion of ice is 1436 cal mole^{-1}. Melting involves the transition of ions or molecules from an orderly crystal lattice to a liquid state of randomness. This transition occurs when the thermal vibration of the atoms overcomes the interionic or intermolecular forces holding the substance in a solid lattice. The latent heat of fusion is the energy required to accomplish this transition without a change of temperature.

A substance with a high heat of fusion has a high melting point. A crystal that is held together by the weak van der Waals force has a low melting point and a low heat of fusion. A sample of paraffin with a melting point of 52° has a heat of fusion of 35.1 cal g^{-1}. In comparison, sodium chloride, a crystal held together by strong ionic interaction, has a melting point of 801° and a heat of fusion of 124 cal g^{-1}. Intermediate between ionic and van der Waals bonding is dipole-dipole interaction. Ice, which is held together by hydrogen bonding, has a melting point of 0° and a heat of fusion of 80 cal g^{-1}.

An important use of the melting point is its use as a criterion of purity. If a substance is pure, the melting point is sharp. If a small amount of compound B is mixed with compound A, the melting point of the mixture is lower than that of pure A. If the two components form an ideal binary system, their additive properties are linear functions of their composition. The melting-point lowering, ΔT, of A is proportional to the mole fraction, N_A, of A in the mixture and may be mathematically expressed as

$$\Delta T = -\frac{2.303 R T T_0}{\Delta H_f} \log N_A$$

where ΔH_f is the molar heat of fusion, T the absolute equilibrium temperature, T_0 the melting point of pure A, and R the gas constant.

The lowering of the melting point is inversely proportional to the heat of fusion. For compounds that have a very low molar heat of fusion, e.g., camphor and cyclohexanol, a large lowering of melting point is observed in the presence of a small amount of a second component. A substance that has a high molar heat of fusion, eg.., cetyl alcohol or stearic acid, will show little change in melting point with the addition of a second component.

The extent of lowering of the melting point of a compound is a function of its melting point. A compound with a high melting point shows a greater lowering for a given mole fraction of impurity than a compound with a low melting point. Anthracene and capric acid have nearly identical molar heats of fusion, and their melting points are 216° and 32°, respectively. Anthracene, with the higher melting point, has a lowering approximately 2.5 times as great as that of capric acid for 1 mole per cent of an impurity.

A temperature-composition diagram expresses the melting point as a function of composition of all solid phases in a two- or three-component system. The determination of the melting point of a mixture is important in pharmacy. The trivial case is the relationship between two components, e.g., azobenzene and oxalic acid, that are completely insoluble in each other. As neither dissolves any of the other component, no lowering of either melting point occurs. In general, high-melting, highly polar compounds are mutually insoluble in low-melting, nonpolar compounds. This may be encountered when one component is an organic and the other is an inorganic compound. Pharmaceutical preparations that are mixtures of salts and sugars behave in this manner.

Figure 63 shows a diagram for a two-component system in which the two components are completely miscible in the liquid state and do not form a solid solution or an addition compound. The eutectic is the lowest-melting mixture that crystallizes as a physical mixture of the two components. The two melting-point curves express the lowering of the melting point of each pure compound by the addition of the other component. On heating a solid mixture begins to melt at the eutectic melting point, E. At all temperatures above the eutectic melting point only one solid phase can exist along with the melt. On the right portion of the curve the solid phase will be B.

A phase is a definite part of a system which is homogeneous throughout and physically separated by distinct boundaries. In an equilibrium system of ice, liquid water, and water vapor, there are three phases. The major variables that determine the state of equilibrium are temperature, pressure, and concentration; a diagram that relates these variables to the phases is known as a phase diagram.

The phase rule describes the conditions under which the various phases in a system may exist. The phase rule is

$$F = C - P + 2$$

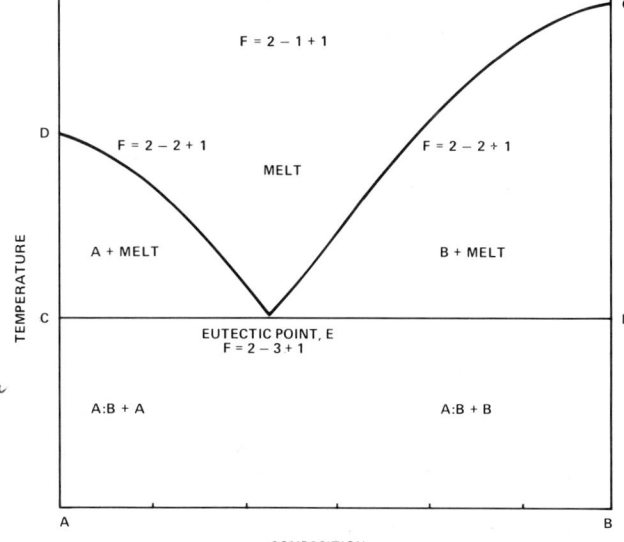

Figure 63. Binary composition diagram of a simple eutectic formation showing the application of the phase rule.

118 • properties of solids

where F is the number of degrees of freedom, C the number of components, and P the number of phases. The number of components is the minimum number of chemical constituents that must be specified to describe the composition of each phase present.

The number of degrees of freedom is the number of independent variables, e.g., temperature, pressure, and concentration, that must be specified to define the system completely. The number 2 is valid only if there are two variables, e.g., temperature and pressure, in addition to concentration. If there were a third variable the phase rule would be

$$F = C - P + 3$$

When camphor and salol are mixed, a eutectic melting point of 10° is obtained at atmospheric pressure. As pharmacists are working under atmospheric pressure, the pressure is considered fixed. Thus, the only variable in addition to composition is temperature, and the phase rule is

$$F = C - P + 1$$

Application of the phase rule to the area above the melting curves of the two-component system in Figure 63 shows that temperature and composition can be varied without a change in the number of phases; that is, there are two degrees of freedom,

$$F = 2 - 1 + 1 = 2$$

Along the melting curves DE and EG, fixing the temperature or composition defines the system; i.e., there is one degree of freedom,

$$F = 2 - 2 + 1 = 1$$

At the eutectic point where both A and B appear together, any change in concentration or temperature results in the disappearance of one of the two solid phases or the liquid phase. Then

$$F = 2 - 3 + 1 = 0$$

While the pharmacist is preparing solid pharmaceuticals, a formulation may be encountered in which the melting points of the constituents are lowered by other drugs until liquefaction occurs at room temperature. Obviously, it would be difficult to prepare a capsule, tablet, or a divided powder with a melt. Common drugs exhibiting this effect are acetanilid, aminopyrine, antipyrine, betanaphthol, chloral hydrate, menthol, phenol, thymol, and the salicylates. The eutectic temperatures of some binary mixtures are given in Table XX.

In examining Figure 63 it is apparent that at room temperature certain compositions are liquid and certain compositions are solid. By referring to this phase diagram the pharmacist compounding a prescription of A and B would know if the particular composition would be liquid or solid. Unfortu-

Table XX Eutectic Temperature of Some Binary Mixtures

Binary System	Eutectic Temperature (°C)
Clopane hydrochloride (114°) and acetanilid (115°)	30
Resorcinol (110°) and acetanilid	33
Pyrocatechol (104°) and acetanilid	37
Sparteine hydrochloride (103-105°) and acetanilid	47
Aspirin (130-136°) and acetanilid	81
Phenacetine (135°) and acetanilid	90
Aspirin (130-136°) and phenacetin (135°)	97
Phenolphthalein (263°) and sodium acetate (328°)	142

nately, the availability of phase diagrams is limited by the large number of possible combinations of drugs in dosage forms. In practice the pharmacist recognizes probable offenders and compounds them as if liquefaction would occur.

Any drug having low intermolecular forces as indicated by a low melting point, a soft crystalline structure, or ready sublimation probably will liquefy when triturated with a chemical of similar nature. Medicinal chemicals which fall in this category are often aldehydes, ketones, or phenols.

As the atmospheric pressure is fixed and the temperature does not vary greatly, the composition of a mixture is the most important factor in determining its physical state. In addition to the therapeutic agent, most pharmaceutical dosage forms have additives, which may influence the properties of the preparation. If liquefaction of the therapeutic agents occurs, there may be a sufficient amount of higher-melting-point additives to effectively sorb the liquid. Small amounts of liquefying ingredients may be mixed and the resulting liquid taken up in the pores and on the surface of other ingredients.

30. Salicylic acid   0.5 g
    Phenol   0.1 g
    Eucalyptol   0.1 ml
    Menthol   0.1 g
    Thymol   0.1 g
    Zinc sulfate   12.5 g
    Boric acid, powdered   86.6 g

    Sig.: Dust on dermatosis

The phenol, eucalyptol, menthol, and thymol are triturated until liquefaction occurs. The zinc sulfate and salicylic acid are triturated to a fine powder. The liquefied drugs are added to the zinc sulfate and salicylic acid and blended. The boric acid is added and the mixture is triturated until uniform. The powder is then passed through a 100-mesh sieve.

If the amount of liquefying substances is too large to be sorbed, each of the liquefying drugs is mixed separately with an inert, high-melting-point protective, and then they are lightly blended. The protective tends to function as a mechanical barrier or coat to prevent contact between the lower-melting ingredients. In addition, if any liquefaction occurs, the liquid is sorbed on the large surface of the protective ingredient.

31. Chloral hydrate   0.25 g
    Aminopyrine   0.25 g

    M. ft. Caps. XXIV

    Sig.: Two at bedtime

Upon trituration the aminopyrine and chloral hydrate readily liquefy. An attempt to sorb this liquid on an inert substance produces too great a bulk for a capsule. To prevent liquefaction each drug is separately mixed with kaolin or talc. Mix approximately 100 mg of kaolin with each of the drugs in a capsule; then lightly blend the two mixtures and place in a No. 00 capsule.

In pharmacy kaolin, magnesium oxide, and magnesium carbonate have traditionally been employed as inert protectives. Magnesium carbonate is preferred to the oxide, which may react with other ingredients, water, or carbon dioxide to form a hard, insoluble mass. The desired characteristics of a protective are therapeutic and chemical inertness, a high melting point, and a large specific surface.

The mechanical coating may be illustrated by a consideration of a camphor-salol system in which magnesium carbonate with a melting point of 350° is used to surround the particles of camphor and salol. In preparing a prescription for 100 capsules each containing 0.1 g of camphor and 0.1 g of salol, a pharmacist would expect liquefaction because of the low melting points, i.e., camphor (176°) and salol (43°). Separate trituration of the drugs would reduce the particle size to d_{av} = 200 μ. The

120 • properties of solids

densities of camphor, salol, and magnesium carbonate are 1.0, 1.25 and 3.1 g cc^{-1}, respectively. Magnesium carbonate has d_{av} = 20 μ. From this information, assuming the particles are spherical, the amount of magnesium carbonate required to coat or surround 10 g of camphor may be calculated.

1. The surface area of a single spherical particle of camphor is

$$A_i = \pi d^2 = \pi (2 \times 10^{-2})^2$$

2. The area covered by a single particle of magnesium carbonate is its cross-sectional area, i.e., $\frac{1}{4}d^2$,

$$A = \frac{\pi d^2}{4} = \frac{\pi}{4}(2 \times 10^{-3})^2$$

3. The number of particles of magnesium carbonate required to coat one particle of camphor is

$$\frac{A_i}{A} = \frac{\pi(2 \times 10^{-2})^2}{(\frac{1}{4}\pi (2 \times 10^{-3})^2)} = 400$$

4. The weight of a single particle of camphor is equivalent to the product of its density and volume, i.e., $V = 1/6 \, \pi d^3$,

$$W_i = \rho V = \frac{\pi}{6} d^3 \rho = \frac{\pi}{6}(2 \times 10^{-2})^3 = 4.19 \times 10^{-6} \text{ g}$$

5. The total number of particles in 10 g of camphor is

$$\frac{10}{W_i} = \frac{10}{4.19 \times 10^{-6}} = 2.4 \times 10^6$$

6. The number of particles of magnesium carbonate required to coat all the particles of camphor is the product of the number of particles of camphor and the number of particles of magnesium carbonate required to coat one particle of camphor, or

$$2.4 \times 10^6 \times 400 = 9.6 \times 10^8$$

7. The weight of a single particle of magnesium carbonate is

$$W = V\rho = \frac{\pi}{6} d^3 \rho = \frac{\pi}{6}(2 \times 10^{-3})^3 (3.1) = 1.3 \times 10^{-8} \text{ g}$$

8. The weight of protective needed to coat 10 g of camphor is the product of the number of particles of protective and the weight of a single particle, or

$$1.3 \times 10^{-8} \times 9.6 \times 10^8 = 12.5 \text{ g}$$

9. In a like manner, the amount of protective needed to coat 10 g of salol is found to be 9.9 g.

10. The total weight of magnesium carbonate to coat both the camphor and salol is 22.4 g.

The camphor is triturated to a powder and 12.5 g of magnesium carbonate is added and mixed until uniform. The powdered salol is mixed with 9.9 g of magnesium carbonate until uniform. The two mixtures are then blended by light trituration or tumbling in a blender. Four hundred and twenty-four milligrams of the mixture is placed in an appropriate-sized capsule.

A substance has its peculiar physical properties chiefly as a consequence of its molecular weight and its intermolecular forces. The spatial configuration of a molecule may affect its physical properties. In chemistry it is recognized that for a given isomeric, aliphatic hydrocarbon series the linear molecule has a greater opportunity for van der Waals intermolecular attraction than the branched hydrocarbons.

properties of solids • 121

The linear molecule in a series will therefore have a higher melting point than the branched compounds of equivalent molecular weight.

The spatial arrangement of the hydroxybenzoic acids affects their physical properties. Salicylic acid has a hydroxyl group in a position ortho to the carboxy group. This ortho position permits an intramolecular hydrogen bond to be formed. As the hydroxyl groups, which are intramolecularly hydrogen bonded, do not bond with adjacent molecules, the intermolecular force between the salicylic acid molecules is less than the other isomers. This is reflected in a lower melting point, as shown in Table XXI. Other examples of intramolecular hydrogen bonding are shown in Figure 64.

Salts that are held together by strong ionic bonds have high melting points. In general, with an increase in interionic distance between the oppositely charged ions there is a decrease in melting

Table XXI Effect of Intramolecular Hydrogen Bonding on Melting Point

Isomer	Melting Point (°C)	Hydrogen Bonding
o-Hydroxybenzoic acid	159	Intra
m-Hydroxybenzoic acid	201	Inter
p-Hydroxybenzoic acid	213	Inter
o-Hydroxybenzamide	138	Intra
m-Hydroxybenzamide	170	Inter
p-Hydroxybenzamide	162	Inter
o-Chlorophenol	7	Intra
m-Chlorophenol	33	Inter
p-Chlorophenol	43	Inter

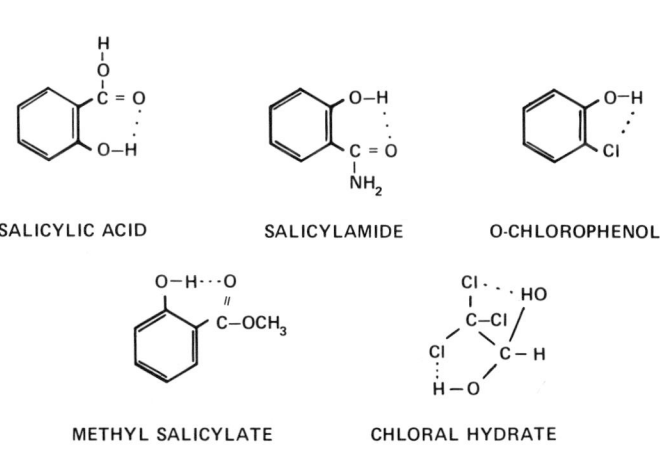

Figure 64. Some pharmaceutical compounds with intramolecular hydrogen bonding.

122 • properties of solids

point. As shown in Table XXII, for a given cation as the size of the anion increases the melting point decreases. With salts of similar interionic distances, those in which the ions have a greater charge have a higher melting point. Calcium oxide has the same interionic distance as sodium fluoride but, owing to its higher charge, its melting point is approximately 2.5 times higher.

Table XXII Effect of Interionic Distance and Charge on the Melting Points of Salts

Salt	Interionic Distance (Å)	Melting Point (°C)
NaF	2.31	977
NaBr	2.90	755
NaI	3.11	651
NaF	2.31	997
CaO	2.39	2580

Some organic compounds, e.g., ascorbic acid, sugar, amino acids, alkaloids, and amides, are unstable at their melting points and decompose; however, most organic compounds crystallize easily and quickly on cooling. If supercooled with liquid air most organic melts solidify in the amorphous form or as a glass. A few compounds, e.g., phenobarbital and quinine, may solidify in the amorphous form even at room temperature. The amorphous solid has no definite repeating structure. Any existing pattern extends only a short distance from a given atom or molecule, and the overall arrangement is a random one. Amorphous substances have no sharp melting point but soften over a temperature range.

Volatility

The volatility of a liquid or a solid is its ability to pass into the vapor phase. Quantitatively, volatility is expressed in terms of vapor pressure of the substance. The pressure at which a liquid or a solid and its vapor are in equilibrium at a given temperature is the vapor pressure of a substance. As the temperature increases, the vapor pressure increases.

Sublimation is the conversion of a solid to a vapor without passing through a liquid phase. There is no single sublimation temperature. A substance sublimes only at a faster or slower rate as the temperature rises or falls. Certain pharmaceuticals, e.g., benzoic acid, iodine, and sulfur, can be purified by sublimation because their high vapor pressure makes the rate of sublimation rapid enough for practical use.

"Dry ice" is one of the best known examples of sublimation. At its melting point, i.e., -56°, solid carbon dioxide has an equilibrium vapor pressure of 5 atm. Solid carbon dioxide cannot be converted into a liquid unless this pressure is exceeded; therefore, at atmospheric pressure solid carbon dioxide passes directly into a gas at all temperatures.

The change from a solid to a vapor requires energy to disrupt the crystalline structure. This energy is acquired by absorbing heat from the environment. The amount of heat required to convert 1 mole of a solid directly into a vapor is known as the heat of sublimation, ΔH_{sub}. At a given temperature and pressure the heat of sublimation is equal to the sum of the heat of fusion and heat of vaporization. Any substance that has a vapor pressure at its melting point that exceeds atmospheric pressure will sublime. From the practical viewpoint, at room temperature only a few substances have a vapor pressure that is greater than atmospheric pressure and will sublime.

The relation of vapor pressure of a solid to temperature is expressed by the Clapeyron-Clausius equation,

$$\frac{dp}{dT} = \frac{\Delta H_{sub}}{T(V_v - V_s)} = \frac{l_s}{T(v_v - v_s)}$$

where dp/dT is the rate of change of vapor pressure with temperature, V_v and V_S the molar volumes of the vapor and solid state at absolute temperature T, l_S the heat of sublimation per gram, and v_v and v_S specific volumes of vapor and solid state. As V_S is small compared to V_v, it may be neglected. For an ideal system the above equation may be derived to

$$\frac{d \ln p}{dT} = \frac{\Delta H_{sub}}{RT^2}$$

where p is the vapor pressure and R the gas constant.

In compounds held together by van der Waals force, the heat of sublimation is less than in those compounds also held together by dipole-dipole interaction. In general, as the bonding forces of a substance become stronger, the heat of sublimation and the melting point increase. Some examples are shown in Table XXIII.

Lyophilization, the removal of water from the thermolabile products by freezing and vaporizing at low pressures, is a sublimation operation. Figure 65 will aid in understanding lyophilization. In each

Table XXIII Effect of Type of Bonding Force on Heat of Sublimation and Melting Point

Compound	Molar Heat of Sublimation (kcal mole^{-1})	Melting Point (°C)	Molecular Weight (g mole^{-1})	Bonding Force
Acetamide	13.6	81	59	Hydrogen bonding
Phenol	16.1	41	94	Hydrogen bonding
Urea	21.0	137	56	Hydrogen bonding
Benzoic acid	21.8	122	122	Hydrogen bonding
p-Hydroxybenzoic acid	27.8	213	138	Hydrogen bonding
Benzene	10.5	5	78	Van der Waals
Naphthalene	13.2	80	128	Van der Waals
Docosane		44	310	Van der Waals

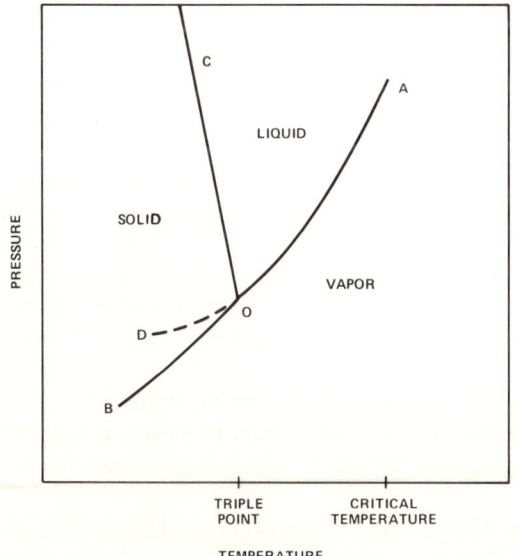

Figure 65. Schematic pressure-temperature phase diagram

of the three general areas labeled, only one phase can exist. Along the vapor-pressure curve *AO*, water and its vapor are in equilibrium. The melting curve *OC* shows how the melting point changes with pressure. Along the sublimation curve *BO*, ice and vapor are in equilibrium. Above *BO* is ice and below *BO* is vapor.

At *O* all three phases are in equilibrium; this is the triple point. For water the triple point is 0.0099°. The freezing point of ice and water exposed to the atmosphere is 0°. This difference is caused by the dissolved air lowering the freezing point 0.0024° at atmospheric pressure and by the increase over the water-vapor pressure of 4.57 mm of mercury to 1 atm, which lowers the freezing point 0.0075°.

During lyophilization the temperature and pressure are reduced so that the process is carried on to the left of the triple point. No liquid phase can exist, so the ice sublimes during the drying process.

In dispensing solid dosage forms, i.e., powders, capsules, and tablets, that contain volatile ingredients, the pharmacist should package them in airtight glass containers to minimize loss. Divided powders may be heat sealed in a cellophane envelope or double wrapped with an inner waxed paper and a bond paper.

    32. Methenamine   0.5 g
           Sodium biphosphate 0.5 g

           Make 10 powders

           Sig.: One q.i.d.

Commercially prepared tablets and capsules are coated to retard the loss of volatile drugs.

Polymorphism

The capacity for a substance to crystallize in more than one crystalline form is known as polymorphism. Sulfathiazole has been prepared in three crystalline forms, progesterone has been prepared in five crystalline forms, and nicotinamide has been prepared in four crystalline forms. Some properties of the five polymorphs of cortisone acetate are compared in Table XXIV. It is possible that all compounds can crystallize in different crystal forms or polymorphs.

By convention polymorphic forms are designated by Roman numerals. Form I is generally the most stable at room temperature. Other forms are numbered in order of their discovery, which often follows their order of stability. The color, hardness, melting point, solubility, and other properties of a compound depend on the polymorphic form. The effect of these properties on the physical characteristics of solid dosage forms has been known for many years; however, it is only recently that the effect of polymorphism on physiological response has been appreciated. The efficacy of a drug depends on its solubility in the blood or in the gastrointestinal fluids, and the solubility and rate of dissolution may vary from one crystalline form to another for a given drug.

Polymorphism results from different arrangements of molecules in the solid state. The molecules may be of different shape in two polymorphs; however, this shape change is limited to resonance structures, rotation of parts of molecules about certain bonds, and minor distortions of bond distances and angles. These limited distortions of molecular shape arise from polarizability effects of one molecule on another due to the change in relative positions of adjacent molecules in the two different crystalline arrangements. Two polymorphs will have different crystal lattices, but their liquid and vapor states are identical.

In broad terms, the mechanisms of polymorphic transformation may be expressed on the basis of structural change. Transformations of secondary coordination occur by bending but not breaking of the lattice or by breaking and reforming into a new lattice. The former occurs rapidly and the latter occurs slowly.

Transformations of disorder occur by a rotational disorder transformation in which some weak bonds are broken while the stronger bonds remain, and then parts of the molecule may rotate about the

Table XXIV Some Characteristics of Cortisone Acetate Polymorphs*

Form	Melting Point (°C)	Optics	System	Density (g cc^{-1})	Number of Molecules Per Unit Cell	Hydration
I	241-245	Opaque needle	Monoclinic	1.25	6	Anhydrous
II	235-238	Flat plate	Orthorhombic	1.21	4	Anhydrous
III	251-233	Prism	Orthorhombic	1.25	4	Anhydrous
IV	245-237	Column with spear-shaped ends	Orthorhombic	1.26	4	Two molecules of water
V	238-242	Transparent needle	Monoclinic	1.25	2	Two molecules of water

* R. K. Callow and O. Kennard, *J. Pharm. Pharmacol. 13,* 723 (1961).

fixed structure. This is a rapid transformation. Substitution transformations of disorder occur slowly if two different atoms in the structure can occupy the same lattice points and have the same valence and ionic radius.

Transformations of first coordination occur rapidly with small shifts in position with a change in coordination number or slowly if the lattice is broken and reformed, involving the first coordination.

Transformation may occur by a basic change in bond structure as is the case with graphite and diamond.

Polymorphic changes may be more readily understood by use of phase diagrams. In a system of two forms there is only one liquid-vapor or boiling-point curve because both polymorphs have identical liquid phases upon melting. As shown in Figure 66, each form has its solid-vapor or sublimation curve. Usually the two sublimation curves cross. The liquid-vapor curve may intersect the two solid-vapor curves above or below their intersection. In some compounds, e.g., betanaphthol, the three curves intersect at the same point and the melting points of the two polymorphs are the same. A complete phase diagram as shown in Figure 67 also contains the melt-vapor, solid-vapor, and solid-melt curves.

The transition point is the temperature at which the two polymorphs are in equilibrium. At the transition point they have identical energy, vapor pressure, and stability. If the change from one form to another is reversible, the system is enantiotropic. Figure 66 shows a typical two-form enantiotropic system with a definite transition temperature below the melting points of both forms. Below temperature T_1 form I is stable. At the transition point T_1 both forms are in equilibrium. From T_1 to T_2 form II is stable. Above temperature T_2 there are no polymorphs, as melting has occurred.

In the monotropic system the hypothetical transition point lies above the melting points of both polymorphs. As shown in Figure 68, form I cannot be converted to form II without passing through the liquid or vapor phase. Thus, at atmospheric pressure only one polymorph is stable.

The metastable polymorph has a higher vapor pressure, a higher free energy, a greater solubility, and a lower melting point than the stable polymorph. In an enantiotropic system a metastable form may be prepared by maintaining a crystal in the temperature range of the desired polymorph until transformation occurs. All forms may be obtained by supercooling the melt below the melting points. The first form to crystallize is the metastable form. If allowed to stand at room temperature this will

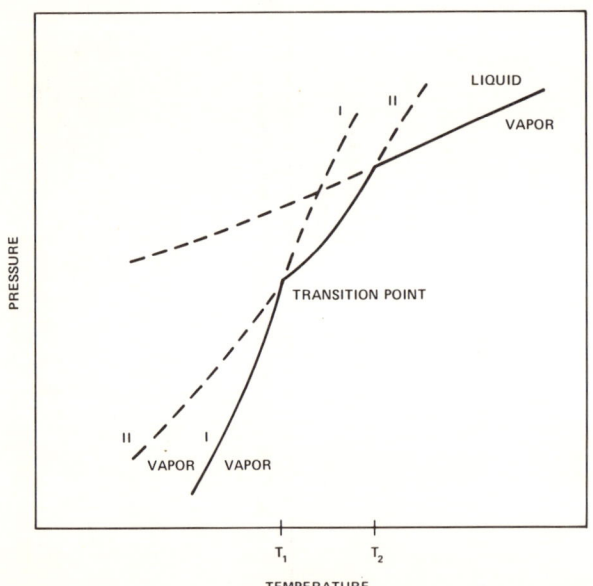

Figure 66. Sublimation and boiling-point curve for an enantiotropic two-form system.

properties of solids • 127

Figure 67. Melting-point and transition-temperature curves added to Figure 66 for an enantiotropic two-form system. (Adapted from W.C. McCrone, *Fusion Methods in Chemical Microscopy,* Wiley-Interscience, New York, 1957.)

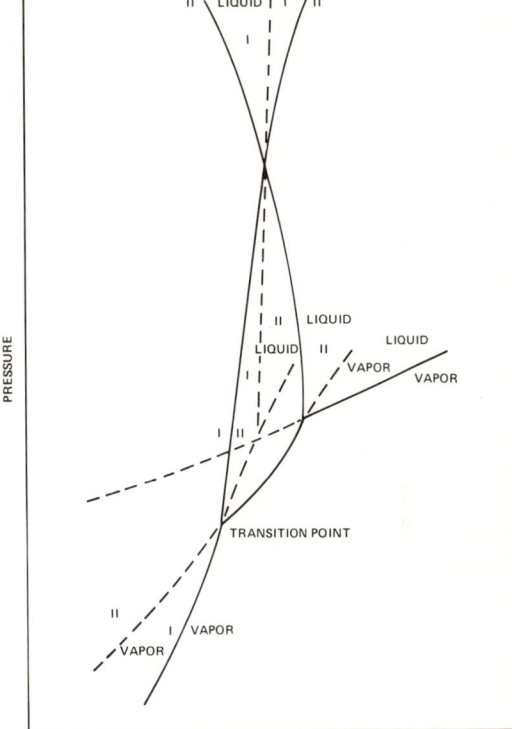

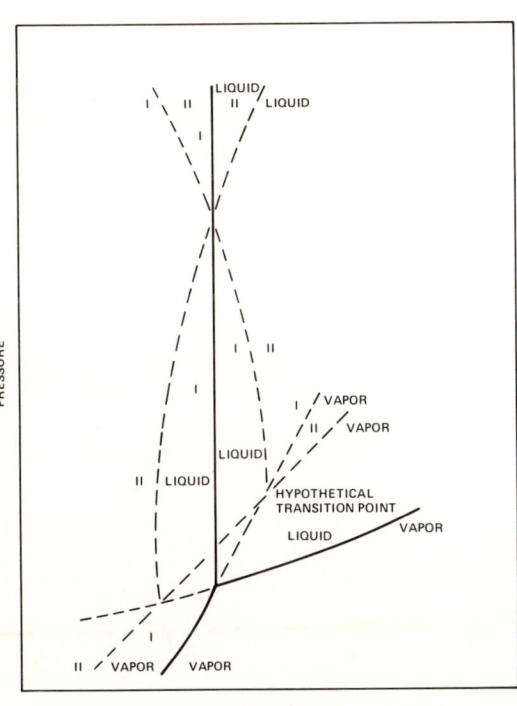

Figure 68. Pressure-temperature phase diagram for a monotropic 2 form system. (Adapted from W.C. McCrone, *Fusion Methods in Chemical Microscopy,* Wiley-Interscience, New York, 1957.)

successively pass to more stable forms until converted to the most stable form. A metastable form may also be prepared by crystallization from a supersaturated solution. The polymorph produced depends on the temperature, the solvent, and the rate of cooling of the supersaturated solution.

The solid-solid transformation of a metastable polymorph at room temperature may require a few seconds, e.g., acetanilid and picric acid, or a lifetime, as in the case of diamond. Many drugs, e.g., barbital, cinchophen, estrone, mafenide, progesterone, and sulfathiazole, are used in the metastable form. These drugs have a slow rate of transformation and are utilized before appreciable transformation occurs. It has been suggested that the rate of transformation to the stable form may be retarded by the inclusion of an additive. If the dimensions of the additive permit it to fit in only one lattice of a polymorphic compound, transformation to a stable form becomes more difficult, as the voids in the stable lattice cannot contain the impurity without being subjected to high stress.

Occasionally one polymorph may be clinically more effective than the other forms. This is due to the differences in solubility, partition coefficient, and in rate of dissolution, which effect the absorption and ultimate therapeutic response of a drug administered in the solid state. Riboflavin is reported to exist in three forms having solubilities of 60, 80, and 1200 mg liter^{-1}. In solid dosage forms absorption would be facilitated by using the most soluble polymorph. In rats it has been demonstrated that the absorption rate of methyl prednisolone from a subcutaneous implant is 1.7 times greater from the more soluble form II than from the stable form I. The use of a metastable polymorph is feasible if the rate of transformation to a stable form is slow. Activated carbon has been prescribed in dyspepsia to reduce hyperacidity, and although graphite and diamond are chemically identical no one would recommend their use in a therapeutic capacity!

Although the metastable form may be desirable clinically, the stable form is preferred from the viewpoint of physical and chemical stability. In a pharmaceutical suspension the rate of polymorphic transition depends on the solubility of each form and the rate of diffusion of the molecules in solution. As the solubility and the difference in solubility between the polymorphs increases, the rate of transformation increases. An increase in viscosity of the liquid slows diffusion and the rate of transformation. In a suspension containing two polymorphs, the more stable form is less soluble, and particles of the more stable form grow at the expense of particles composed of the more soluble metastable form. This process will continue until the transformation is completed, and often this transformation is accompanied by caking and a change in flow characteristics of the suspension. Upon prolonged contact with water all forms of cortisone acetate change to form I with considerable caking. Thus, in manufacturing a cortisone acetate suspension the drug should be converted to form I before preparation to avoid an increase in particle size and caking of the suspension. In compressed tablets both forms I and II have been used.

The effect of polymorphism on the physical characteristics of pharmaceuticals is clearly illustrated by the widely used fatty acids, waxes, and glycerides. Fatty acids and fats expand when they are heated, but they contract if there is a transition from a metastable to a stable polymorph. Flash cooling often produces metastable polymorphs. Polymorphism may be detected by flash cooling a melt and determining its specific volume as the temperature is slowly increased. As the temperature rises a substance will expand in a smooth curve until completely melted, as shown for polyethylene glycol in Figure 69. If there is a polymorphic change as shown for theobroma oil between 20 and 24°, it is indicated by a decrease in specific volume, as a result of the less dense, unstable form being converted into the more dense stable form.

The effect of temperature and rate of change in temperature on polymorphs is shown by tristearin. Tristearin, a typical glyceride, is monotropic and progressively transforms to more stable polymorphs. Its crystalline form depends mainly on the rate of cooling. As the tristearin melt is cooled, the hydrocarbon chains arrange themselves parallel. This arrangement in the liquid is postulated to extend for perhaps 100 molecules and initiates nucleation. If the tristearin melt is cooled rapidly to below 54°, the α polymorph is formed. The hydrocarbon chains of tristearin are packed normal to the basal plane and free to rotate in the α form. Less rapid cooling to a temperature about 5° above the melting

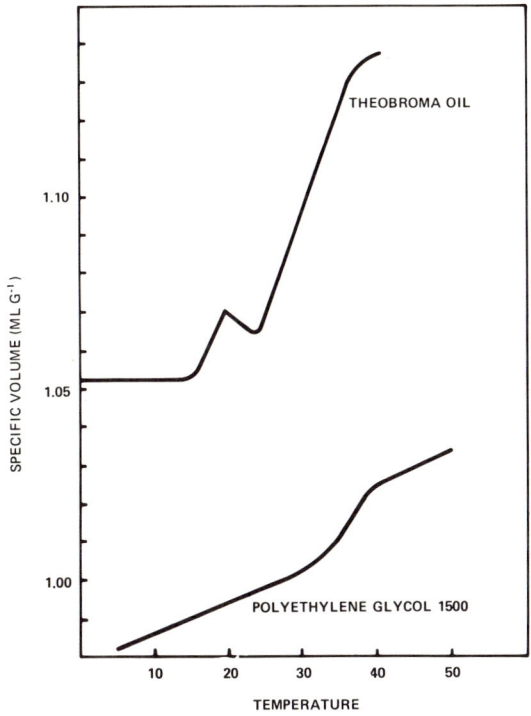

Figure 69. Effect of flash cooling on theobroma oil and polyethylene glycol. [Adapted from L.J. Ravin and T. Higuchi, *J. Am. Pharm. Assoc.* **46**, 736 (1957).]

point of the α form will produce the β' form, which melts at 64°. In the β' form the hydrocarbon chains are tilted. Very slow cooling allows maximum freedom for molecular orientation, and subsequent crystallization occurs in the most stable, or β, form with a melting point of 71.5°.

With compounds containing long hydrocarbon chains, the molecular end groups associate with each other to form planes. The distance between planes in the crystal correspond to integral multiples of molecule or chain length. Often tilting of long chains occurs with respect to end-group planes. Triglyceride polymorphs are caused by differences in angles of tilt of the hydrocarbon chains with reference to the terminal planes. As van der Waals force is insensitive to slight changes of mutual orientation of long chains of adjacent molecules, a large number of lattice structures with minor energy differences can exist. Polarity and geometry of the molecule determine if spacing is in single or multiple lengths of the chain.

Among practicing pharmacists theobroma oil is probably the most widely known substance commonly exhibiting polymorphism. Theobroma oil is a bland, yellowish mixture of triglycerides which liquefies around 30° and melts at 35°. It is thought to consist of liquid triglycerides entrapped in a lattice of solid triglycerides. As listed in Table XXV, theobroma oil is composed chiefly of symmetrically disaturated glycerides with 2-oleopalmitostearin as the most abundant constituent.

When theobroma oil is heated above 40°, all polymorphic forms are melted. If this melt is flash cooled to below 15°, it crystallizes in the γ form with a melting point of 15°. If the γ form is gradually warmed, it is transformed into the α polymorph with a melting point of 22°. Upon further gradual warming the α form is transformed into the β' form with a melting point of 28°. Final warming transforms the β' form into the stable β form with a melting point of 34.5°.

When theobroma oil is used as a suppository base, it must be in a form that is firm enough at room temperature to permit insertion but which will melt at body temperature. If the theobroma oil is heated to 40° and quickly cooled in a chilled suppository mold, the mass solidifies as a mixture of unstable polymorphs. When removed from the mold, these suppositories are unsatisfactory, as they melt at

Table XXV Composition of Theobroma Oil
(S, stearate; P, palmitate; O, oleate)

Glyceride	Per Cent
CH$_2$O-S (or P) | CH-O-S (or P) | CH$_2$O-S (or P)	2-3
CH$_2$O-P | CH-O-O | CH$_2$O-S	52-57
CH$_2$O-S | CH-O-O | CH$_2$O-S	19-22
CH$_2$O-P | CH-O-O | CH$_2$O-P	4-6
CH$_2$O-P | CH-O-O | CH$_2$O-O	7-8
CH$_2$O-S | CH-O-O | CH$_2$O-O	6-12
CH$_2$O-O | CH-O-O | CH$_2$O-O	1-2

room temperature and cannot be inserted. Flash cooling retards the transformation to more stable higher-melting polymorphs. If the molten theobroma oil is slowly cooled, the γ polymorph formed is rapidly and spontaneously converted into the stable form.

Sorbed and Chemical Water

Water may be physically or chemically attracted and held to a solid pharmaceutical. This attraction may be an important consideration in processing, packaging, and storing of a solid dosage form.

Water of Hygroscopicity. Solids exposed to the atmosphere usually adsorb some water vapor on their surfaces. Water is a polar molecule, and it strongly interacts with ions or polar molecules on the surface of a crystal lattice by dipole-ion or dipole-dipole interaction, respectively. This adsorbed water is called water of hygroscopicity.

The amount of water adsorbed depends on the particle size of a powder. As water of hygroscopicity is held by a surface phenomenon, under a specified set of conditions for a given weight of a substance, a greater amount of moisture will be adsorbed by a sample of the powder with the greater specific surface.

Water-vapor adsorption by pharmaceutical powders is also a function of the humidity to which they are exposed. The relationship between the amount of water vapor adsorbed and the water-vapor pressure is given by a typical adsorption isotherm, as shown in Figures 11 and 70.

Certain polymeric substances, e.g., agar, cellulose, gelatin, and starch, may contain a high percentage of moisture while retaining the appearance of a dry powder. In addition to surface adsorption, the water is held by capillary action in fissures and pores of the solid. Such water, which is held by more than a single mechanism, is known as water of imbibition. As shown in Figure 71, hydroxyethylcellulose contains approximately 1 per cent of water at a relative humidity of 0.1, and 17.5 per cent at a relative humidity of 0.65. With such substances the water content varies considerably with the seasonal humidity unless the substances are stored in moistureproof containers. Equilibrium for water of hygroscopicity is attained rapidly; equilibrium for water of imbibition is attained very slowly.

Dry chemicals and utensils should be used in the preparation of solid pharmaceuticals containing hygroscopic drugs. Double-wrapped divided powders or sealed cellophane envelopes containing powders generally protect hygroscopic substances from moisture during the tenure of an extemporaneous prescription.

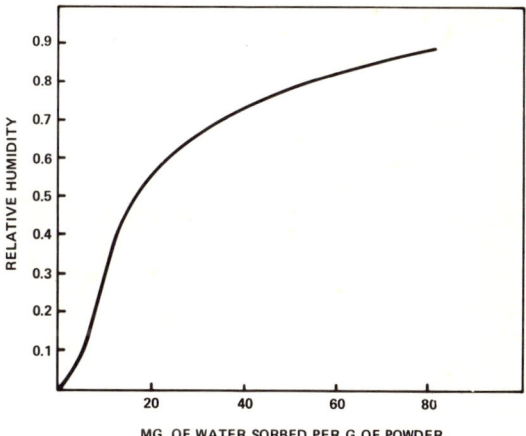

Figure 70. Sorption isotherm at 25° for 100-mesh sodium pentobarbital. [Adapted from W.A. Strickland, *J. Pharm. Sci.* **51**, 310 (1962).]

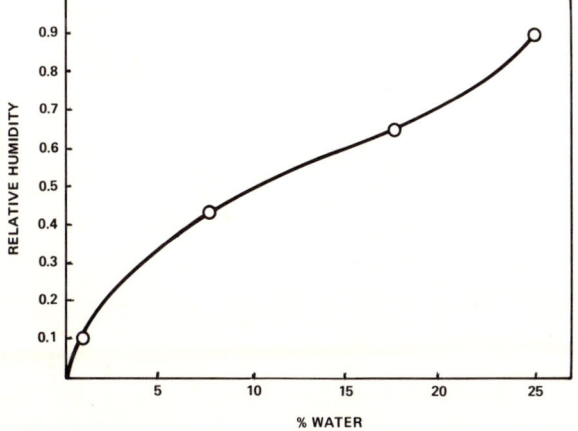

Figure 71. Sorption of water by dried hydroxyethyl cellulose at 25°.

33. Ferric ammonium citrate   0.5 g
    Sodium bromide   0.3 g
    Pepsin   0.2 g

    Make 12 powders

    Sig.: One q.i.d.

34. Sodium salicylate   0.3 g
    Sodium bromide   0.5 g

    Make 24 divided powders

    Sig.: One t.i.d. and h.s.

It has been suggested that hygroscopic powders to be dispensed in a divided powder or a capsule be mixed with a therapeutically inactive substance that has a selective affinity for moisture. Magnesium oxide, magnesium carbonate, starch, and talc have been used for this purpose.

35. Ferric ammonium citrate   0.5 g

    Ft. caps

    Sig.: One with meals

Scale salts, e.g., ferric ammonium citrate, which have been repeatedly exposed to the atmosphere sorb moisture and frequently become sticky when they are triturated in a mortar. Dry ferric ammonium citrate is readily pulverized. The physical stability of the capsule is enhanced if 60 to 100 mg of magnesium carbonate per capsule is blended with the ferric ammonium citrate. The capsules should be dispensed in a moistureproof container.

The uptake of moisture by hygroscopic powders tends to cause the joining and caking of particles. Caked powders do not flow freely and are difficult to fill into capsules and containers. The therapeutic efficacy of dusting powders that have caked is reduced, as the powder does not flow easily or spread uniformly. On occasion caking may be controlled by adding a small percentage of an inert substance, e.g., fumed silica, which has a high specific surface and selectively sorbs moisture. The process of milling and the resulting particle size distribution of the milled material may be influenced by the amount of moisture present.

When the attraction of a hygroscopic drug for moisture is so great that the solid liquefies due to the dissolving of the drug in the adsorbed water, the drug is said to have deliquesced. The strong attraction of choline chloride for moisture as shown in Figure 72 readily produces deliquescence. Since

Figure 72. Sorption isotherm at 25° for 100-mesh choline chloride powder.

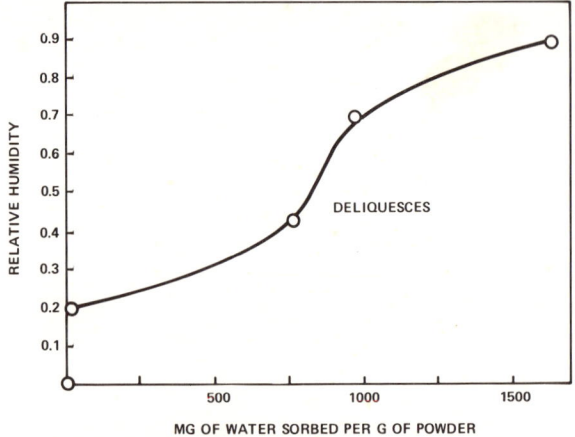

the sorption of moisture is a function of the environmental humidity, a substance cannot be rigorously considered as being deliquescent. For example, potassium acetate at relative humidities less than 0.15 will adsorb moisture and may cake, but it does not dissolve in the adsorbed moisture until higher humidities are involved. Certain drugs are commonly categorized as being deliquescent substances; however, it should be realized that the implication of this statement is that deliquescence occurs with these substances at normally encountered relative humidity, i.e., 0.25 to 0.6.

On rare occasions a deliquescent powder may be dispensed in a cellophane film or a metallic foil. Likewise, a deliquescent powder may be encapsulated and dispensed in a moistureproof vial with a dessicant; however, the deliquescent drugs may abstract moisture from the gelatin capsule, causing it to crack. Deliquescent drugs, e.g., choline dihydrogen citrate, methacholine bromide, potassium acetate, and sodium thiocyanate, are best dispensed as a solution in the form of an elixir or syrup.

Surface moisture and especially imbibed moisture promotes chemical reaction. In the film of water on a solid ester or amide some molecules, e.g., aspirin, dissolve and undergo hydrolysis. Chemical reactions in the surface moisture may influence the physiological availability of a drug. If a layer of an insoluble degradation product is formed on the surface of a drug particle, it may act as a mechanical barrier to body fluids after administration, slowing or preventing dissolution and absorption of the active medicinal compound. Thus, the pharmacist must package a hygroscopic drug in a moistureproof container with a packet of drying agent to ensure not only physical stability but also the chemical stability and physiological availability of the drug.

Crystal Hydrates. A crystal hydrate is a crystalline substance in which water is held in a stoichiometric ratio and a definite pattern in the lattice network. This water is known as water of crystallization.

The shape and size of a water molecule confer important properties on this compound. As shown in Figure 73, the water molecule has two unshared pairs of electrons, which permit interaction with a cation or the positive portion of a polar compound. The water molecule is strongly polar, as it is not a linear structure, but it is a triangular structure with a bond angle of 104.3°. This strong polarity orients and attracts the water molecule to ions. The compact size of the water molecule results in a further strengthening of the ion-dipole interaction, as the force of attraction between opposite charges is an inverse function of the distance separating them. Positive ions are usually smaller than anions, and consequently cations bind water molecules more tightly than anions. The number of water molecules attracted to an ion is called its coordination number or ligancy.

Thus, although the water molecule is a neutral molecule, it may be bound in an ionic structure because of its small size and high polarity. In many hydrates water is coordinated with the cations, and it effectively surrounds them, increasing their effective radii and distributing their charges over a greater space. The difference in size of anions and cations is often too great for simple structures of high coordination to be formed; with a high ionic charge and a large difference in ionic radii, there often is a layer lattice or a purely molecular arrangement. If these cations are coordinated with dipoles of water, they are in effect increased to a size comparable to the anions, and a more stable lattice is formed.

The aluminum ion, which has a radius of 0.57 Å and a +3 charge, is considerably smaller than the chloride ion. The coordination of six molecules of water with the aluminum ion forms an effective

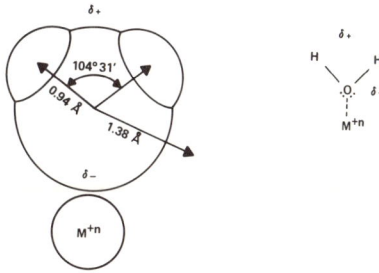

Figure 73. Diagrammatical representations of the dipolar water molecule and its interaction with a cation.

radius of 3.3 Å and widely distributes the cationic charge. This effectively larger cation forms stable structures that are less complicated than the structures smaller, uncoordinated ions would form.

Hydrates are most common and stable among salts, with small, highly charged cations. The coordination water determines the stability of a crystal lattice, and its removal often breaks down the structure, i.e., the anhydrous salt will not necessarily have the same lattice as the hydrate. A few hydrates, e.g., alum, may have the water removed from the lattice without any structural breakdown; however, this type of hydrate is unusual and is said to contain structural water.

As illustrated in Figure 74, aluminum chloride crystallizes with six molecules of water about the aluminum ion. The resulting aluminum chloride hexahydrate has a complex structure with each water molecule adjacent to only two chloride ions. Two schematic representations of copper sulfate pentahydrate are shown in Figure 75. Four of the water molecules are coordinated with the copper ion; the octahedral coordination groups about a copper ion is completed by a fifth water molecule, which is held by hydrogen bonds between water molecules coordinated to the copper ion and the oxygen atom of the sulfate ion. In a similar manner for ferrous sulfate heptahydrate and magnesium sulfate heptahydrate, six water molecules are coordinated with the cation and the seventh is packed nearer the anion. In the alums six of the 12 water molecules are attached to the aluminum ion and the others are nearer the alkali ion.

At a given temperature there exists an equilibrium between the water of crystallization and the water-vapor pressure of the environment. In a two-component salt hydrate system, the equilibrium between the solid and the vapor may be expressed as

$$NaBr \cdot 2 H_2O(s) \rightleftharpoons NaBr(s) + 2H_2O(g)$$

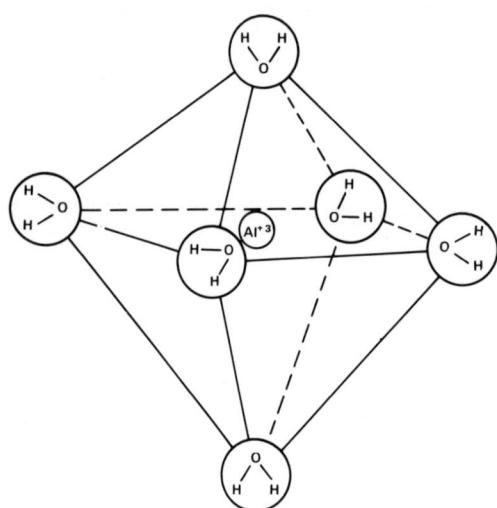

Figure 74. Diagrammatical representation of hydrated aluminum ion.

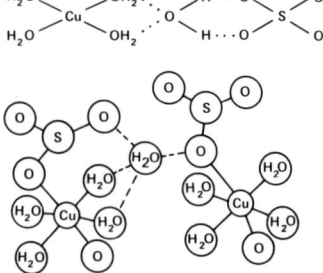

Figure 75. Diagrammatical representations of the water of crystallization in copper sulfate pentahydrate.

If the hydrate is placed at a fixed temperature in a closed vessel with the vapor pressure of water equal to zero, water is given off or effloresces from the hydrate. At equilibrium the water-vapor pressure of the environment is equal to the water-vapor pressure of the hydrate, and it is constant for any mixture of the hydrate and the anhydrous form.

The relation of vapor pressure to composition is shown in Figure 76 for a water-dihydrate-anhydrous sodium bromide system. As increasing amounts of sodium bromide are dissolved in water, the vapor pressure decreases from that of pure water to the relative vapor pressure of a saturated solution, i.e., 0.57. The addition of more sodium bromide does not alter the composition of the saturated liquid phase; therefore, the vapor pressure of a saturated solution is in equilibrium with the vapor pressure of the dihydrate. If the saturated solution is removed, the relative vapor pressure drops to 0.36, which represents the vapor pressure of a mixture of the dihydrate and the anhydrous sodium bromide. When the relative vapor pressure is less than 0.36, water is given off.

The pharmacist is concerned with the effect that atmospheric humidity will have upon his pharmaceuticals. It is customary to express the moisture content of the air in terms of relative humidity, i.e., the ratio of the water vapor pressure of air to that of air saturated with water at the same temperature.

Although increases in temperature increase the vapor pressure, it is the relative humidity that determines the affect of atmospheric exposure on a hydrate because most pharmaceutical procedures are at room temperature. If the relative humidity is greater than 0.57, sodium bromide dihydrate attracts water and forms a saturated solution. After all the solid has dissolved, it will continue to attract moisture until the composition of the solution is such that it has the same relative vapor pressure of the atmosphere. This phenomenon, deliquescence, occurs if the humidity of the atmosphere is greater than the vapor pressure of the saturated solution. The dihydrate has a relative vapor pressure of 0.36, and it will give off water if the atmospheric humidity is less than 0.36. Sodium bromide dihydrate is stable only when stored at relative humidities between 0.36 and 0.57 at 25°. If the relative humidity becomes less than 0.36, the dihydrate will effloresce to the anhydrous sodium bromide.

The U.S. Pharmacopeia states that sodium borate effloresces in warm, dry air and that its crystals are often coated with a white, translucent powder. As a saturated solution of sodium borate at 20° has a relative vapor pressure of 0.99, deliquescence does not occur. The relative vapor pressure of borax is 0.39, when it is in equilibrium with the pentahydrate. If the decahydrate is exposed to the atmosphere with a relative humidity less than 0.39, it effloresces to the pentahydrate. The pentahydrate is stable at relative humidities between 0.39 and 0.25; if the relative humidity becomes less than 0.25, the pentahydrate effloresces to the anhydrous salt. With the loss of water the crystal structure is altered.

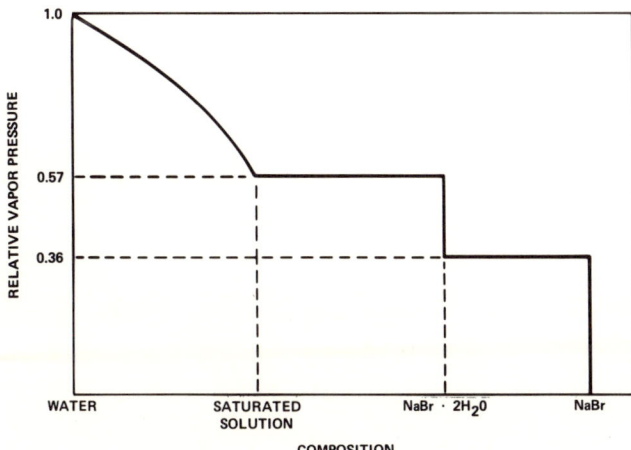

Figure 76. Vapor pressure of water in a water-sodium bromide system.

This change accounts for the powdery layer found on the surface of the effloresced solid. Drugs that effloresce in low humidity and become powdery in appearance include alum, citric acid monohydrate, ferrous sulfate heptahydrate, and terpin hydrate.

The least obvious, yet very significant, way in which atmospheric moisture may affect pharmaceuticals is by a change in the stoichiometry of a hydrate. A crystal hydrate exposed to a dry atmosphere effloresces its water of crystallization. If the effloresced drug is weighed on the basis of the formula weight of the hydrate, an overdose results. Quinine bisulfate effloresces on exposure to dry air. If all the water of crystallization effloresced, there would be a loss of 23 per cent of its weight. Thus, a pharmacist weighing effloresced quinine bisulfate instead of the heptahydrate would be dispensing a 23 per cent greater dose. Conversely, moisture may be incorporated into a solid with the formation of a hydrate containing a greater ratio of water of crystallization. If ignored, this uptake of water would result in an underdose being dispensed.

Water of crystallization may be released from some hydrates by prolonged trituration or grinding. Reduction of particle size will also release water, which has been occluded in the cavities within a crystalline mass.

36.	Magnesium sulfate	80 g
	Sodium phosphate	20 g
37.	Magnesium sulfate	15 g
	Sodium sulfate	15 g
	Sodium potassium tartrate	15 g

Sig.: One teaspoonful in warm water

A wet mass is formed when the salts in formulas 36 and 37 are triturated. A dry powder may be prepared by the use of equivalent amounts of the anhydrous form of the salts. The powder should be packaged in a moistureproof container.

Part II

Solutions

5 | CHARACTERISTICS OF SOLUTIONS

INTRODUCTION

A phase is a definite homogeneous part of a system, and it is physically separated from other parts by distinct boundaries. A solution is a homogeneous one-phase system. A solution is a chemically and physically homogeneous system of two or more substances. Although solutions may be liquid, gaseous, or solid, from the pharmaceutical viewpoint they are generally limited to liquid solutions in which the solute may be a liquid, gas, or solid. The union of biological and physical sciences in pharmacy exposes the pharmacist to numerous means of expressing concentration.

Concentration Expressions

Percentage is probably the most common method of expressing concentration in pharmacy. Percentage by weight (w/w) expresses the number of grams of solute in 100 g of solution. Camphorated parachlorophenol is a 35 per cent w/w solution of *p*-chlorophenol in camphor.

Percentage by volume (v/v) expresses the number of milliliters of solute in 100 ml of solution. Alcohol contains 94.9 ml of C_2H_5OH in 100 ml of solution; with respect to alcohol it is a 94.9 per cent v/v solution.

Percentage weight in volume (w/v) expresses the number of grams of solute in 100 ml of solution. Percentage by weight in volume is peculiar to the health professions, and it disregards the density of the solvent employed. Its use is a matter of convenience. When the physician prescribes and the pharmacist compounds a 0.2 per cent w/v solution, which contains 0.2 g of drug per 100 ml of solution, they know that with each 5-ml teaspoonful taken by the patient he has administered 10 mg of the drug.

By tradition and common consent when the term "per cent" is used without qualification in the practice of pharmacy, it is understood that for mixtures of solids a weight in weight per cent is intended and that for mixtures of liquids a volume in volume per cent is intended. Unqualified per cent for solids or gases in a liquid implies the use of a weight in volume per cent.

Although its use should be discouraged, the term "milligram per cent" appears in the literature of the physician and physiologist. "Milligram per cent" expresses the number of milligrams of solute in 100 ml of solution. If the blood contains 15 mg per cent of a drug, it contains 15 mg of the drug in every 100 ml of blood.

In analytical procedures it is convenient to use solutions that contain a definite number of molecules in each milliliter. A molar solution, M, contains 1 mole of solute in a liter of solution. An aqueous solution containing 55 g of dextrose monohydrate with a molecular weight of 198.2 g mole^{-1} in 1000 ml of solution is 0.28 M.

A normal solution, N, contains the combining or equivalent weight in grams of solute dissolved in 1 liter of solution. In chemical reactions it is the number of charges instead of the number of molecules or ions which are involved in the stoichiometry of the reaction; therefore, it is necessary in using the term normality to specify the reaction under consideration. One milliliter of a normal solution contains 1 milliequivalent of the solute.

The term "milliequivalent" is commonly used to express the concentration of ions in electrolyte solutions for parenteral administration. A milliequivalent may be expressed

$$\text{meq} = \frac{\text{g in 1000 ml} \times 1000 \times \text{valence} \times \text{number of those ions dissociated}}{\text{formula weight}}$$

The milliequivalence of calcium and chloride ion in a solution containing 20 mg of calcium chloride in 100 ml of solution is

$$\frac{0.200 \times 1000 \times 2 \times 1}{147} = 2.6 \text{ meq of Ca}^{++}$$

$$\frac{0.200 \times 1000 \times 1 \times 2}{147} = 2.6 \text{ meq of Cl}^{-}$$

Weight concentrations are used in exacting laboratory procedures so that the concentration does not change with the expansion or contraction resulting from temperature changes as it does with molar and normal solutions. A molal solution, m, contains 1 mole of solute dissolved in 1000 g of solvent. A syrup containing 513 g of sucrose dissolved in 1000 g of water is a 1.5 m solution.

Many properties of solutions are related to the relative number of molecules present. The mole fraction, N, of a substance in solution is the number of moles of that substance divided by the total number of moles of all components of the solution. If a binary solution contains n_2 moles of solute and n_1 moles of solvent, the mole fraction of solute is

$$N_2 = \frac{n_2}{n_2 + n_1}$$

Mole per cent may be obtained by multiplying the mole fraction by 100. The sum of the mole fractions of all constituents is 1. If 100 g of acetone is dissolved in 100 g of water, the mole fraction of acetone may be calculated by the equation

$$N_2 = \frac{\frac{100}{58.1}}{\frac{100}{58.1} + \frac{100}{18}} = 0.236$$

Solubility Expressions

The solubility of a substance at a given temperature is defined as the concentration of the dissolved solute, which is in equilibrium with the solute phase. In a saturated solution in contact with undissolved solid solute, the rate at which molecules or ions leave the crystal surface is equal to the rate at which the solvated molecules or ions return to and become a part of the solid crystal. At a given temperature the solubility or the concentration of solute in solution is a constant, but, owing to the dynamic situation, the identical molecules or ions of the solute do not perpetually exist in the dissolved state. In Figure 77 this is diagrammatically expressed as an equilibrium reaction, where k_s is the rate constant of the dissolution process and k_c is the rate constant of the return to the solid phase. The solubility of a substance is the ratio of these rate constants at equilibrium.

Solubilities are expressed in numerous ways, e.g., grams of solute in 100 g of solvent, grams of solute in 100 ml of solvent, grams of solute in 100 ml of solution, and grams of solute in 100 g of solution.

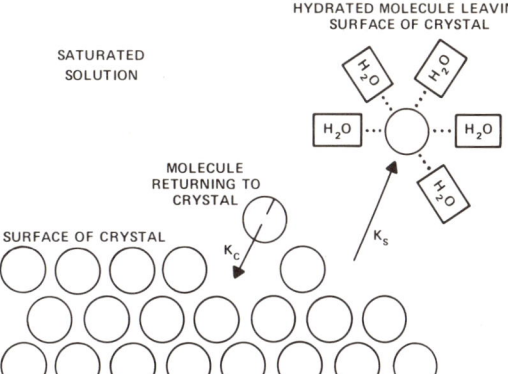

Figure 77. Diagrammatical representation of the equilibrium of a saturated solution of sugar in water.

The U.S. Pharmacopeia expresses solubility in terms of milliliters of solvent required to dissolve 1 g of solute; e.g., 1 g of boric acid dissolves in 18 ml of water. Descriptive terms for solubility are given in the official compendia to aid those who use, prepare, and dispense drugs. The descriptive solubilities are defined in Table XXVI.

The solubility of a very slightly soluble electrolyte may be expressed as a solubility product. If the solute phase is composed of two or more definite ionic species, the solubility may be expressed as the product of the concentrations of the ions in a saturated solution, each concentration in gram-ions per liter being raised to the power corresponding to the number of each species of ion produced. If in a saturated solution

$$C_nA_{m\text{ solid}} \rightleftharpoons C_nA_{m\text{ solution}} \rightleftharpoons nC^+ + mA^-$$

and the solubility product, S, is

$$S = c_{C^+}^n \, c_{A^-}^m$$

where c_{C^+} is the concentration in gram-ions per liter of the cation and c_{A^-} is the concentration of the anion.

By use of the solubility product the maximum concentration of an ion that a given solution will maintain in equilibrium with the solute phase may be calculated. The amount of silver nitrate that

Table XXVI Descriptive Terms of Solubility

Term	Parts of Solvent Required for One Part of Solute
Very soluble	<1
Freely soluble	1-10
Soluble	10-30
Sparingly soluble	30-100
Slightly soluble	100-1,000
Very slightly soluble	1,000-10,000
Practically insoluble, or insoluble	>10,000

can be added to a 1 per cent aqueous solution of procaine hydrochloride before precipitation occurs may be calculated. A 1 per cent procaine hydrochloride solution is 0.036 M with respect to the chloride ions. As the solubility product of silver chloride is 1.56×10^{-10}, the maximum concentration of silver ions that will remain in solution is

$$S = c_{Ag^+} \, c_{Cl^-}$$
$$1.56 \times 10^{-10} = 0.036 \, c_{Ag^+}$$
$$c_{Ag^+} = 4.3 \times 10^{-9} \, M$$

Since the molecular weight of silver chloride is 169.9 g mole^{-1}, the maximum amount of silver nitrate that could be added is

$$4.3 \times 10^{-9} \times 169.9 = 7.3 \times 10^{-7} \text{ g liter}^{-1}$$

If the electrolyte dissociates into more than two ions, the ionic concentration is raised to a power corresponding to the number of that kind of ion. For example, silver phosphate dissolves in water according to the equation

$$Ag_3PO_4(\text{solid}) \rightleftharpoons Ag_3PO_4(\text{solution}) \rightleftharpoons 3Ag^+ + PO_4^{3-}$$

and its solubility product is

$$K_{sp} = (Ag^+)^3 (PO_4^{3-})$$

RATIONALE OF SOLUBILITY

The process of dissolution involves the breaking of interionic or intermolecular bonds in the solute, the separation of the molecules of the solvent to provide space in the solvent for the solute, and the interaction between the solvent and the solute molecule or ion. A review of the forces of attraction among the solvent-solvent and the solute-solute molecules or ions will aid in visualizing the mechanics of dissolution.

Bonding Forces Present In Solvents

The bonding forces present in solids were discussed in Chapter 4. These forces in solids are:
1. Van der Waals force.
2. Dipole-dipole force.
3. Ionic force.
4. Covalent bonding.
5. Metallic bonding.

Only the first two types of forces are found in liquids and gases. Both forces are electrical in origin, and the contribution of each to the total bonding interaction depends on the electronic configuration of the molecule.

Van der Waals Force. A symmetrical molecule with a zero dipole moment is a nonpolar molecule. The condensed state of a nonpolar compound is solely a consequence of van der Waals interaction. Although a nonpolar molecule is electrically neutral, at a given instance a temporary polarity may arise from the electronic movements within the molecule. This internal electronic oscillation induces further oscillation in neighboring molecules, producing an induced dipole. Induced dipoles interact and maintain such compounds as benzene and carbon tetrachloride in a liquid state at room temperature. The induced dipole-induced dipole interaction force is weak as indicated by the low boiling points, e.g., benzene (80°) and carbon tetrachloride (77°).

The induced dipole-induced dipole or van der Waals force exists in all substances. The induced molar polarization, P_i, contributed by van der Waals force is expressed by the equation

$$P_i = \frac{4\pi}{3} N\alpha$$

where N is the Avogadro number and α the molecular electronic polarizability. This induced polarization is due to electronic displacement. Induced polarization is independent of the orientation of the whole molecule and is produced by an external field. The induced molar polarization is independent of temperature.

Dipole-Dipole Interaction. A dipole or a dipolar molecule is one in which the centers of positive and negative electricity do not coincide, although the entire molecule is neutral. A dipole exists because of the inductive effect or the electromeric effect.

When atoms with different affinities for electrons are bonded, the bonding electrons are held to a greater extent by the atom with the higher charge on its kernel. This partial transfer of electrons produces a type of bond polarization known as the inductive effect. For example, in alcohol the electron pair that bonds the hydrogen to the oxygen is closer to the latter atom because of its higher nuclear charge. This inductive effect establishes a dipole with the hydrogen end of each alcohol molecule positive relative to the other end,

$$\underset{C_2H_5-O:H}{\overset{\delta- \quad \delta+}{}}$$

A second mechanism by which a dipole may be formed is the electromeric effect. The electromeric effect is due to the net electronic displacement produced by resonance. In acetone the high charge on the kernel of the oxygen atom tends to attract the bonding electrons resulting in a polarization of the molecule. This dipole formation by virtue of the electromeric effect is represented as

$$\underset{CH_3}{\underset{|}{CH_3-C=O}}$$

Although acetone has a high dipole moment, i.e., 2.88 debye, it possesses a low boiling point, i.e., 56.5°, which indicates weak intermolecular bonding. This weak intermolecular bonding between acetone molecules is due to the fact that the positive portion of the molecule is diffused and does not reside in a hydrogen atom; thus, hydrogen bonding is not possible.

In water the inductive effect is reenforced by the shape of the water molecule, as shown in Figure 73 and Table XXVII. As a consequence of these two effects, water is a very strong dipole and possesses unique properties. Methane, ammonia, and water have approximately the same molecular weight, and if only van der Waals force were operative, they would have approximately the same melting and boiling points. In methane the four bonds formed by the carbon are directed toward the corners of a tetrahedron with the carbon atom at its center. As the bonds in methane are purely covalent and its dipole moment is zero, it is only a weak van der Waals force that maintains methane in a condensed state at lower temperature.

Ammonia has one unshared electron pair and to a limited extent may associate with other ammonia molecules. It therefore has a higher melting point than methane.

The total polarization, P, of a dipolar molecule is the sum of the polarity arising from van der Waals force, P_i, and the polarity contributed by the permanent dipole,

$$P = P_i + P_d$$

The polarity contributed by the dipole is represented by the equation

$$P_d = \frac{4\pi}{3} \frac{N\mu^2}{3kT}$$

144 • solutions

Table XXVII Effect of Molecular Structure on Some Physical Properties

Structure	Molecular Weight (g mole^{-1})	Boiling Point (°C)	Melting Point (°C)	ϵ
CH$_4$	16	-161	-184	0
NH$_3$ (107°)	17	-33	-78	17
H$_2$O (105°)	18	100	0	80

where k is the Boltzmann constant, μ the dipole moment, and T the absolute temperature. This polarity is dependent on the capacity of the molecule to orient itself within an applied electrical field. As the orientation is opposed by thermal agitation, the polarization decreases with an increase in temperature.

As dipoles tend to be oriented in an electric field, they are affected by the fields of neighboring molecules. The positive portion of a water molecule attracts the negative portion of another water dipole in which the positive portion forms an intermolecular bond with the negative portion of yet another water molecule. The association of water molecules is shown in Table XXVIII. In water roughly two-thirds of the total intermolecular forces arise from dipole-dipole or hydrogen-bond interaction. The tendency for alignment is counteracted by thermal agitation to the extent that a solid is not formed at room temperature, but the intermolecular attraction is sufficient to maintain the water in a liquid state. The boiling point of water is greater than would be anticipated from its molecular weight. In addition to the energy necessary to transport a molecule of water from the liquid to the vapor phase, energy is required to disrupt the hydrogen bonds of the liquid water. The high boiling point of water is due to this energy requirement.

Dipole-dipole interaction becomes an appreciable force if the positive center is located in a hydrogen atom, and it is known as hydrogen bonding. The small size of the hydrogen atom allows it to approach much closer to the negative portion of a neighboring dipole than is possible for any other atom. The coulombic principle states that the force between two opposite charges is proportional to the product of the quantities of electricity and varies inversely as the square of the distances between them. This can be expressed by the equation

$$F = \frac{q^+ q^-}{\epsilon d^2}$$

where q^+ and q^- represent the electric fields, d is the distance between them, and ϵ is the dielectric

Table XXVIII Hydrogen Bonding and Some Physical Constants of Pure Liquids

Compound	Molecular Weight (g mole^{-1})	Boiling Point (°C)	ϵ
$\begin{array}{cccc} NH_2 & NH_2 & NH_2 & NH_2 \\ | & | & | & | \\ H\text{-}C\text{=}O & H\text{-}C\text{=}O & H\text{-}C\text{=}O & H\text{-}C\text{=}O \end{array}$	45	211	109
$\begin{array}{ccccc} H & H & H & H & H \\ | & | & | & | & | \\ H\text{-}O & H\text{-}O & H\text{-}O & H\text{-}O & H\text{-}O \end{array}$	18	100	80
$\begin{array}{cccc} & C_2H_5 & C_2H_5 & C_2H_5 \\ H & | & | & | \\ | & & & \\ C_2H_5\text{-}O & H\text{-}O & H\text{-}O & H\text{-}O \end{array}$	46	78	26
$\begin{array}{cccc} CH_3 & CH_3 & CH_3 & CH_3 \\ | & | & | & | \\ H\text{-}C\text{=}O & H\text{-}C\text{=}O & H\text{-}C\text{=}O & H\text{-}C\text{=}O \end{array}$	44	21	21
$\begin{array}{ccc} CH_3 & CH_3 & CH_3 \\ | & | & | \\ H\text{-}N & H\text{-}N & H\text{-}N \\ | & | & | \\ CH_3 & CH_3 & CH_3 \end{array}$	45	7	5

constant. Applying the coulombic principle to hydrogen bonding explains why hydrogen bonding is the strongest type of dipole-dipole interaction. When the negative field resides in a strong proton acceptor such as an oxygen or a nitrogen atom, dipole-dipole interaction is further strengthened. Hydrogen bonding, usually encountered in compounds containing hydroxyl, amino, or imino groups, forms dynamic, intermolecular association complexes which have high melting and boiling points. Hydrogen bonding of some liquids at room temperature is shown in Table XXVIII. Carboxylic acids readily hydrogen bond. The hydrogen bond is so strong in acetic acid that it exists as a dimer in the vapor state.

Hydrogen bonding is responsible for the unusual properties of ice. Solid water, i.e., ice, is less dense than liquid water, whereas most crystals are denser than their liquid. Ice is a hexagonal crystal in in which each water molecule is tetrahedronally surrounded by four other water molecules and connected to them by hydrogen bonds. As ice melts, some of the hydrogen bonds are broken, and the water molecules pack closer together in the liquid water, as indicated by the higher density of the liquid. Be- between 0 and 4° there exists some structure, as a decrease in temperature in this range results in an increase in volume and a decrease in density.

The polarity of a substance has been expressed in terms of dipole moment, which is a measure of the mechanical moment exerted on dipoles by an electrical field. The polarity of a substance is is also related to its dielectric constant. The dielectric constant, ϵ, is the ratio of the capacity of a given condenser filled with a substance to the capacity of that condenser at the same potential with a vacuum.

146 • solutions

Some dielectric constants are given in Table XXIX. As the values of the dielectric constant increase, the polarities of the corresponding compounds increase.

The solvent properties of water are related to its dielectric constant, i.e., 80. The ratio of the dielectric constants of two media expresses the relative energy required to separate two charged bodies. For example, it requires 1/80 as much energy to separate two charged bodies in water as it does in a vacuum. It requires 3.1/80 as much energy to separate two charged bodies in water as it does in olive oil. The solubilities of electrolytes are related to the dielectric constants of the solvent; in general, electrolytes dissolve in solvents having a high dielectric constant. Compounds with a high dielectric constant are generally water soluble; compounds with a low dielectric constant tend to be water insoluble.

Alcohols, aldehydes, acids, and primary and secondary amines are maintained in a condensed state by hydrogen bonds. The extent of hydrogen bonding may be influenced by the spatial arrangement of the molecule. A comparison of the dielectric constants of the butyl alcohols shows that *n*-butyl alcohol has the highest dielectric constant. As shown in Table XXX, in *tert*-butyl alcohol the steric hindrance of the methyl groups decreases the hydrogen bonds, and the lesser dipole-dipole interaction is indicated by the lower dielectric constant and boiling point of the *tert*-butyl alcohol.

In review, liquids may be arbitrarily considered as polar, semipolar, and nonpolar solvents. Polar solvents consist of dipolar molecules strongly associated through hydrogen bonding. Polar solvents, e.g., formamide, glycerin, and water, have a high dielectric constant and dipole moment.

Semipolar solvents consist of strongly dipolar molecules, which are not capable of forming hydrogen bonds, e.g., acetone, or dipoles with an intermediate value for the dielectric constant.

Nonpolar solvents consist of nonassociating weakly dipolar molecules, e.g., chloroform and ether, or molecules with zero dipole moment, e.g., benzene and mineral oil.

The chloroform molecule may be used to illustrate the relativeness of the terms "polar solvent" and "nonpolar solvent." Chloroform has a low dielectric constant, and it is generally classified as a nonpolar solvent; however, it is frequently used in pharmacy as a solvent for alkaloids, e.g., atropine and ergotamine. In these solutions, the chloroform may be considered as semipolar, owing to the inductive effect. The high kernel charge on the three chlorine atoms attracts the electron pairs from the hydrogen atom. The hydrogen atom of the weakly polarized chloroform molecule tends to align itself with the unshared electron pair of the nitrogen atom in the alkaloid. As a result of this dipole-dipole association the alkaloid dissolves in the chloroform.

Table XXIX Dielectric Constants, ϵ, of Some Liquids at 20°

Compound	ϵ	Compound	ϵ
Formamide	109	Aniline	6.9
Water	80.4	Chloral	4.9
Glycerol (18°)	56.2	Chloroform	4.8
Methanol	33.6	Castor oil (18°)	4.5
Ethanol (18°)	26.1	Ethyl ether	4.3
Propanol (18°)	22.5	Octyl alcohol (18°)	3.4
Acetone	21	Olive oil (18°)	3.1
n - Butanol (18°)	19.2	Oleic acid	2.5
sec - Butanol (18°)	15.5	Benzene	2.3
tert - Butanol (18°)	11.4	Carbon Tetrachloride	2.2
Phenol (60°)	9.8	Octane	1.9

Handwritten annotations:

Compound	ϵ
Glycerin	43.0
Benz. alc.	13.1
Methyl Salicylate	9.0
Liquid Petrolatum	2.5

Table XXX Steric Hindrance to Hydrogen Bonding and Its Influence on Some Physical Constants of Butyl Alcohols

Compound	Boiling Point (°C)	ϵ	Solubility (g in 100 ml of water)
H–O–CH$_2$–CH$_2$–CH$_2$–CH$_3$ (n-butyl alc.)	118	19.2	7.9
CH$_3$–CH(OH)–C$_2$H$_5$ (sec. butyl alc.)	100	15.5	12.5
(CH$_3$)$_3$C–OH (tert. butyl alc.)	83	11.4	Miscible

Solute-Solvent Interactions

The actual solubility of a substance represents the total of the various factors involved in the transport of a solute particle from the solid phase to the solution phase. The impelling force in dissolution is chiefly the interaction of the solvent molecules with the solute molecules or solute ions. A discussion of solute-solvent interactions follows.

Induced Dipole-Induced Dipole (London Forces). If the constituents of a solution are molecules with a zero or small dipole moment, the intermolecular force between the solute and solvent molecules is of the van der Waals type. Induced dipole-induced dipole interaction is the force responsible for the dissolution in nonpolar solvents, e.g., wax in carbon tetrachloride, naphthalene in carbon disulfide, and paraffin in petroleum benzin.

The net result of interactions as a solute dissolves is manifested energetically as the heat of solution. The differential heat of solution, ΔH, is defined as the heat absorbed when 1 mole of the solute is dissolved in a quantity of solution so large that the addition of one additional mole of solute does not appreciably change the concentration of the solution.

The relation of heat of solution to interaction energies may be considered stepwise. Assume in the dissolution process that a solute molecule is removed from the solute phase without leaving a void. The energy $\frac{1}{2}E_{2,2}$ associated with the removal of a single molecule is one-half the interaction energy between the two molecules of each interaction pair.

In the next step of the dissolution process a void large enough to receive a solute molecule is formed in the solution phase. Similarly, the energy $\tfrac{1}{2}E_{1,1}$ associated with this is equal to one-half the total interaction energy between a pair of solvent molecules.

Last, the solute molecule is placed in the void in the solution phase. The total interaction energy attributed to the interaction of a single solute molecule with the solvent is $E_{1,2}$.

If the size of the solute and solvent molecules are similar, the observed or net energy from the dissolution process may be expressed

$$E = E_{1,2} - \tfrac{1}{2}E_{1,1} - \tfrac{1}{2}E_{2,2} = E_{1,2} - \tfrac{1}{2}(E_{1,1} + E_{2,2})$$

Multiplying the equation by the Avogadro number expresses the heat of solution in molar quantities.

In nonpolar systems in which the solvent and solute molecules are similar in size and structure, the net energies or heats of solution are zero or very small. Substances that can be mixed with a zero heat of solution are mutually soluble and are often referred to as ideal solutions.

Induced Dipole-Dipole Interaction. As a strong dipole approaches a nonpolar molecule its electrical fields induce a temporary dipole in the nonpolar molecule, which is then attracted to the dipole. The force of interaction depends on the ease of polarization of the nonpolar molecule. A resonating molecule is easily polarized by a dipole; thus, benzene is a solvent for methyl alcohol, but mineral oil, which is not easily polarized, is not a solvent for methyl alcohol.

Other examples of solutions resulting from a dipole-induced dipole interaction are chloral hydrate in carbon tetrachloride, phenol in mineral oil, and tribromoethanol in benzene.

Dipole-Dipole Interaction. Dipole-dipole interaction is responsible for the dissolution of many pharmaceuticals. The solubility of the lower organic acids, alcohols, amides, amines, esters, ketones, sugars, and alkaloids in polar solvents is a result of dipole-dipole interaction. In most cases, hydrogen bonding is involved, as shown in Figure 78.

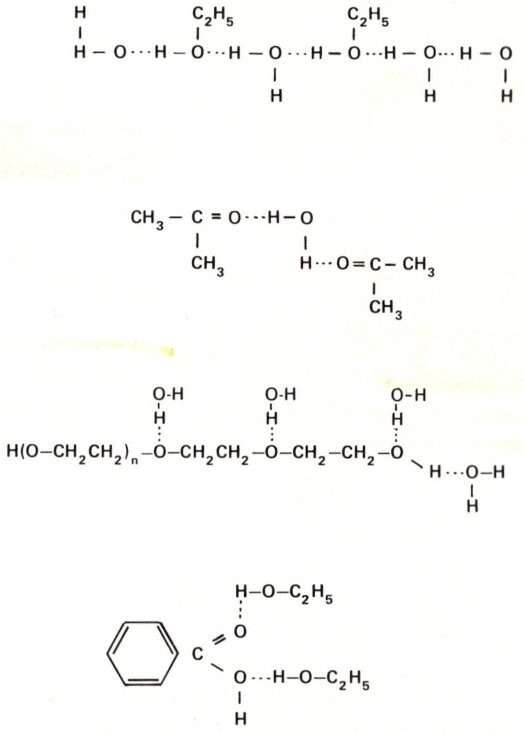

Figure 78. Diagrammatic representation of hydrogen bonding between some solutes and solvents.

Alcohols dissolve in water as a consequence of hydrogen bonding. When the alkyl chain of a monohydric alcohol exceeds five carbon atoms, i.e., amyl alcohol, the polarity is reduced to the degree that these alcohols are not water soluble. These alcohols are capable of dissolving polar solutes, e.g., acids, alkaloids, and phenols, which contain hydroxyl, amino, or imino groups that hydrogen bond with the hydroxyl of the alcohol. Ethyl alcohol is often used by the pharmacist to prevent the precipitation of these substances from aqueous vehicles.

Polyhydric alcohols, e.g., glycerin, glycol, mannitol, and sorbitol, of low molecular weight are polar and highly soluble in water. The dissolution of resorcinol in glycerin is an example of a liquid polyhydric alcohol functioning as a solvent for a polar solute. Sugars, e.g., glucose, fructose, and sucrose, are very water soluble, as these molecules have several hydroxyl groups that affect solution by hydrogen bonding with water.

Phenols dissolve in water, glycerin, and alcohol. As the ratio of the hydroxyl group to the carbon atom content is increased, the solubility is increased. The water solubility of resorcinol is roughly 15 times greater than the solubility of phenol; this is attributed to the additional hydroxyl group, which provides further opportunity for hydrogen bonding.

In a like manner, hydrogen bonding is responsible for the solubility in water and to a lesser degree in alcohol of the lower monocarboxylic acids, the dicarboxylic acids, and the hydroxypolycarboxylic acids.

Aromatic carboxylic acids, e.g., benzoic acid, salicylic acid, and aspirin, are not water soluble, but they dissolve in alcohol and glycerin by a dipole-dipole interaction. The introduction of polar groups into the aromatic nucleus increases the water solubility of the resulting compound. For example, in gallic acid the three hydroxyl groups confer water solubility. Tannic acid is a complex molecule in which some of the hydroxyl groups of glucose are esterified by gallic acid; these many sites for hydrogen bonding make tannic acid very water soluble.

Water-soluble amines dissolve due to the hydrogen bonding between water and the unshared electron pair on the nitrogen atom. Codeine dissolves in alcohol by this interaction.

A dissolution process involves the breaking of solute-solute bonds and solvent-solvent bonds and the formation of solute-solvent bonds. It has been shown that the net energy exchange in a dissolution process for a single solute molecule is

$$E = E_{1,2} - \tfrac{1}{2}(E_{1,1} + E_{2,2})$$

The term $E_{1,2}$ is the solute-solvent interaction, which tends to dissolve the solute. The term $\tfrac{1}{2}(E_{1,1} + E_{2,2})$ represents the solute-solute and solvent-solvent interactions and tends to prevent dissolution.

With strong dipole-dipole interactions, the solute-solvent interaction may exceed both the solvent-solvent and solute-solute interactions, resulting in excess energy, which is evolved as heat. In such cases, the solute is usually highly soluble in the solvent. When polyethylene glycol 6000 is dissolved in water, the solute-solvent interaction energy exceeds the sum of the solute-solute and solvent-solvent interaction energies. As the excess energy is then given off as heat, the dissolution process is an exothermic process. Such a system has a negative heat of solution, because heat of solution is defined as the heat absorbed per mole dissolved and it corresponds thermodynamically to the enthalpy change. See Table XXXI for heats of solution of various substances.

Usually substances with a large negative heat of solution are more soluble than a substance with a smaller negative heat of solution; however, compounds that have a positive heat of solution may be soluble. With certain dipole-dipole interactions the solute-solute and solvent-solvent interaction energies may exceed the solute-solvent energy. To complete the dissolution process thermal energy is absorbed from the environment to supply the deficient energy. This dissolution process is an endothermic process. The heat of solution is positive. Citric acid and sorbitol have positive heats of solution; as they dissolve, the solution becomes cool as thermal energy is absorbed from the surroundings.

Although the heat of solution is indicative of the solubility of a substance, other factors effect the solubility. The spatial arrangement of the solute molecule may hinder the transition from one phase to the other. The heats of solution of inositol and citric acid are 3,400 and 5,300 cal, respectively. Based solely on a comparison of the heats of solution, inositol would be predicted to be more soluble than citric acid; in fact, citric acid is several times as soluble as inositol.

In dissolving, a citric acid molecule leaving the crystal does not require a particular orientation. A citric acid molecule in the solution phase cannot be deposited on the crystal surface unless it is so oriented that upon contact with the crystal lattice dipole-dipole interaction can easily occur between the polar groups on the crystallizing molecule and those comprising the crystal surface. This tends to maintain the citric acid in solution by hindering its crystallization. A symmetrical molecule, such as inositol, can contact the crystal surface without any specific orientation and crystallize.

As a general rule, crystals composed of unsymmetrical molecules are more soluble than those composed of highly symmetrical molecules.

Table XXXI Heats of Solution

Compound	ΔH (kcal mole^{-1})
Endothermic Dissolution	
Ammonium chloride	3.88
Ammonium sulfate	2.37
Boric acid	10.79
Calcium sulfate dihydrate	0.30
Ferrous sulfate heptahydrate	4.51
Magnesium sulfate heptahydrate	3.80
Potassium alum	10.1
Potassium bromide	5.08
Potassium chloride	4.19
Potassium iodide	5.11
Potassium thiosulfate	5.0
Sodium bicarbonate	4.3
Sodium borate decahydrate	25.86
Sodium chloride	1.18
Sodium nitrate	5.03
Sodium sulfate decahydrate	18.76
Exothermic Dissolution	
Aluminum chloride	-76.5
Calcium chloride	-17.41
Calcium hydroxide	-2.79
Calcium iodide	-28.12
Copper sulfate, anhydrous	-15.80
Ferric chloride, anhydrous	-32.68
Magnesium sulfate, anhydrous	-20.28
Potassium acetate	-3.34
Sodium hydroxide	-9.94
Sodium iodide	-1.22
Strontium bromide	-16.11
Zinc chloride	-15.63

Dipole-Ion Interaction. Dipole-ion interaction is the force responsible for the dissolution of electrolytes in polar solvents, e.g., zinc chloride in glycerin and cocaine hydrochloride in alcohol. This attraction of an electrical center of a dipole to an oppositely charged ion often releases energy of the approximate magnitude of ion-ion interactions. This energy of an ion-dipole interaction is partially expended to break the ion-ion bonds in the solid solute. Nonpolar and weakly polar liquids do not have sufficiently strong interaction energies with electrolytes to act as their solvents.

To be a good solvent for electrolytes a compound should have (1) a high dipole moment, which results in the formation of a strong ion-dipole bond; (2) a small molecular size to enable the dipole to approach close to the ions; and (3) a high dielectric constant, which reduces the intensity of electrical interaction between the solvated ions. Water possesses all these characteristics and is an excellent solvent for electrolytes. Acetone with its high dipole moment is a good solvent for iodide and bromide salts of lithium and potassium. Acetone and inorganic salts may form complexes in which the ion-dipole interaction is so strong that the complex may be recovered as a crystalline solvate, i.e., a compound formed by reaction between a solute and its solvent.

In aqueous solution most ions are surrounded or hydrated by as many water molecules as the size of the ion allows. Anions are generally less highly hydrated than cations. The extent of interaction between ions and dipoles depends on the size and charge of the ions. The combined effect of these two factors can be illustrated by a comparison of the solubility of aluminum chloride and sodium chloride. The aluminum ion with a radius of 0.5 Å is more hydrated than the sodium ion with a radius of 0.95 Å. In addition to the size difference, the triple-charged aluminum ion has a charge-to-size ratio of 6, while the charge-to-radius ratio for the sodium ion is 1.05. The attractive force between the aluminum ion and the unshared electron pair of water is so strong that aluminum chloride may dissolve with vigorous boiling in water to the extent of 70 g in 100 ml of water.

As has been discussed, the ion-dipole interaction is so great that the aluminum ion coordinates with six molecules of water, which remain with the cation as water of crystallization upon crystallization. The sodium ion, with its smaller ratio of charge to radius, has an ion-dipole interaction energy of lesser magnitude, as reflected by a solubility of approximately 35.7 g in 100 ml and its positive heat of solution.

Other examples may be taken from Table XXXII. The cations of the alkaline earth metals — beryllium, magnesium, calcium, strontium, and barium — form water-soluble salts with univalent anions and only slightly soluble salts with polyvalent anions. The solubilities may be rationalized on the basis of the ratio of ionic charge to radius. For ions having the same valence, the smaller ion has a more intense electrostatic field, and consequently a greater ion-dipole interaction, which produces a greater solubility in water. In the alkaline earth metals, the salts of beryllium should be more soluble than those of magnesium, the salts of magnesium should be more soluble than those of strontium, and the salts of strontium should be more soluble than those of barium.

The cations of the alkali metals — lithium, sodium, and potassium — form water-soluble salts with univalent and divalent anions. In general, the lithium salts are more soluble than the sodium salts, and the sodium salts are more soluble than the potassium salts. The solubilities of the salts of a given anion increase with an increase in the ratio of ionic charge to radius of the cation. Exceptions to this general statement occur; however, this is not unexpected in view of the complexity of the dissolution process.

Salts formed from univalent ions, e.g., ammonium chloride, potassium iodide, and lithium chloride, have weaker coulombic forces and are more water soluble than salts formed from combinations of polyvalent cations and anions, e.g., barium sulfate, lead borate, and zinc sulfide.

When electrolytes dissolve in water the ion-dipole interaction energy may exceed the sum of the ion-ion and dipole-dipole interaction of the solute and solvent, respectively. The excess energy is evolved as heat. By thermodynamic definition the heat of solution of these electrolytes is negative. Specific examples encountered by the pharmacist are dissolution in water of anhydrous calcium chloride, anhydrous copper sulfate, anhydrous ferric chloride, and sodium hydroxide.

If the sum of the ion-ion and dipole-dipole interaction energy is greater than the ion-dipole interaction energy for a soluble substance, the deficit in energy is acquired by absorbing heat from the surrounding environment. Potassium iodide will absorb heat as it dissolves in water, and the solution will become cool. Other electrolytes that have a positive heat of solution when dissolved in water are ammonium chloride, ferric sulfate heptahydrate, and sodium bromide.

It is interesting to note that the quantity of water of crystallization affects the heat of solution. In a crystal hydrate the ions are largely hydrated, and consequently the ion-dipole interaction energy is considerably less than that of the anhydrous solute during the dissolution process. With a crystal containing the maximum water of crystallization, energy frequently must be absorbed from the environment to complete dissolution. This is reflected in a positive heat of solution as shown in Table XXXIII for copper sulfate, magnesium sulfate, and sodium phosphate.

Table XXXII Relationship of Electrostatic Fields of Some Cations to the Solubility of Their Salts

Charge	Ion	Ionic Radius (Å)	Charge/Radius	Solubility (g in 100 ml of Water) of:	
				Chloride	Sulfate
+1	Li	0.6	1.67	78.0	37.0
	Na	0.95	1.05	35.7	19.5
	K	1.37	0.75	34.7	12.0
	Rb	1.48	0.67	91.2	42.4
	Cs	1.67	0.60	185.7	167.0
+2	Be	0.31	6.45	Very soluble	42.5 (hydrate)
	Mg	0.65	3.07	54.5	26
	Ca	0.99	2.02	74.5	0.21
	Sr	1.13	1.77	53.8	0.011
	Ba	1.35	1.49	37.5	0.0002
+3	B	0.20	15.00	Decomposed	-
	Al	0.50	6.00	69.9	31.3
	Sc	0.81	3.70	Very soluble	10.3

Table XXXIII Heats of Solution of Some Crystal Hydrates

Hydrate	ΔH (kcal mole^{-1})
Magnesium sulfate	-20.3
Magnesium sulfate monohydrate	-13.3
Magnesium sulfate heptahydrate	3.8
Copper sulfate	-15.8
Copper sulfate monohydrate	-9.3
Copper sulfate pentahydrate	2.7
Disodium phosphate	-5.6
Disodium phosphate dihydrate	0.4
Disodium phosphate heptahydrate	11.3
Disodium phosphate dodecahydrate	22.8

IDEAL AND REAL SOLUTIONS
Gaseous Solutions

With the exception of gases that react chemically with each other, most gases can be mixed in any proportions, and the resulting mixture or solution has properties of the individual gases. For example, the total pressure of a solution of gases is equal to the sum of the partial pressures of each gas taken alone in the same volume. This is known as the Dalton law of partial pressure and is expressed as

$$p = p_1 + p_2 + \cdots + p_n$$

where $p_1, p_2,$ and p_n are the partial pressures of the individual gases and p the total pressure.

Experimentally Boyle found that if the temperature remains constant, the volume, v, of a given mass of gas varies inversely as its pressure, p,

$$v = \frac{k_1}{p}$$

Differentiating yields

$$\left(\frac{dv}{dp}\right)_T = \frac{k_1}{p^2} = -\frac{pv}{p^2} = -\frac{v}{p^2}$$

Gay-Lussac and Charles found that at a constant pressure the volume, v, of a gas is directly proportional to its absolute temperature, T,

$$\frac{v}{T} = k_2$$

Differentiating this equation yields

$$\left(\frac{dv}{dT}\right)_P = k_2 = \frac{v}{T}$$

A small change in volume, dv, of a gaseous system, produced by changing the temperature and pressure simultaneously, is equal to the sum of two quantities: (1) the change in temperature, dT, multiplied by the rate at which the volume changes with the temperature alone at a constant pressure, $\left(\frac{dv}{dT}\right)_p$, and (2) the change in pressure, dp, multiplied by the rate at which the volume changes with pressure alone at a constant temperature, $\left(\frac{dv}{dp}\right)_T$. Mathematically, this statement is expressed

$$dv = \left(\frac{dv}{dT}\right)_P dT + \left(\frac{dv}{dp}\right)_T dp$$

Substitution of the differentiated Boyle law and Gay-Lussac law into this expression yields

$$dv = \frac{v}{T} dT - \frac{v}{p} dp$$

or

$$\frac{dv}{v} + \frac{dp}{p} = \frac{dT}{T}$$

The integrated form of this equation is

$$\ln v + \ln p = \ln T + \ln(\text{constant})$$

or

$$pv = \text{constant} \times T$$

If the volume of 1 mole, V, of an ideal gas is considered, this equation, known as the ideal gas equation or equation of state, becomes

$$pV = RT$$

in which R is the gas constant.

Experimentally, the value of the gas constant is determined by measuring the pressures and volumes at different temperatures and solving the ideal gas equation for R. At standard conditions, 1 mole of an ideal gas occupies 22.414 liters. Then,

$$R = \frac{1 \text{ atm} \times 22.414 \text{ liters}}{273.16°} = 0.08295 \text{ liter atm deg}^{-1} \text{ mole}^{-1}$$

The gas constant appears in many equations that are derived as limiting relationships, i.e., dilute to the extent that there is no interaction between molecules. The gas constant may be expressed in other units. The pressure in dyn cm^{-2} is found by multiplying 76 cm of mercury by the density of mercury and the acceleration of gravity. The pressure expressed in dyn cm^{-2} multiplied by the volume in milliliters represents the work in ergs. One joule equals 10^7 ergs. In terms of joules the gas constant is

$$R = \frac{pV}{T} = \frac{76 \times 13.595 \times 980 \times 22,414}{273.16 \times 10^7} = 8.314 \, J \text{ deg}^{-1} \text{ mole}^{-1}$$

Since there are 4.184 J per calorie, the gas constant also equals

$$R = \frac{8.314}{4.184} = 1.987 \text{ cal deg}^{-1} \text{ mole}^{-1}$$

In an ideal gas there is no intermolecular interaction. In a real gas, especially at higher pressures and lower temperatures, there is some attraction between the molecules. To account for this interaction van der Waals suggested the following form of the gas equation:

$$\left(P + \frac{a}{V^2}\right)(V - b) = RT$$

in which a/V^2 compensates for deviations from ideal behavior due to the van der Waal force. The term b corrects for the volume occupied by the molecules of the gas.

Ideal Solutions

An ideal solution is one in which the presence of the solute molecules has no effect on the forces existing between the solvent molecules, and vice versa. Consequently, upon mixing there is no change in properties of the components other than dilution. When two liquids dissolve to give an ideal solution, there is no heat effect, and other properties, e.g., density, volume, refractive index, viscosity, and vapor pressure, can be directly calculated by averaging the properties of the components of the solution.

A fundamental property of a substance is the tendency for its molecules to escape or pass into the surrounding space, e.g., vaporization of a liquid, dissolution of a solid in a liquid, and sublimation. Theoretically this escape tendency is quantitatively expressed in terms of free energy, G. For a pure substance the free energy per mole is known as the molar free energy; for a component of a solution the escape tendency is expressed in terms of partial molar free energy.

The escape tendency of a liquid is reflected by its vapor pressure. When a liquid is placed in an evacuated vessel at a given temperature, the molecules vaporize from the surface of the liquid. Eventually, a condition of equilibrium is attained when the rate of vaporization is equal to the rate of condensation. The pressure exerted by the vapor, which is in equilibrium with its liquid, is known as the vapor pressure. The vapor pressure is increased by an increase in temperature. The logarithms of vapor pressure are a linear function of the reciprocals of the absolute temperature. This relation may be expressed as

$$\log p = \frac{a}{T} + b$$

where p is the vapor pressure and a and b are constants.

The vapor pressure of a pure liquid depends on the rate of escape of the molecules from the surface. If the liquid is mixed with another substance, the concentration is decreased and the rate of escape from the surface is decreased. In an ideal solution, the partial vapor pressure of one component is directly proportional to the mole fraction of that component in the solution. The partial vapor pressure, p_A, of component A may be expressed as

$$p_A = N_A p_A^0$$

where N_A is the mole fraction of component A and p^0 is the vapor pressure of pure A. In an ideal binary solution the partial vapor pressure, p_B^0, of the other component, B, is

$$p_B = N_B p_B^0$$

At 20° the vapor pressures of pure benzene and pure toluene are 74.7 and 22 mm, respectively. If a solution of benzene and toluene is made containing 0.27 mole fraction of benzene, the partial vapor pressure of benzene is

$$p_{benzene} = 0.27 \times 74.7 = 20.1 \text{ mm}$$

The partial vapor pressure of toluene is

$$p_{toluene} = 0.73 \times 22 = 16 \text{ mm}$$

The total pressure is the sum of the partial pressures of all the components of the solution,

$$p = p_A + p_B = 20.1 + 16 = 36.1 \text{ mm}$$

Using dilute solutions of nonvolatile solutes Raoult experimentally confirmed the above relation — that the partial vapor pressure of the solvent is equal to the vapor pressure of the pure solvent multiplied by the mole fraction of the solvent in the solution. This relationship is known as the Raoult law and is usually written

$$p_{solvent} = p_{solvent}^0 N_{solvent}$$

The Raoult law applies to the solvent, but it does not apply to the solute in a real solution. The solute is diluted to such an extent that its properties are considerably different from those of the solute in its pure state. In a real solution the Henry law applies to the solute; it is expressed as

$$p_{solute} = K N_{solute}$$

The partial vapor pressure of the solute is proportional to the mole fraction of the solute; however, K is not the vapor pressure of the pure solute but an experimentally determined constant. The Henry law finds use in quantitatively expressing the effect of pressure on the solubility of a gas.

Real Solutions

Ideal solutions are seldom encountered in pharmacy. In most solutions there are solute and solvent interactions, which cause abnormal changes of properties of the solvent and solute.

The abnormalities in viscosity of an acetone-water solution are shown in Figure 79. In an ideal solution the viscosity would be a linear function of concentration. With acetone and water there is

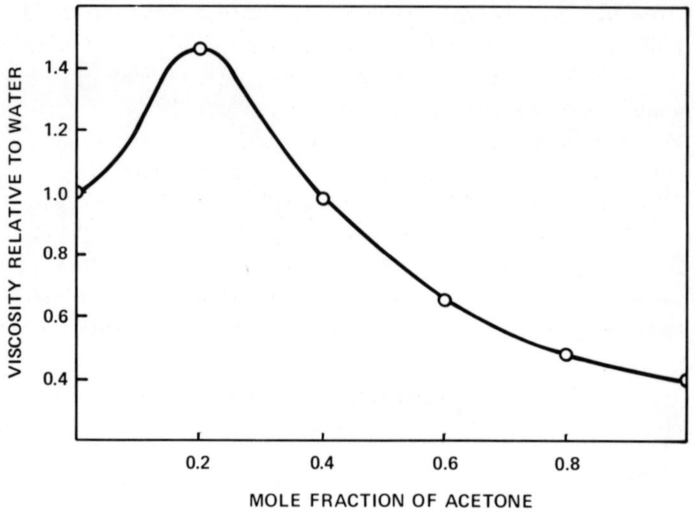

156 • solutions

Figure 79. Real solution in which the greatest extent of hydrogen bonding is reflected in a maximum viscosity.

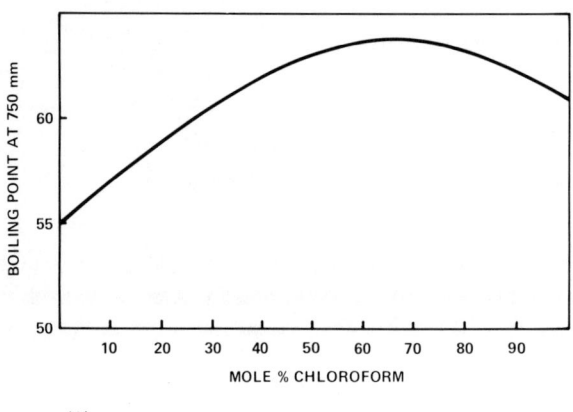

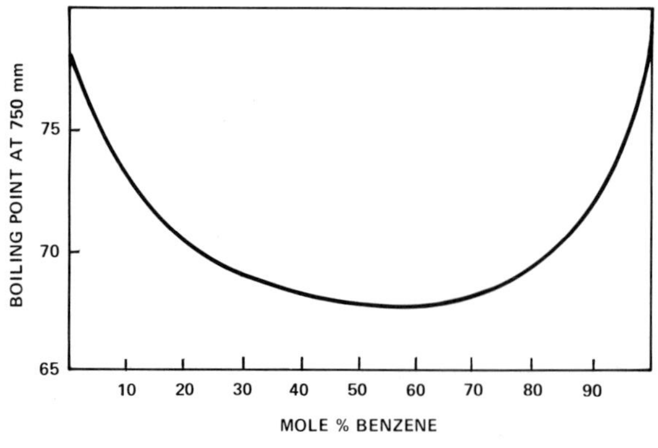

Figure 80. Maximum and minimum boiling points: (a) boiling point-composition curve for the liquid phase of an acetone-chloroform solution showing a maximum; (b) boiling point-composition curve for the liquid phase of a benzene-ethanol solution showing a minimum.

strong hydrogen bonding between the two polar compounds. Maximum viscosity occurs at a concentration of the solute where there is maximum hydrogen bonding and the greatest resistance to flow.

In real solutions departure from ideal behavior may result in maximum and minimum boiling points in the boiling point-composition curves as shown in Figure 80. In a binary solution composed of a polar and a nonpolar liquid, the molecular forces between the solute molecules will be different from the molecular forces acting between the solvent molecules. When the intermolecular attraction between the solute molecules, is stronger than the attraction between the solvent molecules, the escape tendency of the solvent is increased by the presence of the solute molecules. This is shown by a maximum vapor pressure and minimum boiling point at a particular concentration in the vapor pressure-composition and boiling point-composition curves, respectively. Binary solutions exhibiting minimum boiling points at a particular concentration are carbon tetrachloride and alcohol, ethyl acetate and water, and benzene and ethanol.

If two liquid components of a binary solution have a strong solute-solvent interaction, their escape tendency is reduced. This interaction is shown by a minimum total vapor pressure and a maximum boiling point at a particular concentration for the vapor pressure-concentration and boiling point-concentration curves, respectively. In a chloroform-ether system, the chloroform hydrogen bonds with the unshared electron pair of the ether, resulting in a maximum boiling point.

6 | DISSOLUTION PROCESSES

Drugs that are administered as a solid in a dosage form must dissolve in body fluids before they are absorbed and can exert their therapeutic effect. Considering absorption as a free diffusional process, i.e., migration of a substance solely by means of diffusion toward a region of lower concentration, it can be calculated that 600 mg of aspirin, dissolved in 500 ml of fluid in a 100-cm segment of the intestine, will be 85 per cent absorbed in 2 minutes. Only recently has it been appreciated that absorption of a dissolved drug is rapid and that the dissolution rate is not infrequently the rate-limiting step in drug availability.

In the preparation of a prescription it is expedient for the pharmacist to prepare the solution rapidly. In industrial pharmacy the solutes should be quickly dissolved by use of the proper type and rate of agitation without contributing to the product of unwanted properties, e.g., foaming.

The dissolution rate of a solid in a liquid is affected by the following characteristics of the solid: specific surface, particle size distribution, and shape. In regard to the solvent, the dissolution rate is influenced by the agitation, temperature, viscosity, and concentration of the dissolved solute. The dissolution rate is influenced by the ratio of solids to solvent, by chemical reactions, and by the relative densities of the solid, solvent, and solution.

THEORY OF DISSOLUTION

The Noyes-Whitney equation was empirically developed by studying the dissolution of solids in their own solutions, when the surface area of the exposed solid changes negligibly. The equation states that for a given temperature the rate of concentration change, dC/dt, is at any instant directly proportional to the difference between the concentration of a saturated solution, C_S, and the concentration, C, existing in the solution at that time,

$$\frac{dC}{dt} = k(C_S - C)$$

where the constant, k, incorporates all variable factors held at given values for the system. Subsequently, the surface area, S, was incorporated into the equation,

$$\frac{dC}{dt} = k_1 S (C_S - C)$$

The constant, k_1, is dependent on agitation, temperature, vessel, and so on; however, for a given set of conditions k is constant. It was postulated that a thin layer of saturated solution formed at the surface of the solid and that the dissolution rate was a function of the rate at which the dissolved solute diffused through this layer into the bulk of the solution.

The Noyes-Whitney equation may be drived from the Fick law. The Fick law of diffusion at a given temperature is expressed as

$$\frac{dw}{dt} = -DS\frac{dC}{dx}$$

where dw is the quantity of solute that diffuses through an area S in a time, dt, when the concentration changes by an amount, dC, through a distance, dx, at right angles to the plane of S. The diffusion constant, D, is the amount of solute that will cross 1 cm^2 of cross section in unit time, if the change in concentration per centimeter in a direction perpendicular to this cross section is 1. The diffusion constant has the units cm^2 sec^{-1}.

Assuming a layer of saturated solution of a thickness, h, the distance the dissolved solute must diffuse to reach the bulk solution is $dx = h$. The change in concentration, dC, is equal to the difference in concentration of the saturated layer and that of the bulk solution, $(C_s - C)$. Substitution into the Fick equation gives the equation

$$\frac{dw}{dt} = -\frac{DS}{h}(C_s - C)$$

As we are discussing dissolution rate, the negative sign indicating loss of weight of the solute may be incorporated into the definition of dissolution rate. As $C = w/V$,

$$\frac{dC}{dt} = \frac{DS}{Vh}(C_s - C)$$

If $k_1 = D/Vh$, the equation is identical to the Noyes-Whitney equation.

The above relation has been employed to evaluate the effective thickness of the diffusion layer. As the intensity of agitation is increased, the diffusion layer becomes thinner, and the dissolution rate is increased.

The Hixson and Crowell cube-root equation for dissolution kinetics is based on the assumption that (1) dissolution takes place normal to the surface of the solute, (2) there is no stagnation and the agitation is the same on all exposed surface, and (3) the solute particle retains its geometric shape. By appropriate substitution the general form of the cube-root equation expresses the factors related to the solid in terms of weight; this is advantageous, as the surface is constantly changing and is difficult to experimentally evaluate.

Although the general form is cumbersome, it may be greatly simplified by imposing certain restrictions. If the concentration change is negligible, i.e., $(C_s - C)$ is almost constant, dw/dt, the amount dissolved per unit time, is proportional to the surface. This special case is expressed by the equation

$$\frac{dw}{dt} = 3KS = 3Kaw^{2/3}$$

where $a = \alpha_{sv}/\rho^{2/3}$ (see page 3). The integrated form of this equation is

$$Kat = w_0^{1/3} - w^{1/3}$$

where w_0 is the initial weight, w the weight of the solid at the time t and K the rate constant for a given set of conditions.

As dissolution is a surface phenomenon, a given weight of smaller particles of a substance dissolves in a shorter time than larger particles of the same weight by virtue of the greater surface area exposed to the dissolving medium. For example, 1 g of powdered alum dissolves faster than 1 g of lump alum in a given amount of water; however, the dissolution rate is not changed by a reduction of particle size. It should be stressed that dissolution rate is expressed in terms of the amount of solute dissolved per unit time per unit surface, e.g., $g\ hr^{-1}\ cm^{-2}$. If the concentration change is negligible, the dissolution rate is

$$\left(\frac{dw}{dt}\right)_{S=1} = 3K$$

One method of determining the dissolution rate is based on finding the weight of the particle at given times. As shown in Figure 81, a plot of $w_0^{1/3} - w^{1/3}$ against time is linear with a slope of Ka. The dissolution rate as given in the above equation is $3K$.

The special case in which the concentration change is negligible is applicable to pharmacy. If absorption of a dissolved substance from the gastrointestinal tract is rapid and dissolution is the rate-limiting step in drug availability, the drug is absorbed and removed from the gastrointestinal tract as fast as it dissolves. Consequently, there is no change in concentration in the gastrointestinal lumen. Thus, the effect of various factors on the *in vitro* dissolution rate determined with negligible concentration change may be extrapolated to a similar effect of these factors on *in vivo* dissolution rate.

FACTORS INFLUENCING THE DISSOLUTION RATE

Unreacting Additives

When neutral electrolytes and nonionic organic compounds are additives in the solvent phase, the dissolution rate of the solid is linearly dependent upon the solubility of the solid in the solvent system. The dissolution rate of benzoic acid in aqueous solutions of sodium chloride or sodium sulfate decreases as its solubility decreases. The ion-dipole interaction competitively binds the water, so it is not as available for hydrogen bonding with the benzoic acid. As shown in Figure 82, dextrose also decreases the solubility and dissolution rate.

In examining the dissolution rates and solubilities of 55 compounds, it has been found that the ratio of rate to solubility ranged from 1.5 to 3. Thus, the dissolution rate of a new chemical entity or derivative may be roughly estimated by a consideration of its solubility.

As dissolution proceeds, the concentration of a solute in solution is increased, and the concentration gradient is decreased. This results in a slowing of the dissolution rate. Constituents of the gastrointestinal tract and excipients in solid dosage forms may adsorb a drug. If an additive adsorbs the dissolved solute, the concentration gradient $(C_s - C)$ remains large, and the dissolution rate remains rapid.

Viscosity

In most dissolution processes in pharmacy the reaction at the interface of the solid and the solvent occurs much faster than the rate of transport or diffusion of the reactants from the interface to the bulk solution. An increase in viscosity decreases the dissolution rate of a diffusion-controlled process.

Numerous equations have been proposed which show the dissolution rate to be a function of the viscosity raised to a power, where the exponent ranged from -0.25 to -0.8.

Surface Activity

In highly irregular particles with pores and crevices, the total surface area of the pores may be incompletely exposed to the solvent, owing to occlusion by air. In the presence of surface-active agents, the surface tension is lowered and the entire surface is wetted. This increase of surface contact between the solid and solvent, i.e., effective surface, increases the apparent dissolution rate.

Surface-active agents in low concentrations, i.e., below the critical micelle concentration, do not markedly affect dissolution rate. It has been postulated that a slight increase in rate at low concen-

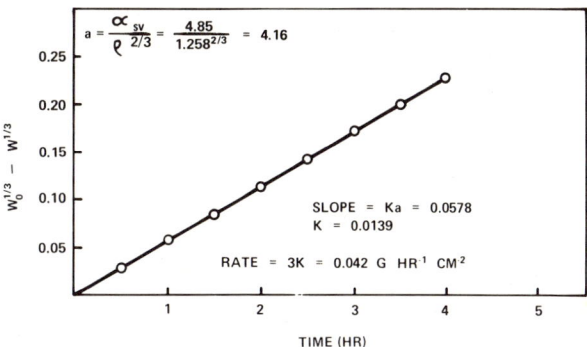

Figure 81. Evaluation of dissolution rate and Ka from the slope of $w_o^{1/3} - w^{1/3}$ against time for a spherical tablet. [Adapted from E.L. Parrott, D.E. Wurster and T. Higuchi, *J. Am. Pharm. Assoc., Sci. Ed.* **44**, 269 (1955).]

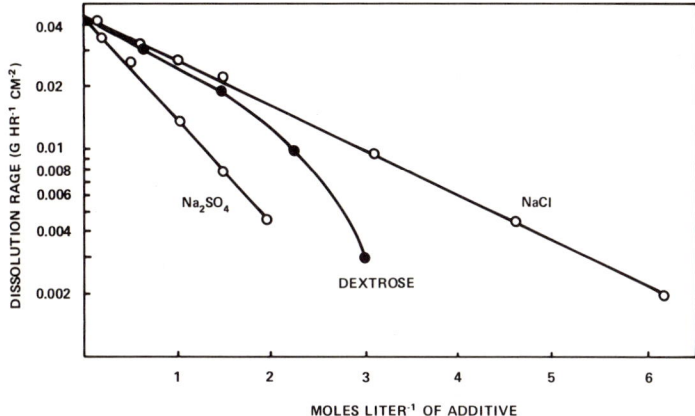

Figure 82. Influence of concentration of neutral additives on the dissolution rate of benzoic acid tablets.

trations can be attributed to the orientation of the dissolved solute between ionized surfactant molecules and the reduction of their repulsive force.

In high concentrations surface-active agents usually increase the dissolution rate. This is probably a consequence of the greater total solubility resulting from the incorporation of the dissolved solute in a micellular structure.

PROCEDURES

Factors directly influencing the solute particle and the solvent during the dissolution process have been briefly considered. In the operational procedures for the production of solutions the influence of temperature and agitation applies directly to the entire system.

Temperature

In general, substances dissolve faster if the system is warmed. If a substance absorbs heat in the dissolution process, its solubility is increased by an increase in temperature. The increase in solubility provides an increased concentration gradient, which results in an increased dissolution rate. The increase in temperature increases kinetic motion and diffusion of the solute through the diffusion layer into the bulk solution, which increases the dissolution rate.

A flow pattern in which the velocity is variable and the path is curved is known as curvilinear flow. In the region of curvilinear flow for each $10°$ rise in temperature, the dissolution rate increases approximately 1.3 times.

Agitation

As most dissolution procedures in pharmacy are accomplished by stirring, this discussion is limited to rotational agitation. The intensity of agitation is one of the most important factors in determining the dissolution rate of a solid. The thickness of the diffusion layer is inversely proportional to the agitation. This has been expressed in the empirically developed relationship

$$K = aN^b$$

where N is the agitation in terms of revolutions per minutes, K represents the dissolution rate, and a and b are constants. For a diffusion-controlled process $b \to 1$. If the dissolution is controlled by an interfacial reaction, the agitation does not influence the dissolution rate and $b \to 0$.

When a stirrer is operated in a liquid so that the only friction is from the walls and bottom of the container and the viscosity of the fluid, the type of agitation is known as free rotational agitation. In free rotational agitation the flow of fluid may be one of three types.

At very low rpm the flow is passive. The solids do not move and the dissolution rate depends on the manner in which the solid is scattered on the bottom of the container. The solid and solution are not transported to the top of the system, and the system has layers of different concentrations. Dissolution does not occur where the particles touch one another in the pile at the center of the tank bottom.

At very high rpm the flow is turbulent. The centrifugal force of the rotating fluid tends to force the particles outward and upward. The cube-root equation does not apply to turbulent or passive flow.

Between these two extremes of flow is the useful curvilinear type of flow. In the curvilinear region shown in Figure 83, the dissolution rate is nearly linearly proportional to the rpm. In curvilinear flow the particles move to the center and pile up, and then they move around circularly to the center. The cube-root equation applies to curvilinear flow.

Container. Good results in industrial mixing are obtained with vertical cylindrical tanks having flat or dished bottoms. The major requirements of mixing equipment for industrial dissolution are shear and volume circulation of the fluid. A high shear is not required, as reduction of particle size is not the function of the mixing equipment; a low shear is required to prevent the formation of a static interface that would reduce the transport of the solute.

To provide the proper shear for dissolution, the ratio of the tank diameter to the impeller diameter should range from 1.6:1 to 3.2:1. The ratio of the tank height to its diameter should range from 1:2 to 2:1. The depth of the fluid generally exceeds the diameter of the tank.

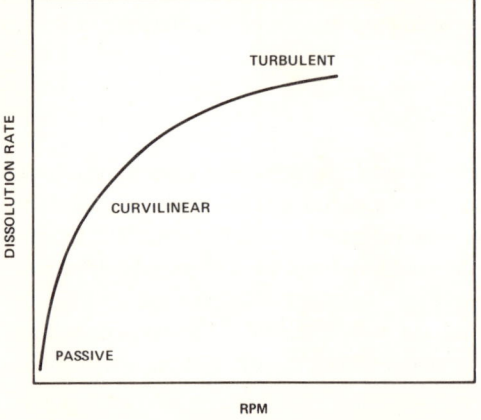

Figure 83. Influence of intensity of rotary agitation on dissolution rate and type of agitation.

Impeller. Although a great variety of rotary impellers are marketed, the flow developed by impellers is one of three basic types: axial, radial, or tangential.

The marine-type propeller is commonly used for laboratory-scale operations. The propeller produces axial flow; i.e., fluid is displaced downward along the axis of rotation. The column of liquid below the propeller tends to rotate with the propeller without horizontal or vertical flow. The proper use of baffles as shown in Figure 84 can convert this motion to horizontal and vertical flow.

The propeller has a more limited circulating capacity than the turbine or paddle impeller. A turbine or paddle impeller may be used in tanks up to 10,000-gal capacity; a propeller mixer is limited to roughly one-third this capacity. To provide two tank turnovers per minute in a 7,000-gal tank would require a 25-hp minimum propeller mixer, but only a 15-hp turbine and probably a 10-hp-maximum paddle mixer. The propeller is generally least effective, because it has a small area and pitch and little lift.

The turbine impeller uses centrifugal force to produce radial flow; i.e., fluid is directed outward from the blades toward the impeller tip, with increasing velocity, at right angles to the axis of rotation. The general flow pattern of a turbine impeller is shown in Figure 85. For a given set of conditions, the turbine impeller gives a faster dissolution rate than the paddle or propeller impeller.

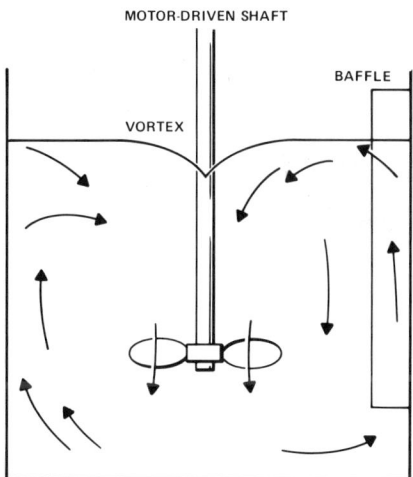

Figure 84. Propeller agitator produces axial-flow pattern shown with and without a baffle.

Figure 85. Turbine impeller produces radial flow shown with and without a baffle.

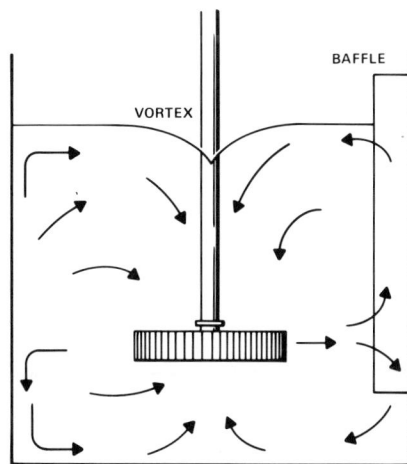

The paddle mixer consists of a shaft with one or more horizontal arms which may or may not be pitched. A multiple-arm paddle is known as a gate mixer. If the rpm and the width of the paddle impeller are held constant, the dissolution rate increases as the length of the paddle is increased up to approximately three-fourths the diameter of the mixing tank. The usual practice is to have the paddle diameter up to 90 per cent of the diameter of the tank with a ratio of impeller width to impeller diameter of 1:8 to 1:12. The dissolution rate is greatest as the paddle impeller approaches the bottom of the mixing tank, and the rate decreases somewhat as the paddle is raised.

Proper agitation produces volume circulation in all parts of the system. Strong vertical flow is desired when heavy solids are to be dissolved; strong lateral flow is desired when miscible liquids of approximately the same densities are to be dissolved.

Any impeller rotating in a smooth, vertical cylindrical tank without stationary objects and in a low viscosity fluid tends to carry the rotational movement of the impeller throughout the liquid with a minimum of axial or radial flow. Such liquid motion is known as a swirl. The laminar circular flow of a swirling liquid tends to carry dissolving particles in stratified streams with inadequate vertical and lateral movement.

The paddle mixer produces liquid movement tangential to the mixing device. This is often accompanied by a swirl with a deep vortex. With a vortex mixing will be minimal for the energy expended. The easiest means of avoiding this condition is by off-center positioning of the impeller. The impeller shaft enters the surface of the liquid to one side of the center line and passes through the fluid at an angle to the vertical. The exact position and angle to prevent a vortex is critical and depends on the size of the tank and the depth of the fluid. Similarly, side-entering impellers may be fitted to the side and near the bottom of the tank.

Baffles should be used with all vertical and center impellers to avoid liquid swirl and to provide top-to-bottom circulation. The baffle arrangement is determined by the viscosity of the fluid. High-viscosity fluids, seldom encountered in pharmacy, may not require baffles, as the inertia of the system aids in the mixing process.

In most pharmaceutical dissolution processes, four baffles of a width equal to 1 in. ft^{-1} of tank diameter are located 90° apart on the tank wall. As the viscosity approaches 7,000 cp, the baffles are set out from the wall to eliminate stagnant pockets in front of them. At this high viscosity the area of the baffle is reduced by pitching them or reducing the actual width.

A properly baffled paddle mixer located approximately 1 in. from the bottom of the tank will provide volume circulation and will sweep the tank bottom to keep the dissolving solids in motion. As the shear of the paddle mixer is low, the dissolving time will be longer than with a turbine impeller.

Manual Operations. Ordinarily, the community pharmacist uses a graduate and a stirring rod to effect the solution of readily soluble substances. Approximately one-half to three-fourths of the required volume of solvent is placed in the graduate and the solid drug is added. The system is stirred until the drug has dissolved, and then sufficient solvent is added to make up to the required volume. If necessary the solution may be filtered through a quantitative grade of filter paper to ensure clarity.

For drugs with a slow dissolution rate, a glass mortar and pestle may be used to effect solution. A glass mortar is used in preparing solutions so that one can see when dissolution is completed. Since the solid is to be dissolved before dispensing to the patient, the fine particle size obtained by use of a porcelain mortar is not necessary as for ingredients in a solid dosage form. The solid drug is crushed in the mortar, and a portion of the solvent is added while stirring with the pestle. When the solid has dissolved, the solution is transferred to a graduate and brought to final volume with the solvent.

With gums, colloids, and scale salts, e.g., colloidal silver chloride, ferric ammonium citrate, and mild silver protein, the solid is sprinkled onto the surface of the solvent. As the solute dissolves the more dense solution settles to the bottom of the container and is replaced by more solvent. If these colloids and gums are triturated in a mortar, they tend to form sticky clumps that dissolve very slowly.

It is generally good practice to have the solute divided to facilitate more rapid dissolution; however, the solid may be so finely pulverized that its high surface energy attracts and adsorbs gaseous molecules from the atmosphere. The layer of occluded air hinders contact of the solid surface with the solvent and hinders dissolution. Boric acid is available in crystalline, granular, and powdered form. If an aqueous solution is to be prepared the powdered form should not be used. The powdered form is occluded by air, floats, and is difficult to wet.

Heat may be employed to effect dissolution, but care must be taken to avoid the formation of a metastable or supersaturated solution. A solution of boric acid is sometimes used as an eye wash. If the solution were prepared by heat, and a metastable solution were formed inadvertently, this might later deposit crystals which would be injurious if introduced into the eye. It is interesting to note that pharmacy has long recognized this problem in the preparation known as boric acid solution. The solution, which is dispensed by the pharmacist, is a 5 per cent solution of boric acid known as a "saturated solution," although boric acid is saturated at 5.3 per cent. This medicinal solution is undersaturated, to minimize the possibility of crystal formation.

Heat is to be avoided if the product or prescription contains a volatile or thermolabile drug.

38. Potassium iodide   100 g
    Purified water, q.s.   100 ml

    Sig.: gtt. vi

Dissolve the salt in 68 ml of hot purified water. Cool to room temperature and add sufficient purified water to make 100 ml.

39. Aqueous mild silver protein, 25%   30 ml

    Sig.: Instill in eye

A 25 per cent w/v solution is prepared by sprinkling 7.5 g of mild silver protein on approximately 20 ml of water in a graduate. After dissolution sufficient water is added to bring the volume to 30 ml.

40. Ephedrine sulfate   0.80 g
    Codeine phosphate   0.24 g
    Terpin hydrate elixir, q.s. 120   ml

    Sig.: ℨ i q. 4 hr

DISSOLUTION IN A REACTIVE MEDIUM

The discussion has been concerned with dissolution of a solid in a nonreactive medium. This is applicable to the preparation of solutions and the dissolution of drugs which do not undergo chemical reaction in body fluids. With these slightly soluble nonreacting drugs, e.g., chloramphenicol and griseofulvin, an increase in specific surface of the administered solid is a practical means of decreasing the time required for the drug to dissolve and to speed up onset of therapeutic activity. As physiological conditions are not neutral, acidic and basic drugs react to the various pHs of the gastrointestinal tract with marked changes in solubilities and dissolution rates.

Theory

During the dissolution of a solid acid in an aqueous alkaline medium, there exists a diffusion layer adjacent to the solid surface. Within this layer it may be assumed that there is a concentration gradient of the reactants and products as shown in Figure 86. The solid dissolves as previously discussed and diffuses toward the bulk solution; simultaneously the base diffuses from the bulk solution toward the solid surface. There occurs neutralization and the formation of a salt, which in turn diffuses toward the bulk solution. The distance from the solid surface at which neutralization occurs is represented by

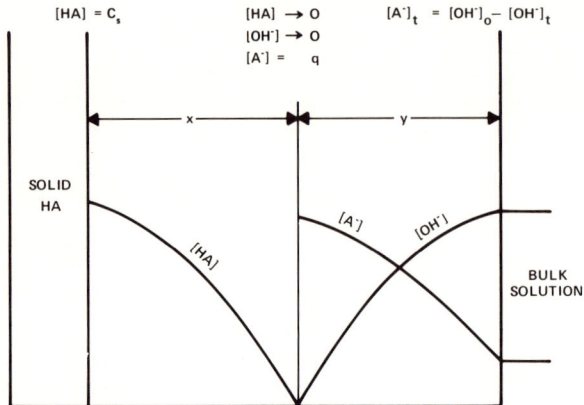

Figure 86. Dissolution of a solid, monocarboxylic acid in an aqueous monohydroxyl base. [HA], [A⁻], and [OH⁻] represent the molar concentrations in various regions of the diffusion layer of the acid, anion, and hydroxyl ion, respectively. C_s is the solubility of the acid in water. $[A^-]_t$ is the total solubility of the anion or salt formed in the alkaline medium by reaction with hydroxyl ion $[OH^-]_t$, where $[OH^-]_0$ is the initial concentration of hydroxyl ion. At the point of neutralization [HA] = [OH⁻] = 0 and the concentration of [A⁻] = q.

x. The distance that the base must diffuse from the bulk solution to the neutralization zone is y. The distance that the neutralization product or salt must diffuse to the bulk solution is also y. The total thickness of the diffusion layer is $x + y$.

The concentration of the acid and base decreases to zero in the neutralization zone as the reaction occurs. Thus, there are concentration gradients of dissolved acid and base, which are probably not linear, as the neutralization zone is not necessarily defined by a single plane as drawn. At any time, the overall dissolution rate of the acid depends on (1) the rate of diffusion of the dissolved, unreacted acid through the solution of the product that has been formed, and (2) the rate of diffusion of the base through the solution of the product, which in itself has a concentration gradient between the zone of neutralization and bulk solution. This oversimplified interpretation applies well to systems involving a reaction equilibrium that lies far to the right.

At a constant alkalinity, an increase in agitation decreases the thickness of the diffusion layer. The dissolution rate is increased.

Pharmaceutical Formulation

The dissolution rate in reactive medium is decreased as the viscosity is increased. The dissolution rate is slowed by the addition of other solutes, which compete for the solvent molecules and effectively decrease the solubility of the drug. Conversely, if the solubility of the drug in the diffusion layer is increased, the dissolution rate of the drug is increased. The solubility of acidic and basic drugs may be increased by modifying the pH of the diffusion layer.

The total solubility of a weak acid, HA, is the sum of the concentration of the un-ionized acid, [HA], and the ionized acid, [A⁻],

$$C_S = [HA] + [A^-]$$

The ionization of a weak acid in an aqueous medium is expressed by its ionization constant, K_a, which is defined by the equation

$$K_a = \frac{[H^+][A^-]}{[HA]}$$

in which the brackets indicate the concentration of the species in moles liter⁻¹. This may be rearranged to

$$[A^-] = K_a \frac{[HA]}{[H^+]}$$

Substituion results in the expression for total solubility of

$$C_S = [HA] + K_a \frac{[HA]}{[H^+]} = [HA]\left(1 + \frac{K_a}{[H^+]}\right)$$

When $[H^+]$ is very small compared to K_a, this equation approaches

$$C_S = K_a \frac{[HA]}{[H^+]}$$

or, expressed in the logarithmic form,

$$\log C_S = \log K_a + \log [HA] - \log [H^+]$$

Using the notation $pH = -\log [H^+]$ and $pK_a = -\log [HA]$, the logarithmic form may be written

$$\log C_S = \log [HA] - pK_a + pH$$

Substituting the C_S term in the Noyes-Whitney equation (see page 28), the dissolution rate is given by

$$\left(\frac{dw}{dt}\right)_{S=1} = k\left(K_a \frac{[HA]}{[H^+]} - C\right)$$

An inspection of the above equation reveals that the dissolution rate of a weak, solid acid increases as the pH of the dissolving fluid is increased.

A similar argument may be advanced for the increase in dissolution rate of a weakly basic solid as the pH of the diffusion layer is decreased.

The dissolution of a solid acidic drug may be increased by increasing the pH of the diffusion layer. In the administration of oral dosage forms, antacids may be administered to raise the pH of the stomach. This method has its limitations and is impractical because of the massive dose of antacid required. Certainly it is an uninspiring method if one is attempting to formulate a product as a single tablet or capsule.

A second method for increasing the dissolution rate of a solid acid is to mix the acid with a solid basic substance, e.g., sodium bicarbonate or sodium citrate. This mixture provides an increased pH of the immediate environment of the acid. In Figure 87 the dissolution rates of several acidic solids are shown as a function of the fraction of acid in the compressed pellet of a mixture of the acid and tribasic sodium phosphate. There is an optimum ratio of the two constituents, depending on the fraction of the total surface of each and the strength of the acid. The maximum dissolution rate of the mixture for a given surface is not as great as the dissolution rate of the true salt.

The most effective and practical means of increasing the pH in the diffusion layer is to use a highly water soluble salt of the weak acid instead of the acid. As the salt dissolves it raises the pH and a higher dissolution rate is obtained. As shown in Table XXXIV, the dissolution rate of the sodium salt of a weak acid in an acidic medium may be many times greater than that of the weak acid itself.

The comparative *in vitro* dissolution rate of several tetracycline derivatives compressed into a pellet with limited surface are tetracycline hydrochloride > tetracycline sodium hexametaphosphate > tetracycline phenolsulfonphthalein > tetracycline. Upon comparing at given times these *in vitro* dissolution rates with the rate of urinary excretion from humans, there appears to be a qualitative correlation as shown in Figure 88. Those derivatives with the faster *in vitro* dissolution rate were excreted at a faster rate, indicating that the dissolution rate controlled the availability of the drug.

After its dissolution as the sodium salt, the drug may be precipitated by the gastric fluid as the free acid. This fact does not nullify this technique, because the drug is precipitated as very fine particles with a large specific surface. This large specific surface maintains a large $(C_S - C)$ value which favors drug dissolution as the drug is absorbed or additional fluids become available.

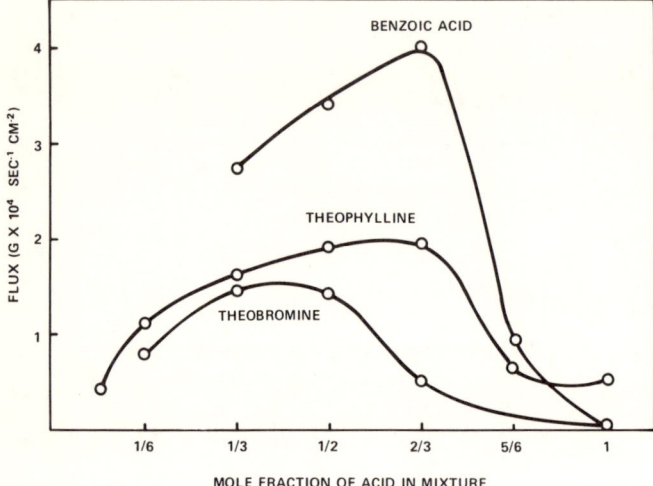

Figure 87. Relationship between dissolution rate and fraction of acid for mixtures of weak acids and tribasic sodium phosphate. [Adapted from E. Nelson, *J. Am. Pharm. Assoc. 47,* 300 (1958).]

Table XXXIV Comparative Dissolution Rates of Weak Acids and Their Sodium Salts in 0.1 N Hydrochloric Acid*

Compound	mg in 100 min (cm^{-2})
Benzoic acid	2.1
Sodium salt	980
Phenobarbital	0.24
Sodium salt	~200
Salicylic acid	1.7
Sodium salt	1870
Succinic acid	2100
Sodium salt	6000
Sulfathiazole	<0.1
Sodium salt	550

* Adapted from E. Nelson, *J. Am. Pharm. Assoc., Sci. Ed. 47,* 297 (1958).

By keeping the dosage form and the surface area constant, this effect has been demonstrated *in vivo* for such drugs as penicillin V, salicylates, and tolbutamide. The gastric absorption of penicillin V and its potassium salt are depicted in Figure 89. The potassium salt with its faster dissolution rate was dissolved and absorbed faster, producing a higher serum level of penicillin V than the acid form.

A chemical reaction may result in products that cause deviations from the dissolution kinetics discussed. If one of the products of the reaction is a gas, e.g., carbon dioxide, this may increase the dissolution rate by producing a greater intensity of agitation by virtue of movement of the bubbles, or this may decrease the dissolution rate by acting as a gaseous barrier between the solid surface and the solvent. The effect cannot be predicted and must be determined experimentally.

A chemical reaction may produce an insoluble product which forms a film on the solid surface. This barrier to the solvent decreases the dissolution rate. This effect has been noted with aluminum aspirin and several amine pamoates and diliturates.

It has been suggested that the rapidity of drug availability is increased by using the most soluble polymorph of a drug. The metastable polymorphs have greater solubilities and dissolution rates than the stable form. Unfortunately, only a few compounds, e.g., methyl prednisolone and riboflavin, have been studied to demonstrate a relation between polymorphism and solubility (and absorption).

dissolution processes • 169

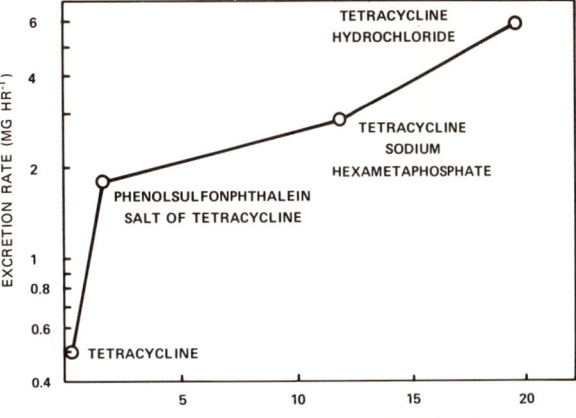

Figure 88. Correlation between excretion rate at 1 hour and *in vitro* dissolution rate when various tetracyclines are taken in the form of pellets. [Adapted from E. Nelson, *J. Am. Pharm Assoc., Sci. Ed. 48,* 96 (1959).]

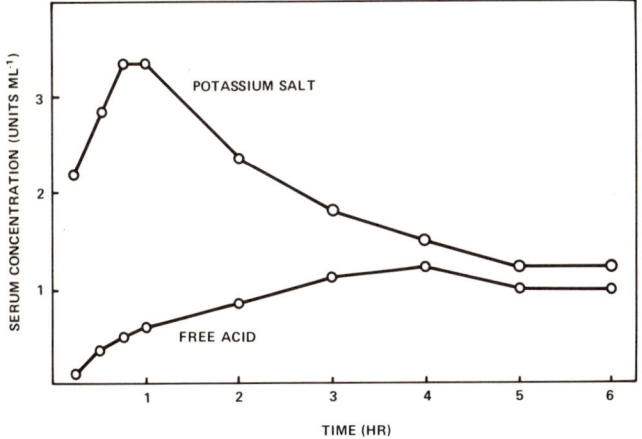

Figure 89. Serum concentration of penicillin V in dogs as a consequence of gastric absorption of the free acid and the potassium salt. [Adapted from C.C. Lee, R.O. Froman, R.C. Anderson and K.K. Chen, *Antibiot. Chemotherapy 8,* 354 (1958).]

7 | AQUEOUS PHARMECEUTICAL SOLUTIONS

Since water is the physiological fluid of the human body, it is not surprising that water is the vehicle in most medicinal solutions. The water used in the preparation and in the completed dosage form depends on the purity required. The U.S. Pharmacopeia recognizes five standards of water.

1) For ablution and extraction of crude drugs and in the operations requiring great amounts of water, tap water conforming to the standards of Water U.S.P. may be used by the pharmaceutical manufacturer. It may contain no more than 0.1 per cent total solids, which consist mostly of inorganic salts, and it meets the U.S. Public Health Service regulations for potable water with respect to bacteriological purity, i.e., not more than one coliform organism per 100 ml sample.

2) Purified Water U.S.P. is water obtained by distillation or by ion-exchange treatment. Freshly distilled water has a pH 5.6; purified water meets specifications if its pH lies between 5 and 7. Purified water may contain not more than 10 parts per million of total solids, and it has a limitation on the amount of oxidizable substances present. Purified water is used in prescriptions and finished manufactured products except for parenteral and ophthalmic products.

3) Water for Injection U.S.P. is intended for use as a solvent for the preparation of parenteral solutions. In addition to conforming to the standards of purified water, it is free of pyrogens, i.e., nonvolatile, fever-producing materials.

4) Sterile Water for Injection U.S.P. is water for injection sterilized and packaged in single-dose containers of Type I or II glass (see page 285) not exceeding 1-liter capacity. The limitations for total solids are: up to 30-ml capacity, 40 parts per million; from 30-ml to 100-ml capacity, 30 parts per million; and for larger sizes 20 parts per million.

6) Bacteriostatic Water for Injection U.S.P. is sterile water for injection containing one or more suitable bacteriostatic agents. In excess of the bacteriostatic agent it may not contain more than 40 parts per million of total solids. It is packaged in a single-dose or multiple-dose container of Type I or II glass with a capacity not exceeding 30 ml.

Solutions have the disadvantage of being bulkier and more liable to degradation and to interactions between constituents than solid dosage forms. Owing to the disagreeable taste of a drug, an oral solution may be difficult to flavor.

The solution has the advantage of being homogeneous and more easily swallowed by some patients than a solid dosage form. With solid drugs having a slow dissolution rate, the action is more rapid with a solution as the drug is dissolved and ready for absorption upon administration.

The same fundamental interactions and characteristics are present in all aqueous solutions; however, it is convenient to classify aqueous solutions according to their use and/or formulation.

AROMATIC WATERS

Aromatic waters are saturated aqueous solutions of volatile oils or other aromatic or volatile substances. An aromatic water may be used as a pleasantly flavored vehicle for a water-soluble drug or as the aqueous phase in an emulsion or suspension. If a large amount of a water-soluble drug is added to an aromatic water, there may be a separation of an insoluble layer at the top. If this layer is taken with a dose of the medication, an irritating and burning taste will be experienced. This separation or salting out may be viewed as a competitive process in which the molecules of the water-soluble drug have more attraction for the solvent molecules of water than the volatile oil molecules; thus, the associated water molecules are pulled away from the volatile oil molecules, which are then no longer held in solution. Formulation 41 is cloudy because of the separation of the peppermint oil caused by the sodium bromide.

    41. Sodium bromide   20 g
           Peppermint water, q.s.   120 ml

           Sig.: $\mathfrak{z}$ i p.r.n.

Aromatic waters are primarily vehicles, as the small amount of aromatic substance present is insufficient to exert a significant therapeutic action. Waters should be stored in tight, light-resistant bottles because loss due to volatilization and degradation from sunlight impairs their flavor and fragrance. Cold temperatures decrease the solubility of the volatile constituents, producing cloudiness.

Aromatic waters may be prepared by three methods — distillation, solution, and alternate solution. Distillation is a universal method, but it is not practical or economical in most products; however, it is the only method of preparing stronger rose water and orange flower water.

In preparing Stronger Rose Water U.S.P. the fresh flowers of the rose are mixed with distilled water and steam distilled. Excessive heat and contact of the flowers with the vessel is avoided to prevent the development of an empyreumatic odor, i.e., odor peculiar to organic substances burned in a closed vessel, resulting from the scorching of the flowers. The excess oil is separated from the distillate; the clear aqueous portion is stronger rose water. Filtration may be necessary. Rose water is prepared by diluting the stronger rose water with an equal volume of purified water.

In the solution method 2 ml or 2 g of the volatile substance is agitated for 15 minutes with sufficient water to make 1000 ml of solution, set aside for 12 hours, and filtered through wetted filter paper. The wetted filter paper prevents the passage of excess oil into the filtrate and eliminates adsorption of the dissolved aromatics. As many fine droplets are formed, it is often difficult to obtain a clear solution by this time-consuming process.

Alternate solution is the most expedient method of preparing waters. The volatile substance is thoroughly mixed with 15 g of an inert adsorptive agent, e.g., talc, purified siliceous earth, and pulped filter paper. A liter of purified water is added and agitated for 10 minutes. The solution is filtered until a clear filtrate is obtained and enough purified water is added to make the product measure 1000 ml. The volatile substance is adsorbed on the inert ingredient, increasing the total area of volatile substance exposed to the water, thus facilitating the formation of a saturated solution. The adsorptive agent also acts as a clarifier in filtration, as the undissolved volatile material remains adsorbed and does not pass through the filter.

SYRUPS

A syrup is a concentrated or nearly saturated aqueous solution of sugar. Syrup U.S.P. contains 850 g of sucrose and 450 ml of water in a liter of syrup; yet, it is not saturated, as 1 g of sucrose dissolves in 0.5 ml of water. The high content of sugar imparts to syrups a moderately high viscosity, e.g., 100 cp, and a high specific gravity, e.g., 1.2 to 1.4.

The sweet taste of syrups makes them pleasant vehicles for the oral administration of medication. Syrups that contain no medicinal agent are known as flavoring syrups, e.g., cherry syrup, cocoa syrup, and tolu balsam syrup. Traditionally it has been suggested that the bitter taste of alkaloids be masked by aromatic eriodictyon syrup or glycyrrhiza syrup and that a saline taste be masked by cherry or raspberry syrup. Although this may be true in many instances, the choice of a masking and flavoring

172 • aqueous solutions

vehicle is unpredictable and must be experimentally determined by a taste panel. Syrups that contain therapeutically active compounds are known as medicinal syrups, e.g., chlorpheniramine maleate syrup, ephedrine sulfate syrup, and piperazine citrate syrup.

42. Hydrocodone bitartrate   0.1 g
    Purified water   5.0 ml
    Cherry syrup, q.s.   100 ml

Sig.: ℨ i for cough

43. Potassium iodide   18 g
    Ipecac syrup   18 ml
    Tolu balsam syrup   18 ml
    Purified water, q.s.   120 ml

Sig.: ℨ i s.o.s.

There are three methods of preparing syrups: (1) agitation, (2) agitation with heat, and (3) percolation. Orange syrup is an example of a syrup prepared by agitation without heat. The sweet orange peel tincture and citric acid are mixed with talc, and purified water is gradually added with agitation. The talc serves to distribute the orange oil and to aid filtration. The mixture is filtered and sucrose is added to the filtrate. Solution is completed by agitation. Heat is avoided, as the flavor would be impaired by a loss of the volatile orange oil. Orange syrup is a slightly acidic, flavored vehicle. It should be stored in a tight container, as the terpines in the orange oil may be oxidized to products possessing a terebinthinate taste.

Syrup U.S.P. is a 85 per cent w/v or an approximately 65 per cent w/w sucrose solution with a specific gravity of 1.313. It is used as a sweetening agent and a vehicle for other syrups. Syrup may be prepared by any of the three methods. Syrup prepared by agitation of sucrose and water is colorless. As the sucrose dissolves and saturation is approached, the dissolution rate becomes slow as the concentration gradient $(C_s - C)$ becomes small. Thus, the preparation of syrups by agitation is not a rapid process.

Syrup U.S.P. may be made by adding sucrose to boiling water. Syrup prepared by the hot method frequently has a pale yellow color. A solution of sucrose undergoes hydrolysis to dextrose and fructose in the presence of mineral acids or heat. While an aqueous solution of sucrose rotates polarized light to the right, a hydrolyzed solution rotates polarized light* to the left. The hydrolysis is consequently known as inversion. Invert sugar is an equimolar mixture of dextrose and fructose. Invert sugar is reputed to be sweeter and more easily fermented than sucrose.

---

*Polarimetric measurements are reduced to a set of standard conditions. The length used as a standard is 10 cm for liquids. The standard wavelength is that of green mercury line (5461 Å), although the sodium doublet (589 Å + 5896 Å) had been widely used in the past. The standard temperature is 20°. The specific rotation, $[\alpha]$, at a temperature indicated by a superscript and at a wavelength indicated by a subscript, is defined as

$$[\alpha] = \frac{100}{dc}$$

where α is the observed rotation in degrees, d the layer thickness of the solution in decimeters, and c the concentration of solute in g per 100 ml of solution.

aqueous solutions • 173

$$+66.4 \qquad +52.3 \qquad -92$$

$$[\alpha]_D^{20°} = -39.7°$$

If a sugar solution is excessively heated, the sweet taste is destroyed and a dark brown liquid is formed. This process is known as caramelization. The hot method cannot be used to prepare a syrup containing a thermolabile or volatile ingredient. When using the hot method the temperature should be carefully controlled to avoid darkening of the syrup.

Syrup U.S.P. may be prepared by percolation. Percolation is the extraction process in which the desired constituents are dissolved from a granulated or powdered drug by the descent at a controlled rate of suitable solvent through a column of the drug. A percolator is a cylindrical or tapered vessel with a lower outlet from which the flow may be controlled (see page 243). The sucrose is packed into a percolator, which has a layer of loosely packed cotton over the lower outlet. Purified water is added and the percolate is regulated to a steady drip. Granulated sugar should be used, because fine sugar upon being moistened tends to clog the percolator. If necessary the percolate is returned to the percolator until all the sucrose has dissolved.

Wild cherry syrup is an example of a syrup prepared by percolation with subsequent solution of sucrose in the percolate. The percolator is prepared by placing a thin layer of cotton across the lower outlet, covering this with a thin layer of washed sand, and placing a close-fitting piece of filter paper on the sand. The coarse wild cherry is moistened with water before placing it in the percolator to permit swelling. If expansion occurred after the drug was packed in the percolator, it might interfere with the flow of the solvent. The moistened wild cherry is packed evenly into the percolator and covered with filter paper. Purified water is added as the menstruum, or solvent. Unless the lower outlet is open during the initial addition of the menstruum, the displaced air will rise forming channels through which the menstruum will flow. When the menstruum has been added and allowed to flow down to the outlet, the lower outlet is closed and a layer of menstruum is maintained above the drug. The drug is allowed to macerate or soak for 1 hour. During this period the glucoside of d-mandelonitrile is hydrolyzed to glucose, hydrocyanic acid, and benzaldehyde by the enzyme emulsin. The benzaldehyde imparts the characteristic flavor to this syrup. Heat is not used, as it would deactivate the enzyme and cause the loss of the volatile constituents. During the maceration period equilibrium is established for dissolution of the soluble constituents. After maceration percolation is allowed to proceed rapidly by opening the lower outlet so that percolation is completed in 4 hours. The percolate is collected in a graduated container, which shows the volume of the percolate and the final volume of syrup. Sucrose is added to the percolate and dissolved by agitation. Glycerin is added to maintain any extracted tannin in solution. Alcohol is added as a preservative.

The great solubility of sugar in water indicates that the hydration or hydrogen bonding between sucrose and water is very strong. This strong association between the solute and solvent prevents to any great extent further association of the water dipoles with additional water-soluble drugs; therefore, syrups have a low solvent capacity for water-soluble drugs that may be added. For this reason it may be difficult or impossible to dissolve a drug in a syrup, although the drug would dissolve in the same volume of water. It is often expedient to dissolve a drug in a small quantity of water and to add the flavoring syrup to this solution.

When a bottle of syrup has been used there is frequently unsightly crystallization around, and sticking of the cap. The use of 20 per cent sorbitol in the syrup reduces this tendency to crystallize and may improve the chemical stability of certain drugs.

Glycerin may be used as a cosolvent to increase the solubility of tannin and vegetable extractives in syrups, e.g., wild cherry syrup and ipecac syrup. Alcohol facilitates the incorporation of color and flavor into syrups, e.g., tolu balsam syrup and glycyrrhiza syrup.

The concentration of sucrose in a syrup is critical in the control of microorganic growth. Dilute sucrose solutions are excellent media for microorganisms. Some syrups do not contain a preservative as the concentration of sucrose approaches saturation and the syrups are self-preserved. A saturated solution is not desired, as fluctuations in temperature might cause crystallization of large crystals, which would be difficult to redissolve. Syrup U.S.P. is a self-preserved solution with a minimum chance of crystallization. Syrups developed for commercial use contain other ingredients to obtain the desired solubility for the drug as well as for improvement of taste, appearance, and stability. In such syrups the additive preservative effects of the ingredients are considered during formulation.

In 1 liter of Syrup U.S.P., 850 g of sucrose preserves 463 ml of water; i.e., 1 g of sucrose preserves 0.54 ml of water. The 850 g of sucrose apparently assumes a volume of 537 ml; i.e., 1 g of sucrose occupies a volume of 0.632 ml.

If a potential product being developed contains 600 g of sucrose per liter, the amount of alcohol that must be added to preserve the syrup can be estimated. The 600 g of sucrose will preserve 600 X 0.54 or 324 ml of water. The total volume of the solution, which would be equivalent to Syrup U.S.P., would be the sum of the volume occupied by the sucrose (600 X 0.632 = 379 ml) and the volume of the water preserved by this amount of sucrose (324 ml), or 703 ml. The free water equivalent per liter of this formulation is 1000 - 703 or 297 ml.

Assuming that water is preserved by 18 per cent alcohol, the free water requires 297 X 0.18 or 54 ml of absolute alcohol. In addition to the 600 g of sucrose the final liter of syrup must contain 5.4 per cent alcohol to prevent fermentation.

In general, when dissolved solids other than sucrose are present, the volume they occupy may be subtracted from the free water volume. If glycerin is present, the per cent by volume may be doubled and this value is subtracted from the free water volume. The preservative effect of propylene glycol is equivalent to that of alcohol.

If 1 liter of a product in the developmental stage contains 200 g of sucrose, 5 per cent glycerin, and 150 g of solids that occupy a volume of 60 ml, the amount of alcohol required to preserve this product may be predicted as shown below. This calculated value is then verified by actual storage tests.

The volume of Syrup U.S.P. to which this is equivalent is the sum of the volume occupied by the sucrose (200 X 0.632 = 126 ml) and the corresponding amount of water in Syrup U.S.P. (200 X 0.54 = 108), or 126 + 108 = 234 ml. The difference between the total volume and the syrup equivalent is the free water equivalent, which is 1000 - 234 = 766 ml. From this volume of free water the volume occupied by the solid (60 ml) and the glycerin (100 ml) is subtracted to leave 604 ml of free water. The alcohol required to preserve this free water is 604 X 0.18 = 109 ml. Thus, 10.9 per cent alcohol is required in the product.

SOLUTIONS

As a class of pharmaceuticals, solutions are liquid preparations which contain one or more solutes and which are not by their method of preparation or ingredients classified within another category. Syrups are solutions, but, by virtue of the sucrose content, they are classified as a distinctive pharmaceutical class of preparations. Nasal, ophthalmic, and parenteral solutions are physically solutions; however, they are classified separately because of their specific use and method of production.

Mouthwashes are solutions used for cleansing the mouth or treating diseased conditions of the oral mucous membrane. Most mouthwashes are used for a cosmetic rather than a therapeutic purpose. They impart a pleasant taste and odor while rinsing the mouth.

44. Boric acid   25.00 g
    Thymol   0.50 g
    Chlorothymol   0.50 g
    Menthol   0.50 g
    Eucalyptol   0.10 ml
    Menthyl salicylate   0.20 ml
    Thyme oil   0.01 ml
    Alcohol   300.00 ml
    Purified water, q.s. 1000   ml

Sig.: N.F. Antiseptic Solution

Mouthwashes frequently contain alcohol or glycerin to aid in dissolving the volatile ingredients. In N.F. Antiseptic Solution the boric acid is dissolved in the purified water and the remaining ingredients are dissolved in the alcohol. The two solutions are mixed and allowed to stand for a minimum of 2 hours to ensure saturation. The solution is cooled to 10° and filtered with talc to yield a clear solution. If this precaution were not taken, storage in a cool place would result in a lower solubility and separation of the volatile components, i.e., a cloudy product.

Special denatured alcohol rendered unsuitable for internal use has been approved by the U.S. Treasury Department for use in N. F. Antiseptic Solution if adjustments are made for the amounts of ingredients in the formula. The use of special denatured alcohols for economical reason is common in commercial products, e.g., rubbing alcohol.

If borates are present in a mouthwash, e.g., N. F. Mouthwash, containing glycerin, a chemical reaction occurs. An aqueous solution of sodium borate may hydrolyze to sodium metaborate and boric acid, which may react with glycerin to form an acidic compound, glyceroboric acid, as postulated in the equation

$$2 \begin{array}{c} CH_2OH \\ | \\ CH\text{-}OH \\ | \\ CH_2OH \end{array} + H_3BO_3 \rightarrow 3H_2O + H^+ + \begin{array}{c} CH_2\text{-}O \\ | \\ CH\text{-}O \end{array}\!\!B\text{-}O\text{-}\begin{array}{c} CH_2OH \\ | \\ CH\text{ O-} \\ | \\ CH_2 \\ | \\ CH_2OH \end{array}$$

The glyceroboric acid then reacts with potassium bicarbonate with the effervescence of carbon dioxide. It should be noted that N.F. Antiseptic Solution is acidic, whereas N.F. Mouthwash is alkaline.

Locally applied solutions which precipitate protein-reducing cell permeability without injury are known as astringent solutions. Grossly, astringents cause constriction with wrinkling of the skin and blanching. As astringents reduce secretions, they are used as antiperspirants. Aluminum acetate solution and aluminum subacetate solution are used as wet dressings in a wide range of contact dermatitis; they are diluted 10 to 40 times for use. These solutions become turbid upon standing as more basic and less soluble salts are formed. The precipitation is minimized by the addition of boric acid, which maintains an acidic solution.

Calcium hydroxide solution is a mild astringent employed in lotions as a reactant and an alkalizer. It is prepared by agitation of purified water and calcium hydroxide for 1 hour. Cold water is used as the calcium hydroxide is more soluble at lower than at higher temperatures. The solution is stored over undissolved calcium hydroxide to keep the solution saturated. As the calcium hydroxide reacts rapidly with the carbon dioxide of the air, forming calcium carbonate, the solution should be stored in well-filled, tight containers. Only a clear solution should be used by the patient, as cloudiness indicates the formation of calcium carbonate and thus reduction of the quantity of dissolved calcium hydroxide.

Antibacterial topical solutions are those solutions which, when applied to the skin or mucous membrane in the proper strength and under appropriate conditions, will kill bacteria. Benzalkonium chloride solution, strong iodine solution, and methylrosaniline chloride solution are topical antibacterial solutions. Instruments and inanimate objects may be disinfected by formaldehyde, isopropyl alcohol, and nitromersol solution. Alcohol in a 70 per cent concentration is a good antiseptic for the skin and inanimate objects.

Quarternary ammonium, cationic surface-active agents, e.g., benzalkonium chloride, benzethonium chloride, and cetylpyridinium chloride, are used in antibacterial solutions of concentrations from 1:500 to 1:10,000. In the higher concentration the solutions of the quaternary ammonium compounds are used for sterile storage of instruments. These solutions are used in genitourinary irrigation in concentrations from 1:2000 to 1:20,000 and as a skin disinfectant in concentrations from 1:750 to 1:5000. As preservatives in maintaining the sterility of ophthalmic solutions, they are employed in the approximate concentration of 1:10,000. Unnecessary agitation should be avoided in preparing and packaging these solutions, as they greatly lower interfacial tension, which may result in foaming if strongly agitated.

Hydrogen peroxide solution finds its chief use in cleansing wounds where the effervesence due to the release of oxygen mechanically removes debris from the wound. It is also used as a mouthwash. Hydrogen peroxide solution is a 3 per cent solution which liberates 10 times its volume of oxygen. In the presence of organic matter, light, and heat the solution degrades rapidly. Small concentrations of acetanilid, oxyquinoline, or tetrasodium pyrophosphate may be added to stabilize the solution.

Iodine solution is an effective, nonirritating germicide and fungicide. Upon the addition of 2.4 per cent sodium iodide, 2 per cent water-insoluble iodine is dissolved as the triiodide ion. This is an example of the use of complex formation to effect solution. The dissolution of iodine in strong iodine solution is also effected by complex ion formation.

Nitromersol solution is among the best of the mercurial local antibacterial agents. The solution is prepared by adding nitromersol to an aqueous solution containing sodium hydroxide and sodium carbonate. In an alkaline medium the ring of the insoluble nitromersol is opened and a water-soluble salt is formed,

Thimerosal is maintained in solution as the sodium salt by the use of sodium borate and ethylenediamine, which maintain the required alkalinity. The ethylenediamine absorbs carbon dioxide from the air, forming a nonvolatile carbonate. Monoethanolamine prevents the development of irritating properties in the solution upon storage.

45. Thimerosal   1.00 g
    Ethylenediamine solution 0.28 g
    Monoethanolamine   1.00 g
    Sodium borate   1.40 g
    Sodium chloride   8.00 g
    Purified water, q.s.   1000   ml

Sig.: Thimerosal solution

Merbromin solution offers another example of the technique of using a soluble salt of an insoluble drug to prepare a solution. If nitromersol solution, merbromin solution, or thimerosal solution is mixed with acidic substances, the salt is destroyed and the less soluble compound precipitates. This can be illustrated by the reaction of merbromin in an acidic medium,

A solution of water-soluble nitrofurazone is prepared by using a mixture of polyethylene glycols as a cosolvent.

46. Nitrofurazone 2.0 g
Polyethylene glycol 1540 325.0 g
Polyethylene glycol 300 325.0 g
Octylphenoxy polyethoxyethanol 3.3 g
Water 344.7 ml

Sig.: Nitrofurazone solution

The nitrofurazone is dissolved in the polyethylene glycol mixture, which has been heated to 70° in a glass or stainless-steel container. The solution of octylphenoxy polyethoxyethanol in water is slowly added to the polyethylene glycol solution at 45°.

Carbol-Fuchsin solution is another example of the use of a cosolvent system to dissolve a compound with limited water solubility. The basic fuchsin is dissolved in a mixture of alcohol and water. This solution is added to an aqueous solution of the remaining ingredients.

FLAVOR

To receive consumer acceptance drug and cosmetic products must be aesthetically appealing. The patient assumes pharmaceuticals to be safe and effective, and he judges a product by its appearance, color, flavor, odor, and package design. Pediatric patients especially insist on a pleasant-tasting medication. Pharmaceutical firms are concerned with flavor because, with the similarity of products marketed, it is often the flavor and patient acceptance that will sell a product.

The organs of taste or the taste buds are modified epithelial cells situated mainly on the tongue. A taste bud responds to a solution of a substance by eliciting one of the four primary tastes: sweet, sour, salty, and bitter. It is believed by some that the four types of taste buds are not equally distributed over the tongue. The receptors sensitive to sweet and salty taste are most abundant at the tip of the tongue, whereas those aroused by bitter substances are toward the base of the tongue. The taste buds responsive to acid are distributed mainly along the margin of the tongue.

Certain substances stimulate more than one type of taste bud. Sodium salicylate produces a sweet taste when applied to the tip of the tongue, but when it is swallowed there is a bitter taste as the sodium salicylate passes the region of the epiglottis. Magnesium sulfate produces a salty taste at the tip of the tongue and a bitter taste at the base of the tongue.

Sour taste is caused by the hydrogen ion. Salty taste is generally caused by an ionized salt of relatively low molecular weight. The correlation of bitter and sweet tastes with chemical structure has been specific and only a few general rules have been advanced. With the limited understanding of flavor chemistry, each flavor problem of the pharmacist must be solved by experimentation.

The flavoring agents used may be chemical compounds, e.g., anethole, methyl salicylate, and vanillin, or volatile oils, e.g., anise oil, cinnamon oil, and spearmint oil. Galenical preparations, e.g., glycyrrhiza fluid extract, compound orange spirit, and vanilla tincture, are used in some oral liquids. Traditional pharmaceutical classes are employed as flavor vehicles, e.g., peppermint water, cherry syrup, and aromatic elixir. A saline taste may be masked or disguised by the use of glycyrrhiza syrup, cinnamon syrup, and raspberry syrup. Cherry syrup and acacia syrup are useful in disguising acid taste. Bitterness may be masked by use of aromatic eriodictyon syrup, raspberry syrup, and cocoa syrup.

The majority of flavors used in commercial products are blends or imitation flavors. These imitation flavors are more uniform and cheaper than the natural flavors.

47.
Vanillin	0.180 g
Indol	0.004 g
Aldehyde C_{16}	0.240 ml
Diacetyl	0.060 ml
Phenyl ethyl alcohol	0.240 ml
Aldehyde C_{14}	0.015 ml
Aldehyde C_{18}	0.015 ml
Aldehyde C_{20}	0.400 ml
Orange flower oil	0.005 ml
Ethyl butyrate	0.120 ml
Benzyl acetate	0.075 ml
Alpha novoviol	0.400 ml
Beta novoviol	0.200 ml
Lemon oil	0.060 ml
Propylene glycol, q.s.	100 ml

Sig.: Imitation raspberry concentrate

The most prevalent technique of flavoring liquid medicinals is to add substances that will disguise the ill taste. Odor as well as taste is considered because the subtle variations of flavor are a composite of the psychological blending of the primary taste with the odor and texture of the product. Ginger is not recognized only by the response of the taste buds but also by the burning sensation in the mouth and its odor. Anyone who has a cold with a blocked nasal passage can affirm the contribution of smell to flavor. Unpleasant odors may be masked by aromatic flavors, e.g., benzaldehyde, maple, and vanilla. Menthol, methyl salicylate, and peppermint oil contribute to disguising ill taste by their ability to partially anesthetize the taste buds.

Sweetness is the first sensation sought in most products. Sucrose, mannitol, and sorbitol are natural sweetening agents. The sodium or calcium salts of cyclamate and saccharin are the most widely used synthetic sweetening agents. Excessive concentrations of the synthetic sweetening agents elicit a bitter taste. A 1:10 ratio of saccharin to cyclamate has been found to provide the maximum sweetening with the least bitter aftertaste.

Blends of several flavors are more successful than a single flavor. The product should not be too strongly flavored because the patient will be repeatedly receiving the medication and a strongly flavored preparation may become distasteful. The flavor may be enhanced by the addition of traces of monosodium glutamate, citric acid, malic acid, and sodium chloride.

The texture of a product influences its flavor. A flavored, chewable tablet or a troche should not yield large, gritty particles which produce an unpleasant sensation. Powdered flavors are available for most solid dosage forms. These dry flavors are prepared by spray drying liquid flavors with acacia. The aftertaste of many drugs is caused by the slow removal of the drug from the taste pore. A viscid liquid clings to the oral mucosa and elicits a taste for a longer time than a less viscous liquid.

A decrease in the solubility of a drug will increase the palatability of the product. Occasionally the solubility of the drug may be decreased by use of high concentrations of sugar or sorbitol which salt out the drug. More effective is the use of a derivative that is insoluble and therefore tasteless. Chloramphenicol palmitate is an insoluble derivative which lacks the bitter taste of chloramphenicol; it is used in the formulation of an oral pediatric suspension. Erythromycin ethylcarbonate and triacetyloleandomycin are similarly used in oral suspensions. In using an insoluble derivative it must be demonstrated that the derivative is therapeutically active or forms an active compound in the body.

Carbonation may be used to mask saline and bitter taste. Magnesium citrate solution is a lemon-flavored solution in which the bitter, saline taste of the magnesium ion has been masked by carbonation. Effervescent granules react to carbonate the water before administration.

Emulsification of two immiscible liquids has been suggested for improving the taste. The unpalatable oil or drug dissolved in oil is emulsified into the internal phase, where it is surrounded by a flavored, aqueous phase. Emulsification also eliminates the unpleasant tactual sensation that oil produces in the mouth.

As different persons respond differently to the same taste stimulus, the use of a taste panel is probably the best method of comparative evaluation of a flavored product. The purpose of a taste panel is not to establish customer taste preference but to compare several formulations and to indicate which has the least undesirable flavor characteristics. The main purpose of a flavoring agent is to mask the unpleasant flavor of the drug; a secondary purpose is to impart a well-balanced flavor to the product.

A taste panel may consist of a dozen persons who are in good health and are not affected by any condition that would interfere with their sense of taste and smell. All samples to be tasted should be at room temperature. The mouth is rinsed with 5 ml of purified water. A teaspoonful of the medication is taken into the mouth and thoroughly rinsed to all regions of the mouth. The sample is then ejected and the mouth is rinsed with purified water. The panelist evaluates the formulation on an arbitrary scale, e.g., a 9-point scale, with 0 indicating the lack of a characteristic and 8 indicating a very strong characteristic.

A suspension may be evaluated for the following characteristics: initial bitterness, aftertaste, and tactual feel. Each of these characteristics is given a numerical rating by the panelist. The average rating of the panel and the standard deviation are calculated and used to select the most acceptable formulation. Some pharmaceutical firms establish maximal values which a formulation must not exceed if the formulation is to be considered.

COLOR

Color enhances the sales appeal of cosmetics and the consumer acceptance of medication. The correct design of the label and its color harmony with the packaged product may influence the sale of cosmetic and nonprescription products. In addition to the improvement of appearance, the coloring of pharmaceuticals may be a safety factor in aiding the patient to identify or distinguish between different medications. When a color is properly used, it will facilitate an associated taste response. The green dye in a mint-flavored liquid will by psychological association enhance the flavor. Color may be used to modify or conceal visual impressions. On occasion a physician may wish to continue a drug in which the patient has lost confidence. The physician may then prescribe the same drug in a product with a different appearance, e.g., Alurate® Elixir is available as a red or green elixir; aspirin tablets are available as white, pink, or green tablets.

Colorants used in foods, pharmaceuticals, and cosmetics are known as color additives. The pharmaceutical colorants can be classified into three groups: natural coloring agents, synthetic dyes, and pigments. The natural coloring agents, e.g., caramel and chlorophyll, have largely been replaced by synthetic dyes.

180 • aqueous solutions

Dyes are defined as colorants that are soluble; pigments are colorants that are insoluble. Lakes or pigments are prepared by the reaction of water-soluble dyes with aluminum or calcium radicals and the precipitation on a substrate of aluminum hydrate.

Certified food colors are a select group of dyes that are investigated chemically, physically, biologically, and clinically and have been shown to be safe for consumption. Each batch is approved by the Food and Drug Administration. The certified dyes are classified into three classes. Those certified for use in food, drug, and cosmetics are known as F.D. & C. dyes, e.g., F.D. & C. Red No. 2. The certified dyes listed in Table XXXV are frequently used as the basic colors for pharmaceuticals. Dyes permitted only in drugs and cosmetics are known as D. & C. dyes. If the dye is permitted to be used only externally for drugs and cosmetics, it is known as an Ext. D.C. dye.

The color additives used in pharmaceuticals are restricted by legal requirements, and before using a color additive its current legal status should be ascertained. With a restricted number of dyes a wide range of hues may be obtained by blending of the dyes. There are three physiological primary hues: blue, red, and yellow. By blending two of the primary hues, a secondary color is obtained; e.g., orange is a secondary color made from red and yellow. The hue selected should be appropriate to the flavor and psychological associations with the product; e.g., cough syrups are traditionally associated with a wild cherry flavor and a brownish-red color.

In preparing aqueous solutions of dyes, it is preferable to make a slurry of the dye with a small volume of water in a glass or stainless-steel container. This is then diluted with water at 70° and stirred until dissolved. The solution is allowed to cool, is diluted to final volume, and is filtered.

Excessive color additives are to be avoided. To color a solution, 0.005 to 0.001 per cent synthetic dyes are required. Emulsions require 0.005 to 0.001 per cent color additive. With emulsions it may be advisable to color each phase using a water-soluble and an oil-soluble dye to achieve a more uniform color.

As the concentration of a dye changes, its hue may change. This is known as heterochromism. A 0.005 per cent amaranth solution is a magenta red, and a 0.0125 per cent solution is scarlet. Upon increasing the amaranth concentration to 0.03 per cent, a reddish-orange color is produced. The hue further varies with the thickness of the color layer in a coated tablet or a colored capsule.

A powder may be tinted by incorporation of 0.1 per cent colorant. Dyes may be added to a solid by use of a volatile solvent which has a limited solvent capacity for the powder. In the production of compressed tablets a solution of the dye is added to the excipient and blended. The wet blend is granulated and dried in an oven. The dry colored blend is then ground to a 100-mesh granulation. A powdered pigment or dye may be blended with the excipient; however, fine grinding is necessary to obtain a uniform color.

Chemical groups responsible for the color of a compound are known as chromophores. The chromophores determine the chemical classification of the dye and its oxidation or reduction potential. The common chromophores are the azo, azoxy, carbonyl, ethenyl, nitro, nitroso, and thio groups. The valence electrons of these unsaturated groups absorb certain wavelengths of visible light, i.e., 400 to 700 mμ. The light of the visible spectrum which is not absorbed by the compound is transmitted or reflected, and the compound has the color of the unabsorbed light. If a substance exposed to white light absorbs the blue wavelength, the substance is orange. Usually more than a single chromophore is necessary to produce a colored molecule. The absorption spectrum of an aqueous solution of F.D. & C. Red No. 3 is shown in Figure 90.

Certain groups, e.g., amino, alkylamino, and dialkylamino, intensify the color of a chromophore-containing molecule. These groups, known as auxochromes, increase the resonance of the dye molecule and cause the absorption of longer wavelengths of light, resulting in a deeper color. The auxochromes determine the reaction of the dye to acid, alkali, and light.

The certified dyes may be classified as azo, indigoid, pyrazolone, triphenylmethane, and xanthene derivatives. The majority employed in pharmaceuticals are of the azo type. Most of the

Table XXXV Frequently Used Certified F. D. & C. Colors

Name	Common Name	Shade	Solubility (g in 100 ml) at 25°		
			Water	Glycerin	Propylene Glycol
F. D. & C. Red No. 1	Ponceau 3R	Cherry red	9.8	5	1.25
F. D. & C. Red No. 2	Amaranth	Magenta red	20	18	1
F. D. & C. Red No. 3	Erythrosine	Bluish pink	9	20	20
F. D. & C. Red No. 4	Ponceau SX	Scarlet	11	5.8	2
F. D. & C. Blue No. 1	Brilliant Blue FCF	Greenish blue	20	20	20
F. D. & C. Blue No. 2	Indigotine	Blue	1.6	1	0.1
F. D. & C. Green No. 1	Guinea Green B	Bluish green	20	20	20
F. D. & C. Green No. 2	Light Green SF Yellowish	Bluish green	20	20	20
F. D. & C. Green No. 3	Fast Green FCF	Bluish green	20	20	20
F. D. & C. Violet No. 1	Wool Violet 5BN	Violet	20	20	20
F. D. & C. Yellow No. 5	Tartrazine	Lemon yellow	20	18	7
F. D. & C. Yellow No. 6	Sunset Yellow FCF	Yellowish orange	19	20	2.2

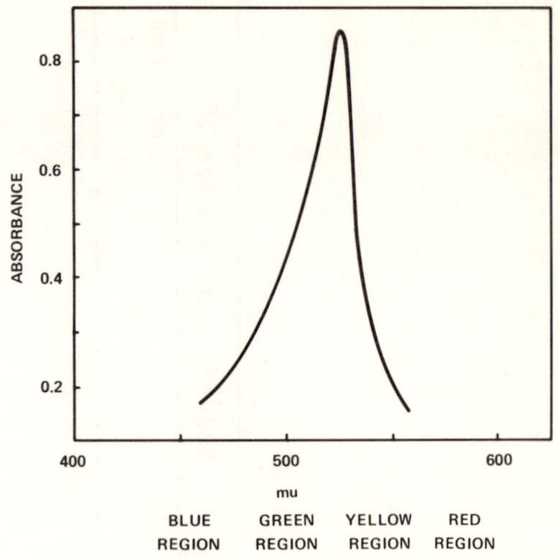

Figure 90. Absorption curve of F.D.&C. Red No. 3 in water at pH 9.

water-soluble dyes are sulfonates or salts of acidic dyes. Although the sulfonic acid salts are not greatly affected by acids, as the sulfonic acid is strongly ionized and soluble, other acidic dyes may have a loss of color or solubility in an acidic medium. The large anion of an acidic dye often forms an insoluble salt by reacting with a large cation, e.g., quaternary ammonium compound or a basic dye. As the concentrations are small, this reaction is often overlooked in the initial steps of product development. The reactions may be illustrated by F.D. & C. Red No. 3, the disodium salt of tetraiodofluorescein,

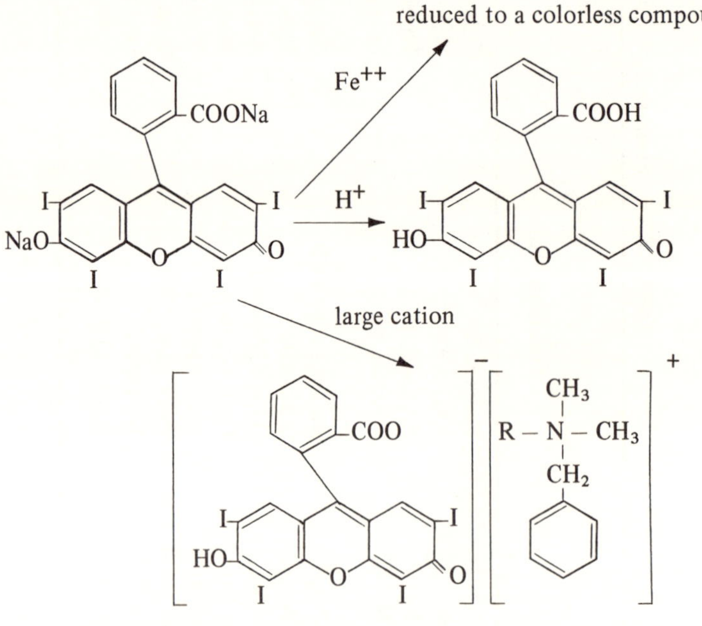

Acidic dyes may lose their color in the presence of trace metallic ions, which function as reducing agents. The components of a formulation may interact with the dye; e.g., in aqueous solution ascorbic acid reduces amaranth with a loss of color. In pan coating a compressed tablet containing an iron salt, the dye may react with the iron to produce a mottled tablet. A coating of shellac before the application of the coloring syrups eliminates this interaction.

The solubility of a dye may be critically affected by a slight lowering of temperature during storage and shipment. Neutral electrolytes physically salt out dyes from some formulations.

Most pharmaceuticals from time of production to utilization are not exposed to sunlight to any significant extent. Amber glass containers afford good protection from light normally encountered. Fading is caused by the visible and ultraviolet light; however, other factors influence the rate and degree of fading. The presence of air and reducing and oxidizing agents accelerate fading.

IONIC PROPERTIES

Since many drugs are electrolytes, which dissociate into ions when dissolved in water, an appreciation of ionic mobility and ionic interactions enables a pharmacist to better understand the properties of medicinal solutions containing electrolytes.

Mobility

A current is conducted in an electrolytic solution by the movement of ions. The movement of the ions produces chemical reactions and a transport of matter to the electrodes. The cation moves toward the negative electrode, where reduction occurs; the anion moves toward the positive electrode, where oxidation occurs.

The cation and anion do not necessarily carry the same fraction of the current. The fraction of the current carried through the solution is a function of the relative velocities with which the cation and anion move. The faster ion carries the larger amount of the current. The fraction of the current carried by an ionic species is known as its transference number. The transference number of the cation, n_c, is

$$n_c = \frac{v_c}{v_c + v_a}$$

where v_c and v_a is the velocity of the cation and anion, respectively. The sum of the transference number of the cation and the anion is 1.

During electrolysis of hydrochloric acid the changes in concentration at the electrodes and the migration of the cations and anions may be visualized by the representation in Figure 91. In each of the imaginary compartments there are seven cations and seven anions. If the current is allowed to flow long enough to deposit six ions, six electrons are removed from the anode and supplied to the cathode; and six cations are discharged at the cathode and six anions are discharged at the anode. At room temperature the hydrogen ion in the hydrochloric acid moves about five times as fast as the chloride ion; i.e., $n_{H^+} = 0.83$. Six ions are discharged at each electrode, but five-sixths of the current is carried by the

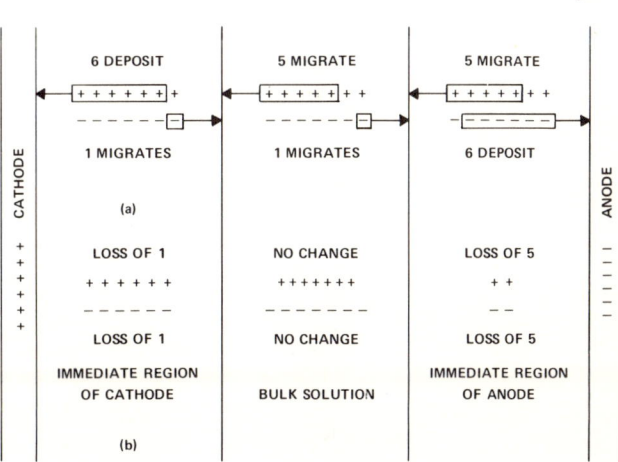

Figure 91. Diagrammatical representation of concentrations in region of the electrodes when the transference number of the cation is 0.83.

hydrogen ions. These changes are indicated in (a) and the net result is shown in (b) of Figure 91. Six hydrogen ions are discharged at the cathode, but five more migrate from the middle compartment with a net loss of one hydrogen ion. One chloride ion is lost because of migration. Six chloride ions are discharged at the anode, but only one migrates to the anode compartment; and the net loss about the anode is five. There is also a loss of five hydrogen ions as a result of their migration to the cathode.

As shown in Table XXXVI, transference numbers vary slightly with concentration. They depend on the relative ionic diameters and the extent of solvation of the ions. Highly solvated ions, e.g., calcium and lithium, move slowly because of the resistance caused by the atmosphere of solvent molecules associated with the ions.

The absolute velocity of ions may be measured by determining the distance traveled in a given time under a definite potential gradient. The velocity of an ion in centimeters per second under a potential gradient of 1 V cm^{-1} is known as its ionic mobility. Some ionic mobilities are given in Table XXXVII. Hydrogen and hydroxyl ions possess abnormally high ionic mobilities. Other ions have ionic mobilities of the order of approximately 3 to 8 × 10^{-4} cm sec^{-1} at 25° under a potential gradient of 1 V cm^{-1}.

Table XXXVI Transference Numbers of Cations at 25°

Electrolyte	Concentration		
	0.01 N	0.05 N	0.1 N
HCl	0.825	0.829	0.831
NaC$_2$H$_3$O$_2$	0.554	0.557	0.559
KNO$_3$	0.508	0.509	0.510
NH$_4$Cl	0.491	0.491	0.491
KCl	0.490	0.490	0.490
KBr	0.483	0.483	0.483
AgNO$_3$	0.465	0.466	0.468
CaCl$_2$	0.426	0.414	0.406
NaCl	0.392	0.388	0.385
LiCl	0.329	0.321	0.317

Table XXXVII Ionic Mobilities at 25° at Infinite Dilution

Ion	Mobility (cm^2 V^{-1} sec^{-1})
H$^+$	0.00362
K$^+$	0.00076
Ba^{++}	0.00066
Na$^+$	0.00052
Li$^+$	0.00040
Cu^{++}	0.00036
OH$^-$	0.00205
SO$_4^{--}$	0.00083
Cl$^-$	0.00079
NO$_3^-$	0.00074
HCO$_3^-$	0.00046

Conductance

The conductance or transmission of a current by the ions of an electrolytic solution is the reciprocal of the resistance. The specific resistance of an electrolyte is defined as the resistance in ohms of a column of solution 1 cm long and 1 cm² in cross section. The specific conductance L is the reciprocal of the specific resistance; it is expressed in ohm⁻¹ cm⁻¹.

The equivalent conductance Λ is the product of the specific conductance and the volume V in milliliters, which contains 1 g-equivalent of the solute,

$$\Lambda = VL = \frac{1000L}{c}$$

These conductance terms may be visualized by a cell 1 cm square and indefinitely high. The two opposing walls act as electrodes. When the cell is filled to a depth of 1 cm with a solution, the conductance measured is the specific conductance. When the cell is filled with a volume of solution that contains 1 g-equivalent of dissolved electrolyte, the solution is V centimeters deep in the cell and the conductance measured is the equivalent conductance.

As the size of the electrodes varies in different conductivity cells, a cell constant for each cell must be determined by use of a standard solution of known specific conductance. Usually a 0.0200 M solution of potassium chloride having $L_{25°} = 0.002768$ ohm⁻¹ cm⁻¹ is used as a standard for calibration of the cell. If r is the measured resistance of the cell when filled with 0.02 M potassium chloride, the conductance is $1/r$. The specific conductance is $k(1/r)$, where k is a constant for that cell. The cell constant at 25° is

$$k = 0.002768r$$

Once the cell constant has been determined, the specific conductance of any solution is obtained from the measured resistance r by the equation

$$L = k/r$$

When a given conductivity cell is filled with 0.02 M potassium chloride at 25°, it has a resistance of 100 ohms as measured by a Wheatstone bridge. When the same cell is filled with 0.005 N solution of an electrolyte, it has a resistance of 300 ohms. The cell constant is

$$k = 0.002768 \times 100 = 0.2768 \text{ cm}^{-1}$$

The specific conductance of the solution is

$$L = k/r = 0.2768/300 = 0.000923 \text{ ohm}^{-1} \text{ cm}^{-1}$$

The equivalent conductance of the 0.005 N solution is

$$\Lambda = \frac{1000L}{c} = \frac{1000 \times 0.000923}{0.005} = 184.6 \text{ cm}^2 \text{ equiv}^{-1} \text{ ohm}^{-1}$$

The equivalent conductance of an electrolyte is increased with a rise in temperature because the ionic mobility is increased. Highly hydrated ions move slowly and have small transference numbers. As the temperature is increased, the highly hydrated ions lose more of the associated atmosphere of water with a proportionately greater increase in velocity than the less hydrated ions.

When solutions of strong electrolytes are diluted, the specific conductance is decreased as the number of ions per unit volume is decreased. Strong electrolytes are completely ionized so that dilution of a solution of a strong electrolyte does not increase the total number of ions carrying a current. The equivalent conductance of a solution of a strong electrolyte increases with dilution, because it is a linear function of the square root of concentration. The equivalent conductance increases upon dilution because the ions move faster, as they are farther apart and are not held back by interactions with oppositely charged ions.

Weak electrolytes are only slightly ionized. Upon dilution the ionization is increased and a greater number of ions is produced. When solutions of weak electrolytes are diluted, the equivalent conductances are increased because of the greater number of ions available to carry the current. As a solution of a weak electrolyte is diluted, the equivalent conductance increases to a limiting value Λ_0 at infinite dilution. Infinite dilution may be considered as the concentration at which the ions are so far apart that there is no interaction between the ions.

A comparison of the equivalent conductances of a strong and a weak electrolyte is made in Figure 92. The Λ_0 of a strong electrolyte can be determined by the extrapolation to infinite dilution of a plot of the equivalent conductance against the square root of concentration. As seen in Figure 92, such an extrapolation cannot be used for a weak electrolyte.

At infinite dilution the ions of an electrolyte behave independently so the equivalent conductance, Λ_0, is equal to the sum of the equivalent conductances of the cation, $l_{0,c}$, and the anion, $l_{0,a}$,

$$\Lambda_0 = l_{0,c} + l_{0,a}$$

This relationship, known as the Kohlrausch law, is useful in calculating the Λ_0 for weak electrolytes. The Λ_0 for acetic acid may be found by the method of differences from the extrapolated Λ_0 values for hydrochloric acid, sodium acetate, and sodium chloride, which are 426.1, 91.0, and 126.5 cm^2 equiv^{-1} ohm^{-1}, respectively.

$$(l_{0,H^+} + l_{0,Cl^-}) + (l_{0,Na^+} + l_{0,CH_3COO^-}) - (l_{0,Na^+} + l_{0,Cl^-}) = l_{0,H^+} + l_{0,CH_3COO^-}$$

$$\Lambda_{0,HCl} + \Lambda_{0,CH_3COONa} - \Lambda_{0,NaCl} = \Lambda_{0,CH_3COOH}$$

$$\Lambda_{0,CH_3COOH} = 426.1 + 91.0 - 126.5 = 390.6 \text{ cm}^2 \text{ equiv}^{-1} \text{ ohm}^{-1}$$

The individual ionic conductance may be calculated by use of transference numbers. The fraction of the total current carried by a given ion is equivalent to the ratio of the conductance of the ion to the conductance of the electrolyte,

$$n_c = \frac{l_c}{l_c + l_a} = \frac{l_c}{\Lambda}$$

and

$$l_c = n_c \Lambda$$

Utilizing the equivalent conductances and transference numbers in the handbooks of chemistry and physics, the Λ_0 for acetic acid may be calculated at 25°:

$$l_{0,H^+} = n_{H^+} \Lambda_{0,HCl} = 0.82 \times 426.1 = 349.4$$

$$l_{0,CH_3COO^-} = n_{CH_3COO^-} \Lambda_{0,CH_3COONa} = 0.45 \times 91 = 40.9$$

$$\Lambda_{0,CH_3COOH} = l_{0,H^+} + l_{0,CH_3COO^-} = 349.4 \times 40.9 = 390.3 \text{ cm}^2 \text{ equiv}^{-1} \text{ ohm}^{-1}$$

At infinite dilution the equivalent conductance is a measure of complete dissociation of a solute into its ions. As a solution of a weak electrolyte is diluted more ions are produced, and the equivalent conductance is increased. Thus, the equivalent conductance at a given concentration represents the number of solute particles present as ions and may be expressed as

$$\Lambda = \alpha l_c + \alpha l_a$$

where α is the fraction of the molecules ionized or the degree of dissociation of a weak electrolyte. From these relationships the degree of dissociation may be calculated from conductance measurements,

$$\frac{\Lambda}{\Lambda_0} = \frac{\alpha(l_c + l_a)}{l_c + l_a} = \alpha$$

aqueous solutions • 187

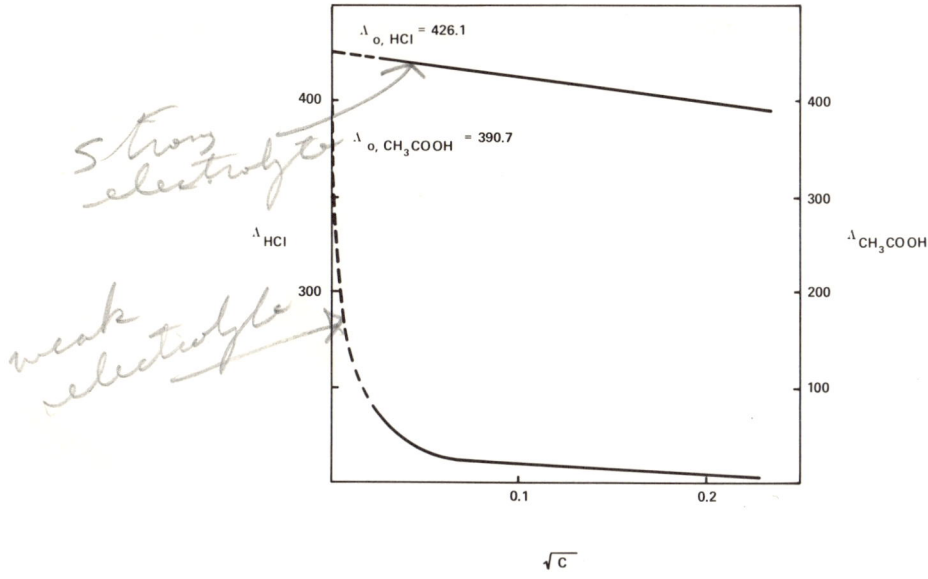

Figure 92. Influence of concentration of a weak and strong electrolyte on equivalent conductance at 25°.

Interaction

The value of an equilibrium constant is constant only for very dilute solutions and for ideal solutions over all concentrations. Electrolytes are ionized, but the ions are associated in some manner by electrostatic attraction so that the ions are incompletely dissociated into free ions. The effective concentration of the free ions is known as the activity of the solute. When activity is used instead of concentration in calculating equilibrium constants, the equilibrium constants are true constants and independent of the concentration of the electrolyte.

The relationship between activities and concentrations may be experimentally determined for a given substance, and then the practical advantage is gained that many simple equations applying to ideal solutions may be applied with exactness by use of activities rather than analytically determined concentrations. This is especially advantageous in solutions of electrolytes where the charge causes a large deviation from ideality.

The activity of a solvent at infinite dilution is considered to be 1; i.e., the activity equals the concentration. As the solution becomes more concentrated in solute, the activity of the solvent generally becomes less. The activity, a, of a volatile solvent can be evaluated from the ratio of the vapor pressure, p, of the solvent in a solution to the vapor pressure of the pure solvent, p^0,

$$a = \frac{p}{p^0}$$

A system in which the constituents behave ideally with the concentration equal to the activity is known as a reference state. The standard state of a constituent in a solution is the state of the constituent at unity activity. A pure liquid at 1 atm and a given temperature is the standard state of a solvent. The standard state of the solute is a hypothetical solution of unit concentration having the properties of an ideal solution or infinitely dilute solution.

As the concentration of a solution of an electrolyte is increased there is greater interionic attraction. The movement of an ion is hindered by an atmosphere of oppositely charged ions and ionic association. The activity of such a solution is generally less than the actual concentration of the solute.

aqueous solutions

The ratio of the activity to the concentration in molality is defined by the activity coefficient, γ,

$$\gamma = \frac{a}{m}$$

Activity coefficients may be considered as proportionality constants relating activity and concentration.

The activity coefficient of a univalent-univalent electrolyte may be defined as the product of the ionic activities,

$$a_{solute} = a_+ \times a_-$$

The ionic activity coefficient γ_+ and γ_- are defined as the ratios of the activities of the ions to their molality,

$$\gamma_+ = \frac{a_+}{m} \;;\quad \gamma_- = \frac{a_-}{m}$$

As yet the activity coefficient of an ion cannot be experimentally determined. The mean ionic activity coefficient can be determined theoretically and experimentally. The mean ionic coefficient of an electrolyte is

$$\gamma = (\gamma_+ \times \gamma_-)^{1/2}$$

In dilute solutions the ionic activities are considered as approximately equal,

$$a_+ = a_- = m\gamma$$

Thus, for a univalent-univalent electrolyte the activity of the solute is

$$a_{solute} = (m\gamma_+)(m\gamma_-) = m^2 \gamma^2$$

As the valence is increased the expressions become more complex. For a divalent-univalent electrolyte such as calcium chloride the activity of the solute is

$$a_{CaCl_2} = a_{Ca^{++}} \, a^2_{Cl^-}$$

When the molality of the calcium chloride is m, the calcium ion concentration is m and the chloride ion concentration is $2m$. The ionic activity coefficients are

$$\gamma_+ = \frac{a_+}{m}; \quad \gamma_- = \frac{a_-}{2m}$$

The mean ionic coefficient is

$$\gamma = (\gamma_+ \times \gamma_-^2)^{1/3}$$

The activity of the divalent-univalent solute is

$$a_{CaCl_2} = (m\gamma_+)(2m\gamma_-)^2 = 4m^3 \gamma^3$$

Strong electrolytes may be classified on the basis of their valences. In the 1-1 electrolytes the cation and anion both have a valence of 1, e.g., sodium chloride and homatropine hydrobromide; in the 2-2 electrolytes the cation and the anion both have a valence of 2, e.g., zinc sulfate and copper sulfate. The first term refers to the cation and the second term to the anion; e.g., aluminum chloride is a 3-1 electrolyte.

In moderately concentrated solutions of strong electrolytes the oppositely charged ions attract each other and cause deviation from ideal behavior. The magnitude of this interionic attraction depends not only on the concentration but upon the valence type. Ions with more than a single charge exert greater interionic attraction and greater deviation than a univalent ion. These two influences can be considered in terms of ionic strength. Ionic strength is defined as

$$\mu = \tfrac{1}{2} \sum_{1}^{n} c_i z_i^2$$

where the summation is the product of the concentration, c_i, of each ionic species and the square of its valence, z_i, from 1 to the nth ionic species. The sum is divided by 2 because the cation-anion pairs contribute to the total electrostatic interaction and the ionic strength refers to the effect of each ion separately.

Normal saline is 0.9 per cent or 0.154 m solution of sodium chloride. Its ionic strength is

$$\mu = \frac{(0.154 \times 1^2) + (0.154 \times 1^2)}{2} = 0.154$$

The ionic strength of a 0.01 m potassium sulfate solution is

$$\mu = \frac{(0.01 \times 1^2) + (0.01 \times 1^2) + (0.01 \times 2^2)}{2} = 0.03$$

The ionic strength of a mixture of electrolytes is the sum of the ionic strength of the individual salts.

There are interionic attractions between the ions of a weak electrolyte; however, the much greater effect of partial ionization makes them relatively unimportant. Although the Arrhenius ionization theory is adequate for weak electrolytes, the Debye-Hückel theory is used to rationalize the effect of valence type and ionic strength in solutions of strong electrolytes.

When ionization is complete, as with strong electrolytes in dilute solution, the activity coefficient of an ion depends only on its valence, the ionic strength, the dielectric constant of the medium, and the temperature. Debye and Hückel expressed the relationship mathematically as

$$-\ln \gamma_i = \frac{e^3 z_i^2}{(\epsilon k T)^{3/2}} \sqrt{\frac{2\pi N \mu}{1000}}$$

where γ_i is the activity coefficient of the ionic species i, z_i the valence of the ionic species, e the charge of an electron, ϵ the dielectric constant of the medium, N the Avogadro number, k the gas constant per molecule, and μ the ionic strength.

When the mean ionic activity coefficient is used for aqueous solutions and numerical values are used for water at 25° for a system of two ionic species, the equation is

$$\log \gamma = -0.509 z_1 z_2 \sqrt{\mu}$$

This equation is satisfactory up to ionic strength of 0.02.

To illustrate the use of this equation the mean ionic activity coefficient of 0.01 M sodium phenobarbital in an aqueous solution of 0.01 M sodium chloride at 25° can be calculated. The ionic strength for the sodium phenobarbital is 0.01 and that of the sodium chloride is 0.01; the total ionic strength is 0.02. The mean activity coefficient is found by solving the equation

$$\log \gamma = -0.509 \times 1 \times 1 \sqrt{0.02}$$
$$= 0.85$$

To be satisfactorily applied to solutions with ionic strength up to 0.2, additional terms are introduced into the Debye-Hückel equation to give it the form

$$\log \gamma = -\frac{0.509 z_1 z_2 \sqrt{\mu}}{1 + aB\sqrt{\mu}}$$

where a is the mean distance of approach of ions called the mean effective ionic diameter and B is a constant depending on the solvent and temperature. Since for aqueous solutions at 25°, B is 0.33 × 10⁸ and a is 3×10^{-8}, the product aB is approximately 1, so the equation becomes

$$\log \gamma = -\frac{0.509 z_1 z_2 \sqrt{\mu}}{1 + \sqrt{\mu}}$$

Colligative Properties

The properties of a solution which are dependent on the number of particles of the solute and are independent of the chemical nature of the solute are known as colligative properties. All colligative properties are interrelated. Osmotic pressure is the colligative property associated with the physiological compatibility of nasal, ophthalmic, and parenteral solutions. As the osmotic pressure is inconvenient to measure, other colligative properties are often measured during the formulation of pharmaceuticals and related to the osmotic pressure.

Lowering of the Vapor Pressure. In most aqueous pharmaceutical solutions the solute is a nonvolatile constituent. The nonvolatile solute does not contribute to the total vapor pressure of the solution except as it affects the escape tendency of the solvent. The total vapor pressure of the solution is provided by the partial pressure of the volatile solvent, i.e., water. The addition of the solute to the solvent decreases the concentration of the solvent and the tendency of the molecules to escape into the gas phase; i.e., the vapor pressure of the solvent is lowered.

The lowering of the vapor pressure is proportional to number of molecules of solute. The Raoult law states that the partial vapor pressure of the solvent is equal to the vapor pressure of the pure solvent multiplied by the mole fraction of the solvent in the solution,

$$p = p^0 N_1$$

where N_1 is the mole fraction of the solvent. In terms of concentration of the solute, this may be expressed as

$$p = p^0 (1 - N_2)$$

where N_2 is the mole fraction of the solute. By rearrangement the lowering of the vapor pressure is

$$p^0 - p = N_2 p^0$$

and the relative vapor-pressure lowering is

$$\frac{p^0 - p}{p^0} = N_2$$

The Raoult law may now be rephrased. In dilute solutions the relative lowering of vapor pressure is proportional to the mole fraction of the solute. To illustrate this relationship the vapor pressure of a solution containing 50 g of dextrose in 1000 g of water may be calculated. At 25° the vapor pressure of water is 23.76 mm of mercury,

$$p = p^0 N_1 = 23.76 \left(\frac{\frac{1000}{18}}{\frac{1000}{18} + \frac{50}{180}} \right) = 23.64 \text{ mm Hg}$$

The vapor-pressure lowering may be calculated as

$$p^0 - p = N_2 p^0 = 23.76 \left(\frac{\frac{50}{180}}{\frac{1000}{18} + \frac{50}{180}} \right) = 0.12 \text{ mm Hg}$$

Elevation of Boiling Point. The boiling point of a liquid is that temperature at which the vapor pressure of a liquid becomes equal to the atmospheric pressure, i.e., 760 mm of mercury. Since the vapor pressure of a solvent is lowered by the addition of a nonvolatile solvent, the solution must be heated to a higher temperature than the pure solvent if both are to have the same vapor pressure. Thus, the boiling point of a solvent is elevated by the addition of a nonvolatile solute, as shown in Figure 93.

In dilute solutions the ratio of the elevation of boiling point, ΔT_b, to the lowering of vapor pressure is approximately constant,

$$\frac{\Delta T_b}{p^0 - p} = k_1$$

or, by rearrangement,

$$\Delta T_b = k_1(p^0 - p)$$

Since the vapor pressure of the pure solvent, p^0, is constant, the elevation of boiling point is proportional to the relative lowering of the vapor pressure,

$$\Delta T_b = \frac{p^0 - p}{p^0} k_2$$

where $k_2 = k_1 p^0$.

According to the Raoult law, the relative vapor pressure is equal to the mole fraction, N_2, of the solute. Therefore,

$$\Delta T_b = k_2 N_2 = \frac{k_2 \, m}{m + \frac{1000}{M_1}}$$

where M_1 is the molecular weight of the solvent and m is the molality of the solute. In dilute solution the number of moles of solute is negligible in comparison to the number of moles of solvent, and the equation may be rewritten as

$$\Delta T_b = k_2 \frac{M_1}{1000} m$$

or

$$\Delta T_b = K_b m$$

where K_b is the molal elevation constant of the solvent defined by the relation

$$K_b = \frac{RT^2 M_1}{1000 \Delta H_{vapor}}$$

where R is 1.987 cal deg^{-1} mole^{-1}, T the absolute boiling temperature, M_1 the molecular weight of the solvent, and ΔH_{vapor} the molar heat of vaporization.

The molal elevation constants for several solvents are given in Table XXXVIII. The K_b may be considered as the boiling-point elevation for an ideal 1 m solution. In practice K_b is the limit of $\Delta T_b/m$, i.e., the ratio of the boiling-point elevation to the molal concentration at infinite dilution. It is determined experimentally by plotting the ratio $\Delta T_b/m$ against m and extrapolating to infinite dilution.

The elevation of boiling point of a solution containing 50 g of dextrose in 1000 g of water is

$$\Delta T_b = K_b m = \frac{0.512 \times 50}{180} = 0.142°$$

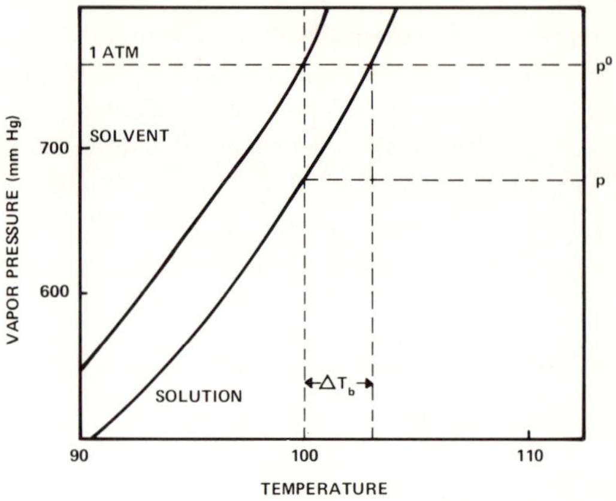

• aqueous solutions

Figure 93. Elevation of boiling point of water by the addition of a nonvolatile solute.

Table XXXVIII Molal Boiling - Point Constants

Solvent	K_b (deg molal^{-1})
Acetic acid	2.93
Acetone	1.71
Benzene	2.53
Carbon bisulfide	2.35
Carbon tetrachloride	5.03
Chloroform	3.63
Ethanol	1.22
Ethyl acetate	2.77
Ethyl ether	2.02
n-Hexane	2.75
Methanol	0.83
Phenol	3.56
Water	0.51

Depression of Freezing Point. The freezing point of a pure liquid is that temperature at which the solid and liquid phase are in equilibrium at 1 atm. The freezing point of a solution is that temperature at which the solid phase of the pure solvent and the liquid phase of the solution are in equilibrium at 1 atm. At the freezing point the liquid and solid have the same vapor pressure. If a solute is added and the temperature is maintained constant, the solid phase passes into the liquid phase; however, a state of equilibrium between the solid and the liquid phase may be maintained by lowering the temperature. The lowering of the freezing point is proportional to the concentration of the solute.

As shown in Figure 94, the vapor pressure-temperature curve of a solid has a greater curvature than that of the corresponding liquid because the heat of sublimation of the solid is greater than the heat of vaporization of the liquid. At the intersection of the two curves, the solid and solvent are in equilibrium, and the corresponding temperature is the freezing point. With an increase in the concentration of the solution, the lowered vapor-pressure curve of the solution intersects the vapor-pressure curve of the solid at a lower freezing-point temperature.

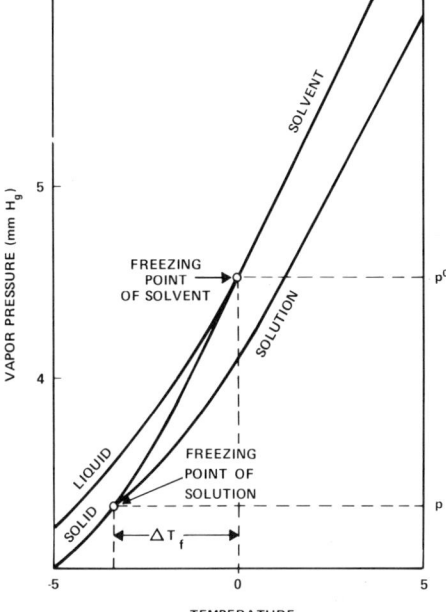

Figure 94. Lowering of freezing point of water by a solute.

For solutions in which the solvent freezes out as a pure solid unmixed with the solute, the relationship between the concentration of the solution and the freezing-point depression, ΔT_f, is

$$\Delta T_f = \frac{RT_0^2 m}{\Delta H_{\text{fusion}} \frac{1000}{M_1}} = K_f m$$

where T_0 is the freezing point of the pure solvent and ΔH_{fusion} is the molar heat of fusion. The molal freezing-point depression constant K_f is a characteristic of the solvent. The K_f for water is

$$K_f = \frac{1.987 \times 273 \times 18}{80 \frac{1000}{18}} = 1.86 \text{ deg mole}^{-1}$$

The molal freezing-point depression constant may be considered as the freezing-point depression for an ideal 1 m solution. In practice K_f is the limit of $\Delta T_f/m$. It is evaluated by plotting the ratio $\Delta T_f/m$ against m and extrapolating to infinite dilution. Some K_f values are given in Table XXXIX.

Table XXXIX Molal Freezing-Point Constants

Solvent	K_f (deg molal^{-1})
Acetic acid	3.90
Benzene	4.90
Formic acid	2.77
Naphthalene	6.8
Phenol	7.40
Stearic acid	4.50
Water	1.86

The freezing-point depression of a solution containing 50 g of dextrose in 1000 g of water is

$$\Delta T_f = K_f m = 1.86 \times \frac{50}{180} = 0.52°$$

The colligative property that can be most easily and accurately measured is the depression of freezing point. The Beckmann molecular-weight apparatus is shown in Figure 95. The inner tube, which is fitted with a Beckmann or differential thermometer readable to $\pm 0.001°$, contains the solvent. The inner tube contains a wire stirrer and has a side arm for introducing the solvent or the solute. The inner tube is surrounded by an air jacket to slow the rate of cooling. This is immersed in a cooling bath approximately 3° below the anticipated freezing point. In most apparatus 20.0 ml of solvent will cover the thermometer bulb and may be pipetted through the side arm so that none adheres to the side of the tube.

Initially the solvent is cooled rapidly until it begins to freeze, and then it is slightly warmed and set into the jacket in the cooling bath fitted with a stirrer. Temperatures are taken at various time intervals. The stationary temperature at which the solid and liquid phases are in equilibrium is the freezing point of the solvent. The rate of cooling should be slow to avoid supercooling.

The solution under investigation is treated in a similar manner. The difference between the freezing point of the solvent and the freezing point of the solution is the freezing-point depression caused by the solute.

Osmotic Pressure. Diffusion is the process by which the solute and solvent molecules migrate. Osmosis is the process by which the solvent molecules pass through a semipermeable membrane from a dilute solution to a more concentrated solution. The pressure that must be applied to the more concentrated solution to just prevent the flow of the pure solvent into the solution is known as the osmotic pressure of the solution.

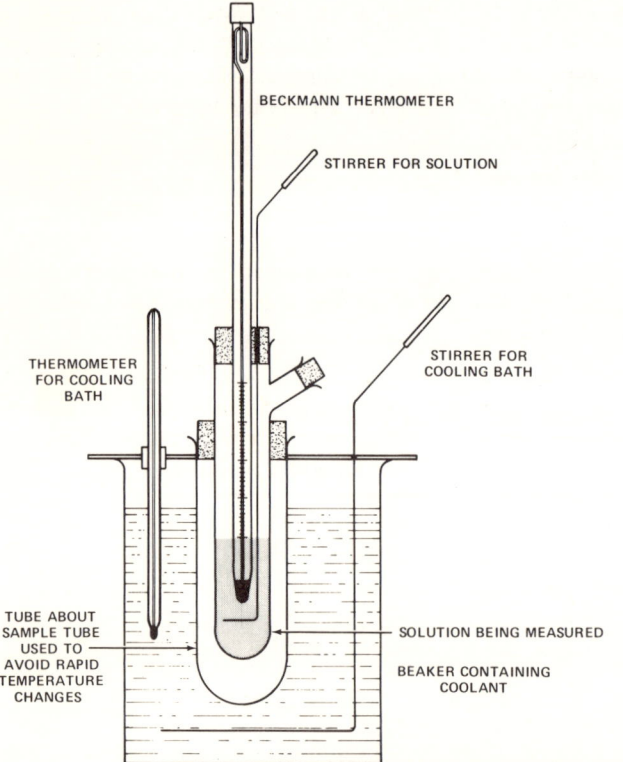

Figure 95. Beckmann freezing-point apparatus.

A semipermeable membrane is a barrier through which only the solvent molecules may pass. The solvent molecules move from a region where their escape tendency is large to a region where their escape tendency is small. The presence of a dissolved solute lowers the escape tendency of the solvent in proportion to its concentration.

The pressure due to osmosis is independent of the nature of the semipermeable membrane. If any of the solute diffuses through a membrane, it is not a semipermeable membrane, and such a process is not to be confused with osmosis. In experimental work different membranes appear to give different pressures; however, if the membranes do not leak and adequate time is allowed for the attainment of equilibrium, the osmotic pressures will be the same. The nature and area of the semipermeable membrane determines the speed of osmosis.

In dilute solutions there appears to be a parallelism between osmotic pressure and the properties of gases. The product, Pv, of the osmotic pressure in atmospheres and the volume of the solution in liters is porportional to the absolute temperature and the number of moles, n, of the solute. This relationship has the same form as the ideal gas law,

$$Pv = nRT$$

In more concentrated solutions, calculations agree better with experimentally measured osmotic pressure if v is taken as the volume of the solvent in liters. The osmotic pressure of a solution of 50 g of dextrose in 1000 g of water is

$$P = \frac{50 \times 0.08205 \times 298}{180 \times 1} = 6.8 \text{ atm}$$

If $n/v = c$, the equation using a concentration term c is

$$P = cRT$$

The best agreement between experimentally measured and calculated osmotic pressure is obtained by introducing the van't Hoff term i,

$$Pv = inRT$$

The i term expresses the extent of deviation of the solution from ideality regardless of the reason for the deviation. The value of i for any solution may be determined by comparing the measured colligative property to that of an ideal solution. Therefore,

$$i = \frac{p}{p_{\text{ideal}}} = \frac{p^0 - p}{(p^0 - p)_{\text{ideal}}} = \frac{\Delta T_f}{(\Delta T_f)_{\text{ideal}}} = \frac{\Delta T_b}{(\Delta T_b)_{\text{ideal}}}$$

SOLUTIONS OF ELECTROLYTES

The osmotic pressure of solutions of various nonelectrolytes is the same for a given concentration. A solution containing 18.2 g of mannitol in 1000 g of water has the same molality as a solution containing 34.2 g of lactose in 1000 g of water. Both of these 0.1 m solutions have the same osmotic pressure and other colligative properties. Thus, the freezing-point depression of a 0.1 m solution of a nonelectrolyte in water is

$$\Delta T_f = K_f m = 1.86 \times 0.1 = 0.186°$$

Solutions of electrolytes exert osmotic pressures that are higher than those of nonelectrolytes. This is due to the ionization of the electrolyte, and each of the ions act as a separate particle and exerts its pressure effect. A sodium chloride solution as a result of ionization has twice as many particles as a nonelectrolyte solution of the same molality. Thus, the freezing-point depression of a 0.1 m solution of sodium chloride is

$$\Delta T_f = iK_f m = 2 \times 1.86 \times 0.1 = 0.372°$$

where for a dilute solution of a strong electrolyte i represents the number of ionic species.

For a uni-univalent electrolyte solution at infinite dilution, the depression of freezing point is twice that of a nonelectrolyte, i.e., $i = 2$. A uni-divalent electrolyte at infinite dilution ionizes into three ions; e.g., potassium sulfate ionizes into two potassium ions and one sulfate ion, which cause a depression of freezing point that is three times that of a nonelectrolyte, i.e., $i = 3$.

At infinite dilution the value of i approaches the number of ions into which the electrolyte ionizes, as shown in Figure 96. The value of i decreases as the concentration of the electrolyte is increased. This is a consequence of more frequent ionic collision and greater interionic attraction, which cause a greater departure from ideality. The i value of a 0.0167 m potassium sulfate solution is 2.70. The freezing-point depression of this solution is

$$\Delta T_f = iK_f m = 2.7 \times 1.86 \times 0.0167 = 0.08°$$

For some electrolytes the i value decreases at high concentrations. This is believed to be caused by hydration of the ions, which decreases the activity of the solvent and enhances the colligative properties.

In a more general interpretation, the van't Hoff term i may be considered to express any deviation from ideality, whether it be caused by ionic interaction, degree of dissociation of weak electrolytes, or associations of nonelectrolytes. The term i may be evaluated by the ratio of any measured colligative property to that of an ideal solution.

Isotonic Solutions

Solutions intended for instillation in the eye or nasal passage or for parenteral injection are less irritating if they have the same osmotic pressure as the corresponding body fluid. Solutions that have the same osmotic pressure as the body fluid are said to be isotonic with the body fluid.

The effect of osmotic pressure on erythrocytes may be shown by suspending the erythrocytes in a 3 per cent saline solution which is hypertonic, i.e., has a higher osmotic pressure. The water in the erythrocyte passes through the semipermeable cell membrane and dilutes the saline solution. As a consequence of the loss of water, the cell shrinks and presents a wrinkled appearance. This phenomenon is known as crenation.

If erythrocytes are suspended in distilled water, the water passes through the cell membrane into the cell, causing it to swell and rupture with the release of hemoglobin. This process is known as hemolysis. The water is hypotonic with respect to the blood and has a lower osmotic pressure.

When erythrocytes are suspended in a 0.9 per cent solution of sodium chloride, the cells are unchanged. This solution is known as physiological saline or normal saline solution. It is isotonic with blood, i.e., has the same osmotic pressure.

These effects make it desirous to have large-volume intravenous solutions isotonic with blood. Aqueous solutions for intravenous injection are often hypotonic with respect to blood, and they may be adjusted to isotonicity by the addition of dextrose or sodium chloride.

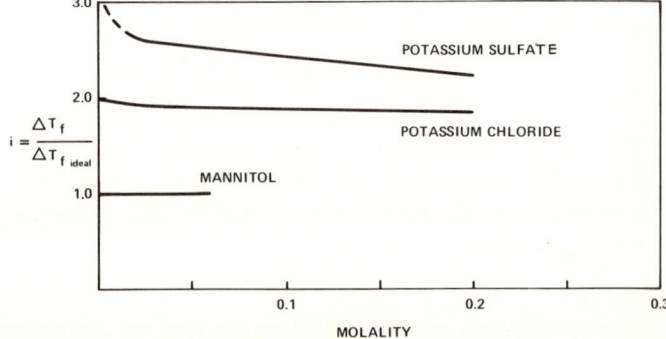

Figure 96. Influence of dilution on the value of i.

Similar changes occur in the eye with the instillation of hypotonic and hypertonic solutions. Prolonged contact causes irritation and pain. To minimize pain and to increase the comfort of the patient ophthalmic solutions may be adjusted to be isotonic with lacrymal fluid. Hypotonic ophthalmic solutions may be adjusted to isotonicity by the addition of boric acid or sodium chloride.

In preparing solutions to be isotonic with body fluids, the physiology of the cell membrane cannot be ignored. The cell membrane of the erythrocyte is not a semipermeable membrane for all drugs. It permits the free diffusion of ammonium chloride, alcohol, boric acid, glycerin, propylene glycol, and urea. Thus, a 1.9 per cent solution of boric acid is isoosmotic, but it is not isotonic with blood, as it causes hemolysis.

In the eye the cell membrane of the tissue is semipermeable to boric acid. Thus, a 1.9 per cent solution of boric acid is an isotonic ophthalmic solution.

Any of the colligative properties may be used to determine the tonicity of solutions; however, the ease and accuracy of the determination of freezing-point depression make it the most useful property to be measured in the determination of tonicity. The freezing point of human blood and tears is -0.52°. An aqueous solution that has this freezing point is isotonic with blood and tears. A 0.9 per cent saline solution has a freezing point and an osmotic pressure that are the same as body fluids. Some convenient methods based on freezing-point depression for calculating the concentration of adjusting solute follow.

L Method. The amount of solute which must be added to adjust a hypotonic solution of a drug to isotonicity can be calculated by means of the thermodynamically derived equation

$$\Delta T_f = K_f m$$

As previously discussed, the introduction of the term *i* will correct for deviations from ideality,

$$\Delta T_f = iK_f m$$

Over an extreme range of concentration *i* will vary. For convenience in pharmaceutical systems where the solutions are dilute and the molar concentration is used interchangeably with molal concentration, the depression of freezing point is represented by

$$\Delta T_f = Lc$$

The value of **L** varies over a wide range of concentration; however, L_{iso} represents the value when the concentration of the substance is such that the solution is isotonic with body fluid. These values have been experimentally determined and are tabulated in Table XL for convenience.

To calculate the amount of solute to be added to a hypotonic solution of a drug, one calculates the difference between the freezing point of the body fluid and that of the hypotonic solution of the drug. This difference is the lowering of freezing point to be contributed by the adjusting solute. Using this difference and the **L** of the adjusting solute, the concentration of the adjusting solute can be calculated.

48. Procaine hydrochloride 1%
    (make isotonic with sodium chloride) 1000 ml
    Sterile purified water, q.s.

    Sig.: For infiltration anesthesia

The depression of freezing point is equal to the **L** of procaine hydrochloride multiplied by the molarity of the drug in soltuion,

$$\Delta T_f = Lc = 3.4 \times \frac{10}{272.8} = 0.125°$$

198 • aqueous solutions

Table XL Molal Freezing-Point Depression in Water at Concentrations Approximately Isotonic with Blood Serum

Substance	L_{iso}	Substance	L_{iso}
Antipyrine	1.9	Morphine sulfate	4.3
Atropine sulfate	4.3	Neosynephrine hydrochloride	3.4
Boric acid	1.9	Phenacaine hydrochloride	3.4
Calcium chloride	4.8	Physostigmine salicylate	3.4
Calcium nitrate	4.5	Physostigmine sulfate	4.3
Camphor	1.9	Pilocarpine hydrochloride	3.4
Chloral hydrate	1.9	Pontocaine hydrochloride	3.4
Chlorobutanol	1.9	Potassium bromide	3.4
Citric acid	2.0	Potassium chloride	3.4
Cocaine hydrochloride	3.4	Potassium phosphate (monobasic)	3.2
Dextrose	1.9	Potassium sulfate	4.2
Emetine hydrochloride	4.8	Potassium tetraborate	7.4
Ephedrine hydrochloride	3.4	Procaine hydrochloride	3.4
Ephedrine sulfate	4.3	Silver nitrate	3.3
Epinephrine hydrochloride	3.4	Sodium acid phosphate	3.4
Ethylhydrocupreine hydrochloride	3.4	Sodium bicarbonate	3.5
Ethylmorphine hydrochloride	3.4	Sodium bromide	3.4
Ferric chloride	6.0	Sodium chloride	3.4
Fluorescein sodium	4.3	Sodium citrate	5.2
Homatropine hydrobromide	3.4	Sodium iodide	3.6
Hyoscine hydrobromide	3.4	Sodium phosphate (dibasic)	4.3
Hyoscine hydrochloride	3.4	Sodium sulfate	4.3
Lactose	1.9	Sodium thiosulfate	4.2
Magnesium chloride	4.9	Sugar	1.9
Magnesium sulfate	2.0	Tartaric acid	2.0
Menthol	1.9	Tutocaine hydrochloride	3.4
Mercuric chloride	1.8	Zinc acetate	4.7
Mercuric cyanide	1.9	Zinc chloride	4.9
Methenamine	1.9	Zinc nitrate	4.9
Metycaine hydrochloride	3.4	Zinc phenosulfonate	4.8
Morphine hydrochloride	3.4	Zinc sulfate	2.0

Since the freezing point of body fluids is -0.52°, the sodium chloride to be added as an adjusting solute must lower the freezing point 0.52 - 0.125 = 0.395°. The concentration of sodium chloride to be added is

$$\Delta T_f = Lc = 0.395 = 3.4c$$
$$c = 0.116$$

To express in terms of weight the molarity is multiplied by the molecular weight of sodium chloride,

$$58.5 \times 0.116 = 6.786 \text{ g liter}^{-1}$$

49. Ethylmorphine hydrochloride   1.5%
    Purified water, q.s.   30 ml
    Prepare isotonic solution

    Sig.: Instill in eye as directed

The depression of freezing point caused by the drug is found by multiplying the **L** value of ethylmorphine hydrochloride by its molarity,

$$\Delta T_f = Lc = 3.4 \times \frac{15}{386} = 0.132°$$

The depression required to obtain a freezing point of -0.52° is 0.52 - 0.132 = 0.338°. The concentration of sodium chloride to be added to contribute this depression is

$$\Delta T_f = Lc = 0.388 = 3.4c$$
$$c = 0.114$$

To express in terms of grams of sodium chloride for 30 ml of solution the molarity is multiplied by the molecular weight and the fraction of a liter to be prepared,

$$0.114 \times 58.5 \times \frac{30}{1000} = 0.199 \text{ g for 30 ml}$$

For dilute solutions utilized in collyria the interionic attractions are approximately the same for a given type of electrolyte. Thus, the practicing pharmacist who does not have available a table of **L** values can prepare acceptable solutions based on the easily remembered values shown in Table XLI.

Sodium-Chloride-Equivalent Method. Another method suggested to facilitate the calculations involved in the preparation of isotonic solutions is the sodium-chloride-equivalent method. The sodium chloride equivalent is the weight of sodium chloride that will produce the same osmotic or freezing-point effect as 1 unit weight of a drug. Antistine hydrochloride has a sodium chloride equivalent, **E**, of 0.19; i.e., 0.19 unit weight of sodium chloride and 1 unit weight of antistine hydrochloride have identical colligative properties.

For the drug,

$$\Delta T_f = L_d c_d$$

and for sodium chloride,

$$\Delta T_f = L_{NaCl} c_{NaCl}$$

By definition the freezing-point depression for 1 g of drug is equal to that of **E** grams of sodium chloride; therefore,

$$\Delta T_f = L_d c_d = L_{NaCl} c_{NaCl} = \frac{3.44 E}{58.8}$$

and as **E** is being calculated in relation to 1 g of the drug,

$$\frac{L_d \times 1}{M_d} = \frac{3.44 E}{58.5}$$

Thus, the sodium chloride equivalent is expressed in terms of the molecular weight of the drug, M_d, and the molal freezing-point depression constant of the drug, L_d,

$$E = \frac{58.5 \, L_d}{3.44 \, M_d} = 17 \frac{L_d}{M_d}$$

The sodium chloride equivalent of atropine sulfate may be calculated if the **L** and molecular weight are known:

$$E = 17 \times \frac{4.3}{695} = 0.11$$

aqueous solutions

Table XLI Approximate L_{iso} Values

Type of Solute	L_{iso}	Examples
Nonelectrolyte	1.9	Benzyl alcohol, chlorobutanol, dextrose
Weak electrolyte	2.0	Boric acid
Di-divalent electrolyte	2.0	Zinc sulfate
Uni-univalent electrolyte	3.4	Pilocarpine hydrochloride, sodium acid phosphate, sodium chloride
Uni-divalent electrolyte	4.3	Atropine sulfate, disodium phosphate, physostigmine sulfate
Di-univalent electrolyte	4.8	Calcium chloride, emetine hydrochloride
Uni-trivalent electrolyte	5.2	Sodium citrate
Tri-univalent electrolyte	6.0	Ferric chloride

In using the sodium-chloride-equivalent method, the amount of the drug is multiplied by the sodium chloride equivalent to obtain the amount of sodium chloride osmotically equivalent to the drug. This is subtracted from the sodium chloride equivalent of the isotonic solution. The difference is the amount of sodium chloride yet to be added to make an isotonic solution. If the adjusting solute is other than sodium chloride, the amount of sodium chloride required is divided by the **E** of the solute to obtain the weight of adjusting solute to be added. Sodium chloride equivalents are given in Table XLII.

Table XLII Sodium Chloride Equivalents *

Drug	Experimental Range In Which Sodium Chloride Equivalent Determined	
	1%	3%
Acriflavine	0.10	0.09
Adrenaline hydrochloride	0.27	0.22
Alum (potassium) N.F.	0.18	0.15
9-Aminoacridine hydrochloride	0.17	
Aminophylline U.S.P.	0.17	
Amiodoxyl benzoate	0.20	0.20
Ammonium chloride U.S.P.	1.12	
Amobarbital sodium U.S.P.	0.25	0.25
Amphetamine phosphate N.F.	0.34	0.27
Amphetamine sulfate U.S.P.	0.22	0.21
Amprotropine phosphate	0.18	0.16
Amydricaine hydrochloride	0.24	0.18
Amydricaine nitrate	0.19	0.17
Amylocaine hydrochloride	0.22	0.19
Antazoline hydrochloride	0.23	
Antazoline phosphate N.F.	0.20	0.17
Antimony potassium tartrate U.S.P.	0.18	0.13
Antipyrine N.F.	0.17	0.14
Apomorphine hydrochloride	0.14	
Aranthol	0.23	0.23
Arecoline hydrobromide N.F.	0.27	0.24
Ascorbic acid U.S.P.	0.18	0.18

* After E. Hammarlund and K. Pedersen-Bjergaard, *J. Am. Pharm. Assoc., Sci. Ed.* **47**, 107 (1958).

Atropine methyl nitrate	0.18	0.15
Atropine sulfate U.S.P.	0.13	0.11
Aurothioglucose N.F.	0.03	0.03
Bacitracin U.S.P.	0.05	0.04
Barbital sodium N.F.	0.30	0.29
Benoxinate hydrochloride U.S.P.	0.18	0.14
Benzalkonium chloride U.S.P.	0.16	0.14
Benzethonium chloride U.S.P.	0.05	0.02
Benzyprinium bromide N.F.	0.20	0.18
Benzyl alcohol N.F.	0.17	0.15
Bismuth sodium tartrate	0.09	0.06
Boric acid U.S.P.	0.50	
Bromodiphenhydramine hydrochloride	0.17	0.10
Butacaine sulfate	0.20	0.13
Butethamine formate	0.26	0.21
Butethamine hydrochloride N.F.	0.25	
Caffeine U.S.P.	0.08	
Caffeine and sodium benzoate U.S.P.	0.26	0.23
Caffeine and sodium salicylate	0.21	0.17
Calcium aminosalicylate N.F.	0.27	0.21
Calcium chloride U.S.P.	0.51	
Calcium chloride (6H$_2$O)	0.35	
Calcium chloride anhydrous	0.68	
Calcium gluconate U.S.P.	0.16	0.14
Calcium lactate N.F.	0.23	0.21
Calcium levulinate	0.27	0.25
Calcium pantothenate U.S.P.	0.18	0.17
Carbochol U.S.P.	0.36	
Cetyltrimethyl ammonium	0.09	0.09
Chiniofon N.F.	0.13	0.11
Chloramine-T	0.23	0.22
Chlorocyclizine hydrochloride U.S.P.	0.17	0.09
Chlorobutanol hydrated U.S.P.	0.24	
Chloresium	0.10	0.06
Chlorpheniramine maleate U.S.P.	0.17	0.12
Chlorpromazine hydrochloride U.S.P.	0.10	0.05
Chlortetracycline sulfate	0.13	0.10
Citric acid U.S.P.	0.18	0.17
Cocaine hydrochloride U.S.P.	0.16	0.15
Codeine hydrochloride	0.15	0.15
Cornecaine	0.18	0.15
Cyclomethycaine sulfate	0.13	0.10
Cyclomethycaine hydrochloride	0.36	
Cyclopentolate hydrochloride U.S.P.	0.20	0.18
Decamethonium bromide	0.25	0.20
Dextroamphetamine phosphate	0.25	0.25
Dextrose U.S.P.	0.16	0.16
Dextrose, anhydrous	0.18	0.18
Dibucaine hydrochloride U.S.P.	0.13	0.11

Dibutoline sulfate	0.16	0.15
Dichlorophenarsine hydrochloride	0.55	
Dicyclomine hydrochloride	0.18	0.17
Dihydrocodeinone enolactate hydrochloride	0.14	0.13
Dihydrohydroxycodeinone	0.14	0.13
Dihydromorphinone hydrochloride U.S.P.	0.22	0.17
Dihydrostreptomycine sulfate U.S.P.	0.06	0.05
Diphenhydramine hydrochloride U.S.P.	0.28	0.20
Diphenmethanil methylsulfate N.F.	0.15	
Emetine hydrochloride U.S.P.	0.10	0.10
Ephedrine hydrochloride N.F.	0.30	0.28
Ephedrine sulfate U.S.P.	0.23	0.20
Epinephrine bitartrate U.S.P.	0.18	0.16
Epinephrine hydrochloride	0.29	0.26
Ergonovine maleate U.S.P.	0.16	
Erythromycin glucoheptonate	0.07	0.07
Ethaverine hydrochloride	0.12	
Ethylenediamine	0.44	
Ethylhydrocupreine hydrochloride	0.17	0.11
Ethylmorphine hydrochloride N.F.	0.16	0.15
Ethylnorepinephrine hydrochloride	0.32	0.28
Ferrous gluconate U.S.P.	0.15	0.12
Ferrous lactate	0.21	
Fluorescein sodium U.S.P.	0.31	0.27
D-Fructose N.F.	0.18	0.18
Galactose	0.18	0.18
Gallamine triethiodide	0.08	0.08
D-Glucuronic acid	0.20	0.19
L-Glutamic acid	0.25	
Glycerin U.S.P.	0.35	
Glyphyllin	0.12	0.10
Guanidine hydrochloride	0.65	
Heparin sodium U.S.P.	0.08	0.07
Hexamethonium bromide	0.22	0.19
Hexamethonium chloride	0.27	0.27
Hexobarbital sodium N.F.	0.26	0.24
Hexylcaine hydrochloride N.F.	0.26	0.22
Hippuran	0.16	0.15
Histalog	0.51	
Histamine phosphate U.S.P.	0.25	0.23
Histidine monohydrochloride	0.29	0.26
Holocaine hydrochloride	0.20	
Homatropine hydrobromide U.S.P.	0.17	0.16
Homatropine methylbromide U.S.P.	0.19	0.15
Hydralazine hydrochloride N.F.	0.37	
Hydrastine hydrochloride	0.15	0.12
Hydroxyamphetamine hydrobromide U.S.P.	0.26	0.25
Hydroxyquinoline sulfate U.S.P.	0.21	0.14
Hyoscyamine hydrobromide N.F.	0.19	0.16

Hyoscyamine sulfate N.F.	0.14	0.12
Intracaine hydrochloride	0.23	0.20
Iodophthalein sodium N.F.	0.17	0.12
Iodopyracet	0.11	0.11
Isoniazid U.S.P.	0.25	0.22
Lactic acid U.S.P.	0.41	
Lactose U.S.P.	0.07	0.08
Lidocaine hydrochloride U.S.P.	0.22	0.21
Lobeline hydrochloride	0.16	
Magnesium sulfate U.S.P.	0.17	0.15
Mannitol N.F.	0.17	0.17
Menadione diphosphate	0.25	0.22
Menadione sodium bisulfite U.S.P.	0.20	0.18
Meperidine hydrochloride U.S.P.	0.22	0.20
Mephenteramine sulfate U.S.P.	0.22	0.20
Mephenesin N.F.	0.19	
Merbromin N.F.	0.14	0.11
Mercaptomerin sodium U.S.P.	0.18	0.18
Mercuric cyanide	0.15	0.14
Mercurophylline N.F.	0.13	0.10
Mercury bichloride N.F.	0.13	0.12
Mersalyl N.F.	0.12	0.11
Methacholine chloride N.F.	0.32	
Methadone hydrochloride U.S.P.	0.18	0.14
Methantheline bromide N.F.	0.15	0.09
Methamphetamine hydrochloride N.F.	0.37	
Methapyrilene hydrochloride N.F.	0.19	0.18
Methenamine N.F.	0.23	0.24
Methionine N.F.	0.28	
Methoxamine hydrochloride U.S.P.	0.26	0.24
Methylatropine bromide	0.14	0.13
Monoethanolamine N.F.	0.53	
Morphine hydrochloride U.S.P.	0.15	0.14
Morphine nitrate	0.19	0.15
Morphine sulfate U.S.P.	0.14	0.11
Naphazoline hydrochloride N.F.	0.27	0.24
Narcotine hydrochloride	0.10	0.08
Neomycin sulfate U.S.P.	0.11	0.09
Neostigmine bromide U.S.P.	0.22	0.19
Neostigmine methyl sulfate U.S.P.	0.20	0.18
Nicotinamide U.S.P.	0.26	0.21
Nicotinic acid U.S.P.	0.25	
Nikethamide N.F.	0.18	0.16
Oxytetracycline hydrochloride U.S.P.	0.13	0.08
Papaverine hydrochloride U.S.P.	0.10	
Pentobarbital sodium U.S.P.	0.25	0.23
Pentolinium tartrate	0.17	0.15
Pentylenetetrazole N.F.	0.22	0.19
Phenindamine tartrate U.S.P.	0.17	0.12

Pheniramine maleate N.F.	0.16	0.14
Phenobarbital sodium U.S.P.	0.24	0.23
Phenol U.S.P.	0.35	
Phenylephrine hydrochloride U.S.P.	0.32	0.30
Phenylephrine tartrate	0.19	0.16
Phenylpropanolamine hydrochloride	0.38	
Physostigmine salicylate U.S.P.	0.16	
Physostigmine sulfate	0.13	0.12
Pilocarpine hydrochloride U.S.P.	0.24	0.22
Pilocarpine nitrate U.S.P.	0.23	0.20
Piperocaine hydrochloride U.S.P.	0.21	0.19
Piridocaine hydrochloride	0.24	
Polymyxin B sulfate U.S.P.	0.09	0.06
Potassium chloride U.S.P.	0.76	
Potassium iodide N.F.	0.34	
Potassium nitrate N.F.	0.56	
Potassium penicillin G U.S.P.	0.18	0.17
Potassium phosphate N.F.	0.46	
Potassium phosphate, monobasic	0.44	
Potassium sulfate	0.44	
Pramoxine hydrochloride	0.18	0.15
Procainamide hydrochloride U.S.P.	0.22	0.19
Probarbital calcium	0.25	
Probarbital sodium	0.32	0.29
Procaine hydrochloride U.S.P.	0.21	0.19
Promethazine hydrochloride U.S.P.	0.18	0.10
Propylene glycol U.S.P.	0.45	
Pyridoxine hydrochloride U.S.P.	0.37	0.29
Pyrilamine maleate U.S.P.	0.18	0.11
Quinidine gluconate N.F.	0.12	0.10
Quinidine sulfate U.S.P.	0.10	
Quinine dihydrochloride	0.23	0.19
Quinine hydrochloride N.F.	0.14	0.11
Quinine and urea hydrochloride N.F.	0.23	0.21
Racephedrine hydrochloride N.F.	0.31	0.30
Resorcinol U.S.P.	0.28	0.27
Scopolamine hydrobromide U.S.P.	0.12	0.12
Scopolamine methylnitrate	0.16	0.14
Secobarbital sodium U.S.P.	0.24	0.23
Silver nitrate U.S.P.	0.33	
Mild silver protein N.F.	0.17	0.17
Strong silver protein	0.08	0.05
Sodium acetate, anhydrous	0.77	
Sodium acetate N.F.	0.46	
Sodium aminosalicylate U.S.P.	0.29	0.28
Sodium ascorbate	0.33	0.30
Sodium benzoate U.S.P.	0.40	
Sodium bicarbonate U.S.P.	0.65	
Sodium biphosphate, anhydrous	0.46	

Sodium biphosphate U.S.P.	0.40	
Sodium bisulfite U.S.P.	0.61	
Sodium borate U.S.P.	0.42	
Sodium cacodylate	0.32	0.28
Sodium carbonate, monohydrated U.S.P.	0.60	
Sodium chloride U.S.P.	1.00	1.00
Sodium citrate U.S.P.	0.31	0.30
Sodium iodide U.S.P.	0.39	
Sodium lactate	0.55	
Sodium metabisulfite	0.67	
Sodium nitrate	0.68	
Sodium nitrite U.S.P.	0.84	
Sodium penicillin G U.S.P.	0.18	
Sodium phosphate exsiccated N.F.	0.53	
Sodium phosphate N.F.	0.29	0.27
Sodium phosphate, dibasic ($2H_2O$)	0.42	
Sodium phosphate, dibasic ($12H_2O$)	0.22	0.21
Sodium propionate N.F.	0.61	
Sodium riboflavin phosphate	0.08	0.08
Sodium ricinoleate	0.10	0.09
Sodium salicylate U.S.P.	0.36	
Sodium sulfate, anhydrous	0.58	
Sodium sulfate N.F.	0.26	0.23
Sodium sulfite, exsiccated	0.65	
Sodium thiosulfate	0.31	
Streptomycin calcium chloride complex	0.20	0.19
Streptomycin hydrochloride	0.17	0.16
Streptomycin sulfate U.S.P.	0.07	0.06
Strychnine hydrochloride	0.18	
Strychnine nitrate	0.12	
Succinylcholine chloride U.S.P.	0.20	0.20
Sucrose U.S.P.	0.08	0.09
Sulfacetamide sodium U. S. P.	0.23	0.23
Sulfadiazine sodium U.S.P.	0.24	0.22
Sulfamerazine sodium U.S.P.	0.23	0.21
Sulfapyridine sodium	0.23	0.21
Sulfathiazole sodium N.F.	0.22	0.20
Sulfisoxazole diethanolamine U.S.P.	0.18	0.15
Sympocaine hydrochloride	0.18	0.15
Synthenate tartarate	0.19	0.17
Tannic acid N.F.	0.03	0.03
Tartaric acid N.F.	0.25	0.23
Tetracycline hydrochloride U.S.P.	0.14	0.10
Tetracaine hydrochloride U.S.P.	0.18	0.15
Tetraethylammonium bromide	0.33	0.28
Tetraethylammonium chloride	0.34	
Tetrahydrozoline hydrochloride N.F.	0.28	0.23
Theophylline N.F.	0.10	
Thiamine hydrochloride U.S.P.	0.25	0.22

206 • aqueous solutions

Thiopental sodium U.S.P.	0.27	0.26
Tolazoline hydrochloride U.S.P.	0.34	0.30
Trasentine hydrochloride	0.22	0.15
Tripelennamine hydrochloride U.S.P.	0.30	0.20
Tropacocaine hydrochloride	0.25	0.20
Tuaminoheptane sulfate N.F.	0.27	0.27
Tubocurarine chloride U.S.P.	0.13	0.10
Urea N.F.	0.59	
Urethan U.S.P.	0.31	
Vinbarbital sodium	0.26	0.25
Viomycin sulfate N.F.	0.08	0.07
Zinc chloride N.F.	0.61	
Zinc phenolsulfonate N.F.	0.18	0.17
Zinc sulfanilate	0.21	0.19
Zinc sulfate U.S.P.	0.15	0.13

50. Ephedrine hydrochloride   1.2 g
     Chlorobutanol   0.3 g
     Sodium chloride, q.s.
     Purified water, q.s.   60 ml

   Make isotonic

   Sig.: Two drops as directed

The osmotic equivalent of 1.2 g of ephedrine hydrochloride is

$$0.3 \times 1.2 = 0.36 \text{ g of sodium chloride}$$

The osmotic equivalent of 0.3 g of chlorobutanol is

$$0.24 \times 0.3 = 0.072 \text{ g of sodium chloride}$$

The total osmotic equivalent of the ephedrine hydrochloride and the chlorobutanol is 0.432 g of sodium chloride. Since an isotonic saline solution contains 0.9 per cent sodium chloride, 60 ml of an isotonic solution of sodium chloride contains 60 x 0.009 = 0.54 g of sodium chloride. The amount of sodium chloride required to make an isotonic solution of the two drugs is 0.54 - 0.432 = 0.108 g.

If dextrose had been selected as the adjusting solute, the amount of sodium chloride to make the solution isotonic would be divided by the E of dextrose,

$$\frac{0.108}{0.16} = 0.68 \text{ g of dextrose}$$

An interesting feature of the sodium-chloride-equivalent method is that the amount of the drug may be expressed in any weight unit, e.g., gram, grain, or percentage.

51. Ethylmorphine hydrochloride   2.5%
     Sodium chloride, q.s.
     Purified water, q.s.   30 ml

   Make isotonic solution

   Sig.: 1-2 drops to produce chemosis

The drug in solution is osmotically equivalent to

$$2.5 \times 0.16 = 0.4\% \text{ sodium chloride}$$

A 0.9 per cent sodium chloride solution is isotonic with body fluids; therefore, the percentage of sodium chloride to be added to make an isotonic solution is

$$0.9 - 0.4 = 0.5\%$$

The weight of sodium chloride to adjust the 30 ml of solution is

$$30 \times 0.005 = 0.15 \text{ g}$$

Cryoscopic Method. The cryoscopic method, using tables of the freezing-point depression of 1 per cent solutions of the drugs, is based on the assumption that the extent of freezing-point depression is proportional to the percentage of the solute. Although this is not a fact over a large range of concentration, it is acceptable within physiological tolerance for the dilute solutions used in pharmaceuticals. For example, a 1 per cent solution of phenylephrine hydrochloride depresses the freezing point of water $0.17°$; it is assumed that a 2 per cent solution of phenylephrine hydrochloride depresses the freezing point of water twice as much as a 1 per cent solution, i.e., $0.34°$.

52. Phenylephrine hydrochloride   0.5%
    Sodium chloride, q.s.
    Purified water, q.s.   100 ml

    Adjust to isotonic solution

    Sig.: Two drops in nose

Assuming a direct proportionality, and knowing the depression caused by 1 per cent of the solute, a ratio may be set up to calculate the depression of freezing point of water produced by 0.5 per cent phenylephrine hydrochloride,

$$\frac{1}{0.17} = \frac{0.5}{x}$$

$$x = 0.085°$$

The depression to be contributed by the sodium chloride is $0.52 - 0.085 = 0.435°$. The percentage of sodium chloride to provide this freezing-point depression is calculated by means of a ratio using the fact that a 0.9 per cent solution of sodium chloride lowers the freezing point of water $0.52°$,

$$\frac{0.9}{0.52} = \frac{x}{0.435}$$

$$x = 0.753\%$$

These calculations may be incorporated into a single equation,

$$x = \frac{0.52 - A}{B}$$

where x is the number of grams of adjusting solute for 100 ml of solution. A is the freezing-point depression of water produced by the drugs, and B is the freezing-point depression of water produced by a 1 per cent solution of the adjusting solute.

53. Pilocarpine hydrochloride   2%
    (make isotonic with boric acid)
    Purified water, q.s.   100 ml

    Sig.: Gtt. i-ii o.s.

aqueous solutions

From Table XLIII the freezing-point depression produced by 1 per cent pilocarpine hydrochloride is 0.13° and that of 1 per cent boric acid is 0.29°. Substitution yields

$$x = \frac{0.52 - (2 \times 0.13)}{0.29} = 0.9 \text{ g of boric acid for 100 ml}$$

In most humans, solutions of sodium chloride ranging from 0.6 to 1.5 per cent concentration do not cause pain or damage to the corneal ephithelial. The majority of extemporaneous ophthalmic solutions would probably be acceptable if dispensed in a 0.8 per cent saline vehicle; however, for industrially produced collyria and parenteral solutions, appropriate calculations should be made during formulation and the solution should be experimentally tested for tonicity.

Table XLIII Freezing-Point Depression of a 1 per cent Solution

Drug	Freezing-Point Depression (°C)
Antipyrine	0.10
Atropine sulfate	0.07
Boric acid	0.29
Calcium chloride dihydrate	0.30
Camphor	0.12
Chlorobutanol	0.14
Citric acid	0.10
Cocaine hydrochloride	0.09
Dextrose	0.09
Emetine hydrochloride	0.06
Ephedrine hydrochloride	0.18
Ephedrine sulfate	0.11
Epinephrine hydrochloride	0.17
Ethylhydrocupreine hydrochloride	0.10
Ethylmorphine hydrochloride	0.09
Fluorescein sodium	0.18
Homatropine hydrobromide	0.10
Hyoscine hydrobromide	0.07
Lactose	0.04
Magnesium chloride hexahydrate	0.24
Magnesium sulfate	0.10
Menthol	0.12
Mercuric chloride	0.08
Mercuric cyanide	0.09
Methenamine	0.13
Metycaine hydrochloride	0.12
Morphine hydrochloride	0.09
Morphine sulfate	0.08
Neosynephrine hydrochloride	0.17
Phenacaine hydrochloride	0.09
Physostigmine sulfate	0.08
Pilocarpine hydrochloride	0.13
Potassium chloride	0.45
Potassium phosphate (monobasic)	0.25
Procaine hydrochloride	0.12

Silver nitrate	0.19
Sodium acid phosphate	0.24
Sodium bicarbonate	0.38
Sodium borate	0.25
Sodium bromide	0.36
Sodium chloride	0.58
Sodium citrate	0.17
Sodium iodide	0.23
Sodium phosphate dihydrate	0.25
Sodium sulfate	0.15
Sodium thiosulfate	0.18
Sugar	0.05
Tartaric acid	0.14
Zinc chloride	0.37
Zinc phenolsulfonate	0.11
Zinc sulfate heptahydrate	0.09

ACID-BASE EQUILIBRIA

According to the original Arrhenius theory, upon ionizing in water, an acid liberates hydrogen ions and a base liberates hydroxyl ions. The Brønsted-Lowry theory defines acids and bases in a broader sense, and it applies to aqueous and nonaqueous systems. An acid is a substance that donates protons and a base is a substance that accepts protons. Thus, the dissociation of an acid, HA, always produces a base, A^-,

$$HA \rightleftharpoons H^+ + A^-$$

Here HA and A^- are referred to as a conjugate acid-base pair, i.e., an acid and a base that differ in their structure by a proton and are in equilibrium. The proton of the acid does not exist free in solution, but it is in combination with the solvent. In water the hydrated proton is known as a hydronium ion. As the exact extent of hydration is unknown, the symbol H^+ is generally used to represent the hydrated hydrogen ion. In nonaqueous systems the solvent accepts the proton, which becomes solvated. There is no direct comparison between the properties of the hydrogen ion in different solvents because their environments are so different.

The relative strengths of acids and bases are determined by the ability of these substances to donate or accept protons. In water HCl gives up protons more readily than acetic acid and consequently HCl is a stronger acid. The affinity of the solvent for protons also determines the strength of an acid. An acid such as HCl may dissociate completely in liquid ammonia and very slightly in glacial acetic acid. Thus, HCl is considered a strong acid in liquid ammonia and a weak acid in acetic acid.

The Lewis electronic theory defines an acid as a molecule or ion that accepts an electron pair from some other atom. A base is a substance that donates a pair of electrons which will be shared with an acid. Thus, amines that do not contain hydroxyl ions are bases due to the unshared electron pair. Since the Lewis concept is broader than is necessary in considering pharmaceutical and biological systems, which are primarily aqueous, the Brønsted-Lowry theory will be used.

Although ionization and dissociation are often used synonymously, there is a subtle difference between the terms. Ionization refers to the complete separation of the ions of a crystal lattice when the salt is dissolved. The ions in solution may be associated by interionic attraction and may not exist as individual ions; the separation of these ions in solution is known as dissociation.

Dissociation Constants

The dissociation of weak electrolytes is a reversible process, and the equilibrium may be expressed by the law of mass action. The law of mass action states that the rate of a chemical reaction is proportional to the product of the concentration of the reacting substances, each raised to a power equal to the number of moles of that substance in the equation. The dissociation of a weak acid in water may be written as

$$HA \rightleftharpoons H^+ + A^-$$

The dynamic equilibrium between the simultaneous forward and reverse reaction is indicated by the arrows. By the law of mass action, the rate of the forward reaction is

$$R = k_1 [HA]$$

and the rate of the reverse reaction is

$$R' = k_2 [H^+] [A^-]$$

The brackets indicate that the concentration is expressed in moles or g-ions liter^{-1}. At equilibrium the rates are equal and

$$k_1 [HA] = k_2 [H^+] [A^-]$$

Solving for the ratio of the rates, the equilibrium expression for the dissociation of a weak acid HA in water may be written

$$K_a = \frac{k_1}{k_2} = \frac{[H^+][A^-]}{[HA]}$$

which defines the acid dissociation constant, K_a. Since strong acids and bases are completely ionized, no equilibrium expression can be written for them, and no dissociation constants are defined.

In the dissociation of a weak acid in water, the total molar concentration of the acid may be represented by c. The hydrogen ion concentration at equilibrium is $[H^+]$. Since for monoprotic acids the hydrogen ion and anion are formed in equimolar concentrations, $[H^+]$ numerically represents the molar concentration of the anion. At equilibrium the concentration of the undissociated acid is $c - [H^+]$. The dissociation constant may be written in these terms,

$$K_a = \frac{[H^+]^2}{c - [H^+]}$$

The solution of this quadratic equation may be avoided if the weak acid is only slightly dissociated. With only slight dissociation c is large in comparison with $[H^+]$, and the term $c - [H^+]$ may be replaced by c without appreciable error:

$$K_a = \frac{[H^+]^2}{c}$$

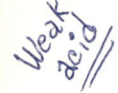
Weak acid

By rearranging and taking the square root, a convenient expression is obtained for calculating the hydrogen ion concentration of a solution of a weak acid,

$$[H^+] = \sqrt{K_a c}$$

At 25° acetic acid has $K_a = 1.75 \times 10^{-5}$. The hydrogen ion concentration of a 0.01 M solution of acetic acid is

e.g. Acetic Acid
Salicylic Acid

$$[H^+] = \sqrt{1.75 \times 10^{-5} \times 0.01}$$
$$= 4.19 \times 10^{-4} \text{ g-ion liter}^{-1}$$

As the [H$^+$] is greater than K_a and is less than 5 per cent of the total acid concentration the use of the approximate equation is justified. The assumption used to derive this convenient expression must be considered in applying it to the calculation of hydrogen ion concentration. The error introduced by the assumption becomes greater as the concentration of the acid becomes smaller and as the K_a becomes larger.

Salicylic acid has $K_a = 1.06 \times 10^{-3}$. If the hydrogen ion concentration of a 0.01 M solution were calculated by the approximate equation,

$$[H^+] = \sqrt{1.06 \times 10^{-3} \times 0.01}$$
$$= 3.26 \times 10^{-3} \text{ g-ion liter}^{-1}$$

As [H$^+$] is of the same magnitude as the K_a and is approximately one-third of the concentration of the undissociated acid, the assumption used in deriving the approximate equation is not attained, and the simplified equation cannot be used. The hydrogen ion concentration must be calculated by means of the equation

$$K_a = \frac{[H^+]^2}{c - [H^+]}$$

which in the general quadratic form is

$$[H^+]^2 + K_a[H^+] - K_a c = 0$$

The solution to this quadrateic equation (see Appendix: Algebra) is

$$[H^+] = \frac{-1.06 \times 10^{-3} \pm \sqrt{(1.06 \times 10^{-3})^2 + (4 \times 10.6 \times 10^{-3} \times 0.01)}}{2}$$

$$= 2.77 \times 10^{-3} \text{ g-ion liter}^{-1}$$

The dissociation of a weak base may be expressed using the K_a expression for the conjugate acid of the base. The conjugate acid is the acid that is formed when a proton reacts with the base. For a base, B, which does not contain a hydroxyl group

$$BH^+ \rightleftharpoons H^+ + B$$

and the dissociation constant for the reaction is

$$K_a = \frac{[H^+][B]}{[BH^+]}$$

For bases it has been traditional to define a base dissociation constant for the reaction of a weak base,

as

$$B + H_2O \rightleftharpoons OH^- + BH^+$$

$$K_b = \frac{[OH^-][BH^+]}{[B]}$$

By reasoning similar to that used for approximating the hydrogen ion concentration in a solution of a weak acid, the hydroxyl ion concentration of a solution of a weak base may be approximately expressed as

$$[OH^-] = \sqrt{K_b c}$$

Ephedrine has a $K_b = 2.3 \times 10^{-5}$ and a molecular weight of 165 g mole^{-1}. The hydroxyl ion concentration of a 1 per cent solution may be calculated as

$$[OH] = \sqrt{2.3 \times 10^{-5} \times 10/165}$$
$$= 1.18 \times 10^{-3} \text{ g-ion liter}^{-1}$$

The degree of dissociation of a weak acid or base is the fraction of the initial un-ionized acid or base that has dissociated. If the initial molar concentration is represented by c and the concentration of the dissociated electrolyte is represented by x, the degree of dissociation is

$$\alpha = \frac{x}{c}$$

The degree of dissociation of a 1 per cent ephedrine solution is

$$\alpha = \frac{1.18 \times 10^{-3}}{0.061} = 0.02$$

Only 2 per cent of the ephedrine in this solution is dissociated into hydroxyl and ephedrine ions; 98 per cent of the ephedrine is in the undissociated form.

One of the methods of measuring the dissociation constant utilizes the equivalent conductance of the electrolyte solution. The molar concentration of ions from a weak acid is equal to the total concentration of the acid multiplied by the fraction that is dissociated, i.e., $x = \alpha c$. Substitution into the equation, which defines K_a, yields

$$K_a = \frac{(\alpha c)(\alpha c)}{c - \alpha c} = \frac{\alpha^2 c}{1 - \alpha}$$

If the equivalent conductance at infinite dilution, Λ_0, is known and the equivalent conductance of the solution is measured, the degree of dissociation is Λ/Λ_0. Substitution into the preceding equation provides the relationship

$$K_a = \frac{\Lambda^2 c}{\Lambda_0 (\Lambda_0 - \Lambda)}$$

The calculation of K_a may be illustrated by considering a 0.005912 N acetic acid solution which at 25° has an equivalence conductance of 20.9 cm² equiv⁻¹ ohm⁻¹. The literature value of Λ_0 for acetic acid is 390.6 cm² equiv⁻¹ ohm⁻¹. The dissociation constant is

$$K_a = \frac{(20.9)^2 (0.005912)}{390.6 \, (390.6 - 20.9)}$$

$$= 1.8 \times 10^{-5}$$

Certain compounds may donate or accept more than one proton, and they will consequently have more than one dissociation constant. The carbonates, which are important in the buffer system of the blood plasma, dissociate in two steps. The first step is

$$H_2CO_3 \rightleftharpoons H^+ + HCO_3^-$$

for which the dissociation constant is

$$K_1 = \frac{[H^+][HCO_3^-]}{[H_2CO_3]} = 4.3 \times 10^{-7}$$

The second step is

$$HCO_3^- \rightleftharpoons H^+ + CO_3^{--}$$

for which the dissociation constant is

$$K_2 = \frac{[H^+][CO_3^{--}]}{[HCO_3^-]} = 4.7 \times 10^{-11}$$

With the negative charge on the HCO_3^- it becomes difficult for the water to remove a second proton; thus, K_2 is very small and very little CO_3^{--} exists in a solution of carbonic acid.

Basic compounds and alkaloids may dissociate in more than one step. Quinidine is an example of an alkaloid that has two dissociation constants. The first step of dissociation is

$$C_{20}H_{24}N_2O_2 + H_2O \rightleftharpoons C_{20}H_{24}NH^+NO_2 + OH^-$$

for which the dissociation constant is

$$K_{b_1} = \frac{[C_{20}H_{24}NH^+NO_2][OH^-]}{[C_{20}H_{24}N_2O_2]} = 3.7 \times 10^{-6}$$

The second step of dissociation is

$$C_{20}H_{24}NH^+NO_2 + H_2O \rightleftharpoons C_{20}H_{24}NH^+NH^+O_2 + OH^-$$

for which the dissociation constant is

$$K_{b_2} = \frac{[C_{20}H_{24}NH^+NH^+O_2][OH^-]}{[C_{20}H_{24}NH^+NO_2]} = 1 \times 10^{-10}$$

pH and Hydrogen Ion Concentration

Hydrogen ion concentrations are determined to very small values, and to avoid the nuisance of writing many zeros to describe the concentrations, an exponential notation has been adopted. The pH is defined as the negative exponent of 10, which equals the hydrogen ion concentration. Thus,

$$[H^+] = 10^{-pH}$$

or

$$pH = -\log[H^+] = \log \frac{1}{[H^+]}$$

The hydrogen ion concentration of a solution with a pH 4 is

$$[H^+] = 10^{-4} = 0.0001 \text{ g-ion liter}^{-1}$$

The interconversion of pH and hydrogen ion concentration is often required in pharmacy. The pH of blood of a healthy human is 7.4. The hydrogen ion concentration is calculated (see Appendix: Logarithms)

$$pH = -\log[H^+] = 7.4$$
$$\log[H^+] = -7.4 = (-8.0 + 0.6)$$
$$[H^+] = \text{antilogarithm } 0.6 \times \text{antilogarithm } -8.0$$

From the logarithmic tables the antilogarithm of 0.6 is 3.98 and the antilogarithm of -8.0 is 10^{-8}. The hydrogen ion concentration is

$$[H^+] = 3.98 \times 10^{-8} \text{ g-ion liter}^{-1}$$

To illustrate the conversion of hydrogen ion concentration to pH consider a solution that has $[H^+] = 2 \times 10^{-5}$ g-ion liter^{-1}. Since the logarithm of a product is equal to the sum of the logarithms of the numbers to be multiplied,

$$pH = -\log[H^+] = -\log(2 \times 10^{-5})$$
$$= -(\log 2 + \log 10^{-5})$$

From the logarithmic tables the logarithm of 2 is 0.3, and by definition the logarithm of 10^{-5} is -5.0. Thus,

$$pH = -(0.3 - 5.0) = 4.7$$

The convenience of using pH values should not obscure an appreciation of the magnitude of changes in hydrogen ion concentration. When the pH decreases from 6 to 5, the hydrogen ion concentration increases from 10^{-6} to 10^{-5}, or 10 times its initial value. When the pH falls from 5 to 4.7, the hydrogen ion concentration increases from 10^{-5} to 2×10^{-5}; thus, a fall in pH of 0.3 unit means that the hydrogen ion concentration has doubled.

pH of Solutions of Weak Acids or Bases

Water is a very weak electrolyte which dissociates according to the reaction

$$H_2O \rightleftharpoons H^+ + OH^-$$

An equilibrium constant, which is based on the law of mass action, expresses the equilibrium of this reaction,

$$K = \frac{[H^+][OH^-]}{[H_2O]}$$

As the molecular water exists in great excess in comparison to the concentration of hydrogen and hydroxyl ions, the denominator is constant and is usually incorporated into the ionization constant, K_w, which is known as the ion product of water,

$$K_w = [H^+][OH^-]$$

In pure water at 25° the hydrogen and hydroxyl ion concentratons are equal with a value of 10^{-7} g-ion liter^{-1}. The dissociation of weak electrolytes varies slightly with temperature. This effect is illustrated in Table XLIV for the ion product of water.

Table XLIV Ion Product of Water

Temperature (°C)	$K_w \times 10^{14}$	pK_w
0	0.114	14.94
10	0.292	14.53
20	0.681	14.17
25	1.008	13.99
37	2.57	13.59

Since K_w remains constant at a given temperature, the increase in hydrogen ions upon the addition of an acid to water is offset by a decrease in hydroxyl ions. If an acid with a $K_a = 1.75 \times 10^{-5}$ is added to water to make a 0.01 M solution, the hydroxyl ion concentration may be calculated. The hydrogen ion concentration of the solution of the weak acid is

$$[H^+] = \sqrt{K_a c}$$
$$= \sqrt{1.75 \times 10^{-5} \times 0.01}$$
$$= 4.19 \times 10^{-4} \text{ g-ion liter}^{-1}$$

and the hydroxyl ion concentration is

$$[OH^-] = \frac{K_w}{[H^+]} = \frac{10^{-14}}{4.19 \times 10^{-4}}$$
$$= 2.4 \times 10^{-11} \text{ g-ion liter}^{-1}$$

If the negative logarithms of the equation for calculating the hydrogen ion concentration of a solution of a weak acid are taken,

$$-\log[H^+] = -\tfrac{1}{2}\log K_a - \tfrac{1}{2}\log c$$

In the same manner that the symbol pH is used for the term $-\log [H^+]$, the symbol pK may in general be used to represent $-\log K$, regardless of the constant that K represents. If pK_a represents $-\log K_a$, the equation may be written

$$pH = \tfrac{1}{2} pK_a - \tfrac{1}{2} \log c \qquad \text{Weak Acid}$$

Barbital has a $pK_a = 7.9$ and a molecular weight of 184.2 g mole^{-1}. The pH of a 0.5 per cent solution of barbital is calculated by

$$pH = (\tfrac{1}{2} \times 7.9) - (\tfrac{1}{2} \log 5/184.2)$$
$$= 3.95 + 0.78 = 4.73$$

In a like manner an equation may be derived to calculate the pH of an aqueous solution of a weak base. It has been shown that the hydroxyl ion concentration of a solution of a weak base is represented by the expression

$$[OH^-] = \sqrt{K_b c}$$

Rearrangement of the equation defining the ion product of water and substitution for hydroxyl ion concentration yields

$$\frac{K_w}{[H^+]} = \sqrt{K_b c}$$

which may be rearranged to

$$[H^+] = \frac{K_w}{\sqrt{K_b c}}$$

If the negative logarithms of the equation are taken,

$$-\log [H^+] = -\log K_w + \tfrac{1}{2} \log K_b + \tfrac{1}{2} \log c$$

which in terms of pK symbols becomes

$$pH = pK_w - \tfrac{1}{2} pK_b + \tfrac{1}{2} \log c \qquad \text{Weak Base}$$

Codeine base has a $pK_b = 6.1$ and a molecular weight of 299.4 g mole^{-1}. The pH of a 0.3 per cent aqueous solution at 25° is

$$pH = 14 - \frac{6.1}{2} + \tfrac{1}{2} \log \frac{3}{299}$$
$$\cong 10$$

The dissociation constants of some acids and bases at 25° are shown in Tables XLV and XLVI.

Table XLV Dissociation Constants for Acids in Aqueous Solutions at 25°

Compound	K_a	pK_a
Acetic	1.75×10^{-5}	4.76
Acetylsalicylic	3.27×10^{-4}	3.49
Adipic	3.72×10^{-5}	4.43
a-Alanine	9×10^{-10}	9.05
Aluminum hydroxide	6.3×10^{-3}	12.20
L-Arginine *	3.3×10^{-13}	12.48

216 • aqueous solutions

Arsenic		5×10^{-3}	2.30
		8.3×10^{-8} (2H)	7.08
		6×10^{-10} (3H)	9.22
Arsenious		6×10^{-13}	12.22
L-Aspartic *		1.38×10^{-4}	3.86
		1.51×10^{-10} (2H)	9.82
Barbituric		1.05×10^{-4}	3.98
Barbituric			
	Allylbenzyl	6.2×10^{-8}	7.21
	Diallyl	1.6×10^{-8}	7.78
(Barbital)	Diethyl	1.2×10^{-8}	7.90
	Ethylisopropyl	1×10	8.01
	Ethyl-1-methylbutyl	8×10^{-9}	8.11
	Phenylethyl	3.9×10^{-8}	7.41
Benzoic		$\sim 6.3 \times 10^{-5}$	4.20
Benzyl penicillin		1.74×10^{-3}	2.76
Boric		5.8×10^{-10}	9.24
n-Butyric		1.5×10^{-5}	4.82
Carbonic		4.31×10^{-7}	6.37
		5.6×10^{-11} (2H)	10.25
Chloracetic		1.4×10^{-3}	2.86
o-Chlorobenzoic		1.197×10^{-3}	2.82
m-Chlorobenzoic		1.506×10^{-4}	3.82
p-Chlorobenzoic		1.04×10^{-4}	3.98
o-Chlorophenylacetic		8.6×10^{-5}	4.07
m-Chlorophenylacetic		7.24×10^{-5}	4.14
p-Chlorophenylacetic		6.45×10^{-5}	4.19
Cinnamic			
	trans	3.7×10^{-5}	4.43
	cis	1.32×10^{-4}	3.88
Citric		8.7×10^{-4}	3.06
		1.8×10^{-5} (2H)	4.74
		4×10^{-6} (3H)	5.40
L-Cystine *		1×10^{-9}	8.00
		5.63×10^{-11} (2H)	10.25
Dichloracetic		5×10^{-2}	1.3
Diiodo-L-tyrosine *		3.3×10^{-7}	6.48
Formic		1.76×10^{-4}	3.75
Fumaric		9.3×10^{-4}	3.75
		3.4×10^{-5} (2H)	3.03
Gallic		4×10^{-5}	4.40
L-Glutamic *		8.5×10^{-5}	4.07
		3.4×10^{-10} (2H)	9.47

aqueous solutions • 217

Glutaric	4.54×10^{-5}	4.34
Glycerophosphoric	3.4×10^{-2}	1.47
	6.4×10^{-7} (2H)	6.19
Glycine	4.5×10^{-3}	2.35
	1.67×10^{-10} (2H)	9.78
Hippuric	2.3×10^{-4}	3.64
L-Histidine *	6.6×10^{-10}	9.18
Hydrocyanic	7.2×10^{-10}	9.14
Hydroxy-L-proline *	8.3×10^{-13}	12.08
Hypochlorous	3.5×10^{-8}	7.46
Iodic	1.67×10^{-1}	0.78
p-Iodophenylacetic	6.64×10^{-5}	4.18
Isobutyric	1.55×10^{-5}	4.81
DL-Isoleucine *	1.75×10^{-10}	9.76
Isovaleric	1.46×10^{-4}	3.84
Itaconic	1.46×10^{-4}	3.84
	2.8×10^{-6} (2H)	5.55
Lactic	1.387×10^{-4}	3.86
DL-Leucine *	1.8×10^{-10}	9.74
L-Lysine *	2.95×10^{-11}	10.53
Maleic	1.0×10^{-2}	2.00
	5.5×10^{-7} (2H)	6.26
Malic	4×10^{-4}	3.40
	9×10^{-6} (2H)	5.05
Malonic	1.397×10^{-3}	2.85
	8×10^{-7} (2H)	6.10
Mandelic	4.29×10^{-4}	3.37
DL-Methionine *	6.17×10^{-10}	9.21
	6.1×10^{-4}	3.21
α-Naphthonic	2×10^{-4}	3.70
β-Naphthonic	6.9×10^{-5}	4.16
Nicotinic	1.34×10^{-5}	4.87
Nitrous (18°)	4×10^{-4}	3.40
Oxalic	6.5×10^{-2}	1.19
	6.1×10^{-5} (2H)	4.21
Periodic	2.3×10^{-2}	1.64
Phenol	1.3×10^{-10}	9.89
Phenolphthalein	2×10^{-10}	9.70
Phenylacetic	4.88×10^{-5}	4.31

DL-Phenylalanine *	5.76×10^{-10}	9.24
Phosphoric	7.5×10^{-3}	2.12
	6.2×10^{-8} (2H)	7.21
	4.8×10^{-13} (3H)	12.32
Phosphorous	1.6×10^{-2}	1.80
	7×10^{-7} (2H)	6.15
Phthalic	1.26×10^{-3}	2.89
	3.1×10^{-6} (2H)	5.51
Picric	4.2×10^{-1}	0.38
L-Proline *	2.5×10^{-11}	10.6
Propionic	1.343×10^{-5}	4.87
Pyromucic (furoic)	7.1×10^{-4}	3.15
Pyrophosphoric	1.4×10^{-1}	0.85
	1.1×10^{-2} (2H)	1.96
	2.1×10^{-7} (3H)	6.68
	4.06×10^{-10} (4H)	9.39
Pyrotartaric	8.5×10^{-5}	4.07
Saccharin	2.5×10^{-2}	1.60
Salicylic	1.06×10^{-3}	2.97
DL-Serine *	7.1×10^{-10}	9.15
Succinic	6.4×10^{-5}	4.19
	2.7×10^{-6} (2H)	5.57
Sulfadiazine	3.3×10^{-7}	6.48
Sulfamerazine	8.7×10^{-8}	7.06
Sulfapyridine	3.6×10^{-9}	8.44
Sulfathiazole	7.6×10^{-8}	7.12
Tartaric	9.6×10^{-4}	3.02
	2.9×10^{-5} (2H)	4.54
Trichloracetic	1.3×10^{-1}	0.89
Tryptophan *	4.06×10^{-10}	9.39
L-Tyrosine *	8×10^{-10}	9.11
Uric	1.3×10^{-4}	3.89
Valeric	1.56×10^{-5}	4.81
DL-Valine *	1.9×10^{-10}	9.72

* Dissociation constant at the isoelectric point.

aqueous solutions • 219

Table XLVI Dissociation Constants of Bases in Aqueous Solution at 25°

Compound	K_b	K_a	pK_a
Acetanilide	1×10^{-13}	1×10^{-1}	1.0
Aconitine	1.3×10^{-6}	7.7×10^{-9}	8.11
Ammonium hydroxide	1.77×10^{-5}	5.55×10^{-10}	9.26
Arecoline (15°)	1.4×10^{-7}	7.14×10^{-8}	7.16
Atropine (15°)	4.47×10^{-5}	2.2×10^{-10}	9.65
Benzocaine (15°)	6×10^{-12}	1.67×10^{-3}	2.78
Benzoylecgonine (15°)	1.7×10^{-12}	5.88×10^{-3}	2.23
Berberine (15°)	3.4×10^{-3}	2.9×10^{-12}	11.53
Brucine	9×10^{-7} 2×10^{-12} (2OH)	1.1×10^{-8} 5×10^{-3}	7.95 2.3
Caffeine (40°)	4.1×10^{-14}	2.4×10^{-1}	0.61
Cevadine (15°)	7.2×10^{-6}	1.4×10^{-9}	8.85
Cinchonidine	1.6×10^{-6} 9.3×10^{-11} (2OH)	6.2×10^{-9} 1.2×10^{-4}	8.20 3.97
Cinchonine	1.4×10^{-6} 1.2×10^{-10}	7.14×10^{-9} 9×10^{-5}	8.15 4.08
Cocaine (15°)	2.6×10^{-6}	3.9×10^{-9}	8.41
Codeine (15°)	9×10^{-7}	1.1×10^{-8}	7.95
Colchicine	4.5×10^{-13}	2.2×10^{-2}	1.65
Coniine	7.5×10^{-4}	1.3×10^{-11}	10.9
Cupreine	2.7×10^{-7}	3.8×10^{-8}	7.43
Cytisine	8.3×10^{-7} 8.4×10^{-14}	1.2×10^{-8} 1.2×10^{-1}	7.92 0.92
Ecgonine (15°)	6×10^{-12}	1.67×10^{-3}	2.78
Emetine	1.7×10^{-6} 2.3×10^{-7} (2OH)	5.88×10^{-9} 4.3×10^{-8}	8.23 7.36
Ethanolamine	2.77×10^{-5}	3.6×10^{-10}	9.44
Ethylmorphine (15°)	7.6×10^{-7}	1.3×10^{-8}	7.88

220 • aqueous solutions

Hydrastine	1.7×10^{-8}	5.88×10^{-7}	6.23
Hydrastinine (15°)	2.4×10^{-3}	4.1×10^{-12}	11.38
Hydrochinine (15°)	4.7×10^{-6}	2.1×10^{-9}	8.67
Isopilocarpine (15°)	6.76×10^{-8}	1.5×10^{-7}	6.83
Isoquinoline	2.5×10^{-9}	4×10^{-6}	5.4
Morphine	7.4×10^{-7}	1.3×10^{-8}	7.87
Narceine	2×10^{-11}	5×10^{-4}	3.3
Narcotine	1.5×10^{-8}	6.6×10^{-7}	6.18
Nicotine (15°)	7×10^{-7}	1.4×10^{-8}	7.85
	1.1×10^{-10} (2OH)	9×10^{-4}	3.04
Papaverine	8×10^{-9}	1.24×10^{-6}	5.90
Pelletierine (15°)	1.78×10^{-5}	5.6×10^{-10}	9.25
✓ Physostigmine	7.6×10^{-7}	1.3×10^{-8}	7.88
	5.7×10^{-13} (2OH)	1.7×10^{-2}	1.76
Pilocarpine	7×10^{-8}	1.4×10^{-7}	6.85
	2.7×10^{-13} (2OH)	4×10^{-2}	1.43
Procaine	7×10^{-6}	1.4×10^{-9}	8.85
Pseudotropine (15°)	1.6×10^{-4}	6.2×10^{-11}	10.20
Quinidine	3.7×10^{-6}	2.8×10^{-9}	8.6
	1×10^{-10} (2OH)	1×10^{-4}	4.0
Quinine	1×10^{-6}	1×10^{-8}	8.0
	1.3×10^{-10}	7.6×10^{-5}	4.11
Quinoline	3.2×10^{-10}	3×10^{-5}	4.5
Sarcosine	1.8×10^{-12}	5.5×10^{-3}	2.26
Solanine (15°)	2.2×10^{-7}	4.5×10^{-8}	7.34
Sparteine	5.7×10^{-3}	1.8×10^{-12}	11.76
	2.8×10^{-10}	3.8×10^{-5}	4.54
Strychnine	1×10^{-6}	1×10^{-8}	8.0
	2×10^{-12} (2OH)	5×10^{-3}	2.3

Thebaine	9×10^{-7}	1.1×10^{-8}	7.95
Theobromine (18°)	1.3×10^{-14}	7.7×10^{-1}	0.12
Tropacocaine (15°)	1.9×10^{-5}	5×10^{-10}	9.68
Urea	1.5×10^{-14}	6.6×10^{-1}	0.18

pH of a Salt Solution

A strong acid and a strong base react to form a salt, which is completely ionized. When the salt is dissolved it dissociates into anions and cations, and as no change occurs in hydrogen or hydroxyl ions, the solution is neutral.

If the salt of a weak acid and a strong base is dissolved in water, an alkaline pH results, because the anions of the salt react with the water to form the weak acid and hydroxyl ions. This hydrolysis can be illustrated for sodium acetate:

$$NaA \rightleftharpoons Na^+ + A^-$$
$$H_2O \rightleftharpoons OH^- + H^+$$
$$\qquad \Updownarrow \qquad \Updownarrow$$
$$\qquad NaOH \quad HA$$

The sodium and hydroxyl ions attract each other, but as the sodium hydroxide is strongly dissociated, there is no decrease in concentration of hydroxyl ions. The acetate and hydrogen ion react to produce undissociated molecules of the weak acetic acid. As the reaction progresses, more of the water dissociates to supply hydrogen ions for the production of acetic acid molecules. When equilibrium is attained, there is a definite excess of hydroxyl ions over hydrogen ions.

Such a hydrolysis of a salt may be considered as a type of acid-base reaction and is generalized by the equation

$$A^- + H_2O \rightleftharpoons OH^- + HA$$

Na salt of weak acid + H_2O ⇌ weak acid + NaOH

where water and hydroxyl ion are a conjugate pair and the weak acid and the anion are the other conjugate pair. The equilibrium constant for the dissociation of the conjugate base of the weak acid is

$$K_b = \frac{[HA][OH^-]}{[A^-]}$$

If the equation for the dissociation constant of a weak acid is multiplied by the constant for the dissociation of the conjugate base of the weak acid,

$$K_a K_b = \frac{[H^+][A^-]}{[HA]} \cdot \frac{[HA][OH^-]}{[A^-]} = [H^+][OH^-]$$

Thus, for an aqueous solution

$$K_a K_b = K_w$$

and, consequently,

$$pK_a + pK_b = pK_w$$

Although the K_b values have been conventionally used to express the dissociation of bases, the dissociation can be expressed in terms of K_a values of the acids conjugate to the weak bases in aqueous solution. For example, at 25° the pK_b of codeine base is 6.1 and its pK_a is

$$pK_a = 14 - 6.1 = 7.9$$

In biochemistry and physiology it is common practice to express the dissociation of acidic and basic compounds in terms of K_a and pK_a. In pharmaceutical sciences the biological activity is often related to the pK_a of a series of drugs within a therapeutic category. In comparing a series of sulfonamides it has been found that sulfonamides with $pK_a = 6.7$ have a maximal antibacterial action. In comparing a series of amines it has been found that the compounds with $pK_a = 8.6$ had a maximal antagonism to histamine, while the compounds with pK_a greater or less than 8.6 had a lesser activity.

The expression for the pH of a solution of a salt of a weak acid and a strong base may be derived. The equation

$$K_b = \frac{K_w}{K_a} = \frac{[HA][OH^-]}{[A^-]}$$

can be written as

$$\frac{K_w}{K_a} = \frac{[OH^-]^2}{c_S - [OH^-]}$$

where c_S is the initial molar concentration of the salt. Since the undissociated acid and the hydroxyl ion are formed in equimolar concentrations, $[OH^-]$ numerically represents the concentration of both species.

If $[OH^-]$ is small compared to the initial concentration of the salt, the denominator may be replaced by c_S without the introduction of appreciable error and the equation simplifies to

$$\frac{K_w}{K_a} = \frac{[OH^-]^2}{c_S}$$

and

$$[OH^-] = \sqrt{\frac{K_w c_S}{K_a}}$$

This may be expressed in terms of hydrogen ion concentration by substitution of $[OH^-] = K_w/[H^+]$,

$$\frac{K_w}{[H^+]} = \sqrt{\frac{K_w c_S}{K_a}}$$

Incorporation of the K_w term and rearrangement yields

$$[H^+] = \sqrt{\frac{K_a K_w}{c_S}}$$

If the negative logarithms of this equation are taken,

$$-\log[H^+] = -\tfrac{1}{2}\log K_a - \tfrac{1}{2}\log K_w + \tfrac{1}{2}\log c_S$$

or

$$pH = \tfrac{1}{2} pK_a + \tfrac{1}{2} pK_w + \tfrac{1}{2}\log c_S$$

Phenobarbital has a $pK_a = 7.4$. A 0.05 M aqueous solution of phenobarbital sodium at 25° has

$$pH = (\tfrac{1}{2} \times 14) + (\tfrac{1}{2} \times 7.4) + (\tfrac{1}{2} \log 0.05)$$
$$= 10$$

A salt of a weak base and a strong acid in aqueous solution has an acidic reaction, according to the reaction

$$B^+ + H_2O \rightleftharpoons H^+ + BOH$$

By reasoning analogous to that of the preceding derivation, for an aqueous solution of a salt of a weak base and a strong acid, the hydrogen ion concentration is approximately

$$[H^+] = \sqrt{\frac{K_w c_s}{K_b}}$$

and

$$pH = \tfrac{1}{2} pK_w - \tfrac{1}{2} pK_b - \tfrac{1}{2} \log c_s$$

pH of a soln. of a salt of a weak base and a strong acid = acidic pH

Papaverine has a $pK_b = 8.1$. At 25° a 0.01 M solution of papaverine hydrochloride has a

$$pH = (\tfrac{1}{2} \times 14) - (\tfrac{1}{2} \times 8.1) - (\tfrac{1}{2} \log 0.01)$$
$$= 4$$

When a salt of a weak acid and a weak base dissolves in water, the solution may be acidic, basic, or neutral, depending on the strength of the acid and the base. The reaction is

$$BH^+ + A^- \rightleftharpoons B + HA$$

and its equilibrium constant is

$$K = \frac{[B][HA]}{[BH^+][A^-]}$$

Making use of the definition of dissociation constant K_b and K_a and substituting equivalent terms,

$$B = \frac{[BH^+][OH^-]}{K_b}$$

and

$$[HA] = \frac{[H^+][A^-]}{K_a}$$

the equilibrium constant is

$$K = \frac{[BH^+][OH^-]}{K_b[BH^+]} \cdot \frac{[H^+][A^-]}{K_a[A^-]}$$

$$= \frac{[OH^-][H^+]}{K_a K_b}$$

$$= \frac{K_w}{K_a K_b}$$

If the solution of a salt of a weak acid and a weak base produces equal amounts of undissociated molecules of the acid and the base, the concentration, $[B]$, of the weak base is equal to the concentraton, $[HA]$, of the weak acid and may be represented by x:

$$x = [B] = [HA]$$

If the initial concentration in moles per liter of the salt is c_s, at equilibrium $c_s - x$ is the concentration of the unhydrolyzed salt. As the salt is only slightly ionized, x may be neglected in the $c_s - x$ term, and substitution yields

$$K = \frac{[B][HA]}{[BH^+][A^-]} = \frac{x^2}{c_s^2}$$

The degree of hydrolysis, λ, or fraction of salt hydrolyzed at equilibrium is

$$\lambda = \frac{x}{c_s} = \sqrt{\frac{K_w}{K_a K_b}}$$

The concentration hydrolyzed is the product of the initial concentration of the salt and the degree of hydrolysis, or λc_s. The concentration of BH^+ and A^- at equilibrium is equal to the initial concentration of the salt minus the concentration that has been hydrolyzed, $(c_s - \lambda c_s)$. At equilibrum $[B] = [HA] = \lambda c_s$. Thus, the equilibrium constant may be written

$$K = \frac{(\lambda c_s)^2}{(c_s - \lambda c_s)^2} = \frac{\lambda^2}{(1-\lambda)^2}$$

and

$$\frac{\lambda}{1-\lambda} = \sqrt{\frac{K_w}{K_a K_b}}$$

Substituting these terms into the defining equation for the dissociation constant of a weak acid,

$$[H^+] = K_a \frac{[HA]}{[A^-]}$$

it becomes

$$[H^+] = K_a \frac{\lambda c_s}{c_s(1-\lambda)} = K_a \frac{\lambda}{1-\lambda}$$

which upon further substitution gives

$$[H^+] = K_a \sqrt{\frac{K_w}{K_a K_b}} = \sqrt{\frac{K_w K_a}{K_b}}$$

The equation in the form of pK notation is

$$pH = \tfrac{1}{2} pK_w + \tfrac{1}{2} pK_a - \tfrac{1}{2} pK_b$$

The pK_a of acetic acid is 4.76 and the pK_b of ammounium hydroxide is 4.76. The pH of an aqueous solution of ammonium acetate at 25° is

$$pH = (\tfrac{1}{2} \times 14) + (\tfrac{1}{2} \times 4.76) - (\tfrac{1}{2} \times 4.76)$$
$$= 7.0$$

In cases where the K_a and K_b are equal, aqueous solutions of the salt are neutral.

BUFFERS

Buffer solutions are solutions that tend to resist changes in pH when acids or bases are added. Buffer solutions usually contain a weak acid and its conjugate base, i.e., salt, or a weak base and its conjugate acid. If a base is added to a buffer solution containing a weak acid, HA, and one of its salts, MA, the alkali is neutralized by the acid:

$$OH^- + HA \rightleftharpoons H_2O + A^-$$

If an acid is added, the hydrogen ions of the acid react with the anions of the salt, forming the undissociated weak acid,

$$H^+ + A^- \rightleftharpoons HA$$

Buffer Equation

Henderson and Hasselbalch derived an equation by which the pH of a buffer solution consisting of a weak acid and its salt may be calculated. This is based on a consideration of the effect that the common ion of the salt has on the dissociation of the weak acid. The equation defining dissociation constant may be transposed,

$$[H^+] = K_a \frac{[HA]}{[A^-]}$$

The addition of a salt with a common ion will decrease the dissociation of the weak acid to maintain equilibrium, i.e., a constant K_a value. Since the acid is only slightly dissociated, the anions for practical purposes may be considered as coming from the highly dissociated salt, MA; and the term [HA] may be considered to represent the total concentration of acid. The hydrogen ion concentration of the buffer solution is then equal to the product of the dissociation constant and the ratio of the concentration of the acid and the salt,

$$[H^+] = K_a \frac{[HA]}{[MA]}$$

If the negative logarithms of this equation are taken, the pH may be calculated directly:

$$-\log[H^+] = -\log K_a - \log \frac{[HA]}{[MA]}$$

This equation expressed in terms of pK's is known as the Henderson-Hasselbalch equation,

$$pH = pK_a + \log \frac{[MA]}{[HA]}$$

The pK_a of acetic acid at 25° is 4.76. The pH of a buffer solution consisting of equal volumes of 0.1 N acetic acid and 0.1 N sodium acetate may be calculated. As equal volumes are mixed, the final concentrations of acetic acid and sodium acetate are 0.05 N. By substitution into the buffer equation the pH is calculated to be

$$pH = 4.76 + \log \frac{0.05}{0.05} = 4.76$$

The pH of a solution is numerically equal to the pK_a of the acid in a buffer solution, which contains equal moles of a weak acid and its salt. This relation offers a method of determining pK_a. A solution of equal concentrations of the weak acid and its salt is made and the pH is measured. The pK_a is numerically equal to the measured pH.

The buffer equation has certain limitations as a result of assumptions made in its derivation. It does not apply when the weak acid in the form of its salt is less than 10 per cent of the total buffer concentration or when the hydrogen ion concentration is great enough to constitute a significant part of the total ions present. These limitations do not distract from its use in the pH range 4 to 10 commonly encountered in pharmacy.

A comparable relation may be derived for buffers composed of weak bases and the corresponding salt of a strong acid,

$$pH = pK_w - pK_b + \log \frac{[B]}{[BH^+]}$$

Atropine has a pK_b = 4.35. It is recommended that atropine be dispensed at pH 6.8 Using the buffer equation, the percentage of the total atropine that exists in the base form may be calculated for a 1 per cent solution:

$$pH = 6.8 = 14 - 4.35 + \log \frac{[B]}{[BH^+]}$$

$$\log \frac{[B]}{[BH^+]} = -2.85 = 7.15 - 10.00$$

antilogarithm of 7.15 - 10.00 = 0.0014

$$\frac{[B]}{[BH^+]} = \frac{0.0014}{1}$$

Thus, approximately 0.14 per cent of the atropine exists in the base form at pH 6.8.

Since $pK_a = pK_w - pK_b$, if the dissociation constant of the base is expressed as K_a, the preceding equation becomes

$$pH = pK_a + \log \frac{[B]}{[BH^+]}$$

Neutralization Curves and Buffer Capacity

Buffer capacity is the ability of a buffer solution to resist pH change. The smaller the pH change caused by the addition of a given amount of acid or alkali, the greater is the buffer capacity of the solution. Quantitatively buffer capacity may be defined as the number of gram equivalents of an acid or base that changes the pH of a liter of buffer solution 1 unit.

If 1 ml of 0.1 N HCl is added to 99 ml of pure water at pH 7, the hydrogen ion concentration of the solution will be 10^{-3}. The pH of the water has been changed 4 units by the addition of the acid. If 1 ml of 0.1 N HCl is added to 99 ml of a buffer solution containing 0.1 N acetic acid and 0.1 N sodium acetate, the pH changes 0.01 unit. The dependence of the buffer capacity on the ratio of the salt and acid is demonstrated by a neutralization curve for the titration of acetic acid with sodium hydroxide, as shown in Figure 97. At pH 4.76 the acid and salt are in equal concentration and the maximum buffer capacity of this buffer pair is attained.

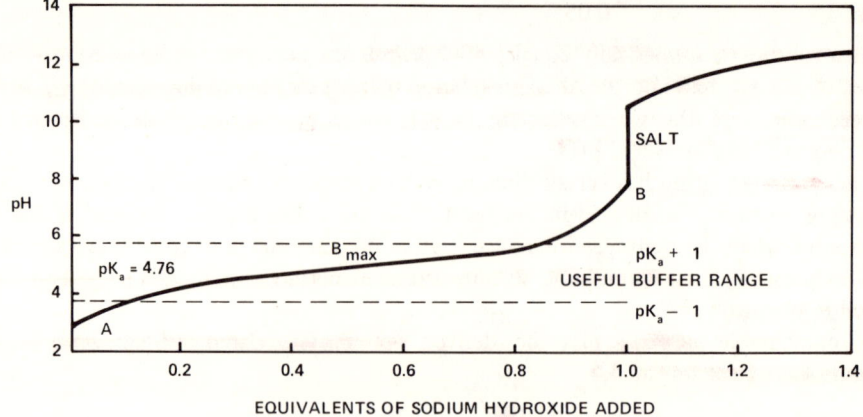

Figure 97. Titration of 0.1 N acetic acid with sodium hydroxide.

Equations which have been presented may be applied to different regions of the titration curve. In Figure 97 the pH of the solution of acetic acid before any sodium hydroxide is added (A) is

$$pH = \tfrac{1}{2} pK_a - \tfrac{1}{2} \log c \quad \text{weak acid}$$

When neutralization is completed (B), the pH is

$$pH = \tfrac{1}{2} pK_w + \tfrac{1}{2} pK_a + \tfrac{1}{2} \log c \quad \text{salt of weak acid and strong base}$$

Between points A and B the pH of the solution is expressed by the buffer equation

$$pH = pK_a + \log \frac{[A^-]}{[HA]}$$

To change the pH 1 unit from the pK_a value, the ratio of salt to acid must be changed tenfold. A greater change in the ratio results in an appreciable change in pH. Thus, the useful limits of a buffer system are usually considered to be $pK_a \pm 1.0$. For an acetic acid-sodium acetate buffer system the limits of its usefulness are from pH 3.7 to 5.7. In Figure 97 it can be seen that in this pH range there is only a slight change of slope as sodium hydroxide is added, resulting in an increase in the $[A^-]/[HA]$.

The buffer capacity is influenced by the concentration of the buffer constituents, because a higher concentration of these provides a greater acid and alkaline reserve. Van Slyke related the buffer capacity, β, to the total buffer concentration, C, where the concentration is the sum of the molar concentrations of the acid and the salt:

$$\beta = 2.3 \, C \, \frac{K_a[H^+]}{[K_a + (H^+)]^2}$$

At pH 4.76 the buffer capacity of a system containing 0.01 M acetic acid and 0.01 M sodium acetate is

$$\beta = 2.3 \times 0.02 \, \frac{1.75 \times 10^{-5} \, (1.75 \times 10^{-5})}{[(1.75 \times 10^{-5}) + (1.75 \times 10^{-5})]^2}$$

$$= 0.011$$

At the same pH maintained by 0.1 M acetic acid and 0.1 M sodium acetate, the buffer capacity is

$$\beta = 2.3 \times 0.2 \, \frac{1.75 \times 10^{-5} \, (1.75 \times 10^{-5})}{[(1.75 \times 10^{-5}) + (1.75 \times 10^{-5})]^2}$$

$$= 0.115$$

Thus, the buffer capacity becomes greater as the concentration of the buffer components increases.

The buffer capacity depends on the value of the ratio of salt to acid form, and it increases as the ratio approaches unity. The maximum buffer capacity occurs when $pH = pK_a$ and is given by

$$\beta_{max} = 0.576c$$

As phosphate buffers occur in biological systems and are used in pharmaceuticals, the dissociation and the titration curve of phosphoric acid are of interest. The first step centered about pH 2.0 is

$$H_3PO_4 + H_2O \rightleftharpoons H^+ + H_2PO_4^-$$

for which the dissociation constant is

$$K_1 = \frac{[H^+][H_2PO_4^-]}{[H_3PO_4]} = 7.5 \times 10^{-3}$$

As shown in Figure 98, when 1 equivalent of sodium hydroxide has been added at approximately pH 4.5, the further addition of a small amount of sodium hydroxide causes a sharp rise in pH. Then as more alkali is added, the second step in dissociation about pH 6.8 is

$$H_2PO_4^- + H_2O \rightleftharpoons H^+ + HPO_4^{--}$$

for which the dissociation constant is

$$K_2 = \frac{[H^+][HPO_4^{--}]}{[H_2PO_4^-]} = 6.2 \times 10^{-8}$$

The law of mass action does not require that H_3PO_4 and PO_4^{3-} be totally absent at pH 6.8. The principal ionic species are $H_2PO_4^-$ and HPO_4^{--}, so K_2 expresses the dissociation. The buffer equation may be used to calculate the ratio of these ions in the blood plasma at pH 7.4:

$$pH = pK_2 + \log \frac{[HPO_4^{--}]}{[H_2PO_4^-]}$$

$$7.4 = 7.2 + \log \frac{[HPO_4^{--}]}{[H_2PO_4^-]}$$

$$\frac{[HPO_4^{--}]}{[H_2PO_4^-]} = \frac{2.5}{1}$$

The final step is

$$HPO_4^{--} + H_2O \rightleftharpoons H^+ + PO_4^{3-}$$

for which the dissociation constant is

$$K_3 = \frac{[H^+][PO_4^{3-}]}{[HPO_4^{--}]} = 4.8 \times 10^{-13}$$

The concentration of HPO_4^{--} in human blood plasma is 0.001 M. The concentration of tertiary phosphate ion is

$$pH = pK_3 + \log \frac{[PO_4^{3-}]}{[HPO_4^{--}]}$$

or

$$7.4 = 12.3 + \log \frac{[PO_4^{3-}]}{0.001}$$

$$[PO_4^{3-}] = 1.3 \times 10^{-8} M$$

This value illustrates the great difficulty with which the third hydrogen ion is formed at physiological pH values.

Solubility as a Function of pH

Buffer solutions may be used to increase the solubility of drugs. Many organic acids are water insoluble, but they dissolve readily in alkaline solution. The enhanced solubility is due to salt formation. The undissolved phase in equilibrium with the saturated solution is composed of unreacted acid. The increase in solubility is not influenced by the solubility of the salts formed.

The dissolution of a relatively insoluble organic acid occurs in two consecutive steps,

$$HA_{solid} \rightleftharpoons HA_{solution}$$

$$HA_{solution} \rightleftharpoons H^+ + A^-$$

aqueous solutions • 229

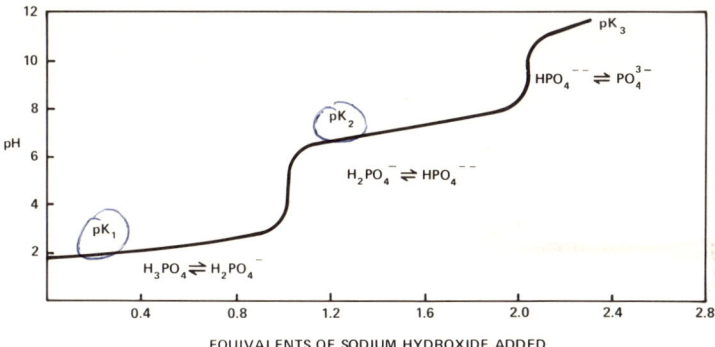

Figure 98. Titration of phosphoric acid with sodium hydroxide.

The solubility of a weak acid in distilled water is

$$S_0 = S'_0 - \frac{K_a}{2}\left(\sqrt{\frac{1 + 4S'_0}{K_a}} - 1\right)$$

where S'_0 is the total solubility in distilled water and the second term of the right side of the equation represents the amount of weak acid existing in the dissociated form. As the degree of dissociation of a weak acid is very small, the dissolved species may be considered to be the undissociated form. Then the equilibrium constant, S_0, corresponds to the solubility of the acid in distilled water.

The equilibrium constant for the second reaction is the dissociation constant, K_a. The total solubility, S_a, of the acidic compound in solution is the sum of the dissociated and nondissociated forms,

$$S_a = [HA] + [A^-]$$
$$= [HA] + K_a \frac{[HA]}{[H^+]}$$

and, as $S_0 = [HA]$,

$$S_a = S_0 + S_0 \frac{K_a}{[H^+]}$$
$$= S_0 \left(1 + \frac{K_a}{[H^+]}\right)$$

Thus, the total solubility of an acid is a function of the hydrogen ion concentration of the solution.

In solutions in which the hydrogen ion concentration is appreciably less than the dissociation constant, $K_a/[H^+]$ becomes the dominant term and 1 is of little significance. Then, as an approximation, the equation

$$S_a = \frac{K_a S_0}{[H^+]}$$

is written. It may be expressed in the equivalent logarithmic form,

$$\log S_a = \log K_a + \log S_0 - \log[H^+]$$

but since $-\log[H^+] = pH$ and $-\log K_a = pK_a$,

$$\log S_a = \log S_0 + pH - pK_a$$

Benzoic acid is soluble in water to the extent of 0.028 mole liter^{-1} and has $K_a = 6.3 \times 10^{-5}$. The total amount of benzoic acid that dissolves in a buffer solution with pH 6 is

$$S_a = \frac{K_a S_0}{[H^+]} = \frac{6.3 \times 10^{-5} \times 0.028}{10^{-6}} = 1.76 \text{ moles liter}^{-1}$$

The equation relating total solubility to pH may be rearranged to

$$pH = pK_a + \log \frac{S_a - S_0}{S_0}$$

which is convenient for calculating the pH at which precipitation of an acid drug from solution will occur. The pH at which 0.5 per cent solution, i.e., 0.035 M, of sodium benzoate begins to form a precipitate may be calculated:

$$pH = 4.2 + \log \frac{0.035 - 0.028}{0.028} = 3.6$$

Corresponding relationships exist for the dissolution of a slightly soluble basic compound, which dissolves in water in two steps,

$$B_{solid} \rightleftharpoons B \cdot H_2O_{solution}$$
$$B \cdot H_2O_{solution} \rightleftharpoons BH^+ + OH^-$$

The dissociation constant of the base is

$$K_b = \frac{[BH^+][OH^-]}{[BH_2O]}$$

The total solubility, S_b, of the basic compound is the sum of the undissociated and the dissociated forms,

$$S_b = S_0 + \frac{K_b S_0}{[OH^-]} = S_0 \left(1 + \frac{K_b}{[OH^-]}\right)$$

Since $K_w = [OH^-][H^+]$, the hydroxyl ion concentration may be expressed in terms of the more commonly used hydrogen ion concentration,

$$S_b = S_0 \left(1 + \frac{K_b [H^+]}{K_w}\right)$$

If the hydroxyl ion concentration of $K_w/[H^+]$ is much less than the dissociation constant, the total solubility is approximately

$$S_b = \frac{S_0 K_b [H^+]}{K_w}$$

or

$$\log S_b = pK_w - pH - pK_b + \log S_0$$

Codeine with a molecular weight of 299.4 g mole^{-1} has a solubility of 1 g in 120 ml of water and a $K_b = 9 \times 10^{-7}$. It is desired to formulate a solution that contains 60 mg of codeine per teaspoonful (5 ml). The pH to which the solution must be buffered to achieve this solubility may be calculated in the following manner:

$$\frac{12}{299.4} = 0.0278 \left(1 + \frac{9 \times 10^{-7} [H^+]}{10^{-14}}\right)$$

$$[H^+] = 4.87 \times 10^{-9}$$

$$pH = -\log(4.87 \times 10^{-9}) = 8.3$$

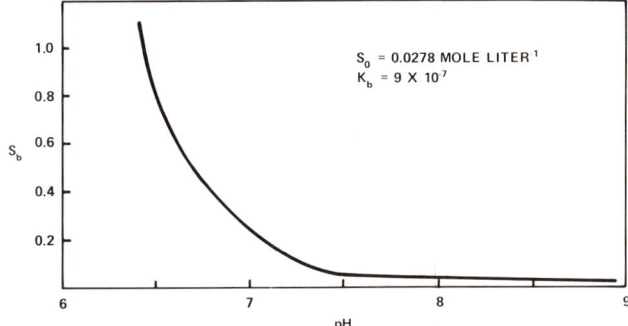

Figure 99. Calculated solubility, S_b, in moles liter^{-1} of codeine as a function of pH.

The relationship of solubility of a basic compound to pH is shown graphically in Figure 99, where the calculated total solubility of codeine is plotted against pH of the solution.

Pharmaceutical Buffer Solutions

The initial step in the development of a buffer system is the selection of a weak acid with a pK_a approximately equal to the pH at which the buffer is to be used. This will provide a high buffer capacity. Then using the pK_a and pH values, the buffer equation is used to calculate the required ratio of the salt and weak acid. The concentrations of the acid and its salt depend on the desired buffer capacity and the effect of this concentration on the particular way in which the pharmaceutical system is to be used. Many buffer systems are possible, but the toxic effects, when administered orally or parenterally, severely limit the number of buffer systems that may be used in pharmaceuticals. Some of the buffer solutions that have been routinely used in pharmacy will be discussed.

Standard Buffers and Indicators. The buffer solutions of Clark and Lubs are used to standardize a pH meter and for research work in which the pH must be constant. The Clark and Lubs system consists of 0.2 M solutions of (1) hydrochloric acid, (2) sodium hydroxide, (3) potassium biphthalate, (4) monobasic potassium phosphate, (5) boric acid and potassium chloride, and (6) potassium chloride. The Clark and Lubs buffer may be used from pH 1.0 to 10.0 by mixing appropriate volumes of these solutions, as shown in Table XLVII. At 25° these values are reproducible to ±0.02 pH unit. The potassium chloride is added to adjust the ionic strength of the buffer solution to 0.1.

The pH is determined by colorimetric method as well as by electrometric method, i.e., pH meter. In the colorimetric method the color of an unknown solution is matched with the color of a standard solution containing the same indicator. The practicing pharmacist most commonly employs indicators in the form of an indicator saturated paper, e.g., pHydrion paper or Alkacid test paper. The color of the paper after immersion in the solution is compared with a color chart to determine the pH.

The indicators function as weak acids or bases and their dissociation may be treated accordingly. The dissociation of an indicator may be written

$$HIn \rightleftharpoons H^+ + In^-$$

(acid color) (alkali color)

At equilibrium

$$K_{In} = \frac{[H^+][In^-]}{[HIn]}$$

The HIn gives the acid color, e.g., colorless for phenolphthalein, and In$^-$ gives the alkali color, e.g., pink for phenolphthalein. If acid is added to a solution of the indicator, the common-ion effect suppresses ionization, and the indicator exists predominantly in the acid form.

Table XLVII Clark and Lubs Buffer

Hydrochloric Acid Buffer *

Place 50 ml of the potassium chloride solution in a 200-ml volumetric flask, add the specified volume of hydrochloric acid solution, then add water to volume.

pH	1.2	1.3	1.4	1.5	1.6	1.7	1.8	1.9	2.0	2.1	2.2
ml of HCl	85.0	67.2	53.2	41.4	32.4	26.0	20.4	16.2	13.0	10.2	7.9

Acid Phthalate Buffer *

Place 50 ml of the potassium biphthalate solution in a 200-ml volumetric flask, add the specified volume of hydrochloric acid solution, then add water to volume.

pH	2.2	2.4	2.6	2.8	3.0	3.2	3.4	3.6	3.8	4.0
ml of HCl	49.5	42.2	35.4	28.9	22.3	15.7	10.4	6.3	2.9	0.1

Neutralized Phthalate Buffer *

Place 50 ml of the potassium biphthalate solution in a 200-ml volumetric flask, add the specified volume of the sodium hydroxide solution, then add water to volume.

pH	4.2	4.4	4.6	4.8	5.0	5.2	5.4	5.6	5.8
ml of NaOH	3.0	6.6	11.1	16.5	22.6	28.8	34.1	38.8	42.3

Phosphate Buffer *

Place 50 ml of the monobasic potassium phosphate solution in a 200-ml volumetric flask, add the specified volume of the sodium hydroxide solution, then add water to volume.

pH	5.8	5.8	6.0	6.2	6.4	6.6	6.8	7.0	7.2	7.4	7.6	8.0
ml of NaOH	3.6	5.6	8.1	11.6	16.4	22.4	29.1	34.7	39.1	42.4	44.5	46.1

Alkaline Borate Buffer *

Place 50 ml of the boric acid and potassium chloride solution in a 200-ml volumetric flask, add the specified volume of the sodium hydroxide solution, then add water to volume.

pH	8.0	8.2	8.4	8.6	8.8	9.0	9.2	9.4	9.6	9.8	10.0
ml of NaOH	3.9	6.0	8.6	11.8	15.8	20.8	26.4	32.1	36.9	40.6	43.7

* See the text, page 231

The pH of an indicator solution is

$$pH = pK_{In} + \log \frac{[base]}{[acid]}$$

The indicator shows its greatest color when pH = pK_{In}, where the ratio [base]/[acid] is unity. An indicator finds its usefulness in the range $pK_{In} \pm 1$, over which the eye cannot discriminate a color change. Thus, phenolphthalein, which has pK_{In} = 9.4, is used to discern a color change that occurs in the pH range from 8.4 to 10.4.

Ophthalmic Buffers. The lacrymal fluid normally has a pH 7.4 with a range pH 5.2 to 8.3. The eye will usually tolerate the instillation of ophthalmic solutions within this pH range because of (1) the small volume of solution being introduced, (2) the buffer of the lacrymal fluid, and (3) the increase in tear production.

Acidity produces pain; a 1 per cent solution of isotonic pilocarpine hydrochloride is tolerated, but further increases in the concentration of pilocarpine hydrochloride progressively increase the irritation. Epinephrine bitartrate solution is more irritating than a solution containing an equivalent concentration of epinephrine hydrochloride, because the tartrate is dibasic and the acidity of the free carboxylic acid group makes it more irritating. Pain caused by the acidity of ophthalmic solutions depends on the acidity of the solution and the volume of lacrymal fluid necessary to adjust the fluid to normal pH range.

The buffer capacity of pharmaceutical buffers used in ophthalmic and parenteral solution should be low. The natural body buffers assimilate and bring medicinal solutions to the pH of body fluids. If buffers with a high buffer capacity were used, they would resist change and interfere with the normal pH and buffer mechanisms of the body. A 1.9 per cent solution of boric acid is frequently used as a vehicle for ophthalmic solutions. It has a pH 5, but it may safely be used in the eye, as it has a low buffer capacity and is rapidly adjusted to the physiological pH of the lacrymal fluid.

Various buffer systems have been suggested for pharmaceutical solutions, and useful ophthalmic buffer systems are given in Tables XLVIII to LII. No one system is suitable in all preparations. For example, Sorensen modified buffer cannot be used with zinc salts because zinc phosphate is precipitated.

It is believed that weakly acidic and basic drugs diffuse across biological membranes primarily in the undissociated form. The pK_a of the drug and the pH of the solution establish the ratio of the dissociated and undissociated form. Thus, weak bases, e.g., amines and alkaloid-type drugs, would be absorbed more effectively at higher pH, because a greater fraction of the basic drug would exist in the undissociated form.

It is doubtful that ophthalmic vehicles buffered near the physiological pH have clinical superiority over acid buffers with a low buffer capacity. The vehicles with a low buffer capacity are rapidly changed by the lacrymal fluid to a normal pH with little opportunity for enhanced absorption, owing to the greater ratio of undissociated compound to dissociated compound initially in the instilled solution.

Ophthalmic drugs frequently are amides and esters that undergo hydrolytic degradation. By buffering at an appropriate pH, their stability is greatly increased. For example, an aqueous solution of atropine at room temperature has its maximum stability at pH 3.8. The actual formulation used in an ophthalmic solution in regard to pH adjustment is a compromise among stability, irritation, and absorption. A phosphate buffer with pH 6.8 is recommended for salts of atropine. Although this does not provide maximum stability, excessively low pH, which would irritate the eye, is avoided while adequate stability is maintained. Ophthalmic vehicles recommended for various drugs are given in Table LIII.

234 • aqueous solutions

Clinical Buffers. The adjustment of pH in or on the body may influence the therapeutic efficacy of a drug. The effectiveness of orally administered methenamine as an urinary antiseptic depends on the liberation of formaldehyde in acidic urine. The urine is adjusted to a pH 5 by the simultaneous administration of an acid-forming salt, e.g., ammonium chloride or sodium acid phosphate.

Diluted sodium hypochlorite solution is used to irrigate wounds as a local antibacterial and to dissolve necrotic tissue. Adjustment of the solution to pH 9 with sodium bicarbonate minimizes the dissolving of blood clots while allowing the removal of unwanted debris.

Buffered ointments and lotions that maintain the normal acidity of the skin and facilitate healing are marketed. Control of pH in ointments not only prevents irritation and promotes stability of the drugs, but it may enhance the activity of the drug. Ammoniated mercury and mercurous iodide ointments have greater antiseptic activity as the pH decreases to an optimum value of approximately pH of 4.

Table XLVIII Atkins and Pantin Ophthalmic Buffer

Acid Stock Solution		Alkaline Stock Solution	
Boric acid	12.405 g	Sodium carbonate, anhydrous	21.2 g
Sodium chloride	7.50 g	Purified water, q.s.	1000 ml
Purified water, q.s.	1000 ml		

ml of 0.2 M Boric Acid Solution	ml of 0.2 M Sodium Carbonate Solution	pH
93.8	6.2	7.6
91.7	8.3	7.8
88.8	11.2	8.0
85.0	15.0	8.2
80.7	19.3	8.4
75.7	24.3	8.6
69.5	30.5	8.8
63.0	37.0	9.0
56.4	43.6	9.2
49.7	50.3	9.4
42.9	57.1	9.6
36.0	64.0	9.8
29.1	70.9	10.0
22.1	77.9	10.2
15.4	84.6	10.4
9.8	90.2	10.6
5.7	94.3	10.8
3.5	96.5	11.0

aqueous solutions • 235

Table XLIX Feldman Ophthalmic Buffer

Acid Stock Solution		Alkaline Stock Solution	
Boric acid	12.368 g	Sodium borate decahydrate	19.07 g
Sodium chloride	2.925 g	Purified water, q.s.	1000 ml
Purified water, q.s.	1000 ml		

ml of Boric Acid Solution	ml of Sodium Borate Solution	pH
100	0	5.0
100	0.4	6.0
95	5	7.0
94	6	7.1
93	7	7.2
91	9	7.3
89	11	7.4
87	13	7.5
85	15	7.6
82	18	7.7
80	20	7.8
76	24	7.9
73	27	8.0
69	31	8.1
65	35	8.2

Table L Gifford Ophthalmic Buffer

Acid Stock Solution		Alkaline Stock Solution	
Boric acid	12.4 g	Sodium carbonate monohydrate	24.8 g
Potassium chloride	7.4 g	Purified water, q.s.	1000 ml
Purified water, q.s.	1000 ml		

ml of Boric Acid Solution	ml of Sodium Carbonate Solution	pH
30	0.05	6.0
30	0.1	6.2
30	0.2	6.6
30	0.3	6.8
30	0.5	6.9
30	0.6	7.0
30	1.0	7.2
30	1.5	7.4
30	2.0	7.6
30	3.0	7.8
30	4.0	8.0
30	8.0	8.5

Table LI Palitzsch Ophthalmic Buffer

Acid Stock Solution		Alkaline Stock Solution	
Boric acid	12.404 g	Sodium borate decahydrate	19.108 g
Purified water, q.s.	1000 ml	Purified water, q.s.	1000 ml

ml of 0.2 M Boric Acid Solution	ml of 0.05 M Sodium Borate Solution	pH
97	3	6.8
94	6	7.1
90	10	7.4
85	15	7.6
80	20	7.8
75	25	7.9
70	30	8.1
65	35	8.2
55	45	8.4
45	55	8.6
40	60	8.7
30	70	8.8
20	80	9.0
10	90	9.1

Table LII Sorensen Modified Phosphate Buffer

Acid Stock Solution		Alkaline Stock Solution	
Sodium biphosphate, anhydrous	8.006 g	Sodium phosphate, anhydrous	9.473 g
Purified water, q.s.	1000 ml	Purified water, q.s.	1000 ml

ml of $M/15$ Sodium Biphosphate Solution	ml of $M/15$ Sodium Phosphate Solution	pH
90	10	5.9
80	20	6.2
70	30	6.5
60	40	6.6
50	50	6.8
40	60	7.0
30	70	7.2
20	80	7.4
10	90	7.7
5	95	8.0

Table LIII Recommended Vehicles for Ophthalmic Solutions

Vehicle	pH	Salts of
Boric acid, 1.9%	5.0	Cocaine, dibucaine, phenylephrine, piperocaine, procaine, tetracaine, zinc
Sorensen modified phosphate	6.8	Atropine, ephedrine, eucatropine, homatropine, pilocarpine, scopolamine

8 | NONAQUEOUS PHARMACEUTICAL SOLUTIONS

Although from their physical properties various solvents may appear to be desirable for use in pharmaceutical products, with few exceptions, organic solvents are irritating or toxic liquids. Aromatic hydrocarbons cause paralysis of the central nervous system and are irritating to the skin. Methyl alcohol is a toxic liquid, and butyl alcohol and amyl alcohol are irritating liquids. Volatile ethers paralyze the central nervous system, and although this effect decreases with an increasing molecular weight, the irritation to mucous membranes increases. Ketones and low-molecular-weight esters are mildly irritating liquids.

Nonpolar solvents used in liquid pharmaceutical dosage forms are mineral oil and vegetable oils, e.g., corn oil, cottonseed oil, olive oil, peanut oil, and sesame oil. Camphor liniment is a solution of camphor in cottonseed oil. Ergocalciferol solution is an example of an orally administered solution which may have a vegetable oil as a solvent. Ophthalmic solutions are usually aqueous, so they are physiologically similar to the lachrymal fluid; however, peanut oil is used as a solvent in isoflurophate ophthalmic solution, because the isoflurophate is rapidly decomposed by water. Carbon tetrachloride, ether, and petroleum benzin are used as solvents in extraction and processing, but they are not used in the finished dosage form. Van der Waals force is the interaction force in nonpolar solvents; consequently, the nonpolar solvents do not dissolve ionic and polar substances.

The polar solvents used for orally administered liquid dosage forms are alcohol, glycerin, and propylene glycol. The use of isopropyl alcohol is limited to external preparations. A solution of diethyltoluamide in isopropyl or ethyl alcohol is applied topically as an anthropod repellant. Alcohol is used as a solvent for coal tar solution, which contains a surface-active agent, polysorbate 80, for the purpose of permitting the aqueous dilution of the coal tar solution without precipitation. Glycerin is the solvent in tannic acid glycerite. Tribromoethanol solution is a solution of tribromoethanol in amylene hydrate. It is a rectally administered anesthetic given as a preliminary to a gaseous anesthetic. The uniqueness of this solution lies in the fact that not only the solute, but also the solvent, functions as a central-nervous-system depressant and contributes to the anesthesia. Acetone and carbon bisulfide are sometimes used as solvents during processing, but they are not used in finished dosage forms.

A cosolvent is a mixture of solvents used to increase the solubility of a drug. Nonaqueous cosolvents are used in a number of pharmaceuticals, e.g., isopropyl alcohol and propylene glycol in monobenzone lotion, and alcohol and ether in collodion. In pharmacy an alcohol and water solution is the most frequently used cosolvent. Miscible liquids, e.g., alcohol and water, and glycerin and water, are those liquids which dissolve in each other in all proportions. Immiscible liquids, e.g., mineral oil and water, are those liquids which are not soluble in any proportion.

ELIXIRS

Elixirs are pleasantly flavored hydroalcoholic solutions intended for oral use. In general, the presence of sugar and alcohol distinguishes the elixir from other categories of pharmaceutical preparations. The alcoholic content of elixirs varies from 5 per cent in sodium bromide elixir to 40 per cent in terpin hydrate elixir. Sufficient alcohol is used to just maintain the drug in solution. Most elixirs become turbid when moderately diluted by aqueous liquids.

Elixirs are prepared by dissolving the ingredients in the appropriate solvent. In general, the alcohol-soluble substances are dissolved in the alcohol and the water-soluble substances in the water. The two solutions are then mixed with stirring by adding the aqueous solution to the alcoholic solution.

54. Compound orange spirit   12 ml
    Syrup   375 ml
    Talc   30 g
    Alcohol
    Purified water, each, q.s. 1000 ml

    Sig.: Aromatic elixir

Sufficient alcohol is added to the compound orange spirit to make 250 ml. The syrup is added gradually with vigorous agitation; the water is then added gradually with vigorous agitation. The talc is mixed with the liquid, and the mixture is filtered through a filter wetted with diluted alcohol until the filtrate is clear. Filtration is slow because of the talc and the syrup, which increases the viscosity of the aromatic elixir. Talc is used as a filtering agent to adsorb any excess volatile oil present. If the excess oil is not removed, the elixir will be turbid. Aromatic elixir may be diluted with water without turbidity. This property makes it a useful vehicle for mixing with aqueous preparations. Red aromatic elixir is an aromatic elixir to which amaranth has been added.

Iso-alcoholic elixir is a vehicle for various medicinals that require solvents of different alcoholic concentrations. It consists of a low-alcoholic elixir containing 8 to 10 per cent alcohol and a high-alcoholic elixir containing 75 to 78 per cent alcohol. By mixing appropriate volumes of the two elixirs an alcoholic content sufficient to dissolve the drugs can be obtained. The alcoholic content of the iso-alcoholic elixir to be used with a single liquid galenical is approximately the same as that of the galenical. When galenicals of different alcoholic concentrations are to be mixed, the iso-alcoholic elixir should be selected to obtain a solution. In general, this is approximately the average of the alcoholic concentrations of the several galenicals. For nonextractive or nongalenical preparations, the iso-alcoholic elixir with a low alcohol content is generally selected.

Elixirs that contain therapeutically active compounds are known as medicated elixirs. Phenobarbital elixir is a medicated elixir; however, at times it is used as a vehicle for other drugs.

55. Phenobarbital   4.00 g
    Orange oil   0.75 ml
    Amaranth solution   10.00 ml
    Alcohol   150.00 ml
    Glycerin   450.00 ml
    Syrup   150.00 ml
    Purified water, q.s. 1000 ml

    Sig.: Phenobarbital elixir

In preparing phenobarbital elixir, the phenobarbital and the orange oil are dissolved in alcohol. The remaining ingredients are then added, and the solution is adjusted to final volume by the addition of water. If all the ingredients were mixed and the phenobarbital were added last, the phenobarbital would dissolve with difficulty. The 15 per cent alcohol in the phenobarbital elixir is not sufficient to maintain the phenobarbital in solution. It is the aqueous alcohol and glycerin solution that maintains the drug in solution. The addition of aqueous solutions to phenobarbital elixir may cause precipitation of the phenobarbital.

nonaqueous solutions

In preparing pentobarbital elixir, water-soluble sodium pentobarbital is used to facilitate dissolution. After dissolution it is converted by the addition of diluted hydrochloric acid to pentobarbital, which remains in solution. This conversion is desirable because the pentobarbital is stable in acidic solution but is hydrolyzed in the alkaline solution of the sodium salt.

In amobarbital elixir, methenamine is used to enhance the solubility of amobarbital. The methenamine is added to the amobarbital dissolved in alcohol, and then the flavoring oils, sodium saccharin, propylene glycol, color, and water are added.

As only 1 g of terpin hydrate dissolves in about 200 ml of water, 40 per cent alcohol is required in terpin hydrate elixir to maintain the 85 mg per teaspoonful in solution. If the elixir is diluted with water, terpin hydrate is precipitated.

Salts have limited solubility in alcohol; therefore, the alcoholic content of salt-containing elixirs, e.g., sodium bromide elixir and three bromides elixir, must be low. Elixirs are not the preferred vehicle for salts, as alcohol accentuates a saline taste.

SPIRITS

Spirits or essences are alcoholic or hydroalcoholic solutions of volatile substances. Some spirits are medicinal spirits, e.g., aromatic ammonia spirit, and many spirits, e.g., compound orange spirit and compound cardamon spirit, are used as flavoring agents.

Spirits are usually prepared by solution of the volatile ingredients in alcohol.

56.
Bergamot oil	15 ml
Lemon oil	8 ml
Rosemary oil	7 ml
Lavender oil	4 ml
Orange flower oil	4 ml
Ethyl acetate	2 ml
Purified water	120 ml
Alcohol	840 ml

Sig.: Perfumed spirit

57.
Peppermint oil	100 ml
Peppermint, coarse powder	10 g
Alcohol, q.s.	1000 ml

Sig.: Peppermint spirit

Peppermint spirit is prepared by maceration and solution. The peppermint leaves are macerated for 1 hour with water to remove tannins and other unwanted water-soluble substances. The leaves are expressed or squeezed out, and while moist they are added to alcohol. The leaves are macerated with agitation in alcohol for 6 hours to extract the chlorophyll, which imparts the green color to the spirit. After filtering the mixture, peppermint oil is dissolved in the filtrate.

Aromatic ammonia spirit upon inhalation produces a reflex circulatory stimulation and is used in cases of fainting. A chemical reaction occurs during its preparation.

58.
Ammonium carbonate, in translucent pieces	34 g
Strong ammonia solution	36 ml
Lemon oil	10 ml
Lavender oil	1 ml
Myristic oil	1 ml
Alcohol	700 ml
Purified water, q.s.	1000 ml

Sig.: Aromatic ammonia spirit

The translucent ammonium carbonate N.F. consists of alcohol-insoluble ammonium bicarbonate and alcohol-soluble ammonium carbamate. Upon exposure to a moist atmosphere the carbamate portion loses NH_3, leaving opaque ammonium bicarbonate. The carbamate also absorbs CO_2 from the atmosphere to form the bicarbonate. If excess bicarbonate is present it would not be changed to normal ammonium carbonate during the reaction of the preparation. The ammonia solution and the ammonium carbonate N.F. are allowed to stand for 12 hours, during which they are converted to the normal ammonium carbonate:

$$NH_2COONH_4 + H_2O \rightarrow (NH_4)_2CO_3$$

$$NH_4HCO_3 + NH_3 \rightarrow (NH_4)_2CO_3$$

Then the ammonium carbonate solution is gradually added to the oils dissolved in alcohol. The spirit is set aside for 24 hours and then filtered. It is a colorless solution which gradually acquires a pale yellow color as oxidation of the oils occurs.

Spirits contain from 50 to 90 per cent alcohol, which maintains the water-insoluble volatile oils in solution. If water is added to a spirit, the oils separate. Spirits should be packaged in tight containers to reduce loss by evaporation.

GALENICAL EXTRACTION

Extraction is the operation by which soluble constituents of crude drugs are dissolved in a suitable solvent and separated from unwanted, insoluble materials. The solvent is known as the menstruum, and the insoluble residue remaining after extraction is known as the marc. An extractive is the preparation obtained by extraction. Pharmaceutical extractives, e.g., extracts, fluidextracts, and tinctures, prepared by the extraction of vegetable drugs are known as galenicals. Extraction is also used to obtain the active constituents of animal tissue, e.g., liver and pancreas.

Vegetable and animal tissues contain a huge variety of substances of which only a few are therapeutically active substances. The purpose of extraction is to separate in a pure or more concentrated form the active substances from cellular tissue and some of the inert substances, e.g., albumin, cellulose, gum, pectin, starch, and sugars.

In extraction from solids equilibrium proceeds very slowly, and extraction is not usually accomplished under equilibrium conditions. When the intact plant cells of a crude drug are in contact with the extracting liquid, a partition ratio is the limiting factor in the extraction of a cellular solute. A cellular solute at equilibrium with the whole cell will be partitioned between the cellular fluid and the lipoidal cell membrane; this particular partition ratio will maintain practically all the solute in the cell fluid. The cellular solute, which has partitioned into the cell membrane, will in turn partition between the cell membrane and the extraction liquid. An equilibrium will be established between the two partitions. The partition from the cell interior into the membrane probably is the limiting coefficient, as demonstrated by the resistance normal plant cells exhibit to penetration.

As a result of being dried, most vegetable drugs have lost moisture, the walls of the cells have shrunken, and the constituents of the cell have precipitated or crystallized. If these plant tissues are soaked in a solvent, the solvent may be transported into the intact cell by osmosis. As the solvent enters the cell, it swells and eventually ruptures, permitting direct solution of its contents. If these were the only mechanisms of the extraction process, extraction would be an impractical operation.

Since diffusion is slow, the drug to be extracted should be ground to provide most intimate contact with the solvent. In milling the cell wall is ruptured, permitting the solvent to come into direct contact with the contents of the cell. If the crude drug were completely free of moisture, extraction from the ruptured cells would be a simple dissolving or leaching of the desired cell solute. A dried crude drug may contain several per cent moisture; therefore, even though the plant cell is ruptured, the solute is in an aqueous phase of the residual moisture, and if the menstruum were a solvent not miscible with water, a partition process would be involved between the two phases. Extraction is a complex process that may involve partition ratios, osmosis, and leaching.

The solvent should extract the maximum amount of the active substances and a minimum amount of the inert substances. The inert extracted substances affect the finished product. Galenical extractives often darken on aging, owing to the oxidation of inert substances. These inert substances may be hydrolyzed to insoluble compounds that precipitate. Thus, the smaller the amount of inert substances that are dissolved in the solvent, the more stable is the finished product.

As a solvent water has the disadvantage of extracting a considerable amount of substances that are liable to hydrolysis or oxidation. Water extracts mucilaginous and carbohydrate materials, which form viscous solutions that are difficult to process and are good media for microbial growth.

Alcohol is a good solvent for alkaloids, glycosides, and resins; it does not dissolve inert gums, sugars, and albumins. Alcohol inhibits enzymatic action and microbial growth.

A hydroalcoholic solvent is most frequently used, as it combines the advantages of alcohol and water without the disadvantages of water. Occasionally extraction of relatively insoluble substances may be facilitated by the addition of an acid or a base that forms a soluble salt with the drug. Acetone, ether, and glycerin have been used as solvents in extraction.

Maceration

Maceration is an extraction process in which the ground drug is soaked in the solvent until the cellular structure is penetrated and the soluble constituents have been dissolved. To prevent loss of volatile solvents by evaporation, maceration is performed with agitation in a closed vessel. The length of maceration varies, depending on the structure of the crude drug, and it is determined experimentally for each drug. After maceration the liquid is decanted, and the marc is expressed or strained to avoid loss. The combined liquids are filtered.

Maceration is preferred for the alcoholic extraction of drugs with no cellular structure, e.g., benzoin and tolu, and for the aqueous extraction of drugs containing mucilaginous and albuminous substances.

Percolation

Percolation is the extraction of soluble constituents from a granulated or powdered drug by the slow passage of a suitable solvent through a column of the drug packed in a cylindrical vessel known as a percolator. As the solvent flows through the layers of the drug, it extracts the successive layers until it is saturated. By means of percolation extraction is achieved with the minimum volume of solvent.

The size to which a crude drug is milled prior to extraction depends on (1) the structure of the drug, (2) the ability of the solvent to penetrate and dissolve the active constituents, (3) the length of time needed to exhaust the powder, and (4) the ratio of the solvent to the drug.

To satisfactorily extract a hard, tough vegetable drug, e.g., cinchona or nux vomica, it must be milled to a finer size than a loose, easily extracted drug, e.g., belladonna or gentian. If the active constituents are sparingly soluble or dissolve slowly, the drug should be milled to a fine state of subdivision so that the solute is exposed to as much solvent as practical.

The powdered drug should be reasonably uniform in size to permit uniform descent of the solvent through the column of the drug. If the size of the powder is not uniform, the solvent flows through the coarser particles, which offer the least resistance, and extraction is incomplete. Within the size limit that will not clog the percolator, the finer the size to which the drug is reduced, the easier it is to achieve satisfactory extraction.

The powdered drug is moistened with solvent before packing it in the percolator. If a dried, powdered drug were packed in a percolator and then moistened, the drug in contact with the solvent would swell against the wall of the percolator and prevent further passage of the solvent. Blocking is avoided by moistening the powder and allowing it to stand and swell for 15 minutes before packing the percolator.

Before packing a small-scale percolator a loose plug of cotton is placed in the bottom to act as a filter when the liquid is percolated. This may be leveled by the addition of a layer of clean sand. The moistened drug is then carefully deposited in successive layers, which are pressed down with equal pressure. When the drug is packed uniformly, the solvent will descend evenly in a horizontal plane. If the drug is packed too firmly, the solvent will not flow. If the drug is packed unevenly, the solvent will flow through the loosely packed portions and will not satisfactorily extract the drug.

To prevent disturbing the surface of the drug packed in the percolator a piece of filter paper, which is held in place by a suitable weight, is placed on the surface of the powder. The solvent is added carefully to avoid producing channels in the powder. The lower orifice is closed when the air has been displaced, as shown by the first drops of percolate. Sufficient solvent is added to leave a layer above the surface of the drug. The drug is allowed to macerate for a period of time that depends on the constituents of the drug and their solubility.

As shown in Figure 100, in small-scale percolation the lower orifice is fitted with a one-hole stopper with a glass tube that is flush with the inner surface of the stopper and extends sufficiently below the stopper so that a rubber tube and screw clamp may be attached. By adjustment of the clamp the rate of flow may be controlled. For 1000 g of powdered drug the rates of flow are defined: slowly, 1 ml min^{-1}; moderate, 1 to 3 ml min^{-1}; rapid, 3 to 5 ml min^{-1}.

After maceration the lower orifice is opened and the rate of flow is controlled. If the flow is too rapid, there is insufficient time for the solvent to penetrate the cells and dissolve the active constituents. If the flow is too slow, the liquid may extract excessive inert materials, which form a viscous liquid that blocks the lower layers of the drug.

Percolation is continued until the final volume of solution is collected. If the preparation is to be standardized, a volume estimated to be equal to 95 per cent of the finished volume is collected. The solution is assayed and then adjusted according to calculations based on the assay.

TINCTURES

Tinctures are alcoholic or hydroalcoholic solutions of chemicals or soluble constituents of crude drugs. Although tinctures vary in concentration up to 50 per cent, tinctures prepared from potent drugs are usually 10 per cent tinctures; i.e., 100 ml of tincture represents the activity of 10 g of the drug. Potent 10 per cent tinctures, e.g., digitalis tincture and belladonna tincture, are assayed before completion and then adjusted to standard potency.

Most tinctures are prepared by an extraction process of maceration or percolation. The selection of a solvent (or menstruum) is based on the solubility of the active and inert constituents of

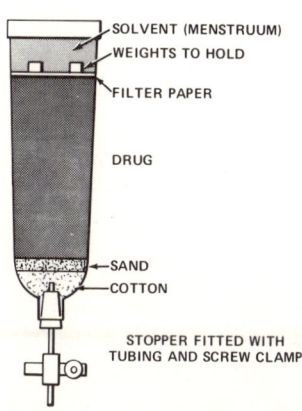

Figure 100. Percolator with screw-cock attachment for regulating flow of percolate.

the crude drug. Ideally only the active ingredient should be extracted by the solvent; thus, it is separated from the unwanted inert materials, which have not been dissolved. Frequently, some unobjectionable, inert material is extracted and allowed to remain in the tincture. If any extracted material is detrimental to the product, it is removed by additional processing. For example, fatty material may be removed by chilling the filtrate or percolate and removing the separated fatty material by filtration. Crude drugs may also be defatted by washing the powder with hexane prior to maceration or percolation. Opium contains lipoid-soluble materials that have a sickening odor. In preparing opium tincture the opium is macerated and percolated with water. The percolate is boiled, and paraffin is added. The offensive lipoid-soluble material dissolves in the melted paraffin and may be removed by filtration.

Tinctures may precipitate inactive constituents upon aging. Glycerin may be added to the hydroalcoholic menstruum to increase the solubility of the active constituent and to reduce precipitation upon storage of the tincture, e.g., aromatic rhubarb tincture, compound cardamon tincture, and compound gentian tincture. In some tinctures, e.g., nux vomica tincture, the solubility of the active ingredient is increased by salt formation so that the extraction is more complete upon the addition of hydrochloric acid to the solvent.

In preparing tinctures percolation is the extractive process of choice for dried crude drugs with a cellular structure. The preparation of belladonna tincture is typical of percolation, or process P. The belladonna leaf is ground to a moderately coarse powder. If the leaf is too coarse, extraction is slow and may be incomplete; if the leaf is ground too fine, it may be packed too tightly in the percolator and obstruct the flow of the solvent. A solvent consisting of 3 volumes of alcohol and 1 volume of water is used. The ground belladonna leaf is mixed with sufficient solvent to wet it evenly. After standing for 15 minutes, it is packed into a percolator. Sufficient solvent is added to saturate the column of drug, and when the solvent is about to drip from the percolator, the lower orifice is closed. The belladonna leaf is macerated for 24 hours. Since belladonna tincture must contain 30 mg of the alkaloids of belladonna, the percolate is assayed. The remaining percolate is adjusted to standard strength with the menstruum as calculated from the assay.

The 70 per cent alcohol in belladonna tincture is a great enough concentration to extract sufficient chlorophyll to impart a pleasant green color and to exclude water-soluble ingredients. When belladonna tincture is added to aqueous solutions, resinous and oily materials are precipitated.

The preparation of tinctures by maceration, or process M, is suitable for gums, resins, and balsams. With sticky, viscous substances, which are difficult to transfer completely, it is recommended that the vessel in which the tincture is to be prepared be tared and the sticky material be weighed directly into it. A volume of alcohol equal to three-fourths of the volume of the finished tincture is added to the drug. In a closed vessel the tincture is macerated in a warm place with agitation for 3 days. Then the mixture is filtered, and the residue is washed with fresh alcohol to remove the liquid retained in the marc. The tincture is adjusted to final volume.

Paregoric, a widely used preparation for treatment of diarrheas, can be prepared by process M.

59. Powdered opium 4.3 g
Anise oil 3.8 ml
Benzoic acid 3.8 g
Camphor 3.8 g
Diluted alcohol 900 ml
Glycerin 38 ml

Sig.: Paregoric

The ingredients are macerated for 5 days with occasional agitation. The mixture is filtered and sufficient diluted alcohol is passed through the filter to make the filtrate measure 950 ml. The filtrate is assayed and adjusted with sufficient diluted alcohol so that each 100 ml contains 0.4 ml of anise oil, 400 mg of benzoic acid, 400 mg of camphor, 4 ml of glycerin, and 40 mg of anhydrous morphine.

Certain tinctures may be prepared by solution of the drugs in the solvent.

60. Green soap   650 g
    Lavender oil   20 ml
    Alcohol, q.s.   1000 ml

Sig.: Green soap tincture

61. Iodine   20 g
    Sodium iodide   24 g
    Alcohol   500 ml
    Purified water, q.s. 1000 ml

Sig.: Iodine tincture

The sodium iodide in the iodine tincture is not added to increase the solubility of iodine, which is soluble in alcohol. The sodium iodide is added to form the triiodide ion, which prevents the formation of ethyl iodide and the corresponding reduction of iodine concentration.

FLUIDEXTRACTS

Fluidextracts are alcoholic solutions that are prepared by percolation so that each milliliter contains the therapeutically active constituents of 1 g of vegetable drug. Fluidextracts are used in the manufacture of other pharmaceuticals, e.g., aromatic eriodictyon syrup and glycyrrihiza syrup. Fluidextracts are not used as a dosage form administered by the patient because of the difficulty of measuring a small dose by means of household measuring devices. For example, an 0.06-ml dose of belladonna fluidextract would be more difficult and less safe to measure than the equivalent 0.6-ml dose of belladonna tincture.

Five modifications of percolation are used to prepare fluidextracts. The most frequently used modification is process A, which consists of percolating the drug with alcohol or hydroalcoholic menstruum. The first 85 per cent of the percolate is set aside and the drug is further percolated. After collection the weak percolate is concentrated by low heat and under reduced pressure. This concentrate is then dissolved in the first percolate. An alcohol-water solution is added to adjust the fluidextract to the required alcoholic content and volume. If the fluidextract is to be adjusted to a standard, the first percolate in which the residue from subsequent percolation has been dissolved is assayed. The solution is then diluted to a volume calculated from the assay results with an alcohol-water solution that will provide the proper concentration of alcohol.

Process B is the same as process A except that two successive solvents are used. The first solvent sometimes contains an acid which forms alkaloidal salts that are more soluble.

Fractional percolation, or process C, is used for drugs containing volatile or thermolabile constituents or in circumstances where suitable equipment for distillation and concentration are absent. No heat or concentration of percolate is required in process C. The ground drug is divided into three portions, i.e., 500 g, 300 g, and 200 g, which are packed in three percolators. The 500 g is percolated, and the first 200-ml of percolate is reserved; then, five successive 300-ml portions of percolate are collected. The 300 g is percolated with the first of the 300-ml portions of percolate, and as percolation proceeds the successive 300-ml portions are added. The first 300-ml of percolate is reserved; then the five successive 200-ml portions are collected. The 200 g is percolated with the first of the 200-ml portions of percolate, and as percolation proceeds the successive 200-ml portions are added. Five hundred milliliters of the percolate is collected and reserved. The three reserved portions are now combined to make 1 liter of fluidextract.

In process D, boiling water is used as the solvent to extract water-soluble constituents. One thousand grams of drug is macerated for 2 hours with about 3000 ml of boiling water in a metallic percolator. The percolate is evaporated on a water bath or in a vacuum still to a specified volume and after cooling alcohol is added as a preservative. After standing for several days the alcohol-insoluble constituents precipitate and may be removed by filtration.

Pressure percolation, or process E, is conducted with a column of small diameter and of such length that extraction is completed by passage of the solvent. This consists of a series of parallel tubes connected by U tubes so the percolate from the bottom of the first passes into the bottom of the second tube, up through the drug and out the top and through a U tube into the top of a third tube, and so on. A reservoir for the solvent is connected to the first tube and a pressure system. Process E may save solvent and eliminates the concentration of the weak percolate.

62.
Cascara sagrada, very coarse powder	1000.00 g
Magnesium oxide	120.00 g
Pure glycyrrhiza extract	40.00 g
Saccharin	2.00 g
Anise oil	0.65 ml
Coriander oil	0.15 ml
Methyl salicylate	0.1 ml
Alcohol	200.00 ml
Water, q.s.	1000 ml

Sig.: Aromatic cascara sagrada fluid extract

The cascara sagrada and the magnesium oxide are mixed and wetted with 2000 ml of boiling water and are macerated for 48 hours. The magnesium oxide neutralizes and partially prevents the extraction of bitter cathartic constituents, so that the fluidextract is more palatable. The mixture is packed in a percolator and percolated with boiling water until the drug is exhausted. The percolate is evaporated at a temperature not exceeding 100° to 750 ml. The glycyrrhiza extract is dissolved immediately in the percolate. When the mixture has cooled, the remaining ingredients are added as an alcoholic solution, and the fluidextract is adjusted to final volume with water. Although the fluidextract is less bitter because the magnesium oxide prevented complete extraction of the drug, it should be realized that the fluidextract is consequently less active physiologically and a proportionately larger dose must be administered than with cascara sagrada fluidextract.

EXTRACTS, RESINS, AND OLEORESINS

Although extracts, resins, and oleoresins are not solutions, they are discussed because they are prepared by extraction procedures. Extracts are concentrated solid, semisolid, or viscous liquid extractives made from crude drugs by extraction, evaporation to dryness or near dryness, and subsequent adjustment to a standard. Extracts are available as a dry powder known as a powdered extract and as a plastic mass known as a pilular extract. From the therapeutic viewpoint the powdered and pilular extracts are interchangeable. The pilular extracts were designed for use in the preparation of pills, ointments, and suppositories. Powdered extracts are used in preparing capsules, powders, and tablets.

In general, extracts are prepared by percolation. The solvent is more alcoholic than that used in the preparation of tinctures and fluidextracts, so there is less inert water-soluble material in the extracts. The percolate is concentrated usually by distillation under reduced pressure without heat. In powdered extracts diluents, e.g., calcium phosphate, glycyrrhiza, lactose, dried starch, or sugar, are added to adjust the extract to standard strength. When white diluents are used, chlorophyll and caramel may be added to approximate the natural color of an extract. Pilular extracts may be diluted to standard with liquid glucose, glycerin, and malt extract.

Pilular belladonna extract is prepared by percolation of belladonna leaf with a mixture of 3 volumes of alcohol and 1 volume of water. The drug is macerated for 16 hours and then percolated at a moderate rate. The percolate is evaporated to a pilular consistency under reduced pressure at a temperature not exceeding 60°. The pilular extract is assayed and adjusted by dilution with liquid glucose so that each 100 g contains 1.25 g of alkaloids of belladonna leaf.

Powdered belladonna extract is prepared by percolation of the belladonna leaf with alcohol. The drug is macerated for 16 hours and then percolated at a slow rate. The percolate is evaporated to a soft extract under reduced pressure at a temperature not exceeding 60°, dried starch is added, and evaporation is continued until the extract is dry. The residue is powdered and assayed. The powdered extract is adjusted to standard by the addition of starch, mixed, and passed through a sieve. Alkaline diluents may not be used, as they hydrolyze the atropine.

The extract may be defatted before adjustment to standard by maceration for 2 hours in hexane. The residue is filtered and washed twice with hexane and dried. Another method of defatting is to wash the extract with three successive portions of hot acidulated water and to skim off the fatty material which rises to the surface. The aqueous liquids are combined, evaporated to dryness, and combined with the residue. The powder is then adjusted to standard.

Extracts should be packaged in tight containers. Powdered extracts exposed to the atmosphere become caked as the result of sorption of moisture. Pilular extracts on exposure to the atmosphere dry out and become hard masses. These physical changes are often accompanied by a change in potency of the extract.

Galenical resins are powders prepared by percolation of a crude drug with an alcoholic solvent, which is removed from the percolate by distillation and evaporation, and the precipitation of the resins by pouring the concentrated percolate into water. The resin prepared in this manner contains the alcohol-soluble and water-insoluble constituents of the crude drug. Galenical resins differ from natural resins. Natural resins, e.g., mastic and rosin, are collected as liquid plant exudates, which upon exposure to the air generally become solid.

Oleoresins are liquid galenical extractives of natural oils and resins extracted by percolation, generally using acetone or ether as a solvent. Fundamentally oleoresins are similar to fluidextracts but differ in the lack of a uniform relationship to the drug, in the solvents used, and in the removal of the solvent after percolation.

LIQUID-LIQUID EXTRACTION

A solute dissolved in one phase, in equilibrium with another immiscible phase, is distributed between the two phases so that the ratio of the concentrations in the two phases is a constant at a given temperature. At equilibrium this constant, K, referred to as the distribution constant or partition coefficient, was defined by Nernst as

$$K = \frac{C_U}{C_L}$$

where C_U and C_L are the concentrations in the upper and lower phases, respectively.

This relationship holds when the molecules in each phase are in the same state of aggregation. If the solute is dissociated or associated, more complex forms of the equation must be applied. It is also recognized that only in an ideal system is the partition coefficient independent of the total solute present; this deviation is so well known that in the literature of chemical engineering the above equation is considered to be a limiting case. In many pharmaceutical extractions the ratio of the concentrations without regard to dissociation or aggregation is used as a practical characterization of the distribution; this value is known as the partition ratio.

In the isolation of alkaloids from crude vegetable extracts, in the separations involved in assays, and in extraction and purification of antibiotics from fermentation broths, it is desired in the extraction to remove a particular solute from a heterogeneous system. The solution left after the extraction is known as the raffinate. At its simplest the number of extractions required to isolate or purify a substance is governed by the partition coefficient and the relative volumes of the two phases. At equilibrium the fraction, U, of the total solute found in the upper layer is

$$U = \frac{K(V_U/V_L)}{K(V_U/V_L) + 1} = \frac{Kr}{Kr + 1}$$

where $r = V_U/V_L$, i.e., the ratio of the volumes of the upper and lower phases, respectively.

The fraction, L, remaining in the lower phase is

$$L = 1 - \frac{Kr}{Kr + 1} = \frac{1}{Kr + 1}$$

At a given temperature and pH 5 the partition ratio of tetracycline between butanol and water is 0.6. With a single extraction of equal volumes of butanol and the aqueous fermentation broth, i.e., $r = 1$, the fraction of the total tetracycline extracted in the butanol is

$$U = \frac{Kr}{Kr + 1} = \frac{0.6}{0.6 + 1} = 0.375$$

The fraction of the total tetracycline remaining in the raffinate is 1 - 0.375, or

$$L = \frac{Kr}{Kr + 1} = \frac{1}{0.6 + 1} = 0.625$$

If the lower phase is reextracted with n successive equal volumes of the upper layer, each nth extraction will contain the fraction U_n of the solute,

$$U_n = \frac{Kr}{(Kr + 1)^n}$$

and the L_n fraction of the solute will remain in the lower layer,

$$L_n = \frac{1}{(Kr + 1)^n}$$

If at pH 5 the tetracycline fermentation broth is extracted with three successive portions of butanol, each having the same volume as the aqueous broth, i.e., $r = 1$, the fraction of the tetracycline remaining in the broth is

$$L_{3rd} = \frac{1}{(0.6 \times 1)^3} = 0.244$$

The fraction of the tetracycline that has been extracted in the butanol is 1 - 0.244 = 0.756. This may also be calculated by totaling the fractions extracted in each successive upper layer. In the first extraction of the total extracted in the upper layer is

$$U_{1st} = \frac{Kr}{(Kr + 1)^n} = \frac{0.6}{0.6 + 1} = 0.375$$

and in the second extraction the fraction extracted in the second upper layer is

$$U_{2nd} = \frac{0.6}{(0.6 + 1)^2} = 0.234$$

and in the third extraction the fraction extracted in the third upper layer is

$$U_{3rd} = \frac{0.6}{(0.6 + 1)^3} = 0.147$$

The three upper layers contain a total of 0.756 of the tetracycline originally in the broth.

The most efficient extraction is obtained with a large number of extractions using small volumes of the extracting solvent. Thus, a more exhaustive extraction is obtained by using a given volume in several portions than in a single extraction. If the same volume is used but in divided portions, the fraction L_n in the lower phase at the nth extraction is

$$L_n = \frac{1}{\left(\dfrac{Kr}{n} + 1\right)^n}$$

where n is the number of equal portions of the extracting solvent.

If the tetracycline broth is extracted with an equal volume of butanol, which is divided into three equal portions for each extraction, the fraction remaining in the broth is

$$L_{3rd} = \frac{1}{\left(\dfrac{0.6 \times 1}{3} + 1\right)^3} = 0.58$$

and 1 - 0.58 = 0.42 of the tetracycline has been removed from the broth. As previously calculated, a single extraction with butanol would remove 0.375 of the tetracycline from the broth.

9 | CHEMICAL STABILITY

The stability of a pharmaceutical must be known to ensure that the patient receives the prescribed dose of a drug and not a therapeutically inactive degradation product. The pharmaceutical manufacturer is responsible for assuring the stability of a marketed product within the limits of its expiration date. The community pharmacist requires a knowledge of the factors affecting stability so that he may properly store prefabricated pharmaceuticals, select the proper containers for dispensing the medication, anticipate interactions when mixing several prefabricated preparations, and inform the patient of any changes that may occur after the medication has been dispensed.

REACTION ORDER

In a unimolecular reaction only one molecule is involved in the chemical change. Examples of unimolecular reactions are the dissociation of bromine at high temperature, the rearrangement of maleic acid to fumaric acid upon heating, and the radioactive disintegration of ^{131}I. In a bimolecular reaction two molecules must collide before the reaction can occur. The inversion of sugar in the presence of hydrogen ion and the alkaline hydrolysis of ethyl acetate are bimolecular reactions. The molecularity of a reaction is defined as the number of reactant molecules that must come together before the reaction can occur. The molecularity is of value in describing the mechanism or steps by which the reaction proceeds.

In considering the chemical stability of a pharmaceutical it is pertinent to know the reaction order, which is obtained experimentally by measuring the reaction rate as a function of concentration of the degrading drug. The overall order of a reaction is the sum of the exponents of the concentration terms of the rate expression. The order with respect to each reactant is the exponent of the individual concentration term in the rate expression.

In pharmacy a definite dose or concentration of a therapeutically active compound is to be present in a product. Thus, chemical stability is considered from the rate of degradation of the active drug and not from the viewpoint of rate of formation of degradation products.

First-Order Reaction

A first-order reaction is one in which the rate of reaction is directly proportional to the concentration of the reacting substance. Mathematically, this may be expressed as

$$-\frac{dC}{dt} = kC$$

where C is the concentration of the reacting material, t the time, and $-dC/dt$ the rate at which the concentration decreases. The constant k is known as the specific reaction-rate constant or the velocity constant. For a first-order reaction it has the dimension of reciprocal time. If, for example, k has a value of 0.001 hr^{-1}, the material is decomposed at the rate of 0.1 per cent per hour.

chemical stability • 251

Integration of the simple differential equation between the limits of concentration C_1 at time t_1 and C_2 at a later time t_2 produces

$$\log \frac{C_1}{C_2} = \frac{k(t_2 - t_1)}{2.303}$$

In pharmacy the initial concentration, C_0, at the time of manufacture of the product and the elapse of time since manufacture are generally utilized, so the form of the equation is

$$\log \frac{C_0}{C} = \frac{kt}{2.303}$$

or

$$\log C = -\frac{kt}{2.303} + \log C_0 \qquad \text{Eq. for a 1st order Rx}$$

As the equation has the form of the equation of a straight line, a plot of the logarithm of concentration against time produces a straight line for a first-order reaction. The slope of such a plot is $-k/2.303$. On occasion it is convenient to use the exponential form of the above equation,

$$C = C_0 e^{-kt} = C_0 10^{-kt/2.303}$$

It is meaningless to attempt to express the time required for all the material to decompose, because theoretically an infinite time is needed. The reaction rate is described by the rate constant or by the half-life period, $t_{1/2}$, i.e., the time necessary for half of a given material to decompose. The half-life is independent of the initial concentration and it is related to the first-order rate constant by

$$k = \frac{2.303}{t_{1/2}} \log \frac{1}{\frac{1}{2}}$$

$$= \frac{0.693}{t_{1/2}} \qquad t_{1/2} \text{ for a 1st order Rx} = \frac{.693}{k}$$

Reactions in which the rate does not depend on the concentration of all the reactants because one of the reactants is present in such a large excess that it remains essentially constant are known as pseudomolecular reactions. Although the inversion of sugar in the presence of hydrogen ion is a bimolecular reaction, the essentially constant concentrations of water and hydrogen ion may be incorporated into the rate constant. As the inversion rate is proportional to the concentration of the sugar, the reaction is said to be an apparent or pseudo-first-order reaction. The rate constant is known as the observed or pseudo-first-order rate constant.

Many degradation reactions of drugs are complex, but they frequently occur in the presence of a great excess of solvent and may be readily characterized as pseudo-first-order reactions. Although two molecules are involved in the hydrolysis of an aspirin solution, the water is in such large excess that only the aspirin appears to change in concentration. The use of first-order reaction-rate calculations may be illustrated with the data given in Table LIV and plotted in Figure 101 for the hydrolysis of an aqueous aspirin solution, which is buffered to pH 5 at 25°. In this plot of concentration against time the concentration of aspirin decreases with time, rapidly at first, then more slowly, and finally approaches zero.

Interpretation of data and the evaluation of the rate constant is more convenient if the logarithm of the concentration is plotted against time, as shown in Figure 102. If the reaction rate is first order, a straight line is produced in accordance with the relation

$$\log C = -\frac{kt}{2.303} + \log C_0 \qquad \text{slope } (-k/2.303)$$
$$\text{y intercept}$$

where C is the concentration at time t and C_0 is the initial concentration; i.e., $\log C_0$ is the intercept

chemical stability

Table LIV Hydrolysis of Aqueous Aspirin Solution Buffered at pH 5 at 25°

Time (hr)	Concentration, C (moles liter^{-1})	log C	$\frac{\Delta C}{\Delta t}$	C_{av} (moles liter^{-1})
0	0.01500	−1.8239		
12	0.01285	−1.8911	0.000180	0.01392
24	0.01107	−1.9560	0.000148	0.01196
36	0.00942	−2.0260	0.000138	0.01024
48	0.00808	−2.0926	0.000112	0.00875
60	0.00692	−2.1600	0.000097	0.00750
72	0.00592	−2.2268	0.000084	0.00642

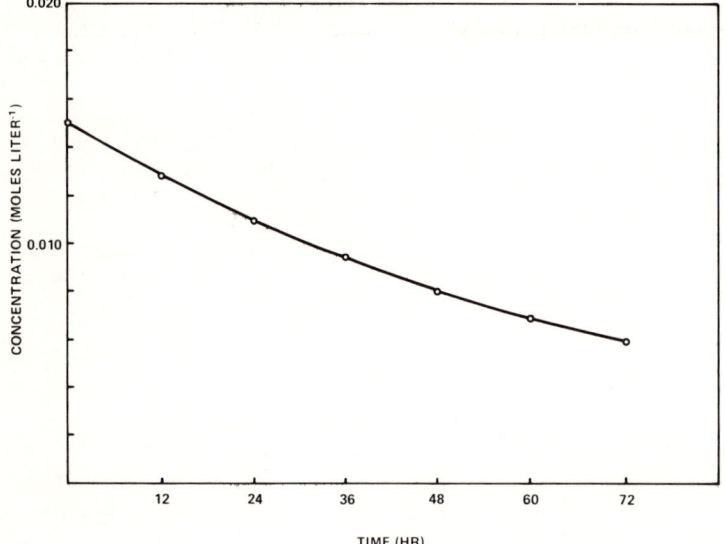

Figure 101. Decrease in concentration of aspirin solution buffered at pH 5 at 25° with time.

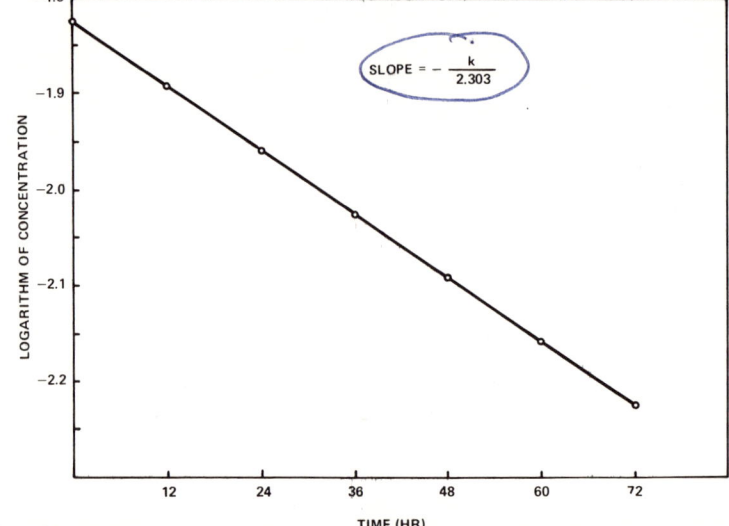

Figure 102. Linear plot of logarithm of concentration against time for the first-order hydrolysis of an aspirin solution buffered at pH 5 at 25°.

SLOPE = $-\frac{k}{2.303}$

with the y axis. The best method of evaluating k is to multiply the slope of the line by 2.303. Selecting the concentration at zero time and 60 hours, the slope of the line in Figure 102 is

$$m = \frac{-2.1600 - (-1.8239)}{60} = -0.0056 \text{ hr}^{-1}$$

The first-order rate constant is numerically equal to 0.0056 X 2.303 = 0.013 hr^{-1}. The half-life is

$$t_{1/2} = \frac{0.693}{0.013} \cong 53 \text{ hr}$$

According to the simple differential equation that expresses a first-order reaction, a plot of $-\Delta C/\Delta t$ obtained by taking increments of concentration and time between successive observations against the average concentration produces a straight line that passes through the origin as shown in Figure 103. Such a curve shows that the rate of decrease in concentration with time is proportional to the concentration. The slope of this straight line is numerically equivalent to k.

The determination of the rate constant allows the calculation of the amount of material remaining unchanged at any time. For example, at 25° and pH 5, the concentration of aspirn may be calculated by means of the equation

$$\log C = -\frac{0.013t}{2.303} - 1.824$$

After 3 days or 72 hours the concentration of aspirin is

$$\log C = -\frac{0.013 \times 72}{2.303} - 1.824$$

$$= -2.2308$$

$$C = 0.0059 \text{ mole liter}^{-1}$$

This loss of 60 per cent of the aspirin in 3 days illustrates the lack of stability of aspirin in the presence of moisture.

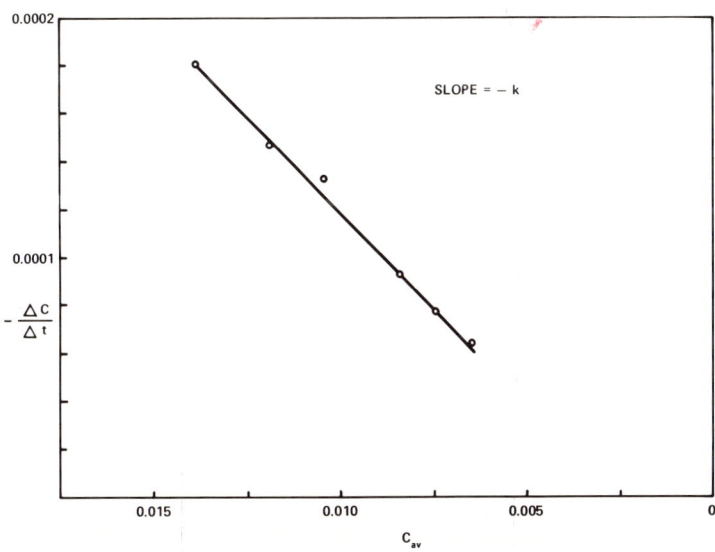

Figure 103. Linear plot of $-\Delta C/\Delta t$ against average concentration for the first-order hydrolysis of an aspirin solution buffered at pH 5 at 25°.

Zero-Order Reaction

Zero-order reactions are reactions in which the rate is independent of the concentration of the reactants. The rate of reaction is determined by other factors, such as absorption of light in certain photochemical reactions or the rate of diffusion in certain surface reactions.

A zero-order rate is mathematically expressed as

$$-\frac{dC}{dt} = k_0$$

where k_0 is the zero-order rate constant, which has the dimensions of concentration divided by time, e.g., moles liter^{-1} hr^{-1}. The above differential equation upon integration yields

$$C = -k_0 t + C_0$$

where C_0 is the initial concentration.

The chemical degradation of drugs in many pharmaceutical suspensions is characterized by a zero-order reaction. Only the dissolved portion of a drug is subjected to degradation, and the dissolved portion is kept constant as the solution is saturated by the suspended drug. Although aspirin in solution hydrolyzes by a first-order process, a suspension of aspirin in a buffered vehicle maintains a saturated solution and its degradation appears to be zero order. The initial concentration is the concentration of the aspirin in the suspension. The zero-order rate constant, k_0, is equal to the product of the solubility of the aspirin and the first-order rate constant at the pH of the suspension. At a pH 5 and 25° the solubility of aspirin is 85.2 g liter^{-1}. Thus, k_0 is 85.2 × 0.013 = 1.108 g liter^{-1} hr^{-1}. For an aspirin suspension containing 0.6 g in a teaspoonful or 120 g liter^{-1} and buffered at pH 5 after 3 days at 25°, the aspirin concentration is

$$C = C_0 - 1.108 t$$
$$= 120 - (1.108 \times 3 \times 24)$$
$$= 40.2 \text{ g liter}^{-1}$$

A plot of the hydrolysis of this aspirin suspension is shown in Figure 104. This is typical of a zero-order reaction for which the slope of the straight line is equal to $-k_0$.

Higher-Order Reactions

When the experimentally determined rate of a reaction is proportional to the concentration of two reactants, the reaction is second order. In the second-order reaction A + B → AB, the rates of the reactions are expressed as

$$-\frac{dC_A}{dt} = -\frac{dC_B}{dt} = k C_A C_B$$

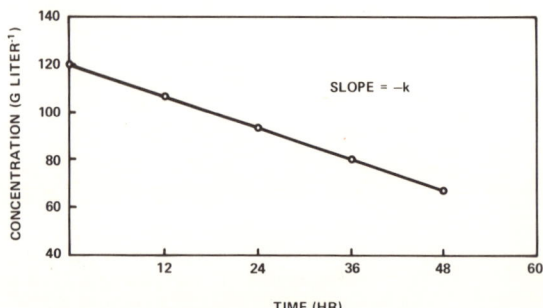

Figure 104. Zero-order hydrolysis of aspirin suspension buffered at pH 5 at 25°.

If a and b represent the initial molar concentration of reactants A and B, and if x represents the number of moles of A or B in each liter reacting in the interval of time t, the rate of the reaction is

$$\frac{dx}{dt} = k(a-x)(b-x)$$

On integration this equation becomes

$$kt = \frac{2.303}{a-b} \log \frac{b(a-x)}{a(b-x)}$$

In the special case where the two reactants are present in equal concentrations, the rate of the reaction is

$$\frac{dx}{dt} = k(a-x)^2$$

which on integration becomes

$$k = \frac{1}{t} \frac{x}{a(a-x)}$$

The graphic method for the evaluation of the second-order rate constant is convenient. When $\log[b(a-x)/a(b-x)]$ is plotted against time, a straight line is produced if the reaction is second order. The second-order rate constant is evaluated by multiplying the slope of the line by $2.303/(a-b)$. A typical bimolecular rate plot for the alkaline hydrolysis of homatropine methylbromide is shown in Figure 105. The second-order rate constant has the units liters mole^{-1} sec^{-1}.

Zero-, first-, and second-order reactions have been discussed, but it should not be assumed that all reactions fit these types. The order of a reaction is determined by the exponents of the concentration terms from which the rate of the reaction is determined. In the reaction A + B → AB, the rate of degradation of A is

$$-\frac{dC_A}{dt} = kC_A^m C_B^n$$

Since most reactions are complex, there is not necessarily any relationship between the stoichiometric reaction and the experimentally determined order. Thus, the exponents may be fractional as well as whole numbers. If m and n are 1.5 and 1, respectively,

$$-\frac{dC_A}{dt} = kC_A^{1.5} C_B$$

and the overall reaction order is 2.5.

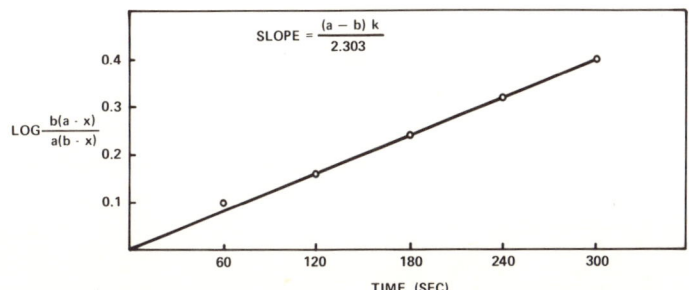

Figure 105. Linear plot for the second-order alkaline hydrolysis of homatropine methylbromide at 25.8°. [J.L. Patel and A.P. Lemberger, *J. Am. Pharm. Assoc. 48,* 106 (1959).]

INFLUENCE OF TEMPERATURE

It is intuitive knowledge that an increase in temperature produces an increase in reaction rate. Arrhenius expressed the relation between temperature and reaction rate as

$$k = s \exp(-E_a/RT)$$

where E_a is the molar activation energy and s the frequency factor.

Molecules do not react until they become activated. The activation energy, E_a, is the amount of energy required to put the molecules in an activated state from which they react to form the products of the reaction. Only a fraction of the total molecules are in an activated state. As the temperature is increased, a greater fraction of the molecules become activated and the reaction rate is faster. The frequency factor, s, embraces the number of colloisions of the molecules and the probability that the orientation of the colliding molecules is such that a reaction may occur.

In the logarithmic form

$$\log k = -\frac{E_a}{2.303R}\frac{1}{T} + \log s$$

which upon differentiation yields

$$\frac{d \ln k}{dT} = \frac{E_a}{RT^2}$$

Integrating between the limits k_1 at T_1 and k_2 at T_2 gives

$$\log \frac{k_2}{k_1} = \frac{E_a}{2.303R}\frac{T_2 - T_1}{T_2 T_1}$$

A straight line is formed when the logarithm of the rate constant is plotted against the reciprocal of the absolute temperature. The rate constants for the hydrolysis of aspirin solutions at pH 5 at various temperatures are given in Table LV and plotted in Figure 106. The slope of this line is $-E_a/2.303R$, and its numerical evaluation, e.g., -3765, from the curve permits the calculation of the activation energy,

$$E_a = 2.303 \times 1.987 \times 3765$$
$$= 17,300 \text{ cal mole}^{-1}$$

When the activation energy and a rate constant for one temperature are known, rate constants may be calculated for other temperatures and the rate of the reaction can be predicted. For example, knowing the activation energy and $k_{25°} = 0.013 \text{ hr}^{-1}$, the rate constant and the stability of an aspirin solution buffered at pH 5 can be calculated for a solution refrigerated at 5°,

$$\log \frac{0.013}{k_{5°}} = \frac{17,300}{2.303 \times 1.987} \frac{298 - 278}{298 \times 278} = 0.9089$$

$$k_{5°} = 0.0016 \text{ hr}^{-1}$$

Utilizing $k_{5°}$ the percentage of the initial aspirin remaining in a solution stored at 5° for 3 days is

$$\log C = \frac{-kt}{2.303} + \log C_0$$

$$= \frac{-0.0016 \times 3 \times 24}{2.303} + \log 100 = 1.9499$$

$$C = 89\%$$

Table LV Hydrolytic Degradation of Aqueous Aspirin Solutions Buffered at pH 5 at Various Temperatures

$t°$	$1/T$	k (hr^{-1})	log k
25	0.003357	0.013	-1.8861
35	0.003247	0.029	-1.5376
50	0.003096	0.127	-0.8962
60	0.003003	0.291	-0.5361

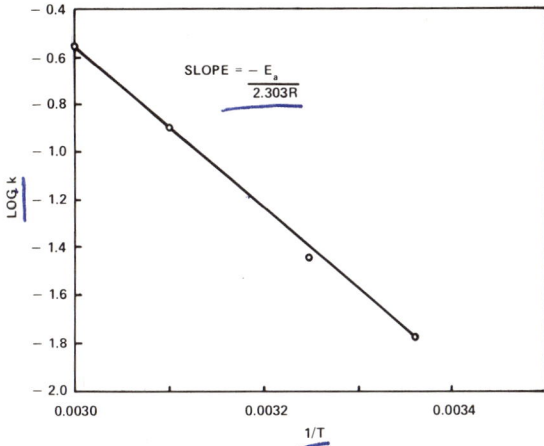

Figure 106. Linear plot of logarithm k against $1/T$ at pH 5 for the hydrolysis of aspirin, from which the activation energy may be calculated.

The activation energy is an important factor in determining the speed of a reaction. In reactions having a high activation energy only a small fraction of the molecules possess this energy, and the reaction is slow. Reactions with an activation energy less than 10,000 cal mole^{-1} proceed very fast. If the activation energy involved in the degradation of a drug is low, one anticipates a rather rapid degradation and stability problems in product development. The activation energy of degradation of many medicinal compounds is in the range 15,000 to 30,000 cal mole^{-1}. The larger the activation energy of a reaction, the more the rate will be affected by a temperature change.

HYDROLYSIS

Since many medicinal compounds are esters, amides, or lactams, hydrolysis is the most frequently encountered type of degradation in pharmaceuticals. Hydrogen and hydroxyl ions are the most common catalysts of hydrolytic degradation in solutions. Catalysis by hydrogen and hydroxyl ions is known as specific acid-base catalysis. The effect of pH on the rate of hydrolysis of an aqueous solution of aspirin is shown in Figure 107. A plot of the rate constant against pH is known as a pH-rate profile. For aspirin the maximum stability is at pH 2.5.

In the general mechanism of acid-base catalysis the observed rate constant is considered to be made up of a number of terms each of which is the product of a concentration and a catalytic coefficient for one of the species present in the reaction medium. The pH-rate profile of aspirin hydrolysis is complex because over the pH range 1 to 12 hydrolysis may take place by six reactions, of which several may occur simultaneously at a given pH.

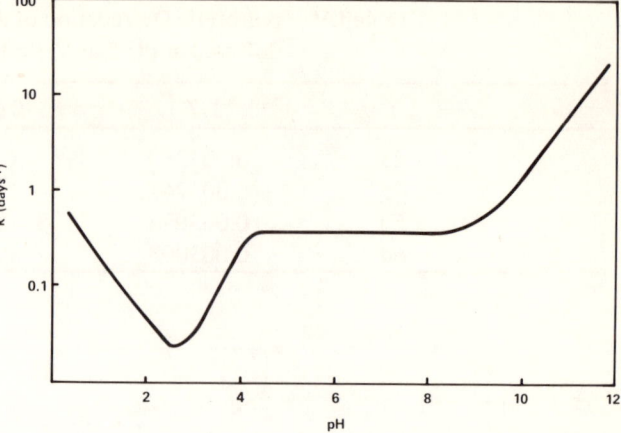

Figure 107. Overall velocity constant for aspirin hydrolysis at 17° as a function of pH. [L.J. Edwards, *Trans. Faraday Soc.* **46**, 723 (1950).]

The effect of pH on hydrolysis is best understood by a consideration of the reaction mechanism. For example, the hydrolysis of N-acetyl-*p*-aminophenol is both an acid-catalyzed reaction,

and a base-catalyzed reaction,

The overall rate equation for its hydrolysis is

$$-\frac{dC}{dt} = k_{H^+}[H^+]C + k_{OH^-}[OH^-]C$$

where C is the concentration in moles liter^{-1} of N-acetyl-*p*-aminophenol, $[H^+]$ and $[OH^-]$ are molar concentrations of hydrogen and hydroxyl ions, and k_{H^+} and k_{OH^-} are the rate constants or catalytic coefficients for acid and base catalysis, respectively. When hydrolysis occurs in an acidic solution in which hydrogen ion is the only effective catalyst, the rate of hydrolysis is

$$-\frac{dC}{dt} = k_{H^+}[H^+]^n C^m$$

where n and m are the order of the reaction in respect to hydrogen ion concentration and concentration of the drug. If the hydrogen ion concentration is maintained constant, the rate of hydrolysis of

N-acetyl-p-aminophenol may be written

$$-\frac{dC}{dt} = k'_{H^+} C^m$$

where $k'_{H^+} = k_{H^+}[H^+]^n$.

By similar reasoning the rate of hydrolysis in alkaline solution is

$$-\frac{dC}{dt} = k'_{OH^-} C^m$$

As shown in Figure 108, a plot of logarithm of concentration against time is a straight line; thus, hydrolysis is first order with respect to concentration of N-acetyl-p-aminophenol.

The order of the reaction with respect to hydrogen ion may be obtained by taking the logarithm of the equation defining k'_{H^+}:

$$\log k'_{H^+} = \log k_{H^+} + n \log[H^+]$$
$$= \log k_{H^+} - n(\text{pH})$$

As this equation has the form of an equation of a straight line, a plot of log k'_{H^+} against pH gives in the strongly acid region a straight line with its slope numerically equal to n. As shown in Figure 109, in the strongly acid region $n = -1$, and the hydrolysis is first order with respect to hydrogen ion concentration.

A similar argument may be presented to show that in strongly alkaline regions, the hydrolysis rate is first order with respect to hydroxyl ion concentration.

In the pH range 4 to 7 more than a single mechanism of hydrolysis is operating and the reaction is not first order but a complex order.

The Arrhenius plot of logarithm k' against the reciprocal of absolute temperature is a straight line with slope $-E_a/2.303$. The activation energy for the hydrolysis of N-acetyl-p-aminophenol in aqueous solutions from pH 2 to 9 is of the magnitude 17,500 cal mole^{-1}. At 90° the first-order rate constant is 0.0008373 hr^{-1} at pH 5. The first-order rate constant at 25° may be calculated as

$$\log \frac{k_2}{k_1} = \frac{E_a}{2.303 R} \frac{T_2 - T_1}{T_2 T_1}$$

$$\log \frac{0.0008373}{k_{25°}} = \frac{17,500}{2.303 \times 1.987} \frac{363 - 298}{363 \times 298} = 2.28565$$

$$k_{25°} = 4.33 \times 10^{-6} \text{ hr}^{-1}$$

The half-life of N-acetyl-p-aminophenol under these conditions is

$$t_{1/2} = \frac{0.693}{4.33 \times 10^{-6}} = 1.6 \times 10^5 \text{ hr}$$

$$= \frac{1.6 \times 10^5}{24 \times 365} = 18.3 \text{ yr}$$

The relationship between the logarithm of half-life and pH is shown in Figure 110. In formulating liquid products containing N-acetyl-p-aminophenol, it is desirable to maintain the pH of the vehicle at pH 5 to 6 to have maximum stability.

The basic structure of a penicillin includes a double-ring thiazolidine β-lactam moiety of which the lactam ring is readily susceptible to hydrolysis in neutral and alkaline media to yield penicilloic acid. The reaction at constant temperature and pH is first order with respect to the penicillin and directly proportional to the hydroxyl ion concentration. In strongly acidic solutions penicillin is rearranged to penillic acid by a first-order reaction.

chemical stability

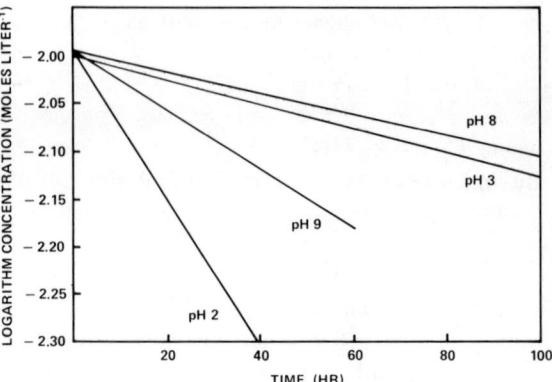

Figure 108. Logarithm of concentration of N-acetyl-*p*-aminophenol against time at 90° at different pHs. [K.T. Koshy and J.L. Lach, *J. Pharm. Sci. 50,* 113 (1961).]

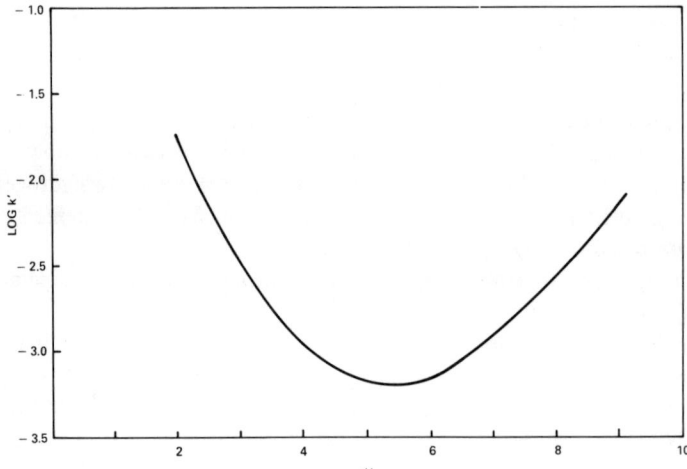

Figure 109. Logarithm k' against pH for the hydrolysis of N-acetyl-*p*-aminophenol at 90°. [K.T. Koshy and J.L. Lach, *J. Pharm. Sci. 50,* 113 (1961).]

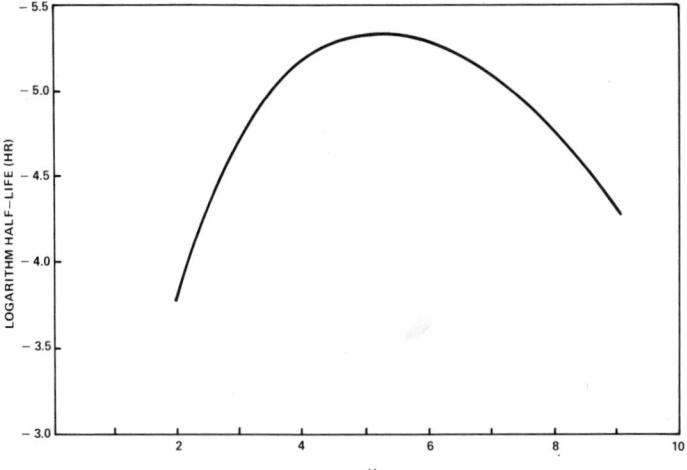

Figure 110. Logarithm $t_{1/2}$ in hours of hydrolysis of N-acetyl-*p*-aminophenol at 25° as a function of pH. [K.T. Koshy and J.L. Lach, *J. Pharm. Sci. 50,* 113 (1961).]

The hydrolytic degradation of the penicillins is better understood by the examination of the hydrolysis of a specific penicillin, potassium phenethicillin. As shown in Figure 111, at a constant temperature and pH the hydrolysis of phenethicillin is an overall first-order reaction. The curvature in the acid region of the pH-rate profile in Figure 112 indicates that more than a single reaction is involved. Phenethicillin is an acid with $pK_a = 2.9$. In an acidic medium it exists as the free acid and the anion that undergo hydrolysis at different rates. The fraction of the phenethicillin existing in the form of an un-ionized acid, f_{PH}, is related to the hydrogen ion concentration by the expression

$$f_{PH} = \frac{[H^+]}{[H^+] + K_a}$$

and the fraction of the phenethicillin existing as the anionic species, f_{P^-}, is related to the hydrogen ion concentration by the expression

$$f_{P^-} = \frac{K_a}{[H^+] + K_a}$$

As the pH is changed, the ratio of un-ionized acid to ionized acid is changed. Since the catalytic effect of hydrogen ion on the degradation of each species is different, the logarithm of the rate constant is not directly proportional to the pH.

The overall rate of hydrolysis for the hydrogen ion catalysis of total phenethicillin, P_t, is

$$-\frac{dP_t}{dt} = k_1 [H^+] [PH] + k_2 [H^+] [P^-] = k'[P_t]$$

where k_1 and k_2 are the rate constants for the acid hydrolysis of the acid and ionic species, respectively; k' the observed or pseudo-first-order rate constant; and [PH] and [P⁻] the molar concentrations of the acid and ionic species, respectively.

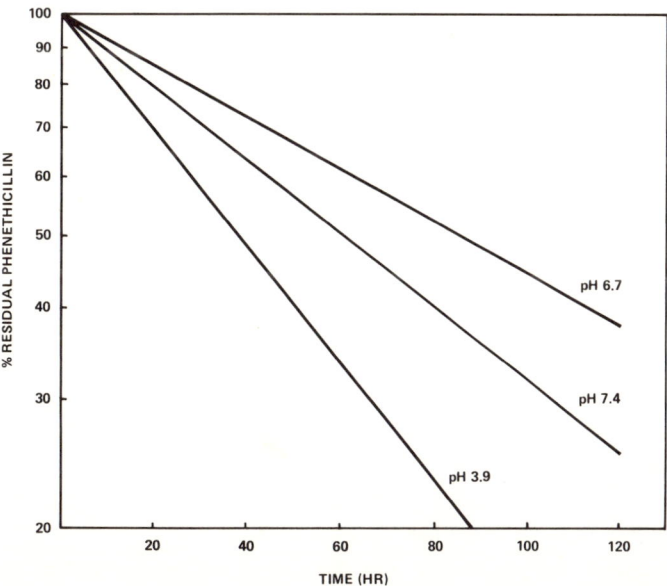

Figure 111. First-order degradation of phenethicillin at 35°. [M.A. Schwartz, A.P. Granatek, and F.H. Buckwalter, *J. Pharm. Sci.* **51**, 523 (1962).]

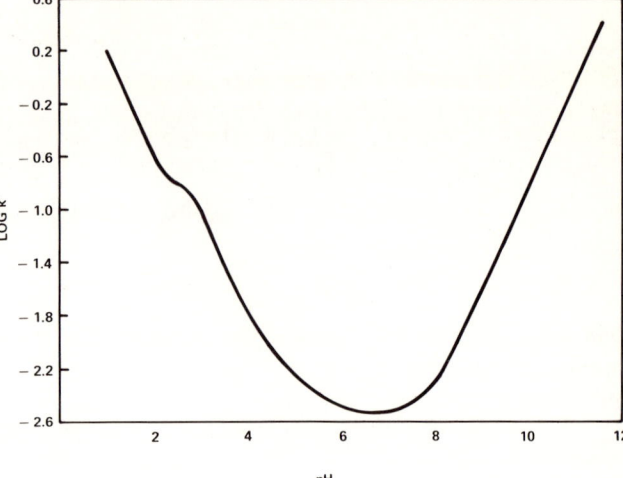

Figure 112. pH-rate profile of the hydrolysis of phenethicillin at 35°. [M.A. Schwartz, A.P. Granatek, and F.H. Buckwalter, *J. Pharm. Sci.* **51**, 523 (1962).]

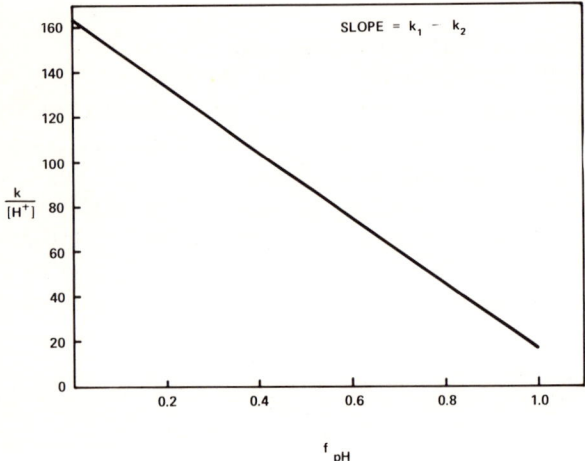

Figure 113. Plot of $k'/[H^+]$ as a function of f_{PH} used to evaluate the rate constants k_1 and k_2 as described in the text. [M.A. Schwartz, A.P. Granatek, and F.H. Buckwalter, *J. Pharm. Sci.* **51**, 523 (1962).]

Dividing the equation by $P_t[H^+]$ and substituting the fractional designation,

$$\frac{k'}{[H^+]} = k_1 f_{PH} + k_2 f_{P^-}$$

Since $f_{PH} + f_{P^-} = 1$, this equation may be rearranged to

$$\frac{k'}{[H^+]} = (k_1 - k_2)f_{PH} + k_2$$

A plot of $k'/[H^+]$ against f_{PH} produces a straight line with a slope of $k_1 - k_2$ and a y intercept of k_2. At 35° as evaluated from Figure 113, k_1 and k_2 are 12.5 and 162 liters mole^{-1} hr^{-1}, respectively. The rate constant k_2 for the hydrolysis of the ionic species is about 13 times greater than k_1, because of the greater affinity of the negatively charged ion for a proton.

In the strongly alkaline region the hydrolysis of phenethicillin is second order. The second-order rate constant for the alkaline hydrolysis is 750 liters mole^{-1} hr^{-1}. In the region pH 8 to 12 the logarithm of the observed rate constant is a linear function of pH. This observed first-order rate constant is actually a product of the second-order rate constant and the hydroxyl ion concentration.

The pH of maximum stability of phenethicillin is 6.7. Although several buffer systems may provide a pH of maximum stability, it is not necessarily a fact that all buffer systems at a given pH provide the same stability. The use of a phosphate buffer at pH 6.7 does not provide stability for a phenethicillin solution, owing to the general base catalysis of the secondary phosphate ion. The pseudo-first-order rate constant k' for the hydrolysis in a phosphate buffer solution is

$$k' = k_2 [H^+] + k_{OH^-}[OH^-] + k_{H_2O} + k_{HPO_4^=}[HPO_4^=]$$

which upon transposition becomes

$$k' - k_2 [H^+] - k_{OH^-}[OH^-] = k'' = k_{H_2O} + k_{HPO_4^=}[HPO_4^=]$$

where k_{H_2O} is the rate constant for the reaction with water, i.e., infinite dilution of all the catalytic species. In the pH range 5.5 to 7, where specific acid-base catalysis is negligible, the base catalysis of the phosphate ion promotes hydrolysis.

A plot of k'' against the concentration of phosphate ion is linear as shown in Figure 114. The slope of the line is equal to $k_{HPO_4^=}$. The rate constant k_{H_2O} is numerically equal to the y intercept. This plot shows that an increase in the concentration of phosphate ion significantly decreases the stability of phenethicillin. With a citrate buffer there is no general acid-base catalysis effect. Thus, in product development not only the effect of pH on stability must be considered, but also any possible effect on the specific ingredients of the buffer system on the stability of the drug.

In the initial development of a liquid product containing a medicinal compound liable to hydrolysis, the influence of pH on stability is a primary consideration. The final pH of the product depends on a compromise between the pH of maximum stability and the pHs of physiological acceptance and therapeutic availability of the drug from the particular dosage form.

Stable suspensions of potassium penicillin G can be made in vegetable oil. The replacement of water by other solvents has been suggested as a method of stabilizing drugs against hydrolysis. This does not always yield a more stable product. For example, penicillin is rendered therapeutically inactive by alcohol and glycerin, probably with esterification of penicilloic acid. The hydrogen-ion-catalyzed degradation of chloramphenicol in a water-propylene cosolvent is increased as the percentage of propylene glycol is increased.

Polar solvents tend to accelerate reactions that form products having higher intermolecular interactions than the reactants. In the hydrolysis of esters, the alcohol and acid are generally more polar than the esters; and the hydrolysis is more rapid in a solvent of higher polarity, e.g., water, than in a solvent of lower polarity, e.g., alcohol. If the products are less polar than the reactants, the reaction is accelerated by solvents of lower polarity and retarded by more polar solvents. The exact influence of the solvent on the rate of hydrolysis cannot be easily generalized.

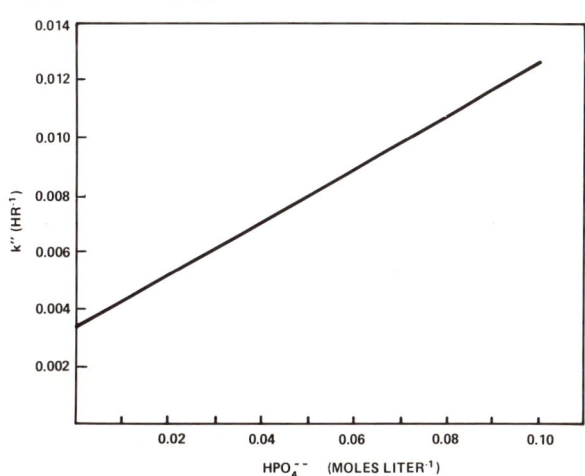

Figure 114. Influence of the general base catalysis by $HPO_4^=$ on the rate of hydrolysis of phenethicillin at 35°. [M.A. Schwartz, A.P. Granatek, and F.H. Buckwalter, *J. Pharm. Sci.* **51**, 523 (1962).]

The stability of a drug in a liquid product may be increased by suppression of its solubility, because only the dissolved drug is degraded. For a saturated solution or a suspension of a drug that is hydrolyzed at a first-order rate, the observed zero-order rate constant is

$$k_0 = kC_s$$

It is obvious from this equation that any decrease in solubility C_s decreases the magnitude of k_0 and slows the rate of degradation.

The solubility may be suppressed by additives that compete with the drug for the solvent molecules. The stability of procaine penicillin G has been increased by the addition of large quantities of sorbitol, dextrose, sodium gluconate, and sodium citrate to the suspension. The addition of procaine hydrochloride, which by its common-ion effect suppresses the dissociation and solubility of procaine penicillin G, further increases the stability of the suspension.

The rate of hydrolysis may be greatly reduced by using an insoluble derivative of the parent drug. Water-soluble penicillins are hydrolyzed rapidly in aqueous solution; however, water-insoluble derivatives, e.g., benzathine penicillin G and hydrabamine penicillin G, are sufficiently stable so that an aqueous suspension may be prepared with a shelf life of at least 12 months. With suspensions both the solubility and the rate of degradation are functions of pH, as shown in Figure 115 for procaine penicillin G.

Complexation has been suggested as another method by which hydrolysis may be retarded. The influence of caffeine on the hydrolysis of benzocaine is illustrated in Figure 116. The complexed benzocaine does not degrade; only the free benzocaine is subject to hydrolysis. Thus, as the concentration of caffeine is increased with a consequential decrease in the concentration of free benzocaine, the stability of the solution is increased; e.g., the half-life of an aqueous solution is increased fivefold by the addition of 2.5 per cent caffeine.

When in an aqueous solution the concentration of a surface-active agent exceeds its solubility, the excessive surface-active agent forms molecular aggregates or micelles of the surface-active agent. Solubilization is the phenomenon by which water-insoluble compounds are dissolved or incorporated within the micelles to produce a colloidal dispersion, which has the appearance of a solution. Solubilized medicinal compounds within the interior of the micelle may be protected from attacking species that cause hydrolysis. As shown in Figure 117, in the presence of 3 per cent Brij® 35 the rate of hydrolysis of benzocaine is reduced to one-fourth of the rate in the absence of the surface-active agent.

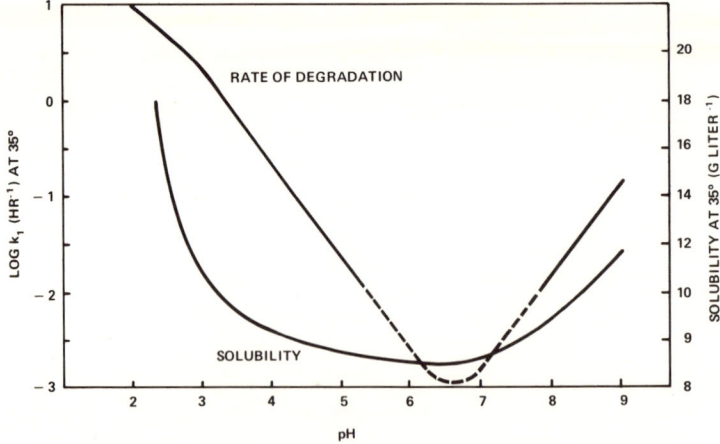

Figure 115. Solubility and rate of degradation of procaine penicillin G as a function of pH. [M.A. Schwartz and F.H. Buckwalter, *J. Pharm. Sci.* **51**, 1119 (1962).]

If other methods for retarding hydrolysis fail, the product may be packaged in a dry form, to which the community pharmacist adds the vehicle at the time of dispensing. Antibiotics are frequently marketed in this fashion. Solid dosage forms acquire moisture from the atmosphere, and any drugs liable to hydrolysis may be degraded; such dosage forms should be packaged with silica gel or another suitable dessicating agent. With troublesome solids it may be necessary to package each individual dosage form in a hermetically sealed aluminum foil.

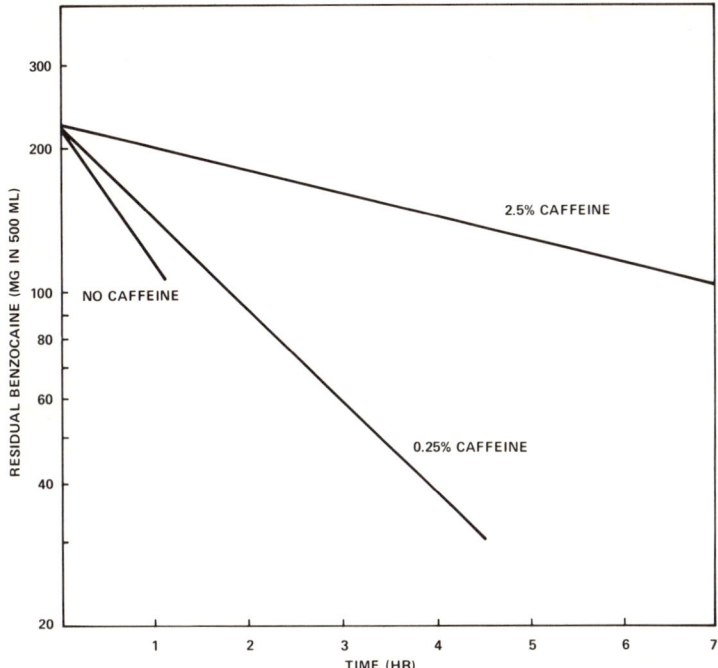

Figure 116. Influence of complexation by caffeine on the rate of hydrolysis of benzocaine at 30° and at 0.04 N hydroxyl ion concentration. [Adapted from T.Higuchi and L. Lachman, *J. Am. Pharm. Assoc.* **44**, 521 (1955).]

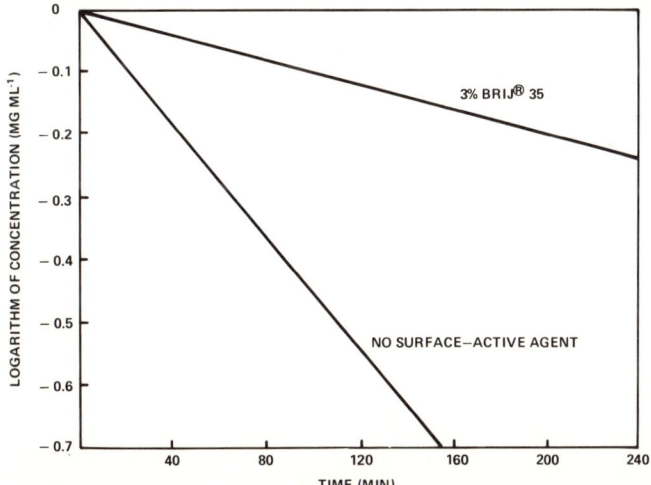

Figure 117. Influence of micellular solubilization by Brij® 35 on the rate of hydrolysis of benzocaine at 30° and at 0.04 N hydroxyl ion concentration. [Adapted from P.B. Sheth and E.L. Parrott, *J. Pharm. Sci.* **56**, 983 (1967).]

ATMOSPHERIC OXIDATION

Autoxidation is the spontaneous reaction under ordinary conditions of a drug with atmospheric or molecular oxygen. It is believed that most oxidation involves a free-radical mechanism and chain reactions. A free radical is an atom or molecule containing one or more unpaired electrons. Free radicals tend to take electrons from other compounds; i.e., they serve as oxidizing agents. As the compound is degraded by more than a single reaction, quantitative kinetic interpretation is not simple.

When the oxygen uptake is measured, it is frequently observed that there is a lag period of little or no oxygen consumption. The oxygen-uptake curve may be straight, but it often shows inflections that are difficult to fit to simple order reactions. This may be caused by traces of metallic ions originating in the drug, solvent, or container. Since metal may initiate oxidation reactions, care is taken to avoid the introduction of metallic ions during manufacture by the use of proper equipment and metal-free solvents. As a precaution, chelating agents, e.g., ethylenediaminetetraacetic acid, may be added to bind any metal present.

Medicinal compounds that undergo autoxidation at room temperature are affected by oxygen dissolved in the solvent and in the void space of their package. The packaging operation should be conducted under an inert atmosphere, e.g., nitrogen or carbon dioxide, to exclude air from the container. The container should be light resistant, as free-radical reactions are promoted by light.

Antioxidants react with the free radicals by providing electrons and easily available hydrogen atoms, and they prevent the propagation of the chain reactions. Some antioxidants used in pharmacy are ascorbic acid, butylated hydroxyanisole, butylated hydroxytoluene, dihydropyrogallol, propyl gallate, nordihydroquaiaretic acid, sodium bisulfite, sodium sulfite, and the tocopherols.

Morphine in aqueous solution undergoes discoloration and precipitates as a result of oxidation of morphine to pseudomorphine and morphine N-oxide. The oxidation is a free-radical reaction which involves the phenolic group and proceeds rapidly in alkaline or neutral solutions. The oxidation of morphine depends on the pH of the solution and the presence of atmospheric oxygen. Solutions of morphine sealed under an inert atmosphere of nitrogen show no evidence of oxidative degradation. In the presence of excess oxygen the rate of oxidation is a function of pH. A plot of the rate constant against pH, as shown in Figure 118, is similar in form to a typical dissociation curve. This indicates that the degradation is dependent on the type of morphine species in solution. In acidic buffers used to prepare solutions of morphine, the existing species are the undissociated and protonated morphine. In the pH range 2.5 to 4 the rate of degradation is approximately constant, because the morphine exists essentially as the protonated species. The undissociated morphine undergoes oxidation more readily than the protonated species. As the pH is increased to 7, the rate of oxidation is increased because an increasingly greater fraction of the morphine exists in the undissociated form.

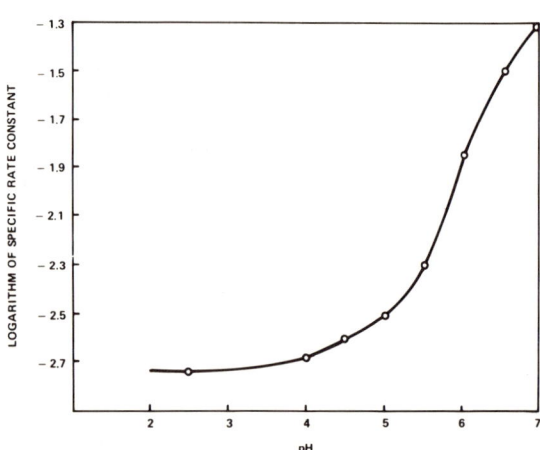

Figure 118. pH rate profile for the pseudo-first-order oxidation of morphine at 95°. [S. Yeh and J.L. Lach, *J. Pharm. Sci.* **50**, 35 (1961).]

The following mechanism has been suggested to describe the oxidation of morphine, in which M represents the undissociated morphine and MH$^+$ represents the protonated morphine. The undissociated and protonated morphine are both oxidized by atmospheric oxygen to form a free-radical semiquinone (MO·) and a free-radical peroxide (HOO·):

$$M + O_2 \underset{}{\overset{k_1}{\rightleftharpoons}} MO\cdot + HOO\cdot$$

$$MH^+ + O_2 \underset{}{\overset{k_2}{\rightleftharpoons}} {}^+HMO\cdot + HOO\cdot$$

This semiquinone radical may react with the undissociated or protonated form of morphine,

$$^+HMO\cdot + M \rightarrow PSM + H\cdot$$
$$^+HMO\cdot + MH^+ \rightarrow PSM + H\cdot$$

to form pseudomorphine, PSM, and a hydrogen free radical, H·. The undissociated semiquinone radical (MO·) may interact with morphine or protonated morphine:

$$MO\cdot + M \rightarrow PSM + H\cdot$$
$$MO\cdot + MH^+ \rightarrow PSM + H\cdot$$

The hydrogen free radical can react with the peroxide free radical to form hydrogen peroxide:

$$H\cdot + HOO\cdot \rightarrow H_2O_2$$

The hydrogen peroxide can react with morphine to form morphine N-oxide (MNO):

$$H_2O_2 + M \rightarrow MNO + H_2O$$

Assuming equilibrium between all the reactions so that the unstable free radicals and intermediates need not be directly considered, the overall rate equation for the oxidative degradation of total morphine, M_t, is

$$-\frac{d(M_t)}{dt} = 3k_1[O_2][M] + 3k_2[O_2][MH^+]$$

where [M] and [MH$^+$] represent the molar concentration of the undissociated and the protonated species, respectively, and k_1 and k_2 are the velocity constants for their respective oxidation. The dissociation of morphine may be written

$$MH^+ \rightleftharpoons M + H^+$$

with the dissociation constant represented by

$$K_a = \frac{[M][H^+]}{[MH^+]}$$

The molar concentration of undissociated morphine is

$$[M] = [M_t]\left(\frac{K_a}{K_a + [H^+]}\right)$$

and the molar concentration of protonated morphine is

$$[MH^+] = [M_t]\left(\frac{[H^+]}{K_a + [H^+]}\right)$$

The overall rate of oxidation may then be written as

$$-\frac{d[M_t]}{dt} = \left[3k_1[O_2]\left(\frac{K_a}{K_a+[H^+]}\right) + 3k_2[O_2]\left(\frac{[H^+]}{K_a+[H^+]}\right)\right][M_t]$$

When oxygen is maintained in excess, the rate equation becomes pseudo first order:

$$-\frac{d[M_t]}{dt} = \left(k'_1 \frac{K_a}{K_a+[H^+]} + k'_2 \frac{[H^+]}{K_a+[H^+]}\right)[M_t]$$

The oxidation of crystalline fumagillin is an example of a second-order autoxidation reaction. Correlation has been demonstrated between the loss of the antibiotic activity of fumagillin and its loss in absorbance. This correlation enables the rate of degradation of crystalline fumagillin to be determined by a spectrophotometric method. As shown in Figure 119, a plot of the reciprocal of absorbance against time is linear; this is typical of a second-order reaction with the slope equal to the second-order rate constant.

In the presence of air the second-order degradation may be explained by the reaction of one molecule of oxygen with two molecules of fumagillin, F,

$$F + O_2 \underset{k_{-1}}{\overset{k_1}{\rightleftharpoons}} FO_2$$

$$FO_2 + F \overset{k_2}{\to} 2FO$$

Consecutive reactions are involved and the first step involves a reversible reaction. The rate of formation of the activated oxygenated fumagillin, FO_2, is

$$\frac{d[FO_2]}{dt} = k_1[F][O_2] - k_{-1}[FO_2] - k_2[FO_2][F]$$

where on the right side of the equation the first term represents its proportionality to the concentration of fumagillin and oxygen, the second term represents the reversible breakdown of FO_2, and the third term represents the consumption of FO_2 in the formation of FO.

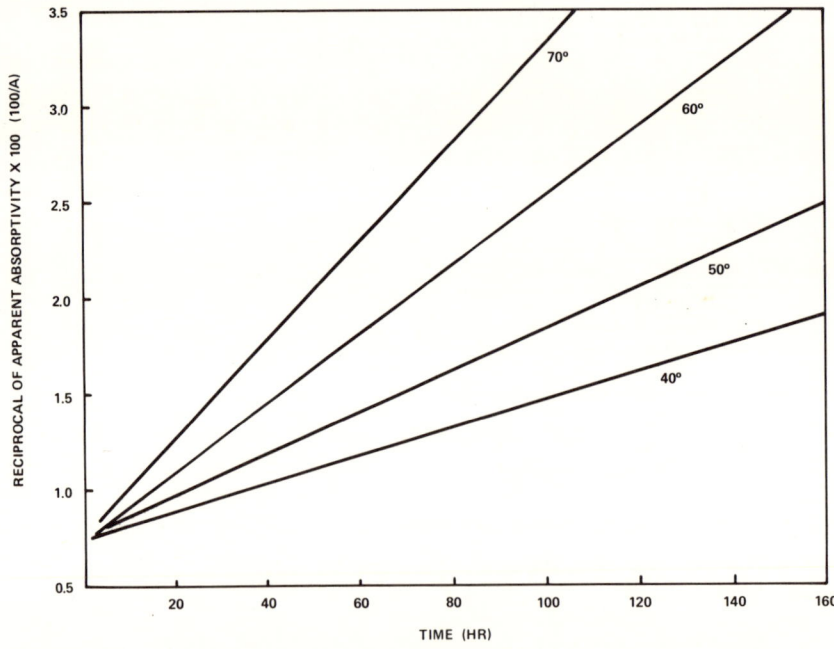

Figure 119. Pseudo bimolecular kinetics of crystalline fumagillin thermal degradation in the presence of air. Plot of 100 times the reciprocal of the apparent absorptivity (100/A with A in liter g-cm^{-1}) at 351 mμ against time in hours for several temperatures. [E.R. Garrett, *J. Am. Pharm. Assoc. 43*, 539 (1954).]

The rate of disappearance of fumagillin depends on the consumption of oxygen represented by the first term on the right side of the equation,

$$-\frac{d[F]}{dt} = k_1[F][O_2] - k_{-1}[FO_2] + k_2[FO_2][F]$$

and the reactions of the activated oxygenated fumagillin represented by the second and third terms. Assuming that the concentration and its rate of change are small, $d[FO_2]/dt = 0$. Substitution and rearrangement shows the rate of degradation of fumagillin to be

$$-\frac{d[F]}{dt} = \frac{2k_1 k_2 [O_2][F]^2}{k_{-1} + k_2[F]}$$

The second reaction in the oxidative mechanism is the rate-limiting step, and the activation-oxygenated fumagillin has a low stability, i.e., $k_{-1} \ggg k_2[F]$, so that

$$-\frac{d[F]}{dt} = \frac{2k_1 k_2 [O_2][F]^2}{k_{-1}}$$

If the oxygen concentration is constant, a constant, $k = \frac{2k_1 k_2 [O_2]}{k_{-1}}$ may be introduced to incorporate all the constant terms; then

$$-\frac{d[F]}{dt} = k[F]^2$$

Thus, the oxidation of fumagillin is second order with respect to fumagillin.

PHOTOLYSIS

Molecules may absorb the proper wavelength of light and acquire sufficient energy to undergo reactions. Photolytic degradation generally occurs upon exposure to light of wavelength less than 400mμ. An amber glass bottle or an opaque container will act as a barrier to this light. A large wraparound label on a flint vial will prevent or retard photodegradation.

The photodegradation of aqueous solutions of chlorpromazine hydrochloride is zero order, as expressed by the equation

$$-\frac{dC}{dt} = kI$$

and its integrated form

$$C = C_0 - It$$

where I is the intensity of the monochromatic light. In Figure 120 a plot of concentration of chlorpromazine against the number of photons per liter absorbed shows a zero-order dependence of the photoreaction.

Photogradation is difficult to study and interpret kinetically, as it may involve several reactions of various orders. Photoreactions often form free radicals, which then initiate oxidation reactions that occur simultaneously.

STABILITY PREDICTION

A product of a pharmaceutical manufacturer must maintain its label potency and initial appearance for the length of its shelf life. The stability of a newly developed product could be

270 • chemical stability

determined by storage at room temperature for a period of its purposed shelf life. Obviously such a method is time consuming, and if the product is unstable, much time is lost before new formulations are undertaken.

The prediction of stability at room temperature can be made from accelerated degradation experiments at higher temperatures by use of the Arrhenius relation. By plotting some expression of concentration as a linear function of time, the rate constants for the degradation at several temperatures are determined. The use of a minimum of four temperatures permits the imposition of finite 95 per cent confidence limits on the rate constants predicted from the Arrhenius equation. The logarithm of the rate constant is then plotted against the reciprocal of absolute temperature to obtain, by extrapolation, the rate constant for the degradation at marketing temperature. Using this rate constant in the appropriate reaction-rate equation, the predicted time that a drug will maintain its required potency can be calculated.

This method is applicable only to chemical reactions with an activation energy of 10 to 30 kcal mole^{-1}. This is the magnitude of the activation energy for many pharmaceutical degradations that occur in solution. With diffusion processes and photolysis the activation energy is only 2 to 3 kcal mole^{-1}. Little is gained by accelerated temperature studies in estimating the stability, because the influence of temperature on rate is small.

The application of chemical kinetics to the degradation of simple systems of drugs has been illustrated by several examples. Since most pharmaceutical liquids are complex mixtures, the accelerated stability analysis would be of limited value if it did not apply to multicomponent systems such as a multivitamin liquid.

63. Ferrous gluconate   43.17 mg
    Calcium glycerophosphate 100.00 mg
    Thiamine hydrochloride   5.45 mg
    Riboflavin   3.47 mg
    Vitamin B_6 1.20 mg
    Nicotinamide   35.00 mg
    d-Panthothenyl alcohol 3.96 mg
    Vitamin B_{12} 4.95 mg
    Tricholine citrate   56.62 mg
    Cobalt (as sulfate)   0.03 mg
    Copper (as sulfate)   0.33 mg
    Manganese (as sulfate)   0.33 mg
    Magnesium (as sulfate)   2.00 mg
    Molybdenum (as sodium molybdate) 0.07 mg
    Zinc (as sulfate)   0.05 mg
    Flavors
    Sugar   60%
    Alcohol   19%
    Tragacanth

    Sig.: Content per 15 ml of liquid

To illustrate the validity of the application of kinetics to complex pharmaceuticals, the predicted stability of the thiamine hydrochloride in the multivitamin liquid is compared to the actual stability upon storage at 30°. The experimental thermal degradation of the thiamine hydrochloride carried out at 40, 50, 60, and 70° is pseudo first order. By utilizing the Arrhenius plot the rate constant for 30° is found and the activation energy is determined to be 25,800 cal mole^{-1}. A comparison of the predicted stability based on these constants to the experimentally determined degradation is shown in Figure 121. The solid line represents the predicted stability, and the dashed line encompasses the

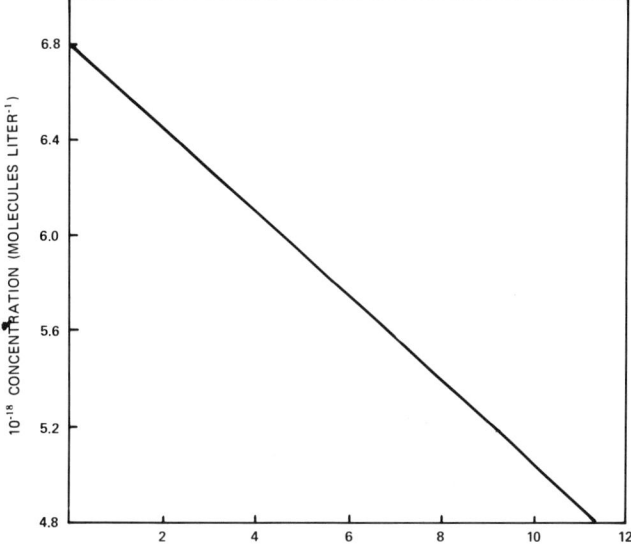

Figure 120. Plot of the concentration of chlorpromazine hydrochloride against the number of photons per liter absorbed showing the zero-order dependence of the photoreaction. [Adapted from A. Felmeister and C.A. Discher, *J. Pharm. Sci. 53,* 756 (1964).]

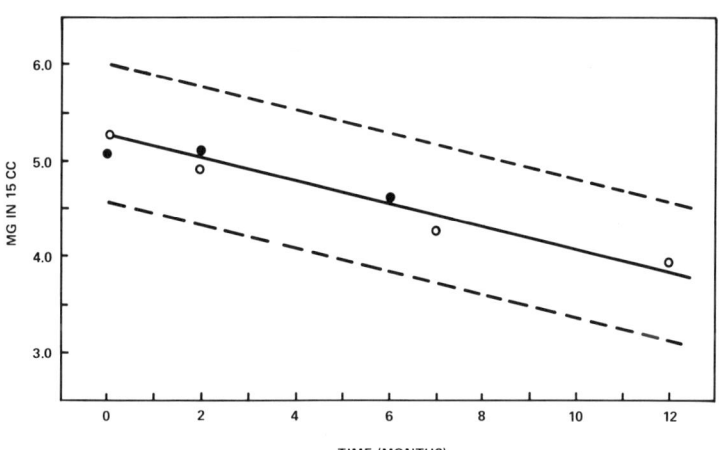

Figure 121. Verification of prediction of thiamine hydrochloride stability at room temperature. The solid line is the predicted thermal degradation rate of thiamine hydrochloride in liquid multivitamin preparation at 30°. The dashed lines encompass the standard error in predicted values and the standard error of a single assay. The open circles are actual data obtained. The closed circles are data obtained on a similar preparation slightly modified in composition and vehicle. [E.R. Garrett, *J. Am. Pharm. Assoc. 45,* 470 (1956).]

standard error in the predicted degradation and 95 per cent confidence limits of a single assay. The open circles are actual values obtained by assay of a multivitamin liquid stored at 30° for 1 year.

Although it is of prime importance that the active ingredient be stable, it is also necessary that pharmaceutical adjuvants, e.g., colorants, flavors, and preservatives, be stable to maintain the elegance and patient acceptance of the dosage form.

A colored product that fades is not pharmaceutically acceptable even if the activity is unchanged. A triple sulfa suspension is colored pink by a blend of F.D. & C. Yellow No. 6 D. & C. Red No. 33, which has an absorption band in the region 480 to 520 mμ. A decrease in the magnitude of this

272 • chemical stability

absorption band causes a visual loss of the pink color. The loss of color at 60° and 500 mμ is a linear function of time, as shown in Figure 122. Thus, by means of a zero-order equation,

$$A_t = A_0 - kt$$

the absorbance A_t at any time t can be predicted.

The zero-order rate constants are evaluated at several elevated temperatures, and the logarithm of the rate constant is plotted against the reciprocal of absolute temperature, as shown in Figure 123. Extrapolation of the straight line provides a value for the rate constant at a selected temperature. The logarithmic form of Arrhenius equation may also be used to calculate the rate constant. The equation corresponding to the curve in Figure 123 for the fading of the pink color is

$$\log k = -\frac{20{,}400}{2.303 \times 1.987} \frac{1}{T} + 10.3$$

In the suspension the initial absorbance, A_0, is 0.470 and from the Arrhenius plot $k_{25°} = 0.0005016$ absorbance decrease per day. Visually an absorbance of 0.225 is not acceptable. The predicted time when the color reaches the unacceptable level of intensity is calculated by the zero-order relationship

$$0.225 = 0.470 - 0.0005015t$$

$$t = 488 \text{ days}$$

This predicted color stability for 1 1/3 years is made without any consideration of the mechanism involved to provide a rapid evaluation of the shelf life of the suspension.

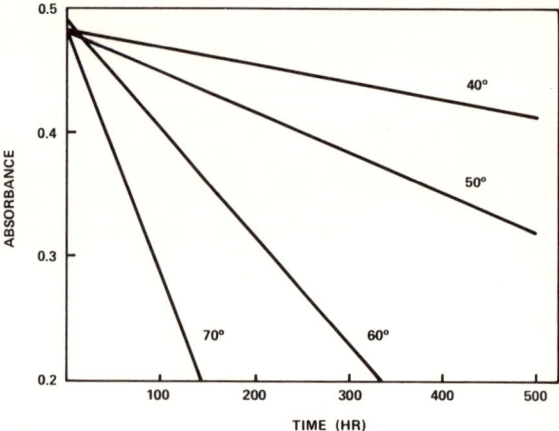

Figure 122. Plot of absorbance against time at various temperatures showing the zero-order color degradation in a triple sulfa suspension. [E.R. Garrett and R.F. Carper, *J. Am. Pharm. Assoc.* **44,** 515 (1955).]

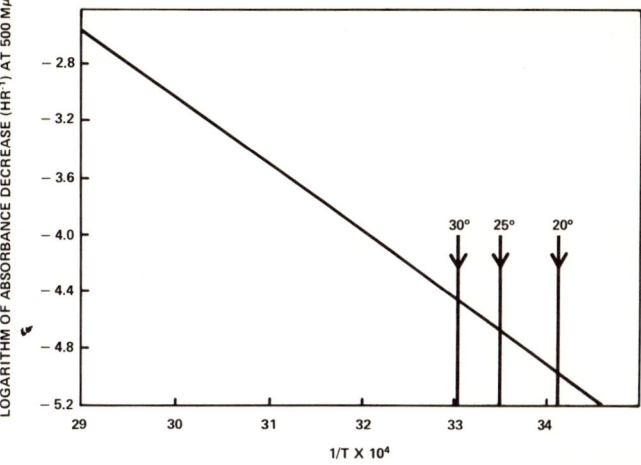

Figure 123. Logarithmic plot of the Arrhenius expression used for predicting the rate of degradation of color in a triple sulfa suspension at lower temperatures. [E.R. Garrett and R.F. Carper, *J. Am. Pharm. Assoc. 44,* 515 (1955).]

10 STERILE SOLUTIONS

Pharmaceutical products that must be sterile include perfusion fluids, injections, collyria, irrigation solutions, topical fluids for use in the operating room, and ophthalmic ointments. Obviously the equipment, glassware, tubing, and gowns used in preparing these products must be sterile.

Sterilization is the process of killing or removing microorganisms and their viable spores. Sterilization may be accomplished by chemical, mechanical, and physical processes. Frequently more than one method is used before the total processing of a sterile dosage form is completed. Aseptic technique is the use of procedures and precautions that prevent contamination by microorganisms. If conventional methods cannot be used to sterilize a pharmaceutical, it may be prepared from its sterile components under aseptic techniques and then packaged in sterile containers.

Microorganisms are destroyed by heat. Death by dry heat is probably caused by dehydration and subsequent oxidation of the microorganism. Moist heat may cause death by denaturation and coagulation of essential protein of the cell. The lethal temperature and the length of time required to sterilize a product depends on the microorganisms, the presence or absence of moisture, and the properties of the product.

Since denaturation of proteins appears to be an unimolecular reaction, the death rate of microorganisms at a given temperature is first order. At other times the death rate of microorganisms follows a sigmoidal pattern, with slowing of the death rate at very low contamination. Regardless of whether the death rate follows an exponential or a sigmoidal pattern, in all methods of sterilization the killing of the microorganisms is a probability function. As the length of the sterilization process increases, the number of surviving microorganism becomes very small and the probability of detecting any living microorganisms is small; however, from the mathematical viewpoint, all the microorganisms cannot be killed.

The efficiency of a sterilization process can be determined by subjecting a microorganism of known thermal death point, i.e., temperature required to kill a culture of the microorganism, to the process for several different intervals of time. From a plot of the logarithm of surviving microorganisms against time, the time required to bring about the proper degree of kill can be found. For practical purposes a reduction of four to five logarithmic phases is necessary.

Sterilization is complicated by the fact that several varieties of microorganisms are present, and even for a given type of microorganism the heat sensitivity may differ at various stages in its life cycle. Pharmaceuticals are not heavily contaminated and do not contain highly resistant microorganisms; most pharmaceuticals to be sterilized do not provide great protection for the microorganisms present.

METHOD OF STERILIZING PHARMACEUTICALS

Steam Under Pressure

In the presence of moisture microorganisms are destroyed at a lower temperature than in dry heat. Steam sterilization under pressure is carried out in an autoclave, which is a jacketed chamber designed to maintain an atmosphere of saturated steam above 100°. Steam is water vapor devoid of air under pressure. At atmospheric pressure it has a temperature of 100°. The pressure in the autoclave permits the attainment of higher moist-heat temperatures; e.g., the temperature of saturated steam at 15 psi is 121.5°.

The steam gives up its latent heat to the object being sterilized and is converted to water at the same temperature. The latent heat is absorbed by the object until it is heated to the same temperature as the steam, after which there is no more heat exchange and no further condensation. This heat exchange by steam is more rapid than by dry heat. Superheated steam is not satisfactory. Although condensation occurs during the initial heating stages with superheated steam, the water is later revaporized, and the sterilization process becomes one of dry heat, for which the conditions are different and the sterilization temperatures are higher.

Because temperature varies directly with pressure, autoclaves are equipped with pressure gauges which indicate the temperature. If the temperature is deduced from the pressure-temperature relation of saturated steam, the presence of air in the autoclave gives an erroneous temperature, because both the air and the steam exert their own partial pressure; e.g., 50 per cent air at 15 psi gives a temperature of 112° instead of 121°.

An autoclave is an airtight, jacketed chamber provided with a door, steam valve, exhaust valve, air entry, gauges to record the pressure and temperature, and a safety valve to prevent explosions. Whether a pressure cooker, a manually operated system, or a fully automatic electronically operated system with preset cycles, the basic design is that shown in Figure 124. The operation of the autoclave in its sterilizing cycle is (1) loading, (2) raising the load to the proper temperature and pressure, (3) sterilizing, and (4) cooling and unloading.

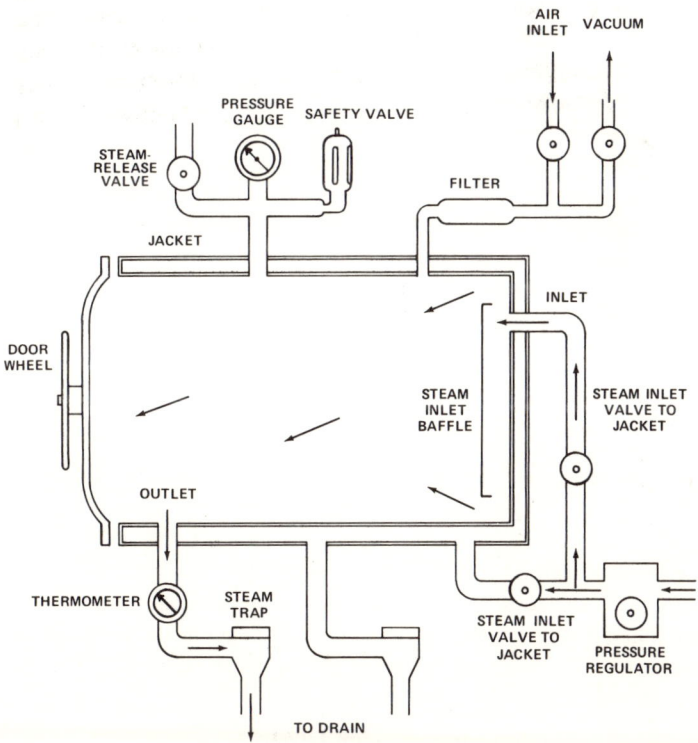

Figure 124. Schematic design of an autoclave.

It is essential that the steam have access to all parts of the load to be sterilized. The load should be loosely packed to allow free flow of the steam. Ampuls should not be piled at random but should be arranged in a tray that does not inhibit the flow of steam.

After the autoclave is properly loaded, steam is admitted to the steam jacket with the connection to the chamber closed. When the pressure is 15 to 20 psi, the steam is admitted to the chamber with the exhaust valve open. In most autoclaves the steam enters from the upper part of the chamber and sweeps the air out through the exhaust valve by downward displacement. The exhaust and the thermometer are located in the lower part of the autoclave to ensure complete evacuation of the air. The removal of air is important because (1) a mixture of air and steam has a temperature lower than that of pure steam at a given pressure, (2) local pockets or layers of air hinders the penetration of steam throughout the load, and (3) the steam jacket at normal sterilization temperatures will cause superheating of an air-steam mixture.

When a heavy flow of steam from the exhaust valve indicates that the air has been displaced and the temperature has reached 100°, the exhaust valve is closed and the pressure is increased to 15 psi. The time required to reach sterilization temperature depends on the size of the load, its heat capacity, and the rate of steam penetration. The time in the autoclave is the sum of the sterilization time and the time required to attain the sterilization temperature. In the pharmaceutical industry temperature probes are placed in several locations within the load, and the temperature is continually recorded during the sterilization process. The presence of the medicinal compound and the preservative may shorten the time required for sterilization. Actually each product is tested for sterility to demonstrate the reliability of the procedure for the individual product. Most pharmaceutical solutions are sterilized by a sterilization time of 20 minutes at 15 psi, e.g., 121°.

After sterilization the exhaust valve is opened gradually to slowly and steadily reduce the pressure to atmospheric pressure, and the steam valve is closed. If the pressure changes suddenly, the rate of loss of pressure exceeds the rate of reduction of temperature and the solution boils vigorously. The vigorous boiling may cause the liquid to froth over or may blow out stoppers.

The rate of heating and cooling of ampuls is fairly rapid because of their high specific surface. Thus, after sterilization of ampuls the autoclave may be opened with little delay. With aqueous solutions in containers not hermetically sealed during the heating process, steam condenses inside them, heating the solution and increasing its volume. If the pressure is gradually reduced after sterilization, this extra volume of water boils off and the volume returns to its original value. The absorption of the latent heat in boiling off this extra water considerably reduces the temperature of the fluid, and generally no further boiling occurs once atmospheric pressure is reached.

In the production of perfusion fluids, where an autoclave may hold 300 one-liter bottles, cooling is prolonged and may require the better part of a day for the temperature to fall so that no pressure exists in the bottle. In large-scale production a very fine mist of water is sprayed on the perfusion bottles at a rate adjusted to the rate of heat transfer so that thermal shock and breakage is minimized. This rapid cooling system not only permits immediate handling and conserves time but is safer, as the bottles removed from the autoclave are not liable to explode. Since the total time at elevated temperature is shortened, the advantage is obtained of less degradation of the product, e.g., discoloration of glucose solution.

Steam sterilization carried out in an autoclave is the most effective and satisfactory method for the sterilization of aqueous solutions, glassware, and rubber articles. It is not satisfactory for sterilizing solutions of drugs that are thermolabile or are liable to degradation in the presence of moisture. Oily liquids and powders cannot be sterilized by means of an autoclave.

Dry Heat

Sterilization by means of dry heat requires higher temperatures and longer exposures than steam sterilization. Dry-heat sterilization is carried out at 160 to 170° for 2 to 4 hours. The exact time and temperature are determined for each product and are dependent on the nature of the product being sterilized, the size of the individual containers, and their distribution in the oven.

The operation of the oven is simple, and the chief problem is to obtain uniform temperature distribution. A fan installed in the oven provides circulation of the hot air; however, unless the fan is properly baffled it may blow about powders that are to be sterilized.

Glassware to be sterilized by dry heat is washed and dried. It is then wrapped in heavy paper or the orifice of the bottle is stoppered with cotton and a piece of paper is tied over the plugged opening. This precaution prevents contamination, as air enters the cooling oven after sterilization and during storage. The oven is loaded in such a way as to allow the hot air to circulate. Heat is applied and the ventilating slide is opened to permit the escape of any residual moisture. When the temperature reaches $110°$, the ventilating slide is closed and the temperature is raised and maintained at the sterilizing temperature for the required time. The slow heating and cooling rate and the high temperature required make dry-heat sterilization a time-consuming method.

Fixed oils and thermostable powders may be sterilized by dry heat. Since the heat transfer is slow, small volumes of oil and thin layers of powder are used to assure proper temperature of the material without prolonging the time to complete the operation.

Bacterial Filtration

Sterilization by filtration is used widely in pharmacy to sterilize thermolabile solutions and biologicals. It is distinct from the other methods of sterilization in that it actually removes the microorganisms from the filtrate, although it does not remove their soluble metabolic products. The types of filter media are unglazed porcelain, compressed siliceous earth, sintered glass, asbestos, and cellulosic materials.

The filtration of particles as small as microorganisms involves interactions associated with electrostatic forces as well as mechanical sieving. Filters frequently have a negative charge. Most bacteria are negatively charged, and they would be repelled by these filters. It is conceivable that the amphoteric protein of a bacterial cell could confer a positive charge to the microorganism and that it would be adsorbed on the filter. As the velocity of flow through a filter is slow, the electrostatic interaction between the filter and the microorganism apparently increases the bacterial retaining property of the filter.

The pores of a filter medium have different sizes and shapes. In the structure of a filter the probability of a series of large holes coinciding for more than a few successive layers with the formation of a continuous pore of appreciable length or through the thickness of the filter is very slight. The structure of the filter is one of an indeterminate number of irregular, short passages of varying size and tortuousness. Consequently, a microorganism is mechanically trapped within the filter by the size, shape, and tortuousness of the void in the filter.

The efficiency and rate of filtration is determined by the maximum pore size of the filter. Any pore size specified for a filter is somewhat arbitrary because of the irregular, complex structure of the filter. Pore size is often considered in terms of bubble pressure. After a filter has been soaked in water until all the air has been removed and the pores filled, air pressure is then applied to the inner surface of the filter until air bubbles just pass through the filter. The minimum pressure required to pass air bubbles is known as the bubble pressure and is related to the pore size. For example, a bubble pressure of 15 psi is minimal for reliable filtration with Berkefeld and Doulton filters, whereas a bubble pressure of 55 psi is required for a Type GS Millipore® filter.

Porcelain Filters. Porcelain filters are manufactured by heating quartz sand and kaolin to a temperature just below their sintering point and shaping into the form of a disk or a hollow cylinder called a candle. The filters are available in a number of grades of porosity. Most of the grades are used to clarify or remove particulate matter from a solution and only a few remove microorganisms.

Porcelain filters can be used repeatedly. They are cleaned with chromic acid or by scrubbing with a brush and rinsing with water. The best method of cleaning is to heat the dry filter in a muffle furnace at 675°, which oxidizes and removes organic matter sorbed on the filter. They are sterilized in an autoclave.

Some commercial porcelain filters are the Pasteur, Chamberland, Doulton, and Selas®. Some properties and uses of various pore sizes of Selas® filters are given in Table LVI.

Siliceous Earth Filter. Siliceous earth filters are manufactured by molding a paste of the material into a candle and firing it in a pottery kiln to give it strength and rigidity. The Berkefeld and Mandler filter candles are examples of siliceous earth filters which are commercially available in several grades of porosity. Berkefeld and Mandler filters having a pore size of approximately 5 μ are successfully in filtration sterilization because adsorption plays an appreciable role in retaining the microorganisms. The siliceous earth filters may be somewhat faster than the porcelain filters.

They are cleaned in a manner similar to porcelain filters, but they are not as durable. Acids cannot be used for cleaning. Both siliceous earth and porcelain candles are provided with threaded nozzles. The joint between the filter medium and the nozzle is a source of weakness in the construction, and care is needed in handling and sterilizing to avoid cracks at the joint. Routine testing is required to detect cracked candles. The candle or the assembled filtration apparatus is sterilized in the autoclave.

Sintered-Glass Filters. Sintered-glass filters are made by heating pulverized glass in a suitable mold to a temperature just below the fusion point so that the particles adhere to form a porous disk, which is sealed into a Buchner funnel used for vacuum filtration. Sintered-glass filters are available in several grades of porosity; however, only the ultrafine grade is suitable for bacterial filtration.

Sintered-glass filters are easily cleaned by acids and are sterilized in the autoclave. Adsorption of constituents of the solution is less than by other nonmembrane filter media.

Asbestos Filters. The Seitz filter pad is composed of asbestos fibers compressed into sheets that are cut into disks or squares. Depending on the degree of compression and the depth of fibers several grades of porosity exist; only the fine Seitz E.K. filter is suitable for bacterial filtration. The soft, pliable pad, especially if wet, is not very strong. Since each filter is discarded after filtration, the use of this medium has the advantage of eliminating cleaning of the medium. The Seitz filter may be sterilized by dry heat or by steam sterilization.

Filtration through an asbestos filter tends to increase the alkalinity and to leach out magnesium compounds, which may precipitate alkaloids from their salts or catalyze degradation of the medicinal compound. If the filter is treated with dilute hydrochloric acid and rinsed with water before use, this problem can be eliminated. As the asbestos filter is fibrous in nature, it tends to shed fibers into the filtrate. This may be remedied by insertion of a fine silk mesh under the pad.

Table LVI Pore-Size Type and Properties of Selas Porcelain Filters

Type	Maximum Pore Diameter (μ)	Mean Pore Diameter (μ)	Bubble Pressure (psi)	General Use
10	8.8	4.4	5.0	Fine crystalline precipitates, initial clarification
01	6.0	3.0	7.0	Polishing
015	2.8	1.4	15.0	Pharmaceutical sterilization
02	1.7	0.85	25.0	Bacteriological filtration, pharmaceutical sterilization
03	1.2	0.6	35	Bacteriological filtration, pharmaceutical sterilization
04, 05, 06				Filtering gases

Membrane Filters. Millipore® filters are cellulose ester membrane filters which are commercially available in 12 grades of pore size, as shown in Table LVII. The filter is thin, i.e., 150 μ, and brittle, so a supporting filter holder is necessary. Approximately 80 per cent of the filter volume is void. The large void and the thinness of the Millipore® filter make its rate of filtration much faster for a given sterilization efficiency than other types of filters. Since the filter is thin, there is no retention of liquid within the filter.

Sterility is achieved by a sieving mechanism which retains particles exceeding the pore size. Adsorption of therapeutic compounds from solution is rare. The cellulose ester is inert and does not contribute ions or particulate matter to the filtrate. As the filter is destroyed by temperatures exceeding 125°, it cannot be sterilized by dry heat and is usually sterilized by means of the autoclave.

Pore size GS is used for sterilizing parenteral solutions and sera. Pore size HA is used to sterilize distilled water that will be used as a solvent for a solution that will be subsequently sterilized, oils, and other products for which previous experience has shown it to be acceptable.

The small pore size of bacterial filters prevents the flow of a solution unless a pressure differential exists. With the Millipore® and Seitz filters, the positive pressure assembly of the type shown in Figure 125 is generally used. The clean, dry apparatus is assembled and sterilized in an autoclave. The hoses should be open, as steam must penetrate into the filter holder to sterilize. After autoclaving for 30 to 45 minutes at 121°, the apparatus is allowed to cool. The filter assembly is then connected to a pressure vessel containing the solution to be sterilized and aseptically to a sterile receiving vessel. The receiving vessel is fitted with a vent to allow the escape of the air being displaced by the filtrate. The vent contains a filter that allows the passage of air but prevents the entrance of microorganisms. To initiate filtration the inlet valve is opened. The vent valve in the top plate of the filter holder is open to allow the displacement of residual air, and it is closed as soon as liquid appears in a steady flow from the vent hole. Most pharmaceuticals will filter satisfactorily at a differential of 20 psi. If the pressure is kept below the bubble pressure, air will not pass through the filter and foaming at the completion of filtration will be prevented.

Small-scale filtration through sintered-glass and porcelain filters often employs a negative pressure or vacuum filtration apparatus of the type shown in Figure 126. A convenient receiving vessel is an aspirating bottle with its lower opening fitted by rubber tubing to a stopcock for delivery of the sterile filtrate into its final container. The entire apparatus is assembled and sterilized in an autoclave. The solution to be sterilized is poured into the glass cylinder surrounding the candle, and a side arm fitted with a cotton plug is connected to the vacuum.

Table LVII Millipore® Filter Pore-Size Type and Filtration Rate at 25° with a Pressure Differential of 13.5 psi

Type	Mean Pore Diameter (μ)	Rate of Flow	
		Water (ml min^{-1} cm^{-2})	Air (liters min^{-1} cm^{-2})
SC	8.0	950	55
SM	5.0	560	35
SS	3.0	400	20
RA	1.2	300	14
AA	0.80	220	9.8
DA	0.65	175	8.0
HA	0.45	65	4.9
PH	0.30	40	3.7
GS	0.22	22	2.5
VC	0.10	3	1.0
VM	0.05	1.5	0.7
VF	0.01	0.5	0.3

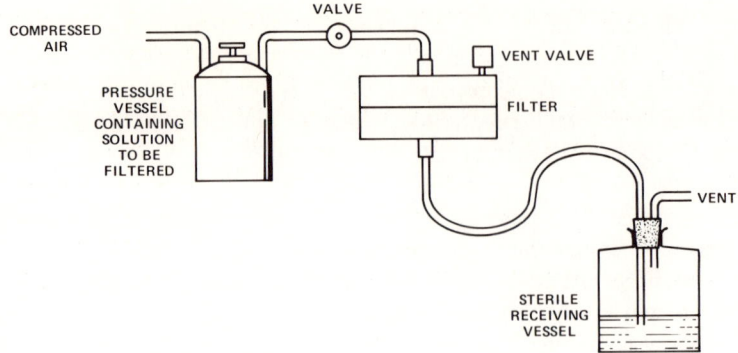

Figure 125. Schematic arrangement for positive pressure filtration.

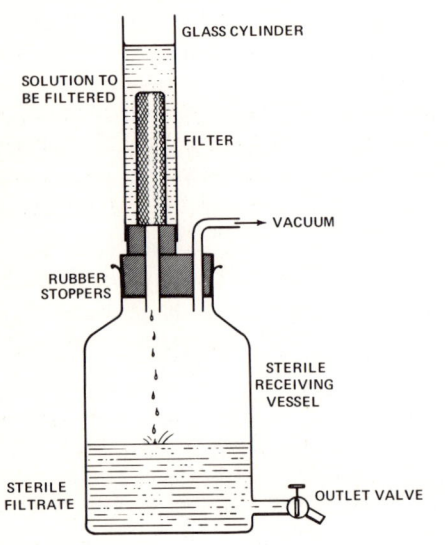

Figure 126. Schematic arrangement for negative pressure or vacuum filtration.

Gaseous Sterilization

Gaseous sterilization is accomplished by exposure to a gas or vapor that kills microorganisms and their spores. Although the gas readily penetrates porous and powdered solids, sterilization is a surface phenomenon and microoganisms occluded within crystals are not killed. Gaseous sterilization is used in pharmacy to sterilize thermolabile materials. The most acceptable bactericidal gas is ethylene oxide. Although the sterilizing vapor damages few materials and is removed from the treated material at the conclusion of the sterilizing cycle, the gas is not inert and its reactivity with the material to be sterilized must be considered; e.g., thiamine, riboflavin, and streptomycin lose potency when treated with ethylene oxide.

Ethylene oxide probably exerts its bactericidal action by alkylation of the acid, amine, hydroxy, or sulfhydryl groups of the cellular enzymes or proteins. Some moisture is necessary for the ethylene oxide to penetrate and destroy the cell. At low humidities, e.g., less than 20 per cent, the death rate is not logarithmic, but the microorganism appears increasingly resistant with decreasing humidity. In practice the humidity in the sterilizer chamber is increased to 50 to 60 per cent and held for a time so that the surfaces and cell membrane sorb moisture before the admission of the ethylene oxide.

Ethylene oxide is explosive when mixed with air. The explosive hazard is eliminated by using a mixture of ethylene oxide and carbon dioxide, e.g., Carboxide®, Oxyfume® 20, or a mixture of ethylene oxide and fluorinated hydrocarbons, e.g., Steroxcide® -12. Both inert diluents have a higher vapor pressure than ethylene oxide and act as a propellant by forcing the ethylene oxide out of the cylinder into the chamber of the sterilizer. The fluorinated compounds have the advantage over carbon dioxide that the mixture can be kept in containers of much lighter weight and that the mixture permits a higher partial pressure of ethylene oxide in the sterilizing chamber at the same total pressure.

Ethylene oxide is a skin vesicant and is toxic when inhaled. Since the gas penetrates easily, the sterilizer must be hermetically sealed to protect the operator. The sterilizer is modified vacuum autoclave which may be used for steam or gaseous sterilization. The operational cycle of a sterilizer is shown in Figure 127. A portable gas sterilizer having a 10 by 16 in. cylindrical chamber and using a 21-oz can of vapor is available.

Gas sterilization is slow. The time of sterilization depends on the extent of contamination, humidity, temperature, and the concentration of ethylene oxide. The minimum concentration of ethylene oxide is 450 mg liter^{-1} at 27 psi; this concentration at 55° and 50 per cent relative humidity requires 4 to 5 hours of exposure. Under the same conditions 1000 mg liter^{-1} requires a sterilization time of 2 to 3 hours. In practice 6 hours of exposure to the ethylene oxide is used to provide a safety margin and to allow time for penetration of the gas into the material. After sterilization the residual gas is removed by a terminal vacuum followed by an air wash of filtered, sterile air.

In addition to being used to sterilize powdered drugs, e.g., penicillin, ethylene oxide has been used to sterilize needles, plastic syringes, and tubing sets. Using ethylene oxide, certain parenteral equipment has been sterilized in the final package, e.g., kraft paper and polyethylene film. Aerosol sprays of ethylene oxide have been used to sterilize small areas in which aseptic manipulations were to be carried out.

Radiation Sterilization

Direct ultraviolet radiation of 2600 Å is lethal to microorganisms in the air and on exposed surfaces; however, it does not penetrate most substances and is useless in the sterilization of drugs, foods, and fabrics. Ultraviolet radiation is useful in substantially reducing the number of airborne microorganisms. In areas for the production of injections the use of ultraviolet lamps in conjunction with aspetic technique is considered to be good manufacturing practice. As ultraviolet radiation has a limited range, the air must pass close to the lamps, which are located in the air ducts and in the immediate vicinity of the sterile operation, to be effective. For small-scale production a dust-free area

Figure 127. Typical sterilizing cycle using Carboxide gas in a concentration of 500 mg liter^{-1} with 50 per cent humidity at 55°.

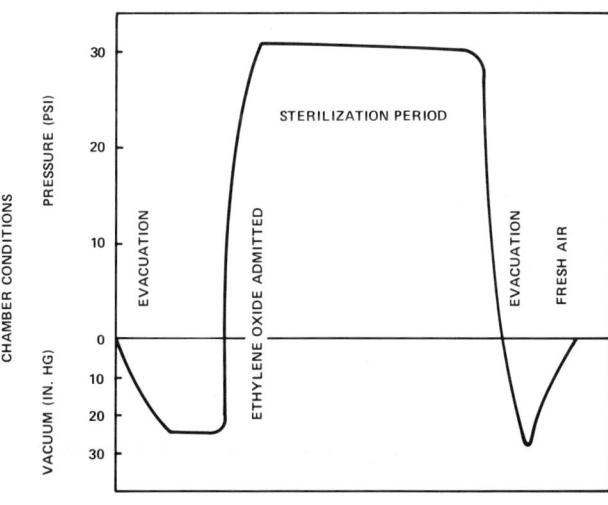

without air currents or microorganisms may be accomplished in a hood fitted with gloves and ultraviolet lamps. Before use the hood should be cleansed with a germicidal solution.

Ionizing radiation, e.g., beta rays, gamma rays, X rays, or accelerated electron beams, may be used to kill microorganisms. When low-energy radiation strikes a molecule, the orbital electrons enter a higher energy level, placing the molecule in an excited or more reactive state. With high-energy radiation orbital electrons are lost from the irradiated molecule, which becomes a positive ion, and gained by another molecule, forming a negative ion. With very high energy radiation the nucleus of the molecule is attacked, resulting in the formation of free radicals. Thus, irradiation is a complex phenomenon in which molecules are excited, ion pairs are formed, and chain reactions are initiated by free radicals. As a result the cellular constituents are degraded at a molecular level, and after a brief period the microorganisms are destroyed.

Since these molecular changes are not limited to the microorganism but may also occur in the constituents of the dosage form, the type of radiation used in sterilization should not cause nuclear changes. The radiation used should have a good penetrating ability, as one of the desired advantages of radiation sterilization is to accomplish sterilization in the finished package. Gamma radiation and highly accelerated electrons appear to be the most practical for sterilization of packaged goods because they sterilize without a nuclear transformation or induction of radioactivity in the product.

A Van de Graaff generator produces a high-velocity beam of electrons, which, owing to the negative charge on the particle, have limited penetrating ability. By use of a microwave linear accelerator the penetration is somewhat improved. Electrons of 8 million eV penetrate water only to a depth of 4 cm. By irradiation from opposite sides, an effective and uniform dose of radiation could be delivered through a material with unit density only to a thickness of approximately 7 cm. Greater penetration could be achieved by increasing the energy of the electrons; however, the risk of residual radioactivity following absorption of the incident energy by atomic nuclei then becomes a significant factor.

Electromagnetic gamma radiation is produced by ^{60}Co, ^{137}Cs, and waste fission products. ^{60}Co has a half-life of 5.26 years and a gamma-ray energy of 1.17 MeV, so there is no danger of residual radioactivity in the irradiated material. Gamma rays are very penetrating; they will sterilize material with unit density, when exposed on opposite sides, to a thickness of 25 cm. Gamma radiation, because of its greater penetrating ability, is preferred to electron beams for sterilizing disposable plastic syringes.

Radiation sterilization depends on the total dose of irradiation, which can be varied by the intensity of radiation or the duration of exposure to a fixed radiation. The radiation-absorbed dose, or rad, is the unit of absorbed energy of any type of radiation in any medium; 1 rad represents an energy absorption of 100 ergs g^{-1}. An exposure of 2.5 Mrads is generally considered to be lethal for all microorganisms and their spores.

Radiation sterilization may be used with thermolabile drugs because the heat released upon the absorption of 1 Mrads is approximately 2 cal. Penicillin, streptomycin, thiamine, and riboflavin have been effectively sterilized by 2 to 4 impulses from a 3-MeV Capacitron; cortisone acetate, chloramphenicol, and exytetracycline have been steriled with gramma radiation. Pharmaceutical products are more likely to be resistant to degradation or change if in a powdered rather than a liquid state. Insulin and heparin solutions are inactivated by radiation. Plasma can be sterilized by gamma radiation, but whole blood cannot, as hemolysis occurs. For each product sterilized by radiation testing it is necessary to demonstrate that there is no loss of potency, formation of toxic or pyrogenic material, or alteration of physical properties. The U.S. Food and Drug Administration considers a drug sterilized by radiation to be a new drug which requires a new drug application to be submitted.

Surgical catgut is now commercially sterilized by irradiation. The greatest potential for the use of radiation sterilization is in disposable metal, plastic, and rubber items. With the high cost of equipment and shielding to protect operators, it seems that radiation sterilization will be limited to large-volume production and will not displace the more conventional sterilization methods used in the preparation of injections.

INJECTIONS

Injections or parenterals are sterile pharmaceuticals that are to be administered through one or more layers of the skin. The injection of a drug may have advantages over oral administration. This route of administration is essential when the gastrointestinal tract cannot be used because of surgery or lack of stability of the drug, e.g., insulin, and penicillin G. The pharmacological response from an injection is often faster and more effective than that from a drug administered orally. In those emergencies in which the patient is unconscious or unable to retain medication given orally, parenteral injections provide an immediate and definite response. An injection may produce a localized effect. The local anesthetic used by the dentist is injected near the trunk of a nerve and relieves the sensation of pain in the immediate area.

To avoid infection parenterals must be sterile and must be aseptically administered. Most individuals dislike receiving an injection. In general an injection is inconvenient, as it requires a trained operator for administration. Care must be taken that intravascular injection does not occur if it is not intended. Sensitivity reactions are more frequent with parenterals than other dosage forms. Parenteral therapy is more costly than other forms because of the cost of administration and manufacture.

Types of Injections

Subcutaneous. A subcutaneous or hypodermic injection is made into the loose tissue beneath the skin. If a large volume of fluid is slowly administered subcutaneously, the process is known as hypodermoclysis. Irritating drugs are not administered subcutaneously, as they may cause sloughing. The absorption of lipid-soluble drugs occurs by diffusion through the capillary membranes into the blood; it is directly proportional to the partition coefficient of the drug. Lipid-insoluble drugs are absorbed into the blood by passage through the aqueous pores in the endothelial membrane; their rate of absorption depends on their diffusion rates in aqueous solution. The rate of absorption is affected by the total area of the absorbing capillary membrane and the solubility of the substance in the interstitial fluid. The enzyme hyaluronidase depolymerizes the hyaluronic acid of the subcutaneous connective tissue and makes the area more fluid. Consequently, the absorption is enhanced because the drug may diffuse through a larger area and is exposed to a greater capillary surface.

Absorption from a subcutaneous injection is frequently slow and provides somewhat prolonged action. Using appropriate pharmaceutical techniques a sustained-action effect may be obtained. The subcutaneous injection of a suspension of a drug in a vehicle in which it is insoluble provides a very slow rate of absorption and a prolonged duration of activity. Insulin injection is a solution which upon subcutaneous injection has its onset of action in 1 hour and its duration of action for 6 hours; insulin zinc suspension has a duration of 24 hours and an onset of action at 2 hours. Certain hormones, e.g., estradiol and deoxycorticosterone acetate, have been subcutaneously implanted as a pellet and have been clinically effective over weeks or months.

Intramuscular. An intramuscular injection is made deep into the layers of muscle. Aqueous solutions of drugs are absorbed rapidly; however, suspensions and oily solutions are slowly absorbed. Maximum blood concentration or level is reached in 15 to 30 minutes after the intramuscular injection of aqueous penicillin solutions, and after 3 to 4 hours the penicillin is barely detectable in the blood. A single intramuscular injection of penicillin G procaine in oil with aluminum monostearate provides therapeutic blood levels for at least 48 hours. Irritating medicinal compounds that cannot be administered subcutaneously may be given by the intramuscular route.

Intravenous. An intravenous injection is made into a vein. With few exceptions only aqueous solutions are administered in this manner. As no absorption process is involved, the exact dose or blood concentration of the drug is obtained with an accuracy and immediacy not possible by any other route of administration. This is the basis for the injection of diagnostic agents, e.g., histamine phosphate injection for gastric function and phenolsulfonphthalein injection for determination of renal function. The immediate response from intravenous injections is essential in emergencies. Plasma is administered to injured persons by intravenous drip or venocylsis. In cases of shock and severe bleeding the only way of rapidly increasing the blood volume and restoring the electrolyte-water balance is by the intravenous administration of Ringer's injection or sodium lactate injection. Comatose patients can be sustained by the intravenous administration of nutrients, e.g., dextrose injection or protein hydrolysate injection.

If necessary, irritating medicinal compounds, e.g., mechlorethamine hydrochloride, vinblastine sulfate, and hypertonic solutions, can be given by intravenous injection. They are injected slowly to permit dilution with the blood. Certain dangers are inherent in the intravenous route. Unwanted reactions are most likely to occur with the intravenous route, and the nature of the intravenous injection makes it virtually impossible to halt the action after injection.

Intraperitoneal. An intraperitoneal injection is made into the peritoneal cavity, i.e., abdominal cavity holding the viscera. The hazards of infection and adhesions are too great to warrant the clinical use of intraperitoneal injection; however, this route is widely used in animal experimentation because the peritoneal cavity is large and provides a large absorbing surface from which the drug is rapidly absorbed into the circulation.

Intrathecal. Injections into the cerbrospinal fluid are known as subarachnoid, subdural, or intrasponal, injections, depending on the region of injection. Usually a volume of cerebrospinal fluid equal to the volume of the solution is withdrawn prior to injection.

Preparation

Physically an injection may be a solution, suspension, emulsion, or a dry solid or concentrated liquid which is dissolved or dispersed in a suitable vehicle prior to administration. All substances that are introduced beneath the protective epidermis of the body must be free of microorganisms, pyrogens, and irritation. With large-volume injections the pH and osmotic pressure of the fluids should be physiologically compatible with body fluids. With small-volume injections the fluid need not be isotonic with body fluids because the fluid is rapidly diluted by the large volume of blood. With small-volume injections a fairly large deviation from physiological pH is tolerated because the blood buffers rapidly adjust and maintain the blood at normal pH.

Vehicles. From the physiological viewpoint water is the most compatible solvent and it is the most common vehicle used in parenterals. The water should not contain pyrogens, e.g., fever-producing, metabolic products of microorganic growth. Water for Injection U.S.P. is used for injections to be sterilized after being filled into their containers. It is pyrogen-free, distilled water that has been recently distilled and is free of microorganic contamination at the time of collection. Production is scheduled so that the solution may be prepared, packaged, and sterilized within a few hours of collection. If it cannot be used at once, Water for Injection U.S.P. may be stored at temperatures above or below that at which bacteria grow.

When a medicinal compound is water-insoluble, e.g., estradiol valerate, and menadione, or degraded by water, it may be dissolved in a nonaqueous solvent that is nontoxic, nonirritating, and nonsensitizing. Obviously, the nonaqueous solvent should have no pharmacologic activity. The viscosity of the nonaqueous solvent should permit easy injection.

Fixed oils, e.g., corn oil, cottonseed oil, peanut oil, and sesame oil, are used as parenteral vehicles. Fixed oils to be used in parenterals must meet rigid specifications. They must have a saponification value of 185 to 200 and an iodine value of 79 to 128, and the limit of fatty acids is that 10 g of the oil must be neutralized by not more than 2 ml of $0.02\ N$ sodium hydroxide. As a few individuals exhibit allergic reactions to specific vegetable oils, the specific oil used in the product must be stated on the label. Mineral oil cannot be used as a solvent, because it is not absorbed from body tissues. Since fixed oils are not miscible with body fluids, an oily suspension of a water-soluble drug may produce sustained release of the drug. Fixed oils are seldom administered intravenously.

The use of glycerin as a parenteral vehicle is controversial; however, because of its high viscosity it is not suitable for easy injection. Glycerin is used as a cosolvent to increase the solubility of medicinal compounds in certain solutions, e.g., deslanoside injection and digitoxin injection. Alcohol is often used in combination with glycerin as a vehicle for digitalis glycosides. A small volume of 50 per cent alcohol may be injected intramuscularly or intravenously; intramuscular injection causes pain.

Propylene glycol has been suggested as a vehicle for compounds that are unstable in water. Solutions of oxytetracycline and sodium salts of barbiturates in propylene glycol have been tested and reported to be suitable for intramuscular and intravenous use.

Cosolvent containing as much as 50 per cent liquid polyethylene glycol have been used to stabilize, e.g., secobarbital injection, and to enhance the solubility, e.g., erythromycin ethyl succinate and reserpine, of intramuscular injections.

Ethyl oleate, benzyl benzoate, and dimethylacetamide have been used in specific products; however, their use is very limited.

Procedure. Parenteral solutions are prepared by the same procedures used to prepare other solutions. Drugs of the highest purity are dissolved in Water for Injection U.S.P. The solution should be free of particulate matter, which indicates the presence of foreign contamination or degradation. The solution may be filtered by means of a glass, porcelain, or membrane filter to remove particulate matter. All parenteral solutions are subjected to individual visual inspection. This is done with a glare-free light against a white and black background.

The solution is sterilized by the most appropriate method (see Table LVIII), which depends on the properties of the drug. The solution is then transferred to filling equipment and filled into its final container. When it is practical, sterilization is carried out in the final container. Since it is impractical to withdraw the entire contents from a container, a slight excess of liquid is placed in the container. The excess volumes recommended are shown in Table LIX.

The area for the preparation of parenterals is an isolated area in which the temperature, humidity, and dust contamination are controlled. The walls are smooth and have rounded corners so they can be easily cleaned with germicidal solutions. The area is under positive pressure and air locks are used to decrease airborne contamination. Recently, laminar air flow has been introduced into production areas. In laminar systems the air flow is directed outward from the working area in parallel lines so that the air is deflected toward the operators and particles shed by the operators are washed away from the work area. The air-filtering system consists of a series of filters. The initial filter is a 1-in. glass-wool filter. This is followed by an electrostatic precipitator and a final filter which removes particles greater than $0.3\,\mu$. Ultraviolet lamps are placed in the air ducts and the working area. Operators wear sterile lint-free caps and gowns, gloves, face masks, and shoe covers. The area is routinely checked by exposure of nutrient plates which are incubated and examined for microorganic growth.

Containers. The package or container for an injection should be easy to sterilize and transport, and it should be convenient to open in an aseptic manner. The containers for parenterals are most commonly made of glass. There are four types of glass: I, II, III, and NP. Type NP is for nonparenteral products. Type I is the best quality and may be used for any parenteral; it is a borosilicate glass and may be repeatedly autoclaved, and it is satisfactory for unbuffered solutions and water. Type II and III are soda-lime glass, which is affected by autoclaving. Type II has been treated with an acidic gas at high temperature to increase its resistance to water and acids; it should be sterilized by dry heat prior to filling under aseptic conditions. Products with a pH less than 7 may be packaged in Type II glass. Type III should not be used for solutions to be sterilized by heat in the final container. Products with a pH

Table LVIII Recommended Methods of Sterilization

Item	Hot-Air Oven	Autoclave	Gaseous	Bacterial Filtration
Glassware (ampul, bottles)	170° for 2 hr	121° for 20 min	-	-
Rubber (stopper, tubing)	-	121° for 30 min	-	-
Metal (apparatus)	-	121° for 30 min	-	-
Nonvolatile, thermostable powder (sulfamerazine, talc, zinc oxide)	150-170° for 1-2 hr	-	-	-
Thermostable, aqueous solution (sodium chloride, morphine, vasopressin)	-	121° for 30 min	-	-
Thermolabile powder (penicillin)	-	-	Ethylene oxide	-
Thermolabile aqueous solution (emetine hydrochloride, physostigmine salicylate)	-	-	-	Include a bacteriostatic agent in solution
Oily liquids (desoxycorticosterone acetate, dimercaprol)	150-170° for 1 hr	-	-	-

Table LIX Excess Volume Fill for Injections

Labeled Size (ml)	For Mobile Liquids (ml)	For Viscous Liquids (ml)
0.5	0.10	0.12
1.0	0.10	0.15
2.0	0.15	0.25
5.0	0.30	0.50
10.0	0.50	0.70
20.0	0.60	0.90
30.0	0.8	1.2
50.0 and greater	2%	3%

greater than 7 should not be packaged in Type III glass; sterile dry powders may be packaged in Type III glass, which should be sterilized by dry heat before filling under aseptic conditions. All glass must be clear, to allow visual inspection of the contents.

Plastic containers are grouped into six classes according to the biological tests used to determine the reaction of living tissue and animals to the presence of portions of the plastic or injections of extracts of the plastic material.

Ampuls are hermetically sealed glass containers holding a single dose of medication. Ampuls have a constricted, elongated neck that permits the ampul to be sealed by heat without affecting the contents. The constricted neck is etched with a file to aid breaking of the neck at the time of withdrawal of the solution. Many ampuls are treated so that they may be evenly broken with manual pressure without use of a file.

Ampuls may be sealed manually by applying the flame of a torch slightly below the tip and pulling off the extra tip by touching it with a glass rod. The fine string of glass that results will melt to a round bead and seal the ampul. On a production scale the ampul is carried by a conveyor to the sealing stage, where it is centered and rotated in a sealing flame until the glass tip melts and forms a bead-like seal. In another design of sealing machine the neck of the ampul is held by grippers which, after the neck is heated, move upward and draw off the tip while exposed to the flame. The contents must be delivered without leaving a droplet on the neck. Such droplets would carbonize and discolor the ampul during sealing. The sealed ampuls are exposed to a dye solution to test for improper seals.

When the ampul is to be sealed under an inert atmosphere, the inert gas is injected into the ampul immediately before the medication. The parenteral liquid then displaces some of the gas and the ampul is sealed before the remaining gas diffuses into the atmosphere. Equipment is also available by which the filling and sealing operation can be carried out in an inert atmosphere under pressure.

Vials are multiple-dose containers, sealed by a rubber or plastic closure that has a small, thin area (known as a diaphragm) in the center. The diaphragm permits the insertion of a hypodermic needle and withdrawal of the contents. It is designed so that a needle may be easily inserted without the detachment of fragments and so that it will reclose upon the withdrawal of the needle. As shown in Figure 128, the sleeve type of stopper has a section that fits into the opening of the vial and a sleeve that fits over the outer lip of the container. The flange type of stopper has a section that fits into the opening of the vial, and the lower edge of the stopper rests on the neck of the vial. Vial stoppers are usually held in place by a metal seal; however, the sleeve type of stopper may be used without a metal seal. Infusion bottles or large-volume parenteral containers are graduated and equipped with a wire hanger to allow the container to be hung upside down while in use. Infusion bottles are closed with rubber stoppers, which permit easy insertion of glass or plastic tubes that are connected to an air-vent device and infusion tubing. The stopper is covered with an aluminum seal.

288 • sterile solutions

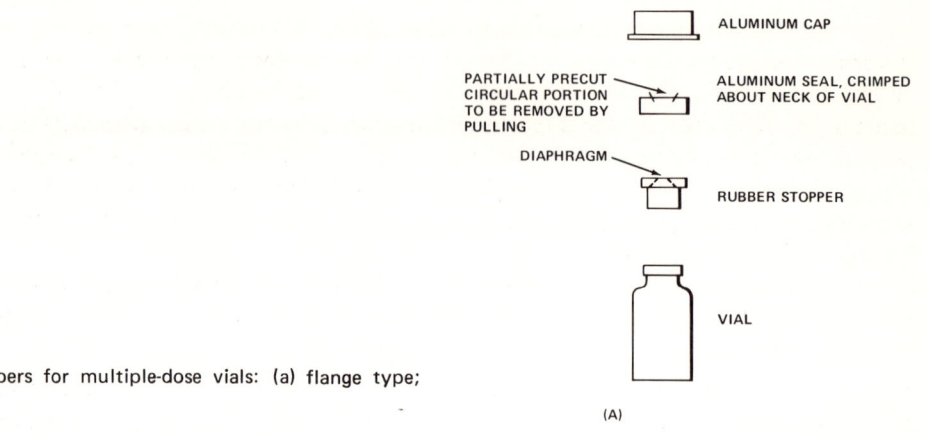

Figure 128. Stoppers for multiple-dose vials: (a) flange type; (b) sleeve type.

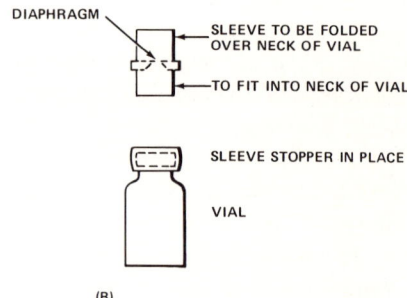

Rubber seems to be the best material for a closure; however, rubber varies in composition and the best closure for a product is determined by experimentation. Stability problems have been encountered with rubber stoppers. Zinc has been leached from certain rubber closures, resulting in incompatibilities with the drug. Sorption of the solvent may cause swelling of the closure. Preservatives or other ingredients may be sorbed by the closure. If the parenteral is sealed under an inert gas, the permeability of the closure to that gas is important. Butyl rubber seems to be the least permeable rubber. If a water-sensitive drug is prepared as a sterile, dry powder, the moisture-vapor transmission of the closure should be minimal.

All containers are cleaned by washing with a hot detergent and rinsing with distilled water. The container is inverted and placed in a tray from which it is drained, dried, and sterilized at 170°. Rubber diaphragms are cleansed of excess sulfur and impurities by boiling for 15 minutes in 2 per cent sodium carbonate containing 0.1 per cent anionic detergent. They are then rinsed with distilled water and dried. If necessary they may be stored in 1 per cent phenol solution. Rubber items are sterilized in an autoclave.

Additives. Parenteral products may contain additives which increase the stability or usefulness of the injection if they are harmless and do not interfere with the therapeutic efficacy. Local anesthetics may contain 1:100,000 epinephrine, which causes vasoconstriction, slows absorption, and prolongs the anesthetic effect of the drug. Repository corticotropin injection contains partially hydrolyzed gelatin, which contributes to its prolonged action. A coloring agent cannot be added solely for the purpose of coloring the finished product.

The chief additives are buffers, preservatives, and antioxidants. For injections packaged in a multiple-dose vial, a suitable preservative must be added to kill and prevent the growth of any microorganisms introduced during withdrawal of a dose. To restrict the number of exposures to possible contamination the maximum volume in a multiple dose container is generally 30 ml. If the injection is to be administered in a volume exceeding 5 ml, care is required in the choice and concentration of the preservative. With mercury and cationic surface-active preservatives the maximum concentration is 0.1 per cent. For chlorobutanol, cresol, and phenol the limit is 0.5 per cent. A single-dose ampul does not require a preservative because it is completely used at the time of administration. Perfusion fluids should not contain a preservative because with the large volumes used the total amount of preservative administered would be harmful.

The maximum amount of antioxidant is 0.2 per cent for sulfur dioxide, sodium bisulfite, and sodium sulfite. If antioxidants and preservatives are used, the names and concentrations employed must be stated on the label.

Testing. In addition to the usual quality-control procedures, those pharmaceuticals which are to be used parenterally must be sterile and free of pyrogens. The purpose of sterility testing is to demonstrate the absence of living microorganisms. It is possible to test a single item for the absence of living microorganisms of a particular class, but it is impossible to test for the absence of all classes of microorganisms. Sterility is easily understood, but it is difficult to experimentally verify. If all items were tested individually, there would be no product to be marketed; therefore, a sample of each batch is taken and if the number of defects or contaminations is below a certain limit, the whole batch is acceptable. If a batch contains a large proportion of contaminated items, a relatively small sample will detect contamination. However, the smaller the percentage of contaminated items in a batch, the larger is the sample size required to detect contamination. Statistically, if ½ per cent defects is acceptable, in a batch of 180 items all items should be tested; in a batch of 5000 to 7000 items 450 items should be tested.

Realistically sterility testing is an estimation of the probability of the absence of microorganisms from a particular batch of a product. In initially designing the specifications of quality control of sterility, a certain level of variation from the average performance, i.e., sterility, is recognized and measured. The size of this variation is based on reasonable judgment by qualified, experienced persons who are satisfied that the production process is functioning well and will produce an article that will satisfy the manufacturer and the consumer. After the variation is measured, a standard deviation is calculated. The quality control can be visualized by a control chart with two pairs of lines or limits drawn at a distance of ±2 and 3 standard deviations from the average. The results of the tests are plotted on the chart. If the values are between the inner and outer limits, the variation is probably due to chance and will require no alteration of procedure. If the test values are outside the limits, the process is faulty and must be corrected.

The U.S. Pharmocopeia states that for liquids which have been sterilized with steam under pressure in the final sealed container, 10 or more vials are selected from each sterilizer load for sterility test. For other liquid products at least 20 vials must be selected from each batch. If the product is aseptically filled, the units are selected at regular intervals throughout the filling operation. The samples are removed aseptically from their container mixed with sterile nutrient medium and incubated at 30 to 32° for at least 7 days in fluid thioglycollate medium, which supports aerobic and anaerobic microorganisms. The sample is also cultured at 22 to 25° for not less than 10 days in fluid Saboruraund medium, which supports yeasts and molds. If no evidence of growth occurs in the culture medium, the product is regarded as sterile. If the product contains a bacteriostatic agent, the agent should be inactivated or the solution diluted sufficiently to eliminate the bacteriostatic effect before sterility testing.

It has been estimated that contamination during sterility testing may be as great as 1 to 2 per cent. A properly designed sterility test procedure should (1) provide an adequate, random sample, (2) allow only minimal accidental contamination during sterility testing and some means of detecting and measuring the accidental contamination, (3) not subject the material to be tested to antimicrobial agents, (4) neutralize any preservative in the product, and (5) include a culture medium that will initiate and maintain growth of a small number of microorganisms.

In the production of parenterals emphasis is placed on the prevention of pyrogen formation rather than pyrogen removal from the product. A clean, well-designed still with adequate baffles is important in avoiding pyrogen contamination. The freshly distilled water is collected in sterile containers that have been rinsed with pyrogen-free water. It is good manufacturing practice to prepare, seal, and sterilize parenteral products as rapidly as practical.

The U.S.P. pyrogen test uses healthy albino rabbits weighing approximately 1500 g. Three rabbits are used for each test. The normal temperature, i.e., 38.9 to 39.8°, of the rabbit is noted. Ten milliliters of the parenteral per kilogram of body weight is injected into an ear vein of each rabbit. The temperature is recorded at 1-, 2-, and 3-hour intervals. The pyrogen test is positive if each rabbit shows an individual rise in temperature of 0.6° of more above its control temperature, or if the sum of the temperature rises of the three rabbits exceeds 1.4°. Although the rabbit pyrogen test is a tedious method, no method has been designed that would satisfactorily replace it.

OPHTHALMIC SOLUTIONS (COLLYRIA)

Medication to be instilled into the eye must be properly formulated and prepared with consideration given to tonicity, pH, stability, viscosity, and sterility. Sterility is desired because the cornea and tissues lining the anterior chamber are good media for microorganisms, and the instillation of a contaminated ophthalmic solution into an eye traumatized by accident or surgery may result in the loss of sight.

The drainage of the conjunctiva into the nose through the nasolacrymal duct washes away gross contaminations that are carried into the eye. In many infections of the conjunctiva the microorganisms grow on the surface and their toxic products produce the pathological effect; few microorganisms pass the intact corneal epithelium. If the corneal epithelium is broken, microorganisms may enter the cornea and cause infections. Corneal ulcerations are readily produced by *Pseudomonas aeruginosa*, which commonly occur on the skin and in the air.

When a physician uses a stock bottle of an ophthalmic solution, it may become contaminated. If the contaminated solution is used to treat a patient with an abraded cornea, the microorganisms may pass into the corneal stroma and into the anterior segment of the eye. Investigations of corneal ulceration due to *P. aeruginosa* led in 1953 to a U.S. Food and Drug Administration regulation that considers a nonsterile ophthalmic solution as being adulterated and misbranded. Although this regulation does not legally apply to extemporaneously prepared collyria, in the interest of public health the community pharmacist should dispense sterile solutions. He should use sterile distilled water in compounding ophthalmic solutions, as distilled water is often heavily contaminated with microorganisms.

For solutions to be instilled in the intact eye it is good practice to prepare sterile solutions which may be packaged in multiple-dose containers. Ophthalmic solutions to be used in an injured eye or during surgery must be sterile and packaged in single-use containers.

Preparation

Ophthalmic solutions are filtered to remove particulate matter. In extemporaneous compounding a lint-free filter paper is satisfactory; in the pharmaceutical industry a sintered-glass, porcelain, or membrane filter is used.

Ophthalmic solutions are generally sterilized by autoclaving or by filtration. Pressure cookers and small bacterial-retaining filters are available for use in sterilizing small volumes of solutions. When the nature of the medicinal compound permits, it is preferable to sterilize by autoclaving in the final container. With the exception of sodium fluorescein or sodium sulfacetamide, most common ophthalmic drugs dissolved in a 2 per cent boric acid vehicle can be autoclaved at 121° for 15 minutes.

In sterilization by filtration the pharmacist must recognize that (1) small amounts of the solution may be retained by the filter, (2) there is danger of a cracked filter, and (3) unless the filter is properly rinsed and stored, it may become a source of contamination. A glass-enclosed chamber having an ultraviolet lamp to sterilize the air and a bacteria-retaining filter can be used with aseptic technique to prepare small volumes of sterile solutions. The simplest extemporaneous procedure is to use a Millipore® membrane filter in a Swinney adapter fitted to a syringe. The entire apparatus as shown in Figure 129 may be sterilized by steam under pressure. Since the membrane is discarded after each solution is prepared, the filter is not a source of contamination.

Ophthalmic solutions are commonly dispensed in dropper bottles for the convenience of the patient. The droppers may be plastic or rubber-fitted glass containers. They should be washed with a detergent solution and rinsed with sterile distilled water to remove particulate matter. Glass and rubber dropper assemblies may be sterilized in an autoclave. Plastic containers generally have a low melting point and cannot be autoclaved.

With all types of droppers the delivery tube is wetted by the solution. After the drop is delivered and the pressure on the container is released, the remaining liquid is withdrawn into the container. If the dropper has touched the infected eye, the solution will probably become contaminated. Contamination during use may be avoided by using sterile, disposable straws to instill the solution to the eye. Another alternative is to incorporate a chemical preservative that will destroy or prevent the growth of microorganisms inadvertently introduced into the solution. A comparison of extensively used preservatives is given in Table LX. Although no single preservative is universally acceptable, benzalkonium chloride is recommended for extemporaneous compounding in a concentration of 1:10,000.

Since preservatives are potentially irritating to the posterior surface of the cornea, iris, and anterior chamber, they are not used in solutions to be applied to the injured eye. In fact, preservatives are not required in solutions to be applied to the injured eye or the eye for surgery, as the sterile solution is packaged in a single-use container and any unused solution is discarded.

64. Naphazoline hydrochloride   0.1%
    Boric acid   1.2   g
    Sodium carbonate   0.0006 g
    Camphor water   20.0   ml
    Phenyl mercuric nitrate   0.0002 g
    Sterile purified water, q.s. 100   ml

    Sig. 1-3 gtt. in O.D.

65. Hydroxyamphetamine hydrobromide   1.0 g
    Boric acid   2.0 g
    Thimerosal   1:50,000
    Sterile purified water, q.s.   100   ml
    Sig. For mydriasis instill 1-2 drops

66. Sodium fluorescein   2.0 g
    Sodium carbonate   3.0 g
    Phenyl mercuric nitrate   1:25,000
    Sterile purified water, q.s. 100   ml

    Sig. Sodium fluorescein ophthalmic solution

Sodium fluorescein solution is prepared by dissolving the sodium fluorescein and sodium carbonate in sterile purified water containing the phenyl mercuric nitrate. The sodium carbonate provides an alkaline pH that will maintain the dye in solution. Sterilization without heat is required, as the dye is thermolabile. The solution is used to detect corneal ulcers, which are colored green by the dye. Sodium fluorescein ophthalmic solution is dispensed in a sterile single-use container or in the form of a sterile impregnated paper strip. When the paper strip touches the eye, it releases sufficient dye to stain any corneal abrasion.

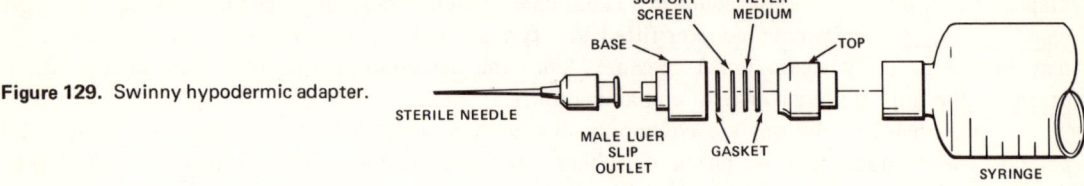

Figure 129. Swinny hypodermic adapter.

Table LX Preservatives for Aqueous Ophtalmic Solutions

Preservative	Concentration (%)	Incompatibilities	Remarks
Benzalkonium chloride	0.01-0.001	Carbonates, nitrates, salicylates, large anions	0.01% sodium ethylene diaminetetracetate increases effectiveness
Chlorobutanol	0.5	Alkaline vehicle	pH-dependent hydrolysis during autoclaving
Methylparaben	0.1	-	-
Phenylmercuric nitrate	0.0001-0.00025	-	Replaces benzalkonium chloride when nitrates and salicylates are present; slow in self-sterilization
Polymyxin B sulfate	1000 units per ml	-	Best antipseudomonal activity

Part III

Polyphasic and Plastic Systems

11 | CHARACTERISTICS OF POLYPHASIC SYSTEMS

A polyphasic dispersion is composed of a particulate phase that is distributed throughout a continuous phase or dispersion medium. Polyphasic dispersions may be classified according to the particle size of the dispersed phase. Polyphasic systems containing aggregates of molecules from 0.001 to 1 μ are known as colloidal dispersions. Suspensions are polyphasic dispersions of solid particles greater than 1 μ. Emulsions are dispersions of liquid particles greater than 1 μ in an immiscible liquid.

The classification based on size is one of convenience. In a solution the molecules or ions are smaller than 5 mμ are are homogeneously distributed throughout a single phase. High-molecular-weight compounds, e.g., carbohydrates, polymers, and proteins, exist in a solvent as a homogeneous molecular solution. However, the size of the macromolecule is so large that the solution may be considered as a colloidal dispersion, and it does possess colloidal properties. Such a solution is frequently referred to as a colloidal solution.

The particles of pharmaceutical suspensions and emulsions often possess a size frequency distribution which includes some particles of colloidal size; therefore, suspensions and emulsions possess characteristics of both colloidal and coarse dispersions.

A colloidal dispersion consists of a dispersed phase, which is also known as a discontinuous or internal phase, and a dispersion medium, which is also known as a continuous or external phase. The physical state, i.e., gas, liquid, or solid, of the dispersed phase and the dispersion medium may be used to classify dispersed systems. Since gases are miscible in all proportions, there are eight systems, as illustrated in Table LXI. A polyphasic system in which colloidal particles are dispersed in a liquid medium is known as a sol. A colloidal system in which a solid or liquid is dispersed in a gas is known as an aerosol.

The validity of classifying a substance as a colloid solely on the basis of its particle size lies in the distinctive properties conferred on the substance by the huge specific surface. A cube of 1-cm edge

Table LXI Classification of Colloidal Systems Based on Physical State

Dispersed Phase	Dispersion Phase	System	Example
Liquid	Gas	Aerosol	Naphazoline hydrochloride nasal spray
Solid	Gas	Aerosol	Iodochlorhydroxyquin insufflation
Gas	Liquid	Foam	Detergent foam
Liquid	Liquid	Emulsion	Sterile phytonadione emulsion
Solid	Liquid	Sol	Mild silver protein sol
Gas	Solid	Foam	Gaseous inclusion in metals
Liquid	Solid	Emulsion	Opal
Solid	Solid	Suspension	Ruby glass

has a surface area of 6 cm² and a volume of 1 cc. If the cube composed of material having a density of 1 g cc^{-1} is repeatedly subdivided into cubes having an edge of 0.1 μ, the specific surface is increased 100,000 times, i.e., from 6 to 6 x 10^5 cm² g^{-1}. Consequently, phenomena, e.g., adsorption, catalysis, and color, associated with a large specific surface are major considerations with colloids.

The adsorption of gases or solutes onto solids depends on the nature of the adsorbent and the adsorbate (see page 21). For a given system the adsorption is a function of temperature, concentration of the adsorbent, and surface area. As colloidal particles have a huge specific surface, an enormous number of surface molecules are exposed to adsorb other substances by van der Waals, dipole, or ion interaction. Adsorption isotherms express the amount of material adsorbed and the equilibrium concentration or pressure at a given temperature. Several mathematical expressions of adsorption isotherms have been discussed in Chapter 2.

OPTICAL PROPERTIES

When a beam of light is directed through a true solution it is not visible when viewed at right angles to the direction of the beam. If a beam of light is directed through a colloidal dispersion, the light is scattered and reflected by the colloidal particles and a cone of light is observed. This effect, known as the Tyndall effect, provides a simple method for distinguishing between a solution and a colloidal sol. The Tyndall effect is utilized in the ultramicroscope to detect colloidal particles and to measure their average size.

When the particles of a colloidal dispersion are observed, they are seen to move in a random, erratic manner known as Brownian movement. Brownian movement is caused by the bombardment of the colloidal particles by the molecules of the dispersion medium. Colloidal sols do not settle, because Brownian movement counteracts the effect of gravity. The rate of movement is inversely proportional to the radius of the particle. In an aqueous medium, as the particles approach a size of 5 μ, the momentum of the molecules of the dispersion medium is not sufficient to move the particles; thus, Brownian movement ceases and the particles will eventually settle upon standing.

The color of a colloidal sol may be a function of the particle size of a colloidal dispersion. A sulfur sol of high dispersion is yellow. As the size of the colloidal sulfur is increased, the sol changes color from orange to violet, to blue, and finally to gray.

ELECTRICAL PROPERTIES

Colloids may be classified as lyophobic or lyophilic colloidal dispersions. Lyophobic colloids have no affinity for the dispersion medium and are not solvated. They are stabilized by a change acquired by preferential adsorption of ions from the dispersion medium. If water is the dispersion medium, they are known as hydrophobic colloids. Lyophilic colloids are highly solvated as well as charged. The charge usually is a result of ionization. If water is the dispersion medium, they are known as hydrophilic colloids. Hydrophobic colloids precipitate if their electric charge is removed; however, hydrophilic colloids remain dispersed after their charge is removed because they are hydrated. Fortunately, most pharmaceutical colloids are of the hydrophilic type and are stabilized by both mechanisms.

The large specific surface of a hydrophobic colloid exposes an enormous number of surface molecules, which are not equally subjected to attractive forces in all directions. Trace ions in the dispersion medium interact with the surface molecules and are strongly held or adsorbed to the surface of the colloid by an ion-induced dipole or ion-dipole interaction. It is the adsorption of trace ions that confers a charge on a hydrophobic colloid. The charged particles repel each other and prevent aggregation and precipitation of the colloidal substance.

The adsorbed ions on the surface of the colloidal particle tend to attract counterions, i.e., oppositely charged ions, and two layers of opposite charge result. The thickness of this double layer is small compared to the diameter of the colloidal particle, and the repulsive force of the charged colloid does not extend beyond the thickness of the double layer.

The diffuse double layer consists of two shells of ions of opposite charge. The inner shell is compact and adheres tightly to the colloidal particle as it moves. The outer shell is wide and diffused with a high concentration of counterions near the inner shell and a progressive decrease in concentration of counterions from inner region of the outer layer to the bulk of the dispersion medium. The outer layer is easily removed as the colloidal particle moves.

Between the surface of the colloidal particle and the bulk of the solution there exists a potential known as Nernst potential. This total potential E may be divided into two parts. The first is the potential between the inner shell and the surface of the colloid, and the second is the zeta or electrokinetic potential. The zeta (ζ) potential is the potential difference between the outer edge of the inner layer of adsorbed ions and the bulk of the dispersion medium.

Figure 130 presents a schematic representation of the double layer about a hydrophobic colloid in the presence of trace sodium and chloride ions. Owing to the attractive force between the surface molecules of the colloidal particle and the ion, the chloride ions are strongly adsorbed to the surface of the particle, conferring a negative charge upon it. The inner shell of adsorbed chloride ions attracts sodium ions in an attempt to achieve electric neutrality. The counterions, i.e., sodium ions, in the outer diffuse layer cause a positive potential, and since the diffused layer does not migrate with the colloidal particle as does the inner shell, there exists a difference in potential. The total potential is measured from the surface of the particle to the bulk of the solution, where there is equal distribution of sodium and chloride ions. The potential that exists between the outer edge of the adsorbed chloride ions and the bulk of the solution is the ζ potential. As the ζ potential is increased, the stability of a hydrophobic colloid is increased.

When an external voltage is applied to a colloidal dispersion, the charged colloidal particles migrate to the oppositely charged electrode. This is known as electrophoresis. Electrophoretic experiments have shown that many colloids are negatively charged, e.g., arsenic trisulfide, gold, silver, sulfur, and bacteria. Many macromolecules, e.g., acacia, algin, and type B gelatin, acquire a negative charge by ionization.

An electrophoretic cell may be used to measure ζ potential. Under the influence of an applied direct current the colloidal particles migrate to the electrode of opposite charge at a velocity dependent on the ζ potential. The mobility of a colloidal particle is defined as the velocity in cm sec^{-1} under a potential of a 1 V. Experimentally the velocity is measured by timing the movement of particle

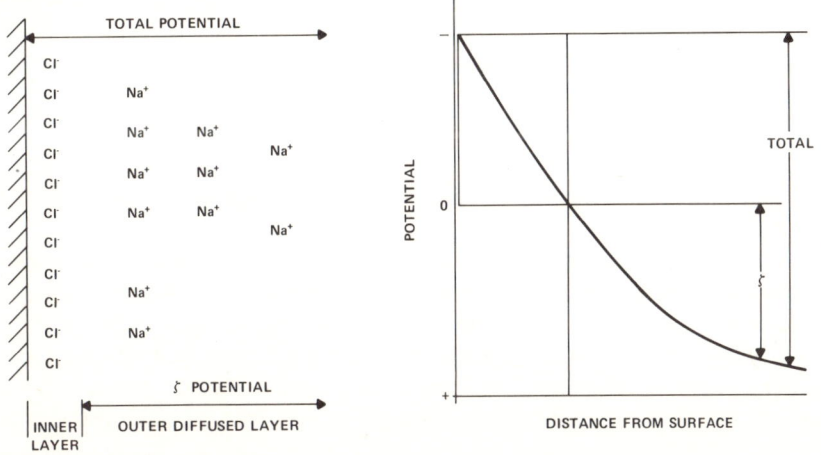

Figure 130. Schematic drawing defining the zeta potential of the double layer of ions around a colloidal particle.

over a given distance at a given potential. The ζ potential expressed in volts is calculated by the relation

$$\zeta = \frac{v}{E} \frac{4\pi\eta}{\epsilon} (9 \times 10^4)$$

where v is the velocity in cm sec^{-1}, E the potential gradient in V cm^{-1}, η the viscosity in poises, ϵ the dielectric constant of the dispersion medium, and the factor 9×10^4 converts electrostatic units to volts.

The factors governing the selective adsorption of ions are not completely known. Colloidal silver iodide formed by mixing dilute solutions of silver nitrate and sodium iodide may be positively or negatively charged. Apparently the charge on the colloidal silver iodide depends on the ion in excess. If a solution of silver nitrate is added to a sodium iodide solution, the iodide ion is in excess and is selectively adsorbed so that the colloid becomes negatively charged. If a solution of sodium iodide is added to a silver nitrate solution, the silver ion is in excess and the colloid becomes positively charged. The sodium and nitrate ions are not adsorbed. Fajans and Paneth suggested that ions which form slightly soluble compounds with the adsorbent are adsorbed rather than those ions which form more soluble compounds; thus, silver or iodide ions are adsorbed on colloidal silver iodide particles rather than sodium or nitrate ions.

The addition of electrolytes to colloidal dispersions alters the charge and mobility of the particles. In a theoretical hydrophobic colloidal system, which contained no ions, the addition of a very low concentration of electrolytes would provide ions that could be adsorbed and would confer a charge on the particles. The charged particles would be more stable, as they would mutually repel one another. This phenomenon is known as deflocculation or peptization.

If the ζ potential is removed or reduced below a critical value, the colloidal particles agglomerate and precipitation occurs. The reduction of ζ potential and the precipitation of hydrophobic colloids usually occurs upon the addition of electrolytes. The electrolyte contributes many ions which promote electric neutrality in the diffuse double layer about the colloidal particle. With the removal of the ζ potential the particles collide or approach close enough for the intermolecular forces to be strong enough to form larger particles, which precipitate. The precipitating ability of an electrolyte is associated with the ion opposite in charge to that of the colloids. The Schulze-Hardy rule states that polyvalent ions having a charge opposite to that of the colloidal particle are more effective in causing precipitation than are monovalent ions. A certain positively charged ferric hydroxide sol is precipitated by 9 millimoles of potassium chloride or by 0.2 millimoles of potassium sulfate. Thus, potassium sulfate is 45 times more effective than potassium chloride as a precipitating electrolyte. Obviously, the divalent ion is more effective than the univalent ion in precipitating the ferric hydroxide sol; however, there is no simple quantitative relation between the valence of the ion and the precipitating concentration.

Hydrophilic colloids acquire a charge by ionization. Most of the plant gums utilized in pharmacy are negatively charged hydrophilic colloids by virtue of a carboxylic or sulfuric acid radical within their structure. Acacia is a typical hydrophilic colloidal material obtained from a vegetable source. Acacia has a macromolecular structure containing *d*-galactopyranose, *d*-glycuronic acid, *l*-rhamnopyranose, and *l*-arabofuranose. Its acidity and negative charge are due to the ionization of the glycuronic acid portion of the structure.

Hydrophilic colloidal proteins are amphoteric and the charge on the protein is dependent on the pH of the dispersion medium. Gelatin is obtained by the partial hydrolysis of collagen, and it is composed of polypeptide chains of various lengths. Gelatin has a positive or negative charge depending on the pH at which hydrolysis occurs. The isoelectric point is the pH at which a substance has no net charge and is known as a zwitterion. At the isoelectric point the ζ potential is zero, the colloid has its minimum stability, viscosity, and electrical conductance. Gelatin derived from an acid-treated precursor is positively charged and is highly hydrated at pH 4 to 4.5; it exhibits an isoelectric point from pH 7 to 9. Gelatin derived from an alkaline treated precursor is negatively charged and highly hydrated at pH 8; it exhibits an isoelectric point between pH 4.7 and 5.

COLLIGATIVE PROPERTIES

The colligative properties of a solution are only slightly affected by the addition of a colloid. Hydrophobic colloidal particles are composed of many molecules, and macromolecules have a high molecular weight, so for a given weight of material colloids contribute few particles to the system in comparision to a solute.

Albumin is the most abundant protein in the human plasma, where it is present to the extent of 4 g in 100 ml. Albumin is colloidal in size and has a molecular weight of 70,000 g mole^{-1}. Assuming no dissociation of albumin, its contribution to the freezing point of blood is

$$\Delta T_f = Lm$$
$$= 1.86 \times \frac{40}{70,000}$$
$$= 0.0011°$$

A dextrose solution of a similar concentration lowers the freezing point of water,

$$\Delta T_f = 1.86 \times \frac{40}{180}$$
$$= 0.413°$$

Polyvinylpyrrolidone is a plasma volume expander for emergency use in hypovolemic shock resulting from extensive loss of body fluids. Polyvinylpyrrolidone with an average molecular weight of 40,000 g mole^{-1} is administered intravenously as a 3.5 per cent solution in normal saline solution. The normal saline vehicle is necessary to provide a solution that has the same osmotic pressure, i.e., 7.4 atm, as the blood, since the osmotic pressure of a 3.5 per cent aqueous dispersion of polyvinylpyrrolidone is

$$P = cRT$$
$$= \frac{35}{40,000} \times 0.08205 \times 310$$
$$= 0.022 \text{ atm}$$

Measurement of osmotic pressure offers a method of determining the molecular weight of a colloidal material by utilization of the van't Hoff equation. The osmotic pressures P of different concentrations of the colloid are measured. The ratio P/c is plotted against the concentration, and the curve is extrapolated to intersect the P/c axis. The numerical value of the intersection as determined by the curve is equivalent to RT/M. This relationship can be solved for the only unknown term, M, the molecular weight of the colloid.

DIFFUSION

The spontaneous movement of particles from a region of higher concentration to a region of lower concentration until the concentration of the system is uniform is known as diffusion. Diffusion is brought about by thermal agitation, i.e., collisional impact of the particles. According to the first law of Fick, the flux, Q, through a plane perpendicular to the direction of diffusion is directly proportional to the concentration gradient, dc/dx,

$$Q = -D\frac{dc}{dx}$$

where D is the diffusion coefficient and has the units cm^2 sec^{-1}. The negative sign indicates that diffusion occurs in the direction of lower concentration. The flux is the quantity of material diffusing per unit time through a unit area; it is expressed in g cm^{-2} sec^{-1}.

For dilute systems of spherical particles the Sutherland-Einstein equation,

$$D = \frac{RT}{6\pi \eta r N}$$

relates the diffusion coefficient D to the viscosity η of the dispersion medium and the radius r of the particles. Since size is traditionally expressed in terms of molecular weight, a relationship may be derived between the diffusion coefficient and molecular weight, M,

$$D = \frac{RT}{6\pi \eta N} \left(\frac{4\pi N}{3 M \bar{v}}\right)^{1/3}$$

where N is the Avogadro number and $\bar{v}$ the partial specific volume, i.e., volume in cm^3 of 1 g of solute. For spherical particles the diffusion coefficient is inversely proportional to the cube root of the molecular weight. At 25° the diffusion coefficient for sucrose is 52.3 X 10^{-7} cm^2 sec^{-1}, and the diffusion coefficient for serum albumin is 6.15 X 10^{-7} cm^2 sec^{-1}.

The diffusion coefficient of serum albumin at 20° in water was experimentally found to be 6.15 X 10^{-7} cm^2 sec^{-1}, and the specific volume is 0.735. The viscosity of water at 20° is 0.010 p. By substituting these values in the above equation the molecular weight of the albumin may be calculated:

$$D = 6.15 \times 10^{-7} = \frac{8.31 \times 10^7 \times 293}{6\pi(6.02 \times 10^{23}) \times 0.010} \left[\frac{4\pi(6.02 \times 10^{23})}{3 \times 0.735\, M}\right]^{1/3}$$

$M = 145{,}000$ g $mole^{-1}$

The albumin molecule is not spherical because the molecular weight determined by a sedimentation method is approximately 50,000 g $mole^{-1}$.

When a solution is separated from the solvent by a semipermeable membrane which is permeable to the solvent but not to the solute, the solvent diffuses through the membrane into the solution. This process is known as osmosis. If a solution of a colloidal electrolyte and a salt are separated from the solvent by a membrane that is permeable to the salt but does not allow passage of the macroions, the measured osmotic pressure is greater than that expected for the colloidal ions alone. This effect is known as the Donnan membrane equilibrium and is caused by the unequal distribution of the salt ions at equilibrium. Owing to the presence of macroions on one side of the semipermeable membrane, the concentration of the small ion on the same side as the macroion is lower on that side of the membrane than in the salt solution; this is compensated for by an increased concentration of the small ion of opposite charge.

If sodium chloride is placed in solution on one side of a semipermeable membrane represented by subscript b and a colloidal electrolyte RNa is placed on the other side, the sodium and chloride ions can diffuse freely but the nondiffusible macroanion R^- cannot. At equilibrium the product of the concentration of sodium and chloride ions must be the same on both sides of the membrane, so that

$$[Na^+]_b\, [Cl^-]_b = [Na^+]\, [Cl^-]$$

and to attain electric neutrality the number of anions and cations must be equal on both sides of the membrane. On the side of the membrane represented by the subscript b

$$[Na^+]_b = [Cl^-]_b$$

and on the other side of the membrane

$$[Na^+] = [R^-] + [Cl^-]$$

Substitution of these two equations gives

$$[Cl^-]_b^2 = ([Cl^-] + [R^-])\,[Cl^-]^2$$
$$= [Cl^-]^2 \left(1 + \frac{[R^-]}{[Cl^-]}\right)$$

which may be rearranged to

$$\frac{[Cl^-]_b}{[Cl^-]} = \sqrt{1 + \frac{[R^-]}{[Cl^-]}}$$

This equation expresses the effect of a macroanion on the equilibrium ratio of concentration of a diffusible anion across a membrane. As the concentration of the macroanion is increased, it drives a greater ratio of the diffusible anion through the membrane.

Absorption from the gastrointestinal tract may be influenced by high concentrations of nondiffusible colloidal electrolytes, e.g., anionic resins and carboxymethylcellulose. If a diffusible drug anion, e.g., benzylpenicillin or salicylate, is represented by D^-, the ratio of concentrations of the drug anion is

$$\frac{[D^-]_b}{[D^-]} = \sqrt{1 + \frac{[R^-]}{[D^-]}}$$

where $[D^-]_b$ is the concentration in the blood and $[D^-]$ is the concentration in the lumen of the gastrointestinal tract. As the ratio of the colloidal electrolyte to the drug anion is increased in the gastrointestinal tract, the ratio of the concentration of drug in blood to the intestinal tract is increased. Thus, the addition of an anionic colloidal electrolyte to a diffusible drug anion enhances the absorption of the drug.

RHEOLOGICAL PROPERTIES

Rheology is the study of the flow properties of matter. Viscosity is the resistance offered when one part of a liquid flows by another. The force required to slip one layer of a liquid past another with a given velocity depends directly on the viscosity of the liquid and on the areas exposed to each other, and inversely on the distances separating the two surfaces. Viscosity may be viewed in terms of a cube of liquid composed of parallel layers of molecules. If the bottom layer of the cube is fixed and the top layer of the liquid is moved at a constant velocity, each lower layer moves with a velocity directly proportional to its distance from the fixed bottom layer. The difference of velocity, dv, between two planes of liquid separated by an infinitesimal distance, dx, is the velocity gradient or rate of shear, dv/dx. The force per unit area, F/A, needed to bring about this flow is known as the shearing stress. Intuitively one realizes that the higher the viscosity of a liquid, the greater is the shearing stress needed to produce a certain rate of shear. Thus, the rate of shear is directly proportional to the shearing stress.

$$F/A = \eta\, dv/dx$$

where η is the coefficient of viscosity, F/A the force per unit area in dyn cm^{-2} acting parallel to the planes, and dv/dx the velocity gradient perpendicular to the planes in sec^{-1}. The dimensions of the coefficient of absolute viscosity are dyn sec cm^{-2} or g cm^{-1} sec^{-1}. For convenience the poise has been designated as the unit of viscosity. A liquid has a viscosity of 1 p when a shearing stress of 1 dyn cm^{-2} is required to maintain a relative velocity of 1 cm sec^{-1} between two parallel planes 1 cm apart. In pharmacy the centipoise, which is equal to 0.01 p is generally used to express viscosity. Fluidity is defined as the reciprocal of viscosity; it is seldom used in pharmaceutical literature.

Absolute viscosity may be determined directly by measuring the time required for a measured volume of liquid to flow through a capillary tube under an applied pressure. Poiseuille developed the expression for the flow of a liquid through a capillary tube,

$$\eta = \frac{\pi r^4 t \, \Delta P}{8 l V}$$

where r is the radius of the capillary tube, t the time of flow, ΔP the pressure head in dyn cm^{-2} by which the liquid flows, l the length of the capillary, and V the volume of the liquid. The pressure head depends on the density of the liquid, the acceleration of gravity, and the difference in heights of the liquid levels in the two arms of the viscometer. The acceleration of gravity is constant, and if the levels in the capillary are maintained constant for all liquids, these terms may be incorporated into a constant. For a given liquid the Poiseuille expression may be written

$$\eta = \frac{\pi r^4 k t \rho}{8 l V}$$

and for a reference of known density, ρ_0, and viscosity, η_0, it may be written

$$\eta_0 = \frac{\pi r^4 k_0 t \rho_0}{8 l V}$$

Division of these equations produces a comparison of the absolute viscosity of the reference to that of the liquid,

$$\frac{\eta}{\eta_0} = \frac{\rho t}{\rho_0 t_0}$$

and permits the calculation of the viscosity of the liquid.

The direct experimental determination of absolute viscosity is difficult, but the measurement of relative viscosity, i.e., ratio of the viscosity of a liquid to that of some reference liquid, is simple and acceptable for most purposes. In practice a capillary viscometer is used with a reference liquid of known density ρ_0 and viscosity η_0. A given volume of the reference liquid is pipetted into the reservoir of the capillary viscometer in a constant-temperature bath. The liquid is drawn up through the capillary tube into the enlarged tube above the upper mark. The liquid is then allowed to flow down the capillary tube and the time t_0 required to flow between the upper and lower mark is measured. The procedure is repeated with the same volume of the liquid for which the viscosity is to be determined. The above equation is then utilized to calculate the viscosity.

At 25° water has a density of 0.99707 g cc^{-1} and a viscosity of 0.00895 p. The time of flow of water in a particular capillary viscometer is 10 seconds. A 65 per cent sucrose solution has a flow time of 890 seconds. If the density of the syrup is 1.313 g cc^{-1}, the viscosity of the syrup may be calculated by means of the above equation:

$$\frac{\eta}{0.00895} = \frac{1.313 \times 890}{0.99709 \times 10}$$

$$\eta = 1.04 \text{ p}$$

The Ostwald type of viscometer as modified by Cannon and Fenske is shown in Figure 131. It is commercially available in several capillary sizes, so a wide range of viscosities as given in Table LXII may be measured. The capillary method may be used to determine the viscosity of Newtonian liquids.

Newtonian liquids are those in which the rate of shear is directly proportional to the shearing stress. A rheogram, i.e., a rheological flow curve of the rate of shear plotted against the shearing stress, of a Newtonian liquid is linear and passes through the origin. The slope of the line is the reciprocal of viscosity. Consequently, a small slope indicates a high viscosity. A single point determination of the viscosity will describe a Newtonian liquid, as the viscosity does not change at different rates of shear.

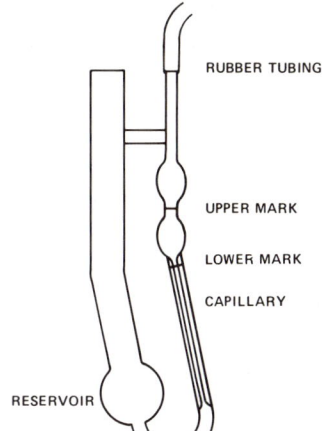

Figure 131. Canon-Fenske modification of the Ostwald viscometer.

Table LXII Viscosity Range of Various Sizes of Cannon-Fenske Viscometer

Series	Efflux Time (sec)	Viscosity Range (centistokes) *
50	300-1500	0.8-3
100	200-700	3-10
200	100-700	10-70
300	100-700	25-175
400	100-700	120-850
500	100-700	800-5600

* Centistoke is the unit of kinematic viscosity and is equal to the absolute viscosity divided by the density of the liquid.

Pure liquids and ideal solutions are Newtonian liquids. In ideal solutions in which no interactions occur, viscosity is additive. Mathematically this may be expressed as

$$\frac{1}{\eta} = \frac{1}{\eta_1} V_1 + \frac{1}{\eta_2} V_2$$

where η is the viscosity of the solution composed of volume fractions V_1 and V_2 of pure liquids 1 and 2 with viscosities η_1 and η_2, respectively.

A solution or a dispersion has a viscosity greater than that of the dispersion medium because of the greater resistance to flow produced by the particles of the dispersed phase. The relationship between the viscosity of the liquid in which the dispersed phase is composed of uniform spherical particles and the volume concentration of the dispersed phase is expressed by the Einstein equation,

$$\eta = \eta_0 (1 + 2.5\phi)$$

where η_0 is the viscosity of the dispersion medium and ϕ is the fraction of the total volume of the liquid occupied by the particles. The Einstein equation is used in various technical fields to define viscosities, as listed in Table LXIII.

The shape of the dispersed particles influences the viscosity. Spherical particles present a smaller specific surface than fibrous or rod-shaped particles. The greater surface and the attending greater frictional resistance of the nonspherical particles produces a higher viscosity. Linear colloidal

Table LXIII Types of Viscosity

Type	Definition	Units
Absolute	$\eta = \dfrac{F/A}{dv/dx}$	Poises
Relative	$\eta_{rel} = \dfrac{\eta}{\eta_o}$	-
Kinematic	$v = \dfrac{\eta}{\rho}$	Stokes
Specific	$\eta_{sp} = \dfrac{\eta}{\eta_o} - 1$	-
Reduced	$\eta_{red} = \dfrac{\eta_{sp}}{C}$	Reciprocal concentration
Intrinsic	$[\eta] = \lim\limits_{c \to 0} \dfrac{\eta_{sp}}{C}$	Reciprocal concentration
Inherent	$\eta_{inh} = \ln \dfrac{\eta_{rel}}{C}$	Reciprocal concentration

particles may entwine to produce much higher viscosities than those predicted by the Einstein equation, which then requires additional terms to adjust for this effect.

The viscosities of most liquids decrease with an increase in temperature. The flow process requires energy, which is more available at higher temperatures. A small change in temperature produces a relatively large change in viscosity because of the exponential relation between the temperature T and the viscosity, *[Viscosity is an exponential function of temperature.]*

$$\eta = A \exp(E/RT)$$

where A is a constant and E is the activation energy for a particular liquid.

In polyphasic pharmaceuticals, e.g., colloidal dispersions, emulsions, and suspensions, the dispersed particles are close enough for interparticular interactions to occur, producing liquids in which the rate of shear is not directly proportional to the shearing stress. Such systems are known as non-Newtonian liquids and are further classified as plastic, pseudoplastic, and dilatant materials.

A plastic material does not flow until a certain minimum shearing stress, which is known as the yield value, is applied. It is postulated that the dispersed particles tend to interact and to entrap the dispersion medium so that the material does not flow until sufficient force is applied to overcome the interparticular forces. After plastic flow begins the apparent viscosity decreases with increasing rates of shear. A typical rheogram of a plastic flow is shown in Figure 132. At low rates of shearing the curve is not linear, and it does not pass through the origin. At higher rates of shearing the curve approaches linearity. Extrapolation of the curve to intersect the abscissa provides a method of evaluation of the yield value, f, which is generally expressed in dyn cm^{-2}. The reciprocal of the slope of the curve is known as the plastic viscosity. The coefficient of plastic viscosity, U, is defined by the expression

$$\dfrac{E-f}{A} = U \dfrac{dv}{dx}$$

The yield value of a plastic system is increased by an increased concentration of the dispersed phase. While standing, many plastic systems form a gel, which upon mechanical agitation breaks down to form a sol. If the sol is left undisturbed, it will reform a gel. This reversible, isothermal gel-sol transformation is known as thixotropy.

A rheogram of a typical plastic material exhibiting thixotropy is shown in Figure 132. Such rheograms are obtained by use of a rotational viscometer, which consists of one cylinder fitted with a very small clearance inside another cylinder. The material is placed in the space between the cylinders and one of the cylinders is rotated at several controllable rates, while the torque on the stationary cylinder is measured. As the shearing stress is successively increased the upcurve is obtained, and as the shearing stress is then successively decreased the down curve is obtained. If the upcurve and the downcurve do not coincide, the plot is known as a hysteresis loop. The area of the hysteresis loop is a measure of thixotropy.

As the rate of shear is increased, the consistency decreases and the thixotropic breakdown increases. Thus, any method of measurement that gives a single value for the viscosity of a plastic system exhibiting thixotropy is not adequate. To properly characterize the rheological pattern of emulsions, ointments, and suspensions requires an evaluation of yield value, plastic viscosity, and thixotropy.

A pseudoplastic material does not possess a yield value, but it flows with the application of force and its viscosity is decreased as the rates of shear are increased. As shown in Figure 133, the rheogram of a typical pseudoplastic material is nonlinear and passes through the origin. An apparent viscosity may be expressed for any given rate of shear; it is the reciprocal of the slope of a tangent to a given rate of shear.

Pseudoplastic flow is exhibited by long-chain or linear polymers, e.g., methylcellulose, sodium alginate, sodium carboxymethylcellulose, and tragacanth. At rest the linear polymers or macromolecules are dispersed at random in the dispersion medium. As shearing stress is applied, the macromolecules tend to become aligned with the long axis parallel to the direction of flow. With this ordered alignment the molecules pass one another with less frictional resistance and the viscosity is decreased. If the shearing stress is decreased, the orientation of the macromolecules becomes more random and the greater frictional resistance to flow is reflected in an increase in viscosity. Since only a molecular alignment is involved, there is no time lag in returning to a more random state, and the upcurve and the downcurve coincide.

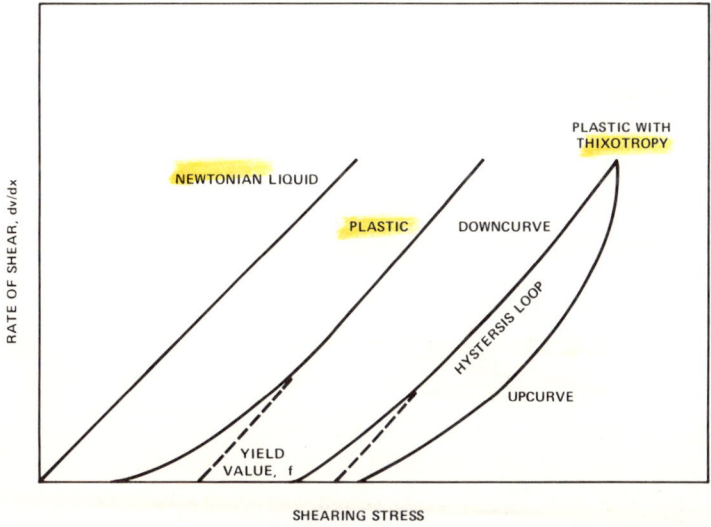

Figure 132. Flow curves of Newtonian, plastic, and plastic with thixotropy materials.

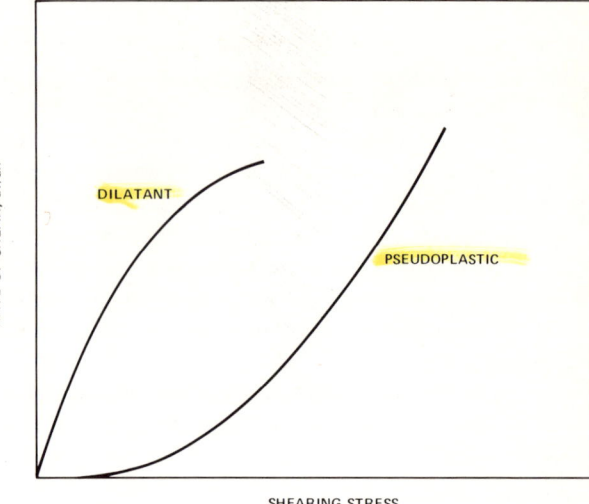

Figure 133. Flow curves of a dilantant and a pseudoplastic material.

A dilatant flow exhibits an increase in viscosity as the shearing stress is increased. Dilatancy is shown by polyphasic systems, e.g., starch suspension and zinc oxide paste, containing a high percentage of irregular particles. It is postulated that in dilatant systems at rest each of the particles is surrounded by a minimum volume of dispersion medium, which decreases the resistance to flow. When shearing stress is applied, the particles are rearranged and the dispersion medium is displaced from around the particles. With an increasing displacement of the dispersion medium from the particles, there is an increased resistance to flow.

SEDIMENTATION

Dispersed particles that have a density greater than that of the dispersion liquid settle under the influence of the gravitational field of the center. The force that causes a particle to settle in a liquid is equal to the acceleration of gravity times its effective mass, i.e., mass of the particle minus the mass of the liquid it displaces. The force retarding settling is the frictional coefficient times the velocity. The frictional coefficient, f, is the force opposing a particle, which is moving with a velocity of 1 cm sec^{-1}. Stokes showed that for spheres falling independently in a nonturbulent flow,

$$f = 6\pi\eta r$$

where r is the radius of the sphere and η the coefficient of viscosity. If the density of the sphere is ρ and the density of the dispersion liquid is ρ_0, the force causing sedimentation is $\frac{4}{3}\pi r^3 (\rho - \rho_0)g$. When the rate of settling, dx/dt, is constant, the retarding force $6\pi\eta r(dx/dt)$ is equal to the force due to gravity,

and

$$\frac{4}{3}\pi r^3 (\rho - \rho_0)g = 6\pi\eta r(dx/dt)$$

$$\frac{dx}{dt} = \frac{2r^2 (\rho - \rho_0)g}{9\eta}$$

In an aqueous medium lyophilic colloids with particles less than 1 μ do not sediment in the gravitational field of the earth. The repulsive force due to the ζ potential on the particles and the random bombardment of the particles by the molecules of the dispersion liquid oppose and overcome the effect of gravity on these small particles.

The Stokes equation may be used to calculate the rate of sedimentation in water of sulfur with an average particle radius of 5.5 μ. The density of sulfur and water at 25° is 1.96 and 0.997 g cc^{-1}, respectively. The viscosity of water at 25° is 0.00895 p. The rate of settling is

$$\frac{dx}{dt} = \frac{2(5.5 \times 10^{-4})^2(1.96 - 0.997)980}{9 \times 0.00895}$$

$$= 7.1 \times 10^{-3} \text{ cm sec}^{-1}$$

The rate of settling is inversely proportional to the viscosity of the system. Substances added to increase the viscosity and slow the rate of settling are known as suspending agents. Natural hydrocolloids, e.g., tragacanth and sodium alginate, and clays, e.g., bentonite and Veegum®, are used as suspending agents in pharmaceuticals. Methylcellulose and sodium carboxymethylcellulose are cellulosic polymers that are popular suspending agents for both internally and externally used dispersions.

In certain dispersions the solid particles are held together by the van der Waals forces in a loose, open structure known as a floccule or floc. If the floc is supported in an open structure by the dispersion medium, it does not settle appreciably. The final volume of sediment is a characteristic of the suspension and it can be used as a measure of the extent of flocculation. The sedimentation ratio is the ratio of the final volume of the sediment to its original volume. If the sedimentation ratio is small, the particles sediment to a compact mass in which the interparticulate forces may be strong enough to cause caking.

INTERFACIAL ADSORPTION

An interface is the region or boundary between two phases. Adsorption is the orientation or collection of a substance at the interface of the solid or liquid phase with which it is in contact. It is the large interface between a colloid and its environment that gives rise to the unique properties of a colloidal system.

The molecules in the bulk of a liquid are subjected equally in all directions to intermolecular attractive forces. At the surface of a liquid, the attractive force between the molecules of the liquid and the air is negligible. As a result on the surface of the liquid there is an unbalanced force which tends to maintain the liquid in a shape possessing a minimum surface area. The magnitude of this force acting perpendicular to a unit length of a line in the surface is called the surface tension. Surface tension is illustrated in Figure 134 by the Dupré frame, in which a film of liquid is stretched on a rectangular framework. If a force, f, is applied to the movable bar of length l, the film of liquid is stretched and the surface

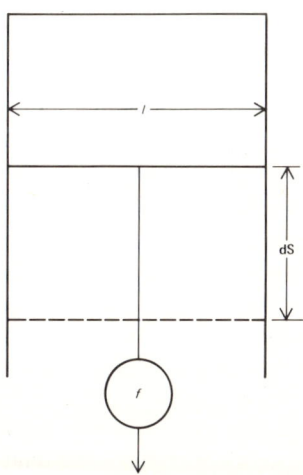

Figure 134. Dupré frame demonstrates the mechanical tension in the surface of a liquid and is used in defining surface tension.

area is increased. The surface tension of the liquid is the force per unit length along the bar required to break the film. Thus, surface tension is defined by the relation

$$\gamma = \frac{f}{2l}$$

where the factor 2 appears because a film has two liquid surfaces. Surface tension is expressed in dyn cm^{-1}.

The ring method is the most widely used technique for measuring surface tension. The DuNoüy tensiometer consists of a platinum-iridium ring supported by a stirrup attached to the beam of a torsion balance. The ring is placed in the surface of the liquid and is pulled upward by turning the torsion wire, which is attached to a calibrated dial from which the applied force is read. The force, f, required to separate the ring from the interface is equal to $4\pi R\gamma$, where R is the mean radius of the ring. Doubling of the circumference arises because there are two boundary lines between the liquid and the wire, i.e., one on the outside and one on the inside of the ring. The surface tension is given by the relation

$$\gamma = \frac{f}{4\pi R} F$$

where F is a correction factor necessitated by the shape of the liquid column, which the ring holds up immediately before breaking from the surface. The shape is a function of R^3/V and R/r, where V is the volume of the liquid held up and r the radius of the wire.

Traditionally, the tension that exists between a liquid and the atmosphere is known as the surface tension, and the tension that exists at the interface between two immiscible liquids is known as the interfacial tension.

An expenditure of energy is required to increase the surface area of a substance. If a force of 250 dyn is applied to the Dupré frame in Figure 134 and it moves a bar of 5 cm length a distance of 10 cm, the work done or the energy expended is 250 X 10 = 2500 ergs. In general, the energy expended, dE, may be expressed as

$$dE = f\,ds$$

where f is the force applied and ds is the distance through which the force is moved. Substituting for force f in terms of the equation defining surface tension gives

$$dE = 2\gamma l\,ds$$

and as $2\gamma l$ is equal to the increase in surface area dA, the energy expended equals the surface tension multiplied by the change in surface area,

$$dE = \gamma dA$$

When a substance is reduced in particle size and its specific surface is increased by the expenditure of energy, dE represents the increase in free surface energy imparted to the surface as a consequence of the work done. It is the large free surface energy that is responsible for the characteristics of a colloidal system. If 1 ml of water is dispersed into spherical droplets 0.01 μ in diameter, its area is 600 m^2. At room temperature the free surface energy for this area is approximately 2.18 X 10^8 ergs, or 10.5 cal. This free surface energy is approximately one-fifth as much as the kinetic energy of vibration of the water molecules.

A system at a high energy level tends to lose energy until it is at the same level as its environment. Oil droplets in an emulsion tend to coalesce, i.e., run together after colloiding, with a reduction in total surface and a decrease in free surface energy. Similarly, solids dispersed in suspensions or colloidal sols are energetically unstable and tend to aggregate.

The addition of a solute to a solvent may change the surface tension. Solutes that reduce surface tension are known as surface-active agents. A surface-active agent is adsorbed or oriented at the surface or interface so that its concentration is greater than in the bulk of the solution. Gibbs quantitatively expressed the adsorption at an interface as

$$\Gamma = -\frac{c}{RT}\frac{d\gamma}{dc}$$

where Γ is the difference in concentration of the solute in the surface layer and the bulk solution in moles cm^{-2}, T the absolute temperature, R the gas constant, and $d\gamma/dc$ the rate of change of surface tension with concentration, c. If a solute causes a decrease in surface tension, $d\gamma/dc$ is negative and Γ is increased; i.e., the solute is adsorbed at the surface.

A solute that causes an increase in surface tension is known as a surface-inactive material, e.g., glycerin, sugar, and sodium chloride. The effect of surface-inactive materials is small, as the solute concentration decreases in the interface, and consequently its effect on surface tension is self-limiting.

When a substance is placed on the surface of a liquid it will spread as a film if the interaction forces between the liquid and the substance are greater than the intermolecular forces of the substance. If mineral oil is placed on water, it assumes a spherical shape and does not spread, because the van der Waals force between the hydrocarbon molecules is greater than any force that may exist between the water and the hydrocarbon.

Slightly soluble molecules, which contain polar and nonpolar groups, spread as a monomolecular layer on the surface of water. Oleic acid is insoluble in water, but it will spread over the surface if dropped on water. The hydrogen bonding between the polar carboxylic acid group and water is sufficient to orient and spread the oleic acid in a monomolecular layer with the alkyl chain oriented toward the atmosphere. This surface orientation of a molecule can be used to determine the dimensions of a molecule. By means of an ultramicro pipet, 0.002 ml of oleic acid is delivered onto a clean surface of water. The area over which the oleic acid spread is 8250 cm^2. The thickness of the film is

$$\frac{0.002}{8250} = 24 \times 10^{-8} \text{ cm}$$

Since the oleic acid is oriented vertically in a monomolecular layer, the thickness of the film represents the length of the oleic acid molecule.

Oleic acid has a density of 0.895 g cc^{-1} and a molecular weight of 282.5 g mole^{-1}. The cross-sectional area occupied by a molecule can be calculated by dividing the area of a monomolecular film by the number of molecules comprising the film. The weight of 0.002 ml of oleic acid is equal to the product of the density and volume,

$$0.895 \times 0.002 = 0.00179 \text{ g}$$

The number of molecules of oleic acid is equal to the number of moles of oleic acid multiplied by the Avogadro number,

$$\frac{0.00179 \times 6.02 \times 10^{23}}{282.5} = 3.8 \times 10^{18}$$

The cross-sectional area of a molecule of oleic acid is

$$\frac{8250}{3.8 \times 10^{18}} = 22 \times 10^{-16} \text{ cm}^2 \quad (\text{or } 22 \text{ Å}^2)$$

The orientation of molecules in a film can be determined by a film balance. A film balance consists of a trough with a horizontal float attached to a torsion wire fitted with calibrated dial and a movable barrier. The material is dissolved in a volatile solvent and is placed on the surface. The solvent evaporates, leaving a film spread on the liquid in the trough. The barrier of the film balance is moved to different positions. At each position the area of the film and the corresponding film pressure is read.

After calculating the area occupied by a molecule, it is plotted against the film pressure. As shown in Figure 135, when the film is spread over an area exceeding 40 Å² per molecule, it exerts little pressure on the float. As the film is compressed into a smaller area by the movable float, the film pressure rises. As the pressure is still further increased, the molecules slip over one another and the monomolecular layer breaks. The cross-sectional area per molecule of closest-packed film at zero pressure is obtained by extrapolation of the linear portion of the curve to the abscissa. Surface-active agents, e.g., cetyl alcohol, stearic acid, and sodium oleate, with an aliphatic alkyl chain have a cross-sectional area of 22 Å². Tristearin, which has three aliphatic alkyl chains, has a cross-sectional area of 66 Å².

In dispersions of mutually insoluble liquids, e.g., water and oil, a surface-active agent is adsorbed at the interface as a result of an approximately equal balance of polar and nonpolar groups. If a molecule is too polar, it will dissolve in the polar liquid and exert no effect on the interfacial tension. If a molecule is very nonpolar, it will dissolve in the nonpolar liquid and exert no effect on interfacial tension.

The hydrophile-lipophile balance, or HLB system, is useful for expressing the ratio of hydrophilic and hydrophobic characteristics of a surface-active agent. The HLB system consists of an arbitrary scale from which experimentally determined HLB values are assigned. Surface-active agents with a low HLB are oil soluble or oil dispersible. A high HLB value indicates water solubility or dispersibility. Sorbitan monooleate is oil dispersible and has an HLB of 4.3. Polysorbate 80 is water soluble and has an HLB of 15.0.

The HLB values are additive, so the HLB value of a blend of surface-active agents is calculated by summing the products of the HLB value of each surface-active agent and its fraction of the total surface-active agents. The HLB value of a blend of equal amounts of polysorbate 80 and sorbitan monooleate 80 is

$$(15.0 \times 1/2) + (4.3 \times 1/2) = 9.65$$

The HLB values for various surface-active agents are shown in Table LXIV. Most surface-active agents produce foam when agitated with air. Foams are generally a nuisance and are avoided. Surface-active agents with an HLB of 1 to 3 are antifoaming agents and may be used to destroy unwanted foams.

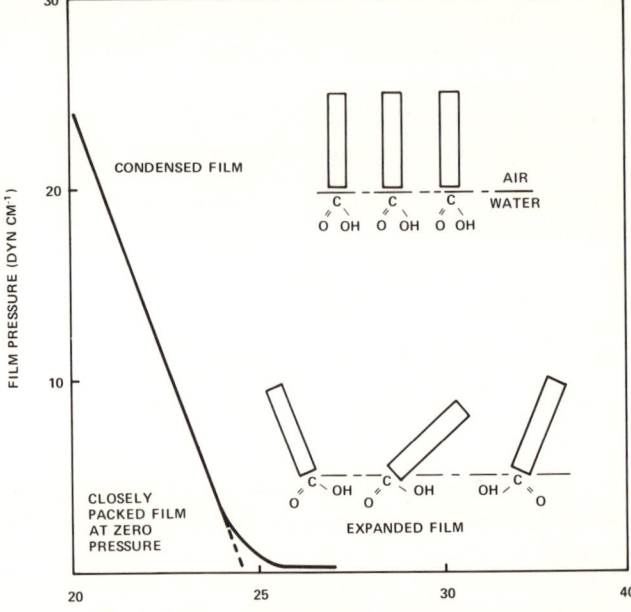

Figure 135. Film pressure-area diagram for stearic acid on water as determined by a film balance.

Table LXIV Average HLB Values of Some Surface-Active Agents

Name	Compound	HLB	Manufacturer*
Acacia		12.0	
Aldol®33	Glyceryl monostearate	3.8	d
Aldol 28	Glyceryl monostearate (self-emulsifying)	5.5	d
Arlacel®85	Sorbitan trioleate	1.8	a
Arlacel 65	Sorbitan tristearate	2.1	a
Arlacel C	Sorbitan sesquioleate	3.7	a
Arlacel 83	Sorbitan sesquioleate	3.7	a
Arlacel 161	Glyceryl monostearate	3.8	a
Arlacel 80	Sorbitan monooleate	4.3	a
Arlacel 60	Sorbitan monostearate	4.7	a
Arlacel 40	Sorbitan monopalmitate	6.7	a
Arlacel 20	Sorbitan monolaurate	8.6	a
Atmul 67	Glyceryl monostearate	3.8	a
Brij®30	Polyoxyethylene lauryl ether	9.5	a
Brij 35	Polyoxyethylene lauryl ether	16.9	a
Emcol®EO-50	Ethylene glycol fatty acid ester	2.7	b
Emcol ES-50	Ethylene glycol fatty acid ester	2.7	b
Emcol PO-50	Propylene glycol fatty acid ester	3.4	b
Emcol PS-50	Propylene glycol fatty acid ester	3.4	b
Emcol PP-50	Propylene glycol fatty acid ester	3.7	b
Emcol PM-50	Propylene glycol fatty acid ester	4.1	b
Emcol PL-50	Propylene glycol fatty acid ester	4.5	b
Emcol DO-50	Diethylene glycol fatty acid ester	4.7	b
Emcol DS-50	Diethylene glycol fatty acid ester	4.7	b
Emcol DP-50	Diethylene glycol fatty acid ester	5.1	b
Emcol DM-50	Diethylene glycol fatty acid ester	5.6	b
Emcol DL-50	Diethylene glycol fatty acid ester	6.1	b
Emulphor®VN-430	Polyoxyethylene fatty acid	9.0	c
Emulphor E1-719	Polyoxyethylene vegetable oil	13.3	c
Emulphor ON-870	Polyoxyethylene fatty alcohol	15.4	c
G-1706	Polyoxyethylene sorbitol beeswax derivative	2.0	a
G-1050	Polyoxyethylene sorbitol hexastearate	2.1	a
G-1704	Polyoxyethylene sorbitol beeswax derivative	3.0	a
G-922	Propylene glycol monostearate	3.4	a
G-2158	Propylene glycol monostearate	3.4	a
G-2859	Polyoxyethylene sorbitol 4.5 oleate	3.7	a
G-1727	Polyoxyethylene sorbitol beeswax derivative	4.0	a
G-917	Propylene glycol monolaurate	4.5	a
G-3851	Propylene glycol monolaurate	4.5	a
G-2139	Diethylene glycol monooleate	4.7	a
G-2146	Diethylene glycol monostearate	4.7	a
G-1702	Polyoxyethylene sorbitol beeswax derivative	5.0	a
G-1725	Polyoxyethylene sorbitol beeswax derivative	6.0	a

* a, Atlas Powder Company; b, Emulsol Corporation; c, GAF; d, Glyco Products Company, Inc.; e, Goldschmidt Chemical Corporation; f, Kessler Chemical Company, Inc.; g, W. C. Hardesty Company, Inc.; h, Dow Chemical Company.

polyphasic systems

G-2124	Diethylene glycol monolaurate (soap-free)	6.1	a
G-2242	Polyoxyethylene dioleate	7.5	a
G-2147	Tetraethylene glycol monostearate	7.7	a
G-2140	Tetraethylene glycol monooleate	7.7	a
G-2800	Polyoxypropylene mannitol dioleate	8.0	a
G-1493	Polyoxyethylene sorbitol lanolin oleate derivative	8.0	a
G-1425	Polyoxyethylene sorbitol lanolin derivative	8.0	a
G-3608	Polyoxypropylene stearate	8.0	a
G-1734	Polyoxyethylene sorbitol beeswax derivative	9.0	a
G-2111	Polyoxyethylene oxypropylene oleate	9.0	a
G-2125	Tetraethylene glycol monolaurate	9.4	a
G-2154	Hexaethylene glycol monostearate	9.6	a
G-1218	Polyoxyethylene esters of mixed fatty and resin acids	10.2	a
G-3806	Polyoxyethylene cetyl ether	10.3	a
G-3705	Polyoxyethylene lauryl ether	10.8	a
G-2116	Polyoxyethylene oxypropylene oleate	11.0	a
G-1790	Polyoxyethylene lanolin derivative	11.0	a
G-2142	Polyoxyethylene monooleate	11.1	a
G-2141	Polyoxyethylene monooleate	11.4	a
G-2076	Polyoxyethylene monopalmitate	11.6	a
G-3300	Alkyl aryl sulfonate	11.7	a
G-2127	Polyoxyethylene monolaurate	12.8	a
G-1431	Polyoxyethylene sorbitol lanolin derivative	13.0	a
G-1690	Polyoxyethylene alkyl aryl ether	13.0	a
G-2133	Polyoxyethylene lauryl ether	13.1	a
G-1284	Polyoxyethylene castor oil	13.3	a
G-1441	Polyoxyethylene sorbitol lanolin derivative	14.0	a
G-7596J	Polyoxyethylene sorbitan monolaurate	14.9	a
G-2144	Polyoxyethylene monooleate	15.1	a
G-3915	Polyoxyethylene oleyl ether	15.3	a
G-2720	Polyoxyethylene stearyl alcohol	15.3	a
G-3920	Polyoxyethylene oleyl alcohol	15.4	a
G-2079	Polyoxyethylene glycol monopalmitate	15.5	a
G-3820	Polyoxyethylene cetyl alcohol	15.7	a
G-1471	Polyoxyethylene sorbitol lanolin derivative	16.0	a
G-7596P	Polyoxyethylene sorbitan monolaurate	16.3	a
G-2129	Polyoxyethylene monolaurate	16.3	a
G-3930	Polyoxyethylene oleyl ether	16.7	a
G-2159	Polyoxyethylene monostearate	18.8	a
G-263	N-Cetyl N-ethyl morpholinium ethosulfate	25-30	a
Glaurin®	Diethylene glycol monolaurate (soap-free)	6.5	d
Igepal®CA-630	Polyoxyethylene alkyl phenol	12.8	c
Methocel®15 cps	Methylcellulose	10.5	h
Myrj®45	Polyoxyethylene monostearate	11.1	a
Myrj 49	Polyoxyethylene monostearate	15.0	a
Myrj 51	Polyoxyethylene monostearate	16.0	a
Myrj 52	Polyoxyethylene monostearate	16.9	a

Myrj 53	Polyoxyethylene monostearate	17.9	a
P.E.G. 400 monooleate	Polyoxyethylene monooleate	11.4	f, g
P.E.G. 400 monostearate	Polyoxyethylene monostearate	11.6	f, g
P.E.G. 400 monolaurate	Polyoxyethylene monolaurate	13.1	f
Pharmagel B	Gelatin	9.8	
Potassium oleate		20.0	
Renex®20	Polyoxyethylene esters of mixed fatty and resin acids	13.5	a
Sodium lauryl sulfate		40	a
Sodium oleate		18	
Span®85	Sorbitan trioleate	1.8	a
Span 65	Sorbitan tristearate	2.1	a
Span 80	Sorbitan monooleate	4.3	a
Span 60	Sorbitan monostearate	4.7	a
Span 40	Sorbitan monopalmitate	6.7	a
Span 20	Sorbitan monolaurate	8.6	a
Tegin®515	Glyceryl monostearate	3.8	e
Tegin	Glyceryl monostearate (self-emulsifying)	5.5	e
Tragacanth		13.2	
Tween®61	Polyoxyethylene sorbitan monostearate	9.6	a
Tween 81	Polyoxyethylene sorbitan monooleate	10.0	a
Tween 65	Polyoxyethylene sorbitan tristearate	10.5	a
Tween 85	Polyoxyethylene sorbitan trioleate	11.0	a
Tween 21	Polyoxyethylene sorbitan monolaurate	13.3	a
Tween 60	Polyoxyethylene sorbitan monostearate	14.9	a
Tween 80	Polyoxyethylene sorbitan monooleate	15.0	a
Tween 40	Polyoxyethylene sorbitan monopalmitate	15.6	a
Tween 20	Polyoxyethylene sorbitan monolaurate	16.7	a

A wetting agent is a surface-active agent that displaces air adsorbed on the surface of a solid and facilitates intimate contact between the solid particles and the liquid in which it is dissolved. In pharmacy wetting agents are used to displace air adsorbed on sulfur and charcoal while dispersing them in water. Wetting agents have an HLB of 7 to 9.

An emulsifying agent is a surface-active agent that reduces the interfacial tension between oil and water and surrounds the dispersed droplets in a tenacious film which prevents coalescence and separation of the dispersed phase. If an emulsifying agent has an HLB value of 3 to 6, it tends to produce a water-in-oil emulsion; i.e., oil is the dispersed phase and water is the continuous phase. If an emulsifying agent has an HLB value of 8 to 18, it tends to form an oil-in-water emulsion.

A detergent is a surface-active agent used for the removal of dirt. The cleansing process consists of initially wetting the dirt and the surface to be cleaned, emulsification of the dirt, and foaming to entrap and wash away the dirt particles. Detergents have an HLB value of 13 to 16.

A solubilizing agent is a surface-active agent capable of dispersing a water-insoluble substance as a hydrocolloid. Solubilizing agents have an HLB of 16 to 18. At low concentrations a surface-active agent exists as individual molecules in solution and as molecules positively adsorbed at the surface. As the concentration of the surface-active agent is increased in excess of its solubility, the excess surface-active agent aggregates into colloidal particles known as micelles. The concentration of surface-active agent at which micelles are formed is known as the critical micelle concentration, CMC. In a hydrocolloidal system the surface-active agent of the micelle is oriented so that the nonpolar portion of the molecule is toward the interior of the micelle and the polar portion is associated with the dispersion medium. At lower concentrations the micelles are probably spherical and composed of approximately 100 molecules. At higher concentrations the micelles may be distorted or laminar. A representation of spherical micelle of sodium stearate is given in Figure 136. Since sodium stearate ionizes, the micelle is negatively charged, and the mutual repulsion between the micelles enhances the stability of the system.

The physical properties, e.g., osmotic pressure and equivalent conductance, of a solution of a surface-active agent change at the CMC. The surface tension of a solution rapidly decreases as the concentration of the surface-active agent is increased until the CMC is attained; further increases in concentration of the surface-active agent beyond the CMC do not significantly decrease the surface tension. In concentrations of surface-active agent exceeding the CMC, the apparent solubility of a water-insoluble compound is a linear function of the concentration of surface-active agent. Solubilization is the process by which a water-insoluble substance is incorporated in the interior of a micelle to produce a colloidal dispersion possessing the appearance of a true solution. Slightly water-soluble compounds with weak polar groups may be oriented with their nonpolar groups toward the interior of the micelle and the polar groups protruding into the aqueous phase.

Surface-active agents in which the ability to lower interfacial tension resides in the anion are known as anionic surface-active agents. Sodium lauryl sulfate and dioctyl sodium sulfosuccinate are anionic surface-active agents. Cationic surface-active agents are those in which the ability to lower interfacial tension resides in the cation. Cationic surface-active agents, e.g., benzalkonium chloride and benzethonium chloride, are not used as emulsifying agents but as antibacterial agents. Nonionic surface-active agents, e.g., polysorbate 80 and octylphenoxy polyethoxyethanol, appreciably lower interfacial tension, but they do not ionize.

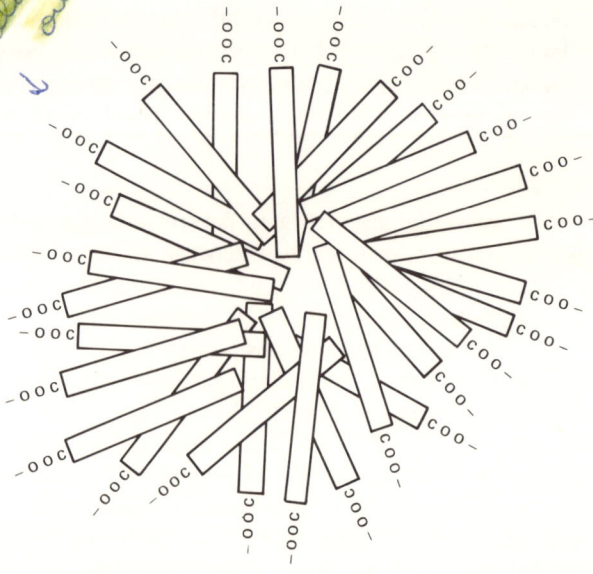

Figure 136. Diagrammatic representation of a spherical micelle formed by an anionic surface-active agent.

STABILITY

A lyophobic sol is unstable from the energy viewpoint. The high free surface energy of the particles tends to cause agglomeration with the accompanying reduction in free surface energy. A lyophobic colloid is not solvated by the dispersion medium, and it is stabilized by the mutual repulsion of the like charges on the particles and Brownian movement. As the lyophobic colloid is not solvated, its viscosity is not much different from that of the pure dispersion medium. Since a lyophobic colloid is stabilized primarily by a charge, it is readily precipitated by small amounts of electrolytes. The ability of an electrolyte to precipitate a lyophobic colloid increases with the increase in valence of the precipitating ion. In precipitating a negative hydrophobic colloid, the cation of the electrolyte is the precipitating ion; thus, aluminum chloride is more effective than barium chloride, which is more effective than sodium chloride. When a lyophobic colloid is precipitated, it cannot be simply redispersed. If a colloidal silver iodide sol is evaporated to dryness, the addition of water to the dry residue will not re-form a sol. Such a colloid is known as an irreversible colloid.

A lyophilic colloid is energetically stable, as it is associated with or solvated by the dispersion medium. Lyophilic colloids that have an affinity for water are known as hydrophilic colloids. Hydrophilic colloidal particles swell or become extended upon hydration. This increases frictional resistance, so that hydrophilic sol has a greater viscosity than the pure dispersion medium.

Moderately high concentrations of electrolytes are required to precipitate or salt out hydrophilic colloids, because in addition to neutralizing the ζ potential, sufficient electrolyte must be added to dehydrate the particles. The greater the interaction force between the added ion and the water molecules, the greater is the ability of the ion to precipitate the sol. A Hofmeister series is a list of ions arranged according to their ability to precipitate hydrophilic colloids. The Hofmeister series for anions is $citrate^{3-} > tartrate^{--} > SO_4^{--} > acetate^- > Cl^- > NO_3^- > Br^- > I^- > CNS^-$. For cations the Hofmeister series is $Th^{4+} > Al^{3+} > Sr^{++} > Ba^{++} > Ca^{++} > Mg^{++} > Li^+ > Na^+ > K^+ > Rb^+ > Cs^+$. In general, the ions that become most highly hydrated, i.e., have the higher hydration energy, are most effective in salting out and precipitating hydrophilic colloids. The smaller ions of the same valence have a more intense electrostatic field than the larger ions. The greater field intensity leads to a greater hydration, which removes the water molecules about the colloid.

The addition of less polar liquids to a hydrophilic sol facilitates precipitation by electrolytes, owing to the reduction in hydration of the colloidal particles. If high concentrations of alcohol are added to an hydrophilic sol, the viscosity decreases and the Tyndall cone becomes definite. Since the alcohol has dehydrated the colloid, a low concentration of electrolyte will remove the ζ potential and cause precipitation.

The stability of hydrophilic colloids which possess both acidic and basic groups in the macromolecule depends on the pH of the system. At low pH, protein molecules exist as cations; at high pH, protein molecules exist as anions. At the isoelectric point the net charge is zero. A colloidal system is least stable at its isoelectric point. If a gelatin sol is evaporated to dryness, the addition of water to the dry residue will re-form the gelatin dispersion. Such a colloid is known as a reversible colloid. Most hydrophilic colloids are reversible colloids. A comparison of the properties of lyophilic and lyophobic colloids is given in Table LXV.

The mixing of two lyophobic colloids of opposite charge results in a loss of stability or precipitation. The addition of a hydrophilic colloid to a hydrophobic colloid may produce a protective effect against precipitation by electrolytes if the hydrophilic macromolecules are adsorbed onto and completely surround the hydrophobic particles. If colloidal silver iodide is prepared in the presence of gelatin, the gelatin is adsorbed onto the surface of the colloidal silver iodide, rendering the system essentially hydrophilic. Such a system is known as a protected colloid because the colloidal silver iodide, which is protected by the gelatin, is reversible and will tolerate moderate concentrations of electrolytes without precipitation. The ability to function as a protective colloid has been expressed in terms of a gold number.

316 • polyphasic systems

The gold number is the weight in milligrams of added material that will prevent a change from red to violet when 1 ml of a 10 per cent sodium chloride solution is added to 10 ml of red colloidal gold sol. Gelatin has a gold number of 0.005 and acacia has a gold number of 0.1; thus, gelatin offers approximately 20 times as much protection as acacia.

If two oppositely charged hydrophilic colloids are mixed, a weak union known as a coacervate is formed between the oppositely charged hydrophilic colloids. If the coacervate separates into a distinct and new phase, the phenomenon is known as coacervation. When a sol of type A gelatin is mixed with acacia dispersion, coacervation occurs between the cationic gelatin and the anionic acacia. The extent of separation and the final charge depends on the proportions of the two hydrophilic colloids. There is a decrease in viscosity proportional to the amount of coacervate formed.

Table LXV Properties of Lyophobic and Lyophilic Colloids

Property	Lyophobic Sol	Lyophilic Sol
Composition of particles	Large number of atoms or molecules	Macromolecules, micelles
Synonyms	Suspensoid, irreversible colloid	Emulsoid, reversible colloid
Optical	Definite Tyndall cone	Diffused Tyndall cone
Viscosity	Roughly same as pure dispersion medium	Often greater than viscosity of pure dispersion medium
Surface tension	Roughly same as pure dispersion medium	Often lower than surface tension of pure dispersion medium
Electrical	Migrates in one direction in electrical field	pH of medium may effect the direction of migration
Stability to electrolytes	Precipitated by low concentrations of electrolytes	Moderately high concentrations required to salt out
Stability	Energetically unstable	Energetically stable

12 | DISPERSION PROCESSES

COLLOIDS

Lyophobic Sol

Lyophobic sols may be prepared by the condensation of molecules, atoms, or ions into colloidal aggregates or by the disintegration of coarse particles into colloidal particles. Mechanical disintegration may be accomplished in a colloid mill or a ball mill in the presence of a liquid. The colloid mill is useful for forming emulsions and breaking up weakly bonded agglomerates of solid particles, but it does not satisfactorily fracture crystals to colloidal size.

Ultrasonic generators of 200,000 cycles per minute can be used to prepare some sols. In an aqueous-liquid metal system the transversal vibrations cause the water to be pushed into the liquid metal. As the water droplet rises to the metal-water interface, it is coated with a fine film of metal. Upon reaching the interface the droplet bursts and the film of metal is colloidally dispersed into the aqueous phase. One advantage of the ultrasonic process is that no extraneous material, which might contaminate the product, is introduced during the process.

In the electric disintegration process an arc is discharged between two electrodes immersed in a liquid or the arc is discharged just above the liquid and the metallic vapor is driven into the liquid by a stream of nitrogen to form a metallic hydrosol.

Lyophobic sols can be prepared by a condensation process that has a high rate of nucleation and a low rate of crystallization. The condensation processes form a supersaturated solution from which molecules will precipitate. Conditions are selected in which there is a high rate of nucleation so that the molecules unite to form colloidal particles and not large crystals. This may be accomplished by a temperature change or by decreasing the solubility by the addition of a second solvent to promote supersaturation, which is followed by the formation of colloidal particles. Colloidal sulfur may be prepared by making a solution of sulfur in hot alcohol and by pouring the solution slowly into water. The hydrosol is stable for only a short time; however, if it is prepared in the presence of a protective colloid it will remain colloidally dispersed.

Lyophobic sols may be prepared by chemical reaction. Salts of weak acids and bases hydrolyze to form colloidal sols. The addition of a solution of ferric chloride to a large volume of boiling water rapidly hydrolyzes the salt to form a red ferric oxide hydrosol:

$$2FeCl_3 + 6H_2O \rightarrow Fe_2O_3 \cdot 3H_2O + 6HCl$$

A silver sol may be formed by the reduction of silver oxide in neutral or alkaline solution by a reducing agent, e.g., hydrogen peroxide, formaldehyde, or hydroquinone. The size of the particles depends on the concentration of the silver salt and the reducing agent. A sulfur hydrosol may be produced by the oxidation of hydrogen sulfide by sulfur dioxide. Double decomposition reactions may produce lyophobic colloids. Mercuric sulfide sols are easily produced by passing hydrogen sulfide through a solution of mercuric cyanide. In the presence of excess hydrogen sulfide, hydrosulfide ions are perferentially adsorbed, forming a stable negative hydrosol of mercuric sulfide.

Lyophobic sols are unstable in the presence of electrolytes. In chemical reactions by which hydrosols are formed, electrolytes are often a side product. To prevent precipitation of the sol, the reaction is carried out with dilute solutions and the reactants are selected so that only monovalent ions are present. If they are to be stable, most lyophobic sols must be dialyzed to remove dissolved electrolytes. In the process of dialysis the colloidal preparation to be purified is placed in a vessel with a semipermeable membrane and is immersed in flowing water. The colloidal particles cannot pass through the semipermeable membrane. The ions and molecules diffuse through the semipermeable membrane into the water, leaving a purified sol within the vessel. Dialysis may be hastened by applying a potential across the semipermeable membrane. The ions migrate out of the dialysis cell under the effect of the electrical attraction superimposed on the diffusion process. This process is known as electrodialysis. Dialysis conducted under an applied pressure is known as ultrafiltration.

Lyophobic colloids, which are protected by a hydrophilic colloid, may be dried in a vacuum. Certain colloidal silver preparations are commercially available in the dried form. They are best dispersed by sprinkling the powder on the water and allowing it to disperse.

Lyophilic Sol

Lyophilic colloids have an affinity for the dispersion medium and they can be dispersed to form sols by the same equipment and procedures used to prepare solutions. The pharmaceutical class of preparations known as mucilages illustrates the method of preparing a hydrophilic sol.

Mucilages are viscous, sticky sols made by dispersing carbohydrate macromolecules in water. Most of the gums used in mucilages are carbohydrate materials obtained from plants, e.g., acacia, agar, and pectin. Since some of the naturally occurring gums used to prepare mucilages are not pure compounds, a small portion of the gum may not form a hydrosol but may be dispersed as a suspension.

    67. Acacia, small fragments   350 g
        Benzoic acid   2 g
        Purified water, q.s.   1000 ml

        Sig.: Acacia mucilage

The acacia is washed with cold water to remove any dust or dirt. The benzoic acid, which is a antimicrobial preservative, is dissolved in warm water. The warm solution is added to the acacia. The mucilage is adjusted to final volume. After dispersion is complete, the mucilage is strained. If a more rapid method is desired, the warm benzoic acid solution is added to the powdered acacia and the mixture is triturated in a mortar until dispersion is completed.

Most of the plant gums require a considerable amount of time to hydrate. Hydration may be more rapid if the powdered gum is blended with a small amount of alcohol or glycerin. The alcohol readily wets and surrounds the particles. Upon the subsequent addition of water, the alcohol and the water hydrogen bond, and the water is drawn through the gum so that each particle is surrounded by water.

Acacia mucilage is acidic and is a negatively charged hydrophilic colloid, owing to ionization of the *d*-glucuronic acid portion of the molecule. It is precipitated by heavy metal ions, which react with the acid groups to form insoluble salts as a stringy precipitation. At concentrations exceeding 40 per cent ethanol, the acacia in acacia mucilage is dehydrated and the sol is precipitated. Other natural gums react in a similar manner.

Methylcellulose is a synthetic, nonionic hydrophilic colloid. Cellulose is insoluble in water because the intermolecular hydrogen bonding between the cellulose molecules does not leave any free hydroxyl groups for hydrogen bonding with water. When cellulose is methylated to the degree of 1.3 to 2.6 methoxyl groups per anhydroglucose unit, the methoxyl groups hinder intermolecular association of the methylcellulose molecules but permit the hydrogen bonding of the remaining hydroxyl groups with water.

A methylcellulose sol is prepared by adding one-half the required volume of boiling water to the powder mixing, and allowing the mixture to stand for several minutes. The thermal agitation ruptures any intermolecular and intramolecular hydrogen bonding so that when the remainder of the water is added as ice or chilled water the hydroxyl groups are available to hydrogen bond with the water to form a colloidal sol. A methylcellulose sol is precipitated by heat.

The mucilaginous hydrosols are used to increase the viscosity of solutions, suspensions, and emulsions. They are used as adhesive excipients in solid dosage forms. Medicinally they are used as demulcents and lubricants.

When the concentration of a surface-active agent exceeds the CMC, aggregates of colloidal size or micelles are formed. The CMC of most surface-active agents is a fraction of 1 per cent concentration; the CMC is reduced by the addition of electrolytes. The shapes of micelles vary from a spherical shape at low concentrations to laminar micelles at high concentrations. In a hydrophilic sol the nonpolar portions of the surface-active molecules are oriented toward the center of the micelle to form their own nonpolar environment, and the polar portions of the surface-active molecules are associated with the external aqueous phase. In a hydrophobic sol the orientation of the surface-active agent in the micelle is reversed. If the surface-active agent is ionic, the micelle will be charged. Counterions surround the micelle in a diffuse layer, and they tend to reduce the charge.

Colloidal dispersions of micelles are used in pharmacy to solubilize water-insoluble materials. Cresol is only soluble in water to the extent of 3 per cent. By use of high concentrations of soap, sufficient micelles are formed to permit the dispersion of 50 per cent cresol in saponated cresol solution. Although this preparation is called a solution, it is actually a colloidal dispersion of cresol within soap micelles. Oil-soluble vitamins are dispensed in aqueous multivitamin liquids as a result of solubilization by nonionic surface-active agents. The effect of the surface-active agent on therapeutic activity must be considered. Orally administered vitamin A is absorbed to a greater extent when given as a solubilized product rather than in oily solution. Although absorption from the gastrointestinal tract may be facilitated by a low concentration of a surface-active agent by virtue of lowering of interfacial tension and increasing the permeability of the cell membrane, it is conceivable that in the presence of a high concentration of a surface-active agent the drug could be held within the micelle and its availability could be decreased.

The solubilization of a substance may improve its chemical stability. Solubilized vitamin A is more stable to autoxidation than its oily solution. Solubilized benzocaine, methantheline, and homatropine are less readily hydrolyzed than their aqueous solutions.

Solubilization presents certain disadvantages. The toxicity of surface-active agents has generally limited those suitable for internal use to the nonionic surface-active agents, of which polyoxyethylene sorbitan fatty acid esters and polyoxyethylene monoalkyl ethers are chiefly used. Many surface-active agents possess an unpleasant taste, which contributes a flavor problem to formulation. Surface-active sols foam easily, and excessive agitation must be avoided in preparing and handling the liquid.

Nonionic surface-active agents in concentrations required for solubilization reduce the efficacy of many antimicrobial preservatives and antiseptics. The parabens or esters of *p*-hydroxybenzoic acid are widely used preservatives in pharmaceutical and cosmetic preparations. Sorbitan esters and polyoxyethylene sorbitan esters greatly reduce the effectiveness of the parabens, sorbic acid, and quaternary ammonium compounds. The inactivating effect of the nonionic surface-active agents is attributed to complexation or micellar solubilization of the preservative, which is then no longer present in sufficient concentration in the aqueous phase to exert an antibacterial effect. The nonionic surface-active agents have no bacteriostatic properties and require an adequate preservative. Hexachlorophene is an anti-infective agent used in preoperative scrubs. In hexachlorophene liquid soap the alkaline potassium soap reacts chemically with one of the phenolic groups to dissolve the hexachlorphene. Nonionic surface-active agents should not be used in preparing scrubbing liquids, as they inhibit the bacteriostatic activity of hexachlorophene by solubilization within the micelles.

Although solubilization of a preservative by a surface-active agent results in loss of preservative activity, the preservative may be used effectively with an increase in the concentration of preservative. In a system containing polysorbate 80 and methylparaben, the free methylparaben in the aqueous phase is in equilibrium with the solubilized methylparaben. At 5 per cent polysorbate 80, only 22 per cent of the total methylparaben is present in the aqueous phase as an effective preservative. The amount of methylparaben required to preserve this system is equal to the desired concentration of free methylparaben in the aqueous phase times the ratio of the total to free methylparaben in equilibrium. If 0.1 per cent methylparaben is required as a preservative for the aqueous phase, the total amount of methylparaben required in a system containing 5 per cent polysorbate 80 is

$$0.1 \times \frac{100}{22} = 0.45\%$$

Gel

A gel is a semisolid, colloidal system in which the movement of the dispersion medium is restricted by an interlacing network of solvated particles or macromolecules of the dispersed phase. The semisolid state is caused by the increased viscosity caused by the interlacing and consequential high internal friction. A gel will often sorb a liquid and swell. The sorption of a liquid by a gel without a measurable increase in volume is known as imbibition. The interaction between the particles of the dispersed phase may be so strong that upon standing the dispersion medium is squeezed out of the gel in droplets. The shrinkage of a gel with a simultaneous extrusion of liquid is known as syneresis.

Although organic gels consist of solvated macromolecules in conceivably a single phase, the macromolecules are held in an interlacing network by strong polar forces. Frequently, a gel may be formed from a hydrophilic sol: by using a higher concentration of the hydrocolloid, by a change of dispersion medium, or by lowering the temperature. As a hot 2 per cent gelatin sol cools, the gelatin macromolecules lose kinetic energy. With a reduction of kinetic energy the gelatin macromolecules are associated through dipole-dipole interaction into elongated aggregates. The number of these associations increases until the dispersion medium is held in the interstices of the interlacing network of gelatin macromolecules, and the viscosity increases to that of a semisolid. Most pharmaceutical gums, e.g., agar, algin, pectin, and tragacanth, form gels by the same mechanism as gelatin.

68.
Ephedrine sulfate	10.0 g
Tragacanth	10.0 g
Methyl salicylate	0.1 ml
Eucalyptol	1.0 ml
Pine needle oil	0.1 ml
Glycerin	150.0 g
Purified water	830.0 ml

Sig.: Ephedrine sulfate jelly

The ephedrine sulfate is dissolved in the water. The glycerin, tragacanth, and other ingredients are added and mixed well. The mixture is kept in a closed container for 1 week with occasional agitation. The hydration and swelling of tragacanth is slow and requires agitation. The viscosity of ephedrine sulfate jelly may vary according to the type of tragacanth used. The temperature and process of manufacture affect the rapidity of hydration and the final viscosity. The viscosity may change upon aging of the gel.

69.
Starch	100 g
Benzoic acid	2 g
Purified water	200 g
Glycerin	700 g

Sig.: Starch glycerite

The starch and benzoic acid are rubbed in the water to a smooth mixture. The glycerin is added and mixed. The mixture is heated on a sand bath to 140° with constant, gentle agitation until a translucent mass forms. The heat ruptures the starch grains and permits the water to reach and hydrate the starch. Starch is composed of linear and branched molecules which upon hydration trap the dispersion medium in the interstices, forming a gel.

Inorganic gels consist of aggregates of inorganic colloidal particles. Bentonite is a colloidal hydrated aluminum silicate that is insoluble in water. Veegum® and bentonite are both a montmorillonite type of clay in which the units in the structure of the clay are held together by weak O-O association. In the presence of water these weak O-O associations are broken to an extent, and the clay sorbs water. As water is sorbed into its structure, the clay swells and effectively the particles are spread out; the interference with particulate movement results in an increase in viscosity. The amount of free water is reduced as the water dipole is oriented in some manner with the swollen particles and is not free to move at random. In concentrations exceeding 4.3 per cent bentonite, these effects produce a thixotropic gel, which makes it a useful suspending agent.

A therapeutic magma is an inorganic gel intended for oral administration. Some of the particles are larger than colloidal size, and upon prolonged standing a supernatant liquid may form. Thus, a magma should be shaken before use. Magmas are made by simple hydration or by chemical reaction. If chemical reaction is employed the solutions should be hot and highly diluted in order to obtain colloidal particles.

70. Bentonite   50 g
    Purified water, q.s.   1000 ml

    Sig.: Bentonite magma

The bentonite is sprinkled on 800 ml of hot purified water. It is allowed to hydrate for 24 hours with occasional stirring. Then purified water is added to make 1000 ml. If a mechanical blender is used, approximately one-half of the water is placed in the blender, and the bentonite is added while the blender is in operation. Purified water is then added to make the volume of 1000 ml, and the blender is operated for 10 minutes.

Bismuth magma is an inorganic gel resulting from chemical reaction.

71. Bismuth   80 g
    Nitric acid   120 ml
    Ammonium carbonate   10 g
    Stronger ammonia solution
    Purified water, each, q.s.   1000 ml

    Sig.: Bismuth magma

The bismuth subnitrate is dissolved in 60 ml of purified water and 60 ml of nitric acid and is converted to bismuth nitrate by heating:

$$Bi(OH)_2 NO_3 + 2HNO_3 \rightarrow Bi(NO_3)_3 + 2H_2O$$

The bismuth nitrate solution is poured into 5000 ml of water containing 60 ml of nitric acid. A solution of ammonium carbonate is prepared in a 12-liter vessel by dissolving the ammonium carbonate in 160 ml of strong ammonia solution diluted with 4300 ml of water. The bismuth nitrate solution is quickly mixed with the ammonium carbonate solution with agitation. A white flocculant precipitate of bismuth hydroxide and subcarbonate is formed:

$$Bi(NO_3)_3 + 3NH_4OH \rightarrow Bi(OH)_3 + NH_4NO_3$$
$$4Bi(NO_3)_3 + 6(NH_4)_2CO_3 + H_2O \rightarrow (BiO)_2CO_3 \cdot H_2O + 12NH_4NO_3 + 4CO_2$$

322 • dispersion processes

After the precipitate has settled it is purified of ammonium nitrate and the excess alkalinity of ammonia water and ammonium carbonate by washing it with water until the washings are no longer alkaline to phenolphthalein. The moist magma is drained and adjusted to 1000 ml with purified water and mixed thoroughly.

Bismuth magma is used as an astringent antacid. Other inorganic gels used as antacids are milk of magnesia, aluminum hydroxide gel, aluminum phosphate gel, and dihydroxyaluminum aminoacetate magma. All gels should be packaged in wide-mouthed containers.

AEROSOLS

An aerosol is a colloidal dispersion of a liquid or a solid in a gas. Nasopharyngeal medication and oral inhalation medication may be administered in the form of an aerosol. Pharmaceutical aerosols may be produced by a manual spray process or from a pressurized package.

Sprays

Various instruments have been used to apply finely divided particles to the nasopharyngeal region and the respiratory tract. An atomizer is an instrument used to disperse a liquid in a fine spray. When the valved rubber bulb of the vacuum atomizer shown in Figure 137 is squeezed, a stream of air moves through the tube. According to the Bernoulli principle, the stream of air moving at a high velocity causes a lowering of pressure at the tip of the dip tube. The liquid is forced up the dip tube by the atmospheric pressure, and it is broken up in to a spray when it meets the air stream from the tube connected to the bulb. The droplets of the spray are coarse, and consequently they are carried only to the nasal passage and the pharynx.

A finer spray is produced by a pressure atomizer. When the rubber bulb of the pressure atomizer shown in Figure 138 is squeezed, part of the air stream produced is directed into the container to produce a pressure greater than the atmospheric pressure. This pressure plus that due to the Bernoulli effect forces the liquid up the dip tube. When the liquid emerging from the tip of the dip tube meets the air stream, it is dispersed as a spray.

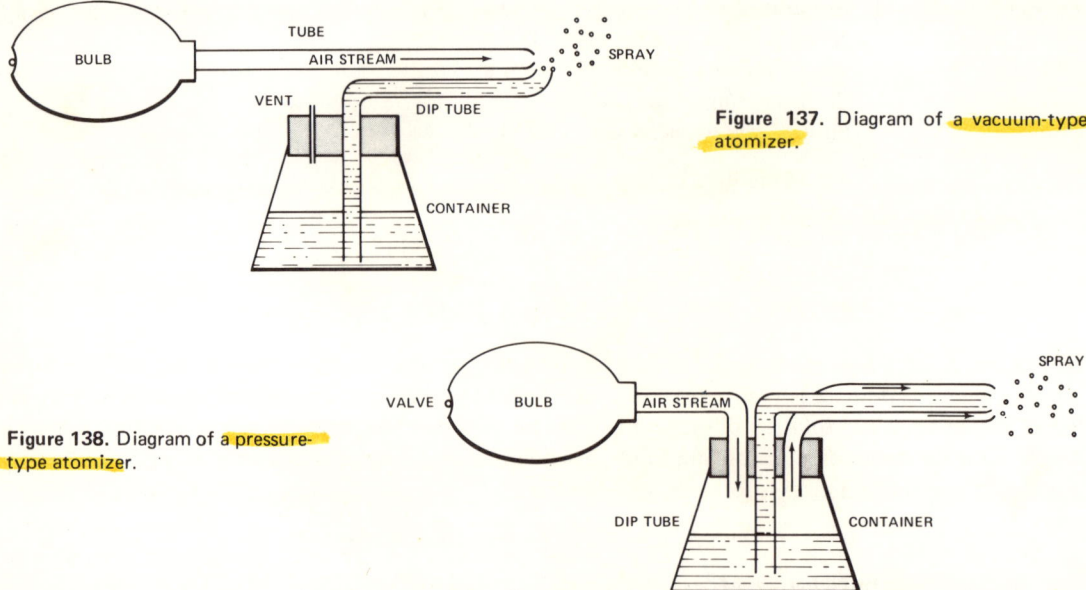

Figure 137. Diagram of a vacuum-type atomizer.

Figure 138. Diagram of a pressure-type atomizer.

Plastic spray bottles dispense a spray in the same manner as a pressure atomizer. When the flexible container is squeezed, the air is compressed. The increased pressure within the container forces the liquid up a dip tube into the tip, where a stream of air is being directed simultaneously.

A powder blower or insufflator consists of a rubber bulb connected to a container and a delivery pipe. When the bulb is squeezed, air is blown into the container and simultaneously causes turbulence in the powder and carries some of the fine particles out through the delivery tube in a stream of air. The size of the solid aerosol depends on the original size of the powder. The solid aerosol may be delivered into the ear or vagina or it may be inhaled through the mouth or nares.

A nebulizer is a small vacuum type of atomizer within a curved chamber. Any large droplets produced strike the chamber and drop back into the container to be processed again. The fine droplets are carried out in the air stream. The nebulizer is placed in the mouth, and the patient inhales as he squeezes the bulb. An inhalation is a preparation to be administered as a nebulized spray which reaches the respiratory tract. If the inhalation is to reach the bronchides, the particles of the spray must be from 1 to 5 μ.

72.
Isoetharine hydrochloride	1.00 g
Phenylephrine hydrochloride	0.25 g
Thenyldiamine hydrochloride	0.10 g
Sodium chloride	0.30 g
Sodium bisulfite	0.30 g
Methylparaben	0.02 g
Propylparaben	0.01 g
Purified water, q.s.	100 ml

Sig.: Asthma inhalation: Spray by use of hand nebulizer

A vaporizer is an electrical instrument that produces moist steam with or without medication for inhalation. It is used to soothe upper respiratory irritations, but it is ineffective in carrying medication to the respiratory tract.

An inhaler is a cylindrical container holding a drug possessing a high vapor pressure. It is fitted with a cap to retard the loss of medication. When it is used, the cap is removed and the inhaler is inserted into a nostril. As the patient inhales, the air passes through the inhaler and carries the vapor of the medication into the nasal passage. This is not a colloidal dispersion but a solution of the vapor in air.

Pressurized Packages

With the widespread use of pressurized packaging the term "aerosol" has become a household word. To the laity an aerosol is a self-contained sprayable product in which the propelling force is supplied by a liquefied or compressed gas. The therapeutic aerosols used in pharmacy are pressurized-package products containing therapeutically active ingredients dissolved, suspended, or emulsified in a propellant or a mixture of a solvent and a propellant; they are intended for either topical administration or for inhalation into the nasopharynegeal region or bronchopulmonary system.

Operation. A liquefied gas sealed in a container is in equilibrium with its vapor phase. The vapor pressure is exerted equally in all directions and is independent of the amount of liquid phase present. When the aerosol valve is opened by pressing the actuator button, the pressure forces the liquid in which the drug is dissolved or dispersed up the dip tube and through the valve orifice. Since the boiling point of the propellant is lower than room temperature, the propellant vaporizes instantly and leaves a spray of colloidal particles when it comes in contact with the atmosphere. The head space, i.e., volume in upper portion of container not filled with liquid, progressively increases as the product is used; however, the remaining propellant vaporizes and maintains a constant pressure.

dispersion processes

A diagram of a two-phase therapeutic aerosol is shown in Figure 139. A two-phase aerosol consists of the vapor phase of the propellant and the liquid phase, which consists of the active ingredients dissolved in the propellant or a mixture of the propellant and a solvent.

73. Octyl nitrite   1%
    Propellants 12/114   99%

    Sig.: Inhale for angina attack

Dissolve the octyl nitrite in the propellants. Fill into a plastic-coated glass vial with a metering valve.

Often the medicinal compound is not soluble in the propellant and a cosolvent must be employed. Such cosolvents must be nontoxic and nonirritating. Alcohol, glycerin, propylene glycol, and ethyl acetate have been used as cosolvents.

In aerosol technology a suspension of a medicinal compound, e.g., antibiotics, steroids, or ergotamine, in a propellant is classified as a two-phase system, although a vapor, liquid, and solid phase exist. In these systems isopropyl myristate is sometimes used as a dispersing agent.

74. Neomycin sulfate   0.50%
    Sorbitan trioleate   0.25%
    Propellants 11/12/114   99.25%

    Sig.: Neomycin aerosol

The neomycin sulfate is mixed with the sorbitan trioleate, which acts as a dispersing agent. It is filled into containers and filled with the propellant.

A three-phase system as shown in Figure 140 usually contains water, which is not miscible with the propellant. A three-phase aerosol consists of the vapor phase of the propellant, the liquid phase of the propellant, and the aqueous solution of the medicinal compounds. The length of the dip tube is adjusted so that it dips into the aqueous layer. Generally a three-phase aerosol operates at 15 psi at 21°. Only a small amount of propellant is used. The absence of propellant from the dispensed solution requires a small valve orifice to mechanically produce a spray.

A foam aerosol consists of a three-phase system in which the liquefied propellant is partially emulsified. When the valve is opened, the emulsion is forced up the dip tube. As the emulsion contacts the atmosphere, the propellant vaporizes and produces a thick foam. In foam aerosols only 6 to 10 per

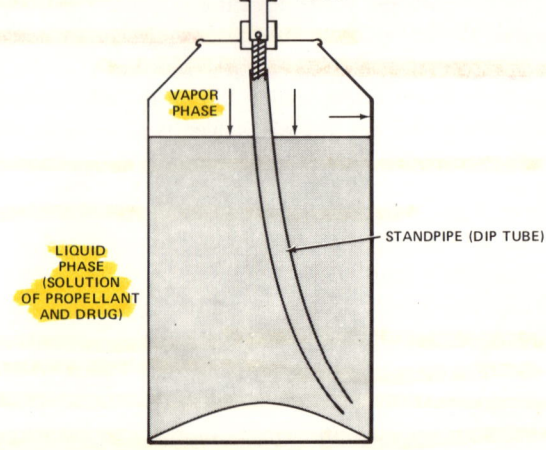

Figure 139. Diagrammatic representation of a two-phase aerosol.

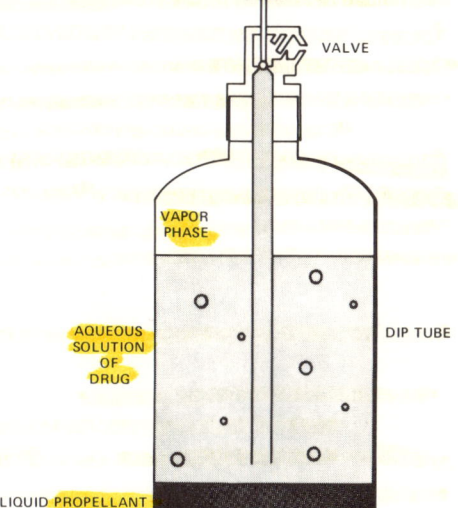

Figure 140. Diagrammatic representation of a three-phase aerosol.

cent propellant is used at 40 psi at 21°. The aerosol should be shaken before use, as it is an emulsion. If the container is used in an inverted position, the dip tube may be eliminated. Medicinal foam aerosols are used to dispense foams topically with little irritation. The following aerosol is formulated to produce a foam that quickly collapses, leaving a thin layer of the solution of the medicinal compounds.

75. Polawax® (stearyl alcohol and a
    condensation product of ethylene
    oxide and a fatty compound) . . . . 1.5% ⎫
    Resorcinol . . . . 3.0% ⎪
    Salicylic acid . . . . 1.5% ⎬ 92%
    Alcohol . . . . 59.0% ⎪
    Water . . . . 35.0% ⎭
    Propellant 12/114 (20:80) 8%

    Sig.: Acne remedy

A recently designed aerosol dispensing system separates the propellant from the product. Its design is based on the Bernoulli effect, and its operation is similar to a vacuum-type atomizer. It consists of a propellant cartridge contained within a nonpressurized outer package that contains the product. The system is controlled by a three-way valve. When the valve is depressed, it releases the propellant vapor from the inner cartridge. The vapor passes through a spray cone, and by the Bernoulli effect the product is siphoned through the dip tube and is carried along in the stream of vapor as a spray. Simultaneously, air enters the outer package, replacing the expelled product. When the valve is released, the system is sealed.

Since the outer package containing the product is not under pressure, a wide variety of materials and designs may be used in the composition of the package. The separation of the product and the propellant avoids incompatibilities and allows the packaging as an aerosol of products with a high water content. As the propellant is not contained in the product and is entirely available to expel the product, the separation of the product and the propellant permits the use of large packages.

The spray pattern of an aerosol may be classified as a space spray, surface spray, or aerated spray. The space spray consists of particles that are less than 50 μ and remain airborne. A space spray is generally used with oral inhalations, bactericides, and room deodorants. The surface spray contains particles that are greater than 50 μ, and it is generally used to deposit a wet surface film. A surface spray is used to apply topical medication, adhesive-tape remover, and hair sprays. The aerated spray consists of a foam; it is widely used in cosmetic aerosols. All three types of spray patterns may be produced by a two-phase system using liquefied gas propellants.

The spray pattern is influenced by the concentration of the propellant, the vapor pressure, and the valve mechanism. In general, a high percentage of propellant produces a space spray, and a low percentage produces a surface spray. Propellant solutions containing a greater percentage of high-boiling propellant tend to produce a surface spray. With foams, propellants with higher vapor pressures tend to produce a stiffer and more elastic foam than with low vapor pressures.

Propellants. The main function of the propellant is to provide the force to expel the material. The characteristics of the expelled material are influenced by the propellant. Propellants may be classified as liquefied gases or compressed gases.

The liquefied-gas propellants have a low boiling point and vapor pressure. With liquefied-gas propellants the pressure within the container is determined by the vapor pressure of the propellant. Thus, liquefied-gas propellants have the advantage over compressed-gas propellants of providing a constant pressure as long as a small quantity of the propellant remains in the container.

The liquefied-gas propellants used in pharmaceutical aerosols are fluorinated chlorohydrocarbons, i.e., substituted methane or ethane derivatives. They are nontoxic and nonirritating; however, each product must be studied for toxicity if it is for oral or inhalation use. Although they are nonflammable, the flammability of the complete formulation must be considered. The wide range of vapor pressures of the propellants permits the attainment of selected pressures by the use of mixtures. Some important physical properties of some of the most common propellants are listed in Table LXVI. The fluorinated chlorohydrocarbons are miscible with most nonpolar solvents, but they are insoluble in water. In aqueous systems alcohol is often used as a cosolvent. Generally a mixture of propellants is used to obtain the best solvent and vapor-pressure properties of the individual formulation.

The nomenclature of the fluorinated chlorohydrocarbons is simplified by the use of three digits. The right digit represents the number of fluorine atoms. The second digit from the right is one more than the number of hydrogen atoms in the compound. The third digit from the right is one less than the number of carbon atoms in the compound. Thus, monofluorotrichloromethane is known as propellant-11. With isomers the most symmetrical compound is only numbered; as the isomers become less symmetrical the number is followed by a letter. If the compound is cyclic, the number is preceded by C.

Although the fluorinated chlorohydrocarbons are relatively inert, propellant-11 is subjected to hydrolysis and alcoholysis, which produce acids that corrode the metal container and valve.

Nitrogen, carbon dioxide, and nitrous oxide are used as compressed-gas propellants. Although compressed gases are used in food aerosols, they are infrequently used in pharmaceutical aerosols. The expansion of the compressed gas in the container forces the contents from the container. The compressed gases do not have the dispersing power of the liquefied gases. Therefore, a mechanical-breakup actuator is used to produce a fine spray. Nitrous oxide and carbon dioxide are soluble compressed gases. If the propellant is soluble in the formulation, an aerated spray or foam is produced. If the compressed-gas propellant is insoluble in the formulation, the material is expelled in a liquid stream having the same consistency as it did in the container. As the aerosol is used, the pressure within the container is progressively decreased. Thus, it is necessary to have a large headspace and a high initial pressure to have sufficient pressure to empty the container.

Nitrogen is the most commonly used compressed-gas propellant. The insolubility of nitrogen permits the dispensing of pharmaceuticals, e.g., multivitamin liquids and cough syrups, in a liquid stream in its original form. Since the nitrogen is insoluble and the product is intended to be dispensed in a stream, the aerosol should not be shaken before use. Nitrogen is a suitable propellant for oral use, as it is nontoxic, colorless, tasteless, and odorless. The chemical inertness of the nitrogen protects the formula-

dispersion processes • 327

Table LXVI Properties of Halogenated Hydrocarbon Propellants

Propellant	Formula	Vapor Pressure (psig) at:		Boiling Point (°C)	Density at $21°$ (g cc^{-1})	Solubility of Water in Propellant at $21°$ (% w/v)	Toxicity*
		21°	55°				
-22	CHClF$_2$	122.5	298.8	-40.8	1.209	0.12	5A
-12	CCl$_2$F$_2$	70.2	181.0	-29.8	1.325	0.08	6
-152a	CH$_3$CHF$_2$	61.7	176.3	-24.0	0.911	0.170	5A
-142b	CH$_3$CClF$_2$	29.1	97.3	-9.4	1.118	0.054	5A
-C318	C$_4$F$_8$	25.4	92.0	-6.1	1.513	0.014	6
-114	CClF$_2$CClF$_2$	12.9	58.8	3.6	1.468	0.008	6
-21	CHCl$_2$F	8.4	50.4	8.9	1.376	0.13	5
-11	CCl$_3$F	2.6	24.3	23.7	1.485	0.009	5A

* Underwriters' Laboratories rating: 6 shows no evidence of toxic effect; groups 5 and lower have progressively greater toxicity.

tion from oxidation and allows the use of aluminum containers. Nitrogen does not produce the cooling effect that occurs with the liquefied gases. In a liquid-stream aerosol nitrogen is used at 90 psi to operate a two-phase system.

Containers and Valves. Pharmaceutical aerosols use metal, glass, and plastic containers. Although steel may be coated with tin or a plastic film to reduce corrosion and prolong shelf life, glass containers are more appealing as they eliminate corrosion and contamination by metal. Glass containers protected by a coat of plastic are popular. The plastic coating adds resilience to the container and lessens breakage. If a plastic-coated bottle breaks, the glass fragments are retained within the plastic coat and a small hole in the plastic allows the gas to escape harmlessly.

The valve promptly controls the start and stop of flow. In regualting the flow the valve influences the characteristics of the spray. A standard valve is suitable for all space and surface sprays if the pressure is not less than 30 psi at 21°. The valve consists of an actuator button, valve core, gasket, and dip tube, as shown in Figure 141. The core is seated in a rubber valve seat. Two orifices, which are 180° apart, extend through the walls of the core into a groove that circles the lower end of the core. The valve seat is connected to the dip tube. The gasket prevents the liquid phase from flowing by sealing the valve when it is closed. The actuator has a spray orifice and provides a means of operating the valve. When the actuator is pushed, the valve core is tilted from the seat at the lower corner. The groove is uncovered and allows the material to rise up the dip tube, pass the orifice, rise through the core, and spray out through the terminal orifice. The size of the terminal orifice determines the fineness of the spray. When the finger pressure is removed from the actuator, the core returns to the closed position due to the elasticity of the rubber seat.

Spray valves have several orifices, which open into a series of expansion chambers. The rate of discharge is controlled by the size of the smallest internal orifice. As the material passes through the first orifice into the expansion chamber, the pressure decreases sufficiently to cause expansion and boiling. As the material passes through the successive orifices, the additional expansion and violent boiling produce colloidal particles that are carried out as a spray. For space spray patterns an orifice of 0.02 in. in diameter is used.

Valves with breakup spray buttons are required for three-phase systems, which are not foams, and for two-phase systems in which the liquid phase consists only of the product. Valves used for compressed gases have a large orifice and dip tube to permit the flow of viscous liquids in an uninterrupted

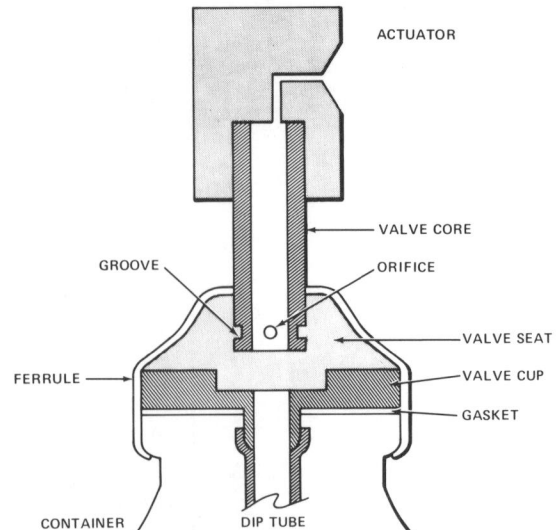

Figure 141. Cross section of an aerosol valve.

stream. A foam valve has one expansion orifice and one expansion chamber, which serves as a delivery nozzle. The orifice of a foam valve may have a diameter as large as 0.3 in. In powder aerosols the material should be insoluble in the propellant so that crystal growth during storage is minimized. To ensure a flow and to prevent clogging a particle size of less than 200 mesh is used and the valve is operated wide open.

Metering valves, which deliver a measured amount of spray, are frequently used for medicinal aerosols. In one type, two valves are separated by a metering chamber. The valves operate together on the upstrokes and downstrokes of the valve controls. On the downstroke the formulation is admitted to the metering chamber and the valve at the dispensing end is closed. On the upstroke the dispensing valve is opened and the other valve is closed. The volume of the metering chamber determines the quantity of the individual spray. In another type of metering valve the dip tube contains a steel ball, which operates between a lower stop and a ball valve seat at the upper level. When the valve is actuated, the expelled material carries the ball up the tube until the ball is seated in the valve seat, at which no more formulation can flow up the dip tube. When the actuator is released, the ball returns to its lower position in the tube.

Filling. A propellant may be liquefied by lowering its temperature below its boiling point or by increasing the pressure. One of these conditions is used in each of the methods of filling aerosol containers. In the cold-fill method, the propellant is cooled below its boiling point to approximately -30 to -40° and the formulation is cooled to approximately -20°. The cooled formulation is quantitatively filled into the container, and then the cooled propellant is added. The temperature is selected so that enough propellant is vaporized to displace the air without excessive loss of propellant. The container is then sealed by crimping the valve in place. In some formulations the propellant and the formulation may be premixed and filled in one operation. The cold-filling method is used in most fluorinated chlorohydrocarbon aerosols. It is faster and offers less chance of entrapment of air than the pressure-fill method. The cold-fill method cannot be used to package aqueous aerosols, as the water would freeze at the low temperatures employed.

In the pressure-fill method the fluorinated chlorohydrocarbon propellant is metered under pressure into the aerosol container through its valve at room temperature. The formulation at room temperature is quantitatively delivered by a filling tube into the container and the valve is inserted and crimped into position. The propellant is metered by volume as a liquid by maintaining it under pressure. In commercial filling the trapped air may be removed by a vacuum system.

In the pressure-fill method using compressed gases, the compressed gas is filled through the valve by a pressure regulator until the desired pressure is obtained. The formulation is quantitatively measured into the container, the valve is crimped to the container, and the gas is added. Air may be removed by a vacuum or be displaced by flushing with the gas prior to sealing the container.

The pressure-fill method can be used with all aerosols. It is a slower process than the cold-filling method. Loss of propellant is insignificant in the pressure-fill method. Since no refrigeration is required, the pressure-fill method is suitable for water-based formulations. Anhydrous filling of aerosols is also done by this method.

Unless the formulation is thermolabile, all aerosols are heated to 55° in a water bath to test the strength of the container and for leakage.

Uses. Pharmaceutical aerosols are compact packages that are ready for instant self-administration with a minimal manual contact with the medication. As the container is sealed, the formulation is protected from any degrading effects of the atmosphere and from contamination by microorganism. An accurate dosage may be delivered by means of a metering valve.

Inhalation aerosols are those used to administer medicinal agents into the respiratory system. The particle size determines the site of deposition and the effectiveness of the inhalation aerosol. Particles larger than 60 μ are deposited in the trachea, and those larger that 20 μ do not reach the bronchioles. Particles of approximately 1 μ often remain airborne and are expired. Sympathomimetic drugs, e.g., isoproterenol and epinephrine, in aerosols are effective in dilation of bronchi for immediate relief by systemic action. Ergotamine tartrate administered as a powder aerosol provides systemic relief from migraine headaches. With drugs absorbed directly from the respiratory system there is no decomposition, which might occur if the drug were given orally.

Most pharmaceutical aerosols are for topical use. Their popularity is probably due to the elimination of much of the waste and messiness associated with the application of topical products. The topical aerosol delivers a thin uniform film without the use of painful application to an injured area. The rapid evaporation and cooling may be therapeutically desirable. For topical use a quick-break foam, which collapses quickly and allows the spread of a thin layer, is used to avoid rubbing. A stabilized foam is used when penetration is to be enhanced by rubbing. In a stabilized foam approximately 2 to 20 times as much surface-active agent is used as in a quick-break foam.

SUSPENSIONS

A suspension or a dispersion of a solid in a liquid is energetically unstable. Systems of high energy tend to lose energy to their environment until an equilibrium is reached where there is no difference in free surface energy. When a solid is reduced to a small particle size, the specific surface is greatly increased and the solid has a high free surface energy. The particles with a high free surface energy tend to clump in a manner that reduces the surface area and the free surface energy. When the particles interact to form clumps or aggregates, the process is known as flocculation or agglomeration. The dispersion of aggregates into individual particles is known as deflocculation. As the aggregates or flocs settle as if they were large single particles, the smaller particles of a deflocculated suspension settle more slowly.

The change in free surface energy, ΔG, upon subdivision of a solid in a liquid is

$$\Delta G = \gamma dS$$

where γ is the interfacial tension between the liquid and the solid phase and dS is the change in surface area. A suspension approaches an energetically stable state as $\Delta G \to 0$. Stability could be obtained by a reduction in specific surface; however, this would result in a loss of valuable pharmaceutical and therapeutical properties of the suspension. Thus, the pharmacist can increase the stability of a suspension by reducing the interfacial tension. The interfacial tension can be reduced by the addition of a surface-active agent; however, it cannot be reduced to zero and the suspension will eventually flocculate. The role of the pharmacist is to develop a formulation that possesses the desired medicinal and pharmaceutical properties and does not aggregate for the duration of its use.

In addition to lowering the interfacial tension, the adsorbed surface-active agent may coat the particles and prevent agglomeration. This mechanical protection is afforded by nonelectrolytes as well as by electrolytes. A surface-active agent may also stabilize a suspension by imparting a charge to the particles without the formation of a protective coat. The interparticular interactions are reduced by the repulsive action of the charge associated with each particle. Soap is an example of an ionic surface-active agent that combines both effects. In aqueous suspensions the charge and the adsorbed protective film contribute to the formation and stability. The agglomeration and caking of such a system involves not only a reduction of ζ potential but also a desorption of the protective film.

Preparation of Suspensions

The first step in the manual preparation of suspensions is to triturate the drugs to a fine powder in a mortar. If the drugs are easily wetted by the vehicle, a small volume of the vehicle is added to the powdered drugs, and the mixture is triturated to a smooth slurry. The slurry is transferred to a graduate. The mortar is rinsed with successive portions of the vehicle, and the rinsings are transferred to the graduate. The suspension is adjusted to final volume by gradually adding the vehicle with stirring.

To obtain a uniform dispersion of the solids, the initial dispersion must be properly done. If a powder is not readily wetted or has adsorbed a layer of air, it will float on the surface of the dispersion medium. Wetting agents are useful in reducing the interfacial tension between the liquid and the solid so that the air can be displaced and the particles wetted. Alcohol penetrates the voids between the particles and displace the air. Then during the blending process the water hydrogen bonds with the alcohol and rapidly gains access to and wets the particles. Glycerin, propylene glycol, and suitable surface-active agents may be used in a similar manner to aid in the rapid dispersion of the particles without producing excessive lumps.

Kaolin mixture with pectin is a suspension that contains two negatively charged, hydrophilic colloids. The pectin and tragacanth are suspending agents that increase the viscosity and slow the rate of sedimentation of the kaolin. The pectin and tragacanth also probably act as a protective colloid; they are adsorbed about the kaolin particles in a mechanical and electrical barrier which reduces interparticular interactions.

76. Kaolin 200.00 g
Pectin 10.00 g
Tragacanth, powdered 5.00 g
Benzoic acid 2.00 g
Sodium saccharin 1.00 g
Glycerin 20.00 ml
Peppermint oil 0.75 ml
Purified water, q.s. 1000 ml

Sig.: Kaolin mixture and pectin

The kaolin is mixed with 500 ml of water. The pectin, tragacanth, and sodium saccharin are triturated with glycerin to hasten hydration without the formation of lumps upon the addition of water. Three hundred milliters of boiling water, which contains the benzoic acid as a preservative, is added with agitation to the suspending agents. After the mixture has cooled, the flavor and the kaolin-water mixture is added and thoroughly blended. Purified water is added to adjust to final volume.

The industrial equipment used in preparing fluid polyphasic systems provides a high-shear mixing. In general, similar equipment, e.g., colloid mill, homogenizer, or turbine mixer, is utilized to manufacture both suspensions and emulsions. The small-scale equipment used in the laboratory often supplies a very high work input compared to production-scale equipment. A laboratory stirrer consisting of one or more propellers on a common shaft will readily prepare a fluid polyphasic system. The Waring Blendor is useful in preparing small volumes of polyphasic liquid, although it incorporates a large amount of air. In industrial production the propeller type of mixer is usually inadequate because the surface-to-volume ratio is low, the speed of agitation is low, the tendency to form a vortex and foam is great, and local overheating may occur.

Turbine Mixer. The use of baffles adjacent to an impeller increases the efficiency of agitation. A turbine mixer consists of a high-speed rotor equipped with impeller vanes or blades and a stator ring or a housing with openings, as shown in Figure 142. A stator ring consists of blades mounted on a ring that has an inner diameter that is slightly larger than the turbine impeller. The centrifugal force of the rotor draws the material downward to produce a continuous top-to-bottom circulation without a large vortex. The material moving at a high velocity from the impeller strikes the stator blades, giving rise to a high degree of shearing action or turbulent eddy currents, which are localized near the center of the mixing vessel. A turbine mixer for the pharmacy has been realized in the Waring Blendor fitted with a Polytron® assembly, which consists of a three-bladed rotor within an eight-slotted stator.

332 • dispersion processes

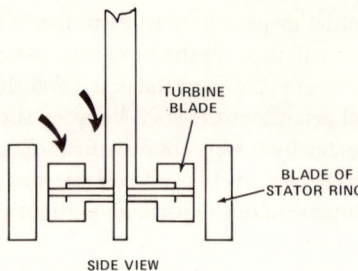

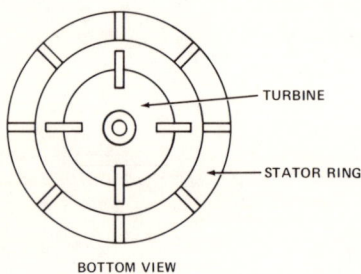

Figure 142. Turbine impeller fitted with a stator ring having blades.

Colloid Mill. A colloid mill consists of a high-speed rotor and stator with a narrow clearance that may be adjusted. In general, the material is fed by gravity to the center of the rotor. Interfacial tension causes part of the liquid to adhere to and to rotate with the rotor. Centrifugal force throws part of the liquid across the rotor onto the stator. At some region between the rotor and stator, as shown in Figure 143, the motion imparted to the liquid by the rotor ceases. In this region hydraulic shear causes the shearing of the particles and the breaking up of aggregates. At peripheral speeds of 7,000 to 20,000 ft min^{-1}, it is not mechanically possible to decrease the clearance between the rotor and stator to less than 0.63 μ. Since the particle size of the dispersed phase that has been passed through a colloid mill is of magnitude 0.1 μ, the shearing action of the mill is not solely due to the mechanical shear of the rotor and stator, which are usually from 0.005 to 0.050 in. apart. The dispersed phase of a product processed by a colloid mill has a narrow size frequency distribution, owing to the fixed clearance. The milled product is discharged through an outlet in the periphery of the housing and is frequently recycled.

Figure 143. Colloid mill with vertical rotor.

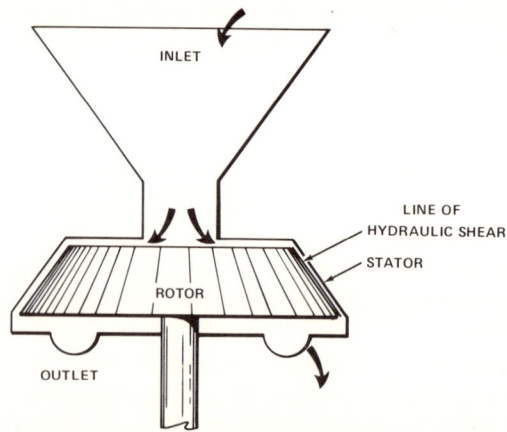

A colloid mill tends to draw in air and disperse it in the polyphasic system. Since the rotor may be operated horizontally or vertically, aeration can be reduced by the use of a vertical rotor, which best seals the point where the rotor shaft enters the housing and keeps the rotor and stator always in contact with liquid. Many variations of the colloid mill exist. The surface of the rotor and stator may be serrated or toothed to increase hydraulic and interparticular shear. There are multiple-rotor mills. Colloid mills are designed so that the liquid flows concurrent with the centrifugal force of the rotor or against it. As a guide, viscous materials up to 10,000 cp are processed in a colloid mill having concurrent flow and are operated between 5,000 and 7,500 ft min^{-1}. A countercurrent flow at a maximum speed of 10,000 ft min^{-1} is common for systems with a viscosity less than 2,000 cp. The size reduction and dispersion by a colloid mill depends on the clearance between the rotor and stator, the peripheral velocity of the rotor, and the viscosity of the polyphasic system.

In any milling process much of the energy expended is wasted as heat. Colloid mills are jacketed so that circulating water can be used to remove excessive heat. Even with cooling the temperature of the polyphasic system may rise from 15 to 25°. Viscous systems passed through a colloid mill with a narrow clearance produce heat. Dilatant materials may flow freely into the mill, but they may stall the mill or overheat the product under the high shearing rate of the mill. A colloid mill should not be used for dilatant materials.

Homogenizer. A homogenizer consists of a high-pressure pump and a spring-seated valve having a small orifice, as shown in Figure 144. At a pressure from 500 to 5,000 psi the liquid passes under the valve seat and may attain a velocity of 57,000 ft min^{-1} as it passes through the orifice. Agglomerates elongate and break up as shear, cavitation, and turbulence are applied. The particles then impinge on the impact

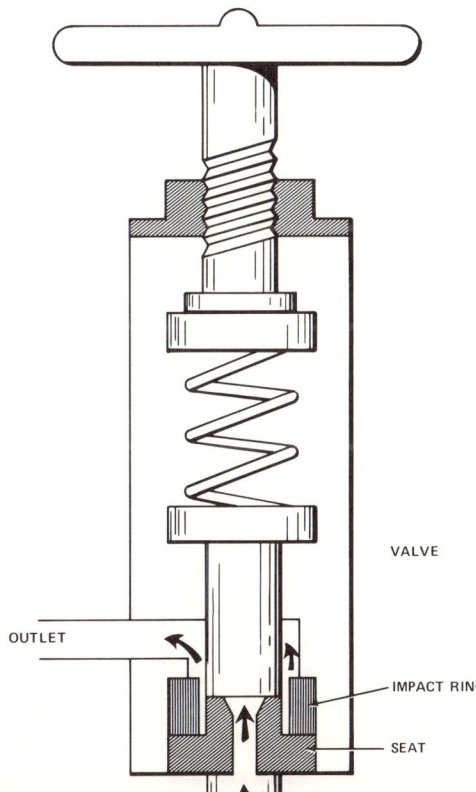

Figure 144. Single-stage homogenizer.

ring and shatter into particles as small as 0.02 μ. Initial homogenization may produce the desired size reduction, but subsequent agglomeration often occurs. A second homogenization at a lower pressure will break up these agglomerates. Two- and three-stage homogenizers are often used in processing pharmaceutical polyphasic systems. Hand-operated homogenizers are available for preparing small volumes of suspensions and emulsions in a pharmacy.

The energy available in a homogenizer is greater than that of a colloid mill. With comparable formulations, homogenizers usually produce a wider size frequency distribution and an average particle size from one-third to one-sixth that of a colloid mill. The temperature rise during homogenization is less, i.e., 5 to 15°, than in a colloid mill. A homogenizer is more efficient at viscosities up to 200 cp and less efficient at viscosities exceeding 1000 cp than the colloid mill. A comparison of the three types of high-shear mixers is given in Table LXVII.

Table LXVII Comparison of High-Shear Mixing Equipment for Processing Suspensions and Emulsions

	Turbine Mixer	Colloid Mill	Homogenizer
Abrasive material	Suitable	Suitable	Ruins valves
Capacity	Fixed	Depends on clearance and viscosity	Constant regardless of pressure and viscosity
Foam	Incorporates air and foams	Incorporates air and foams	Little aeration or foaming
Mechanical speed	High	High	Low
Radio of particle size	12	3	1
Temperature rise	Low	High	Low
Viscosity	Suitable for low viscosity only	Suitable for low and high viscosities	Suitable for low to moderate viscosities

EMULSIONS

An emulsion is a polyphasic system of two immiscible liquids, one of which is dispersed by the aid of an emulsifying agent throughout the other liquid in particles ranging from 0.2 to 50 μ in diameter. When two immiscible liquids are agitated together, the liquids break up into small droplets, with an increase in the total surface area of each liquid. The free surface energy associated with the increased surface area is supplied by the mechanical energy of agitation. The work of dispersion, W, may be expressed as

$$W = \gamma \, dS$$

where γ is the interfacial tension and dS is the change in surface area.

Since the interfacial tension is a measure of the force to be overcome in mixing two immiscible liquids, any substance that lowers interfacial tension facilitates the preparation of an emulsion, as less mechanical energy need be expended to break up the phases. If a pharmacist were to disperse, by means of a mortar and pestle, 500 ml of olive oil with an initial surface area of 600 cm² so that the average diameter of the dispersed oil globule were 10 μ, the work of dispersion may be calculated. The volume of each spherical oil droplet is

$$V_i = \frac{\pi d^3}{6} = \frac{\pi}{6}(10^{-3})^3 = 5.236 \times 10^{-10} \text{ cc}$$

The number of oil globules in the 500 ml of oil is

$$\frac{500}{5.236 \times 10^{-10}} = 9.54 \times 10^{11}$$

Each spherical globule has a surface area

$$S_i = \pi d^2 = \pi(10^{-3})^2 = 3.14 \times 10^{-6} \text{ cm}^2$$

The total surface area of the dispersed phase is the product of the number of globules and the surface area of an individual oil globule,

$$3.14 \times 10^{-6} \times 9.54 \times 10^{11} = 3.0 \times 10^6 \text{ cm}^2$$

The interfacial tension between olive oil and water is 23 dyn cm^{-1}. The work done in dispersing the olive oil is

$$W = \gamma\, dS = 23(3{,}000{,}000 - 600) = 6.9 \times 10^7 \text{ ergs}$$

Ergs may be converted to joules by dividing by 10^7, so the work of dispersion is 6.9 J. Since 1 cal is equal to 4.184 J, the work of dispersion is 1.6 cal.

If 1 per cent polyoxyethylene sorbitan monostearate is added to the system, the interfacial tension is lowered to 3 dyn cm^{-1}. The work of emulsification is then approximately one-tenth as great as that required to disperse the olive oil in the absence of the surface-active agent,

$$W = \gamma\, dS = 3(3{,}000{,}000 - 600) = 9 \times 10^6 \text{ ergs}$$

The work of emulsification in the presence of polyoxyethylene sorbitan monostearate is 0.2 cal.

In addition to facilitating emulsion formation, a surface-active agent stabilizes the emulsion because the lower free surface energy associated with the dispersed phase makes the emulsion energetically more stable.

A surface-active agent collects or is adsorbed at the interface and concomitantly lowers interfacial tension. In an emulsion the nonpolar portion of the surface-active agent is oriented toward the oily phase and the polar portion is oriented toward the aqueous phase. Emulsifying agents are surface-active agents that form a condensed, rigid film about the dispersed particles. This condensed film prevents the coalescence of two colliding globules and increases the physical stability of the emulsion.

There are two types of emulsions. The emulsion in which oil is the dispersed phase in water is known as an oil-in-water emulsion, which is often abbreviated O/W. The emulsion in which water is the dispersed phase in oil is known as a water-in-oil emulsion, W/O. The simplest method of determining the type of emulsion is by stirring it gently with a larger volume of water. If the emulsion disperses easily, it is an oil-in-water emulsion; if it does not disperse readily, it is a water-in-oil emulsion. A dye may be used to determine the type of emulsion. A small amount of an oil-soluble dye is added to the emulsion. If the bulk of the emulsion becomes colored, the external phase is oil, and the emulsion is a water-in-oil emulsion. Since oil does not conduct an electric current, conductivity may be used to determine the type of emulsion. An oil-in-water emulsion conducts a current, but a water-in-oil emulsion does not.

Although the type of emulsion depends on a number of factors, the relative solubilities of the emulsifying agent in the two phases is the most important single factor in determining the type of emulsion formed. In a system with a single emulsifying agent, the water-soluble emulsifying agent forms an oil-in-water emulsion; the oil-soluble emulsifying agent forms a water-in-oil emulsion. The phase in which the emulsifying agent is more soluble generally becomes the external phase. Sodium lauryl sulfate, sodium oleate, and triethanolamine oleate are water-soluble emulsifying agents that form oil-in-water emulsions. Calcium oleate and cholesterol are water-insoluble emulsifying agents that form water-in-oil emulsions. The orientation of several emulsifying agents and the type of emulsion formed are indicated in Figure 145.

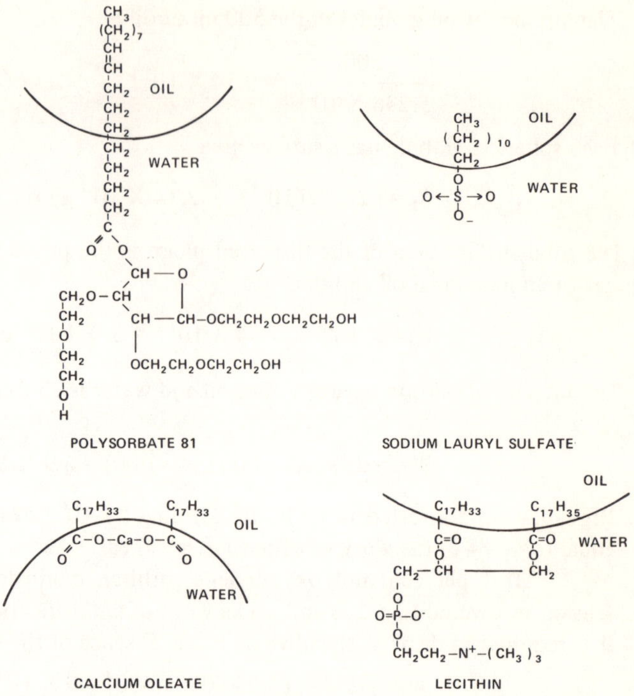

Figure 145. Diagrammatic representation of the orientation of emulsifying agents in emulsions.

POLYSORBATE 81

SODIUM LAURYL SULFATE

CALCIUM OLEATE

LECITHIN

The ratio of the volume of one liquid phase to the volume of the other phase is known as the phase volume ratio. The phase volume ratio may influence the type of emulsion formed. If all other factors are constant, the phase that is present in the greater volume becomes the external phase. Inversion is the process by which one type of emulsion is changed to the other type. During the industrial manufacturing process as the phase volume ratio is changed, emulsions often undergo inversion. When water is gradually added to an oily phase containing a water-soluble emulsifying agents, the oil is present in the greater volume and becomes the external phase, i.e., forms a water-in-oil emulsion. As more water is progressively added until it is present in the greater volume, the inversion point is attained and an oil-in-water emulsion is formed.

The amount of emulsifying agent influences the particle size of the dispersed globules. If a large amount of energy is expended in the dispersion of oil globules in water, the size of the oil globules may be a fraction of a micron. When sufficient amounts of a suitable emulsifying agent are present, it will be adsorbed in a monomolecular film, which protects the oil globules from coalescence. If only a limited amount of the emulsifying agent is present, it cannot form a complete film about all the dispersed oil globules. Coalescence will continue until the surface area of the oil particles has decreased to the value at which the emulsifying agent may form a continuous film about the oil globules.

Knowing that the molecular weight of sodium oleate is 304.4 g mole^{-1} and the molecular cross-sectional area is 22×10^{-16} cm^2, the amount of sodium oleate required to emulsify 100 ml of oil to a globular diameter of 1 μ can be calculated. The volume of each emulsified globule of oil is

$$V_i = \frac{\pi d^3}{6} = \frac{\pi}{6}(10^{-4})^3 = 0.524 \times 10^{-12} \text{ cc}$$

The number of emulsified globules in 1 ml of oil is

$$\frac{1}{0.524 \times 10^{-12}} = 1.91 \times 10^{12}$$

The surface area of each emulsified globule of oil is

$$S_i = \pi d^2 = \pi(10^{-4})^2 = \pi(10^{-8}) \text{ cm}^2$$

The total surface area of all globules of 1 ml of oil is

$$S_{total} = (1.91 \times 10^{12})(3.14 \times 10^{-8}) = 6 \times 10^4 \text{ cm}^2$$

Since the cross-sectional area occupied by a molecule of sodium oleate is 22×10^{-16} cm^2, the number of molecules required to form a monomolecular layer about all the oil globules is

$$\frac{S_{total}}{22 \times 10^{-16}} = \frac{6 \times 10^4}{22 \times 10^{-16}} = 2.72 \times 10^{19}$$

The number of molecules divided by the Avagadro number is the moles of sodium oleate required:

$$\frac{2.72 \times 10^{19}}{6.02 \times 10^{23}} = 0.451 \times 10^{-4} \text{ mole for 1 ml}$$

As 100 ml of oil is emulsified, 0.0045 mole of sodium oleate is needed. The product of the molecular weight and the number of moles required is the weight of the sodium oleate,

$$304.4 \times 0.0045 = 1.37 \text{ g}$$

Similar calculations show that the emulsification of 100 ml of an oil to a diameter of 5 and 25 μ requires 0.27 and 0.055 g of sodium oleate, respectively. Thus, if 0.27 g of sodium oleate is used to emulsify 100 ml of an oil, the diameter of the oil globules cannot be less than 5 μ. If a large amount of energy is expended in dispersing the oil, the globules may be broken up to a fraction of a micron; however, these will coalesce upon standing until a diamter of 5 μ is attained and a monomolecular layer is formed to protect the oil globules from further coalescence.

In an emulsion some of the emulsifying agent may exist as micelles. The film of simple emulsifying agents appears to be monomolecular; however, with complex emulsifying agents there are indications that the film may be greater than a single layer. For these reasons more than the calculated amount of emulsifying agent is used in the actual production of emulsions.

The reduction of interfacial tension is the most important factor in the preparation of an emulsion; however, the rigidity of the adsorbed film of the emulsifying agent is of prime importance in the stabilization of an emulsion. The stability of an emulsion can be best evaluated by size frequency analyses, which measure the rate of coalescence; if the frequency of larger particles increases at a rapid rate, the emulsion is not stable. Thus, an emulsion that has a narrow size frequency distribution needs to be more stable than one with a wide size frequency distribution.

Upon standing, the separation of a layer of emulsified particles may occur because of the difference in densities of the two phases. This separation is known as creaming. If the adsorbed film of the emulsifying agent is rigid and condensed, it will prevent coalescence, and upon being shaken the creamed globules will be redispersed. Thus, an emulsion that creams readily is not necessarily unstable. The rate of creaming is governed by the factors of the Stokes equation, i.e., difference in densities, viscosity, and particle size.

The frequency and force of collisions of the particles influences the stability. An increase in temperature causes an increase in kinetic energy of the particles and a decrease in viscosity of the emulsion, which make the emulsion less stable. A temperature change may also effect the relative solubilities of the emulsifying agent and alter characteristics of the adsorbed film. An increase in viscosity by the addition of a suspending agent or by an increase in phase volume ratio of the internal phase tends to increase stability because it lowers the frequency of collisions and the force of each individual collision.

Most emulsions encountered in pharmacy are the oil-in-water type, in which the emulsifying agent often ionizes and confers a charge to the dispersed globules. The charge affects the tendency to collide, but it has relatively little effect on the strength of the interfacial film. A lowering of the ζ potential increases the collision rate, but it does not necessarily increase coalescence. Many of the pharmaceutical emulsifying agents used for preparing oil-in-water emulsions are hydrophilic colloids that are hydrated in aqueous medium. In such emulsions the stability is decreased by the addition of high concentrations of electrolytes or solvents that strongly associate with water. Coalescence by freezing is attributed to the squeezing together of the oil globules as the liquid aqueous phase is removed in the form of ice.

In general, water-in-oil emulsions have a more rigid film than oil-in-water emulsions, as evidenced by the water droplets being irregular rather than spherical in shape. In water-in-oil emulsions the oil is a nonionizing medium and there is no ionic atmosphere (or counterions) within the oily phase. Usually water-in-oil emulsions are not charged; however, if an electrical double layer exists at the interface it lies within the dispersed aqueous phase and would have little effect in preventing coalescence.

The most effective interfacial films are not generally formed by a single emulsifying agent, but they are composed of several emulsifying agents that differ markedly in their ratio of polar to nonpolar groups. The more stable oil-in-water emulsions are formed when there are present two emulsifying agents, of which one has a high HLB and the other has a low HLB. A satisfactory emulsifying pair forms a stable complex monofilm at the interface. The two emulsifying agents exist side by side in the monofilm with the penetration of one emulsifying agent into the monofilm of the other. A properly selected pair of emulsifying agents form a rigid film and concomitantly markedly lower interfacial tension. A cholesterol-sodium lauryl sulfate blend and a sodium oleate-oleic acid blend produce very stable emulsions.

For a given oil and type of emulsion there is an optimum ratio of the two emulsifying agents at which the emulsion has its maximum stability. The HLB of a blend of emulsifying agents is the sum of the products of the individual HLB values and their fractions of the total blend.

The required HLB value to form the most stable water-in-oil emulsions of mineral oil is 5. Polysorbate 80 and sorbitan sesquioleate have HLB values of 15 and 3.7, respectively. If this pair of emulsifying agents is to be used to prepare a 50 per cent mineral oil-in-water emulsion, the fraction of each to be used in the emulsifying blend may be calculated. If x represents the fraction of the total emulsifying blend composed of polysorbate 80, $(1 - x)$ represents the fraction of sorbitan sesquioleate. Since the blend is to have an HLB value of 5, the fraction of the blend composed of polysorbate 80 is

$$15x + 4.3(1 - x) = 5$$

$$x = 0.115$$

The emulsifying mixture required to form a water-in-oil emulsion consists of 11.5 per cent polysorbate 80 and 88.5 per cent sorbitan sesquioleate.

The same pair of emulsifying agents could be used to prepare an oil-in-water emulsion. The required HLB value to form a stable oil-in-water emulsion of mineral oil is 12. The fraction of each emulsifying agent required in the blend may be calculated as above:

$$15x + 4.3(1 - x) = 12$$

$$x = 0.735$$

The emulsifying mixture required to form an oil-in-water emulsion consists of 73.5 per cent polysorbate 80 and 26.5 per cent sorbitan sesquioleate.

The use of plant gums in the manual preparation of emulsions is classical. In the preparation of an extemporaneous emulsion using acacia as an emulsifying agent, a primary emulsion consisting of 4 parts of oil, 2 parts of water, and 1 part of acacia is prepared. The high viscosity of this primary emulsion hinders coalescence, as the oil globules move less rapidly and allow more time for the emulsifying agent to become properly oriented. After a satisfactory primary emulsion has been formed by rapid trituration in a mortar, it may be diluted with water as required with further trituration. The method is known as the 4:2:1 method, after the ratio of oil, water, and gum.

A classical gum emulsion may be prepared by mixing 1 part of the emulsifying agent with 4 parts of the internal phase, and then 2 parts of the external phase is added all at once with rapid trituration. After a few moments of trituration, a crackling sound indicates the formation of a good primary emulsion. This method in which the water is added at once to the previously mixed gum and oil is known as the continental method.

After the primary emulsion has been formed, other ingredients may be added gradually with trituration. Since electrolytes tend to decrease the ζ potential and/or dehydrate the hydrophilic colloidal gum, they are added last in as high a dilution as practicable. Alcoholic solutions tend to dehydrate and precipitate hydrophilic colloids and should be added in as dilute a form as practicable.

The continental method of preparing a 4:2:1 emulsion is illustrated by liquid petrolatum emulsion.

77. Mineral oil   500 ml
    Acacia   125 g
    Syrup   100 ml
    Vanillin   40 mg
    Alcohol   60 ml
    Purified water, q.s. 1000 ml

Sig.: Mineral oil emulsion

The mineral oil is mixed with the acacia and 250 ml of water is added at once. The mixture is triturated to form a primary emulsion. The syrup, 50 ml of water, and the solution of vanillin in alcohol are mixed and gradually added with trituration to the primary emulsion. Finally, sufficient water is added to make 1000 ml.

Employing the same 4:2:1 ratio of oil, water, and gum, a different order of mixing may be used. In the English method the internal phase is added gradually with trituration to the external phase, which contains the emulsifying agent. If the mixture becomes too viscid, while adding the 4 parts of oil gradually with trituration, a little water may be added with trituration, after which the addition of oil in divided portions is continued. In general, the English method is more time consuming and is less successful for the novice than the continental method.

With the recent advances in the technology of surface-active agents, more synthetic emulsifying agents and fewer naturally occurring gums are being used in pharmaceutical emulsion. Some of the emulsifying agents are formed by chemical reaction during the processing of the emulsion. In oil-in-water emulsions containing soap, the soap is often formed *in situ*. A solution of the alkali is added to the oily phase containing the fatty acid to be saponified. In this way the emulsifying agent content is increased gradually as the water is added. The heat of the reaction may aid diffusion of the emulsifying agent. Benzyl benzoate lotion illustrates an emulsion in which the emulsifying agent is formed *in situ*.

78. Benzyl benzoate   250 ml
    Triethanolamine   5 g
    Oleic acid   20 g
    Water   750 ml

Sig.: Benzyl benzoate lotion

The oleic acid and the triethanolamine are mixed to form the emulsifying agent, triethanolamine oleate. The benzyl benzoate and 250 ml of water are added and mixed to form a primary oil-in-water emulsion. The remainder of the water is added with agitation.

In the industrial preparation of oil-in-water emulsions the emulsifying agent and any oil-soluble ingredients are usually dispersed in the oily phase and the water is slowly added with agitation to form a primary emulsion. If ingredients of the oily phase must be melted, the temperature should not be excessive. The temperature of the oil and aqueous phase should be the same at the time of emulsification. As the water is gradually added to the oily phase, the phase volume ratio favors the formation of a water-in-oil emulsion. As more water is added, the emulsion inverts to the desired oil-in-water type because the phase volume ratio now favors this type and the water-soluble emulsifying agent diffuses into the aqueous phase and promotes the dispersion of oil. After the inversion the water can be added more rapidly. Any water-soluble ingredients are dissolved and added when the emulsion is adjusted to its correct volume. Emulsions prepared by the inversion method have a smaller average particle size than those in which the water is added so rapidly that the emulsion formed immediately is an oil-in-water type. The emulsion is then processed by a homogenizer or colloid mill. The entrapment of air is avoided, as it decreases the stability of the emulsion because the emulsifying agent tends to migrate to the liquid-air interface.

79.
Stearic acid	70 g
Lanolin	5 g
Sorbitan monoleate	5 g
Polyoxyethylene sorbitan monostearate	25 g
Sorbitol solution	50 ml
Methylparaben	1 g
Propylparaben	1 g
Purified water	843 ml

Sig.: Hand lotion

The stearic acid and lanolin are heated with the sorbitan monooleate and polyoxyethylene sorbitan monostearate at 80 to 90°. The methylparaben and propylparaben and sorbitol solution are dissolved in water at 80 to 90°. The aqueous phase is gradually added to the oily phase with agitation. After inversion the remainder of the aqueous phase is added. The emulsion is stirred until it has cooled to 30°.

The equipment used to prepare emulsions is similar to that discussed for the processing of suspensions. The mortar and pestle, the egg beater, and the hand homogenizer can be used manually to prepare emulsions. Small-scale models of motor-driven propellers, turbines, colloid mills, and homogenizers are available.

13 | FLUID PHARMACEUTICAL SUSPENSIONS AND EMULSIONS

A pharmaceutical suspension is a dispersion of finely divided solids in a liquid medium. Certain suspensions are marketed as a dry powder to which a prescribed volume of liquid vehicle is added to form a liquid dispersion before it is dispensed. A suspension may be for ophthalmic, oral, parenteral, or topical use. A pharmaceutical emulsions is a two-phase system in which one liquid is dispersed in the form of small globules through out another liquid. Since suspensions and emulsions are dispersions of particles approaching a colloidal size, many of their properties are similar.

SUSPENSIONS

The chemical stability of suspensions has been discussed in terms of a zero-order degradation in Chapter 9. The physical stability of a suspension is concerned with sedimentation, caking, and resuspension. A suspension should not settle rapidly, and it should be sufficiently fluid to flow easily under the conditions of administration. As a suspension is energetically unstable, the particles that have settled tend to interact to form a cake or hard crystalline network. The pharmacist strives to formulate a suspension in which the caking is minimized so that the particles that have settled may be readily redispersed upon shaking.

Sedimentation and Caking

The rate of sedimentation or settling of rigid, spherical particles in a dilute suspension is expressed by the Stoke equation. Although the Stokes equation is only an approximation for actual suspensions having more than 2 per cent solid particles, it indicates the factors that influence the rate of sedimentation in all suspensions. Since the rate of sedimentation is proportional to the square of the particle diameter, a reduction in particle size contributes greatly to a reduction in sedimentation rate. The rate of sedimentation is inversely proportional to the viscosity of the dispersion medium. Although the viscosity may be increased by the addition of a suspending agent, an excessive viscosity is to be avoided, as the suspension is then difficult to pour from the container and any settled material is difficult to redisperse by shaking. The rate of sedimentation is progressively slowed as the difference in densities of the two phases approaches zero. The adjustment of densities is limited by the solubility of solutes added to the dispersion medium to increase its density and by the fact that most of the dispersed solids have a density somewhat greater than that of the dispersion medium. Thus, the reduction of particle size is the important consideration in developing a suspension, and the increase in viscosity of the dispersion medium is of secondary consideration.

The influence of these factors on the rate of sedimentation can be illustrated by considering a sulfadiazine suspension. Sulfadiazine has a density of 1.5 g cc^{-1} and is available as a powder having an average particle diameter of 2.6μ. According to the Stoke equation the powdered sulfadiazine would settle in water at the rate of

$$\frac{dx}{dt} = \frac{d^2(\rho_i - \rho_e)g}{18\eta}$$

$$= \frac{(2.6 \times 10^{-4})^2 (1.5 - 1.0) 980}{18 \times 0.009}$$

$$= 2.05 \times 10^{-4} \text{ cm sec}^{-1}$$

Microcrystalline sulfadiazine has an average particle diameter of 0.26 μ. If microcrystalline sulfadiazine is used, the rate of sedimentation in water is

$$\frac{dx}{dt} = \frac{(2.6 \times 10^{-5})^2 (1.5 - 1.0) 980}{18 \times 0.009}$$

$$= 2.05 \times 10^{-6} \text{ cm sec}^{-1}$$

Thus, a tenfold reduction of particle size results in a hundredfold slowing of the sedimentation rate. Sorbitol solution has a density of 1.3 g cc^{-1} and a viscosity of 110 cp at 25°. If sorbitol solution is used as a vehicle, both the reduction in the difference in densities and the increase in viscosity retard the rate of sedimentation to

$$\frac{dx}{dt} = \frac{(2.6 \times 10^{-5})^2 (1.5 - 1.3) 980}{18 \times 1.1}$$

$$= 6.7 \times 10^{-9} \text{ cm sec}^{-1}$$

The rate of sedimentation is decreased by the addition of a suspending agent to the water. If the microcrystalline sulfadiazine is dispersed in a 2 per cent methylcellulose, (400 cp) solution, the rate of sedimentation is

$$\frac{dx}{dt} = \frac{(2.6 \times 10^{-5})^2 (1.5 - 1.0) 980}{18 \times 4}$$

$$= 4.6 \times 10^{-9} \text{ cm sec}^{-1}$$

As the rate of sedimentation is inversely proportional to the viscosity in this example, an increase in viscosity by a factor of 444 (4/0.009) results in the decrease of the rate of sedimentation by a factor of 1/444.

In a pharmaceutical suspension the rate of sedimentation must be slowed so that a patient can measure and administer an uniform dose. In deflocculated suspensions the particles settle slowly; however, upon settling the particles slip past each other and form a compact sediment. Caking of the sediment may occur by a physical or chemical reaction. From the energy viewpoint the stability of the system is increased by a decrease in free surface energy. This energy loss is accomplished through an increase in particle size and crystallization between the particles, which produces a hard mass or cake. The hard cake formed when magnesium oxide and sodium bicarbonate are suspended in water is due to the formation of magnesium carbonate crystals, which connect the particles into a hard mass.

In addition to surface energy, electrical forces are functioning in suspensions. The particles, which acquired a charge by ionization or adsorption, are prevented from adhering by electrostatic repulsion. Electrolytes may reduce the ζ potential to the extent that the particles interact to form a flocculated suspension. The flocs settle rapidly, but they can be easily resuspended by shaking. When a negative flocculating agent is gradually added to a suspension of positively charged particles, the ζ potential is decreased. At some concentration of the flocculating agent the ζ potential is reduced to the extent that flocculation occurs. As additional negative flocculating agent is added, the charge on the particle is neutralized, and still further addition of the negative flocculating agent confers a negative charge on the particles. With a high negative or high positive charge on the particles the suspension is deflocculated and may cake after sedimentation. At low ζ potential near neutralization of the charge on the particles, flocculation occurs, and although sedimentation is rapid, caking does not occur.

Inorganic electrolytes, ionic surface-active agents, and hydrophilic polymers may act as flocculating agents. The ionic flocculating agents function by decreasing the ζ potential of the particles. Hydrophilic polymers, e.g., gelatin and methylcellulose, are adsorbed on the surface of the particles. If there is a sufficient concentration of the polymer to completely coat the surface of the particles, the protective film will prevent flocculation by acting as a mechanical barrier toward interparticular interactions. If a limited concentration of the polymer is present, the particles will not be completely coated. Flocculation then occurs when an uncoated portion of one particle contacts the polymer-coated portion of another particle.

A flocculated suspension settles rapidly and leaves an unsightly layer. An elegant suspension is prepared by a compromise between a flocculated and deflocculated system. Frequently the proper selection of a dispersion agent permits the use of fine particles without caking. A small amount of a flocculating agent may be used to produce partial flocculation and prevent caking. A suspending agent is then added to keep the flocs suspended. The increase in viscosity due to the suspending agent also retards crystal growth by slowing the rate of diffusion. Most suspending agents are negatively charged hydrophilic colloids, which are precipitated by positively charged flocculating agents. The phosphate ion is used to flocculate positively charged particles, and it can be used in the presence of negatively charged suspending agents.

During shelf storage a suspension is not subjected to any significant shear. When a suspension is shaken and poured from a container, a shearing rate of the magnitude of 100 sec^{-1} exists. The effect of rate of shear on viscosity is shown in Figure 146 for Newtonian and non-Newtonian fluids. The viscosity of the Newtonian fluid is unchanged by a change in rate of shear. A suspension that behaves as a Newtonian fluid is unsatisfactory, because a viscosity suitable for suspending the particles during storage would be too great a viscosity to permit easy pouring from the container or ready resuspension. The non-Newtonian fluids have a marked change in viscosity with a change in rate of shear. A suspension having pseudoplastic flow possesses a high viscosity at negligible rate of shear and a low viscosity at a high rate of shear; it would settle slowly during storage, but it would be readily poured and resuspended.

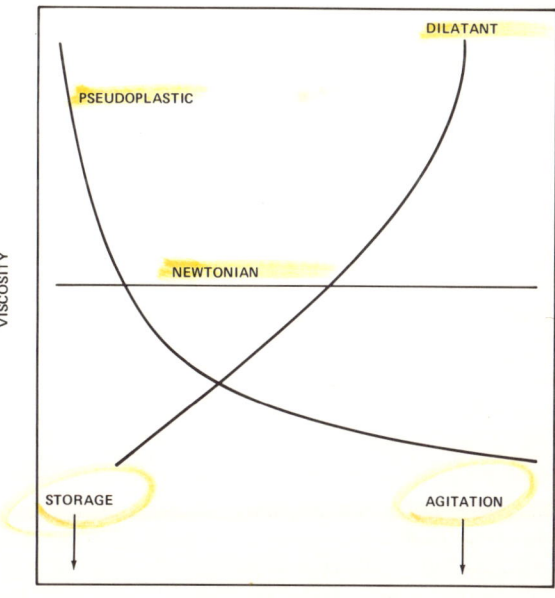

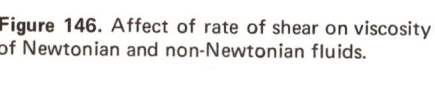
Figure 146. Affect of rate of shear on viscosity of Newtonian and non-Newtonian fluids.

Pseudoplastic materials, e.g., algin, sodium carboxymethylcellulose, and tragacanth, are useful suspending agents in pharmaceuticals. A combination of a pseudoplastic and a thixotropic suspending agent, e.g., sodium carboxymethylcellulose and bentonite, confers desirable characteristics to a suspension. During storage the particles are held in the gel structure; however, upon shaking the suspension becomes fluid enough to pour freely.

Uses of Suspension

Oral Suspensions. An oral suspension is an advantageous dosage form for administration to children or adults who have difficulty swallowing a capsule or tablet. In general, the solid content of a suspension ranges from 250 to 500 mg per teaspoonful. A pediatric drop may be three to four times as concentrated. The vehicle is usually syrup, sorbitol solution, or water thickened with a suspending agent. A suspension provides better dispersion in the gastrointestinal tract than a compressed dosage form because the small particles ranging from 1 to 50 μ are distributed without delay. The patient acceptance of an unpleasant-tasting drug is improved by using a suspension of an insoluble derivative, e.g., chloramphenicol palmitate and triacetyloleandomycin, as only the dissolved molecules stimulate the taste buds. The shelf life of a suspension of a medicinal compound is often greater than that of a solution of the compound. As only an extremely small amount of the medicinal compound is dissolved and subjected to degradation, a suspension of a compound, which is relatively unstable in solution, may possess acceptable shelf life. Drugs, e.g., mystatin and oxytetracycline, that are unstable in liquid form may be prepared as a dry powder or granulation to which the liquid vehicle is added by the community pharmacist at the time of dispensing.

Some of the factors to be considered in the development of a suspension can be appreciated by examination of the formula for an oral penicillin suspension.

80.
Procaine penicillin G	50,000 units/ml	
Sodium citrate	10.00 g	
Sodium gluconate	25.00 g	
Sorbitol	40.00 g	
Saccharin	0.05 g	
Saccharin sodium	0.50 g	
Peppermint oil	0.02 ml	
Chocolate oil, imitation	0.01 ml	
Kaolin	5.00 g	
Tragacanth	0.20 g	
Methylparaben	0.07 g	
Propylparaben	0.01 g	
Purified water, q.s.	100 ml	

Sig.: Oral procaine penicillin G suspension

Procaine penicillin G has a limited solubility and is degraded when it is suspended in water. The stability of a suspension of procaine penicillin G is increased by suppressing its solubility by the addition of sorbitol, sodium gluconate, and sodium citrate. This suspension retains at least 90 per cent potency after storage at room temperature for 6 months. With tragacanth as the suspending agent no separation occurs for several hours after shaking. Upon storage the procaine penicillin G settles, but it does not cake and is readily resuspended upon shaking. A combination of saccharin and sodium saccharin further sweetens the taste of the sorbitol vehicle. The sodium saccharin masks the initial bitterness of the small amount of procaine penicillin G in solution, and the saccharin masks the bitter aftertaste. The flavor is improved by the addition of peppermint and chocolate oils to the sweetened vehicle. The kaolin reduces grittiness and produces a suspension that feels smooth to the tongue. The grittiness could be lessened by using procaine penicillin G particles of 5 to 25 μ; however, the high specific surface favors more rapid dissolution in the mouth and produces a bitter taste. The bitter taste is reduced by using particles from 40 to 60 μ, which is the maximum size that can be used without producing a gritty sensation in the mouth. The parabens act as preservatives from microorganic growth. In addition to suppressing the solubility of procaine penicillin G, sodium citrate adjusts the vehicle to a pH 6.2, near which penicillin G has its maximum stability.

In the suspension known as brown mixture there is no suspending agent.

81.
Glycyrrhiza fluidextract	120.00 ml
Antimony potassium tartrate	0.24 g
Paregoric	120.00 ml
Alcohol	30.00 ml
Glycerin	120.00 ml
Purified water, q.s.	1000 ml

Sig.: Brown mixture

The fluidextract is diluted with the glycerin and 500 ml of water. The antimony potassium tartrate is dissolved in 12 ml of hot water and added to the glycerin-fluidextract solution. The paregoric and alcohol are added, and the mixture is adjusted to final volume by adding water.

All suspensions must be shaken before administration. Many suspensions contain a suspending agent such as Veegum® in the triacetyloleandomycin and triple sulfa suspension.

82.
Triacetyloleandomycin equivalent to oleandomycin	2.50 g
Sulfadiazine	3.33 g
Sulfamerazine	3.33 g
Sulfamethazine	3.33 g
Syrup	80.00 ml
Veegum®	1.30 g
Sodium citrate	1.10 g
Methylparaben	0.25 g
Propylparaben	0.02 g
Citric acid 5% solution adjust to pH 5.6	

Sig.: Triacetyloleandomycin and triple sulfa suspension

The Veegum® is added slowly to the syrup, and the mixture is agitated until smooth. The sodium citrate and the preservatives are added. The blend of sulfa drugs is added and mixed. The suspension is then homogenized. The suspension is adjusted to pH 5.6 by adding the citric acid solution.

Topical Suspensions. Lotions are aqueous suspensions intended for topical application without massage. A lotion may be applied for a cooling effect. In such lotions there is a high alcohol content to increase the rate of evaporation and cooling. In lotions applied to maintain a moist area the glycerin content is high. With some lotions it is desirable to incorporate a suspending agent that upon drying forms a film, which holds the medication in contact with the skin. A lotion should be fluid enough to spread evenly, but it should be viscid enough to adhere. In general, dermatological suspensions contain from 10 to 20 per cent solids. The particles must be small enough so they do not produce a gritty sensation and mechanical irritation when applied to the skin.

83.
Calamine	80 g
Zinc oxide	80 g
Glycerin	20 ml
Bentonite magma	250 ml
Calcium hydroxide solution, q.s.	1000 ml

Sig.: Calamine lotion

The bentonite magma is diluted with an equal volume of calcium hydroxide solution. The calamine and zinc oxide are mixed with the glycerin and approximately 100 ml of the diluted bentonite magma. The mixture is triturated until a smooth paste is formed. The remainder of the magma is gradually added with trituration, and the lotion is adjusted to final volume with calcium hydroxide solution.

84. Zinc sulfate 40 g
    Sulfurated potash 40 g
    Purified water, q.s. 1000 ml

    Sig.: White lotion

White lotion is prepared by mixing filtered solutions of sulfurated potash and zinc sulfate. To facilitate a fine precipitate of zinc sulfide and sulfur the sulfurated potash solution is added slowly to the zinc sulfate solution with agitation. As the precipitate becomes yellow and coagulates, the suspension is freshly prepared prior to dispensing. White lotion does not contain a suspending agent.

In ophthalmology a suspension of microcrystalline cortisone acetate or hydrocortisone acetate is used to treat inflammation of the conjunctiva and anterior ocular segment without producing a systemic effect. Although most individuals do not feel grittiness and irritation in the eye until the particles exceed a size of 50 μ, it is prudent to use particles from 1 to 5 μ in ophthalmic suspensions.

Parenteral Suspension. Parenteral suspensions are injected subcutaneously and intramuscularly; they are not administered intravenously or into the spinal canal. Ideally the diameter of the particles should be less than 5 μ to minimize pain and irritation of the tissue. Size reduction is accomplished mechanically by milling or by crystallization as microcrystals. Parenteral suspensions usually contain less than 5 per cent solids, although there are penicillin suspensions containing 30 per cent solids.

The addition of a wetting agent aids in the dispersion and stabilization of the solid phase. Some surface-active agents that have been used in various parenteral products are lecithin, polysorbate 80, and Pluronic® F-68 (an oxyethylene oxypropylene polymer containing 80 per cent polyoxyethylene in a total molecule of approximately 8,700 g mole^{-1}). A dispersing agent for parenteral use must be nontoxic, nonirritating, nonfebrile, stable, and easily sterilized. These criteria severely limit the number of acceptable dispersing agents. Dispersing agents that have been used in some parenteral products are acacia, gelatin, methylcellulose, polyvinylpyrrolidone, sodium carboxymethylcellulose, and sodium cholate. An ideal dispersing agent should not greatly increase the viscosity of the suspension or form unwanted foam upon shaking.

Since the sterilization of a suspension by heat may alter its physical properties, the constituents are frequently sterilized separately, and the suspension is made under aseptic conditions. The medicinal compound may be purified in a sterile environment so that the final crystallization is sterile. The vehicle, e.g., water for injection or vegetable oil, may be sterilized by heat or filtration. The sterile medicinal compound is wetted with the sterile vehicle, and the suspension is passed through a colloid mill that has been sterilized by steam or ethylene oxide.

When a liquid from a syringe passes through a hypodermic needle, it may be subjected to a shearing rate up to 10,000 sec^{-1}. Syringeability refers to the ability of a liquid to flow from a syringe through a hypodermic needle. Syringeability is reduced by (1) an increase in the viscosity or density of the vehicle, (2) an increase in the size of the particles, and (3) an increase in the solid content of the suspension. Particle shape also affects syringeability. Since a parenteral suspension should be easily redispersed, a flocculated suspension is preferred because it is easily redispersed and does not require an increase in viscosity, which would adversely affect the syringeability. A parenteral suspension should drain cleanly from the walls of its container so that it can be removed from the vial and syringe. Vials may be coated with silicone to facilitate drainage.

Following injection a drug may be rapidly excreted, biotransformed, or degraded. Consequently, to maintain an adequate therapeutic concentration in the body, several injections must be given daily. Since this is inconvenient to the patient and the nurse, pharmaceutical scientists have attempted to provide prolonged duration of a therapeutic effective concentration by proper formulation. A repository or depot parenteral is a product which upon a single injection provides a prolonged therapeutic effect. Penicillin has probably been investigated as much as any other drug with the view to make a repository injection. The absorption of penicillin is influenced by the derivative used; in general, a more soluble derivative is absorbed faster than a less soluble form. For this reason procaine penicillin G has been frequently used in repository intramuscular injections. The vehicle also influences absorption. In general, an oily vehicle provides a more prolonged effect than an aqueous vehicle. A suspension of 300,000 units of procaine penicillin G in peanut oil or sesame oil gelled with 2 per cent aluminum monostearate provides an adequate serum level for approximately 2.5 days.

The effect of the rheological properties of a suspension and the characteristics of the suspended powder on the availability of procaine penicillin G from an intramuscular depot has been demonstrated in the following vehicle.

85.	Sodium citrate	15.00 g
	Polysorbate 80	1.10 g
	Methylparaben	1.00 g
	Propylparaben	0.11 g
	Sterile water for injection	545.00 ml

Sig.: Vehicle for penicillin injection

The important physical factors of the suspension are its structural breakdown point and the percentage of solids. In aqueous suspensions of procaine penicillin G a high solids content of 40 to 70 per cent is usually effective in delaying absorption to provide a repository effect. To ensure a repository effect the breakdown point or yield value of the suspension must be greater than 100,000 dyn-cm. The important physical properties of the powder are its specific surface and its particle size distribution. To be syringeable the powder used in the suspension must have a specific surface greater than 10,000 cm^2 g^{-1} and a relatively broad size distribution. If the breakdown point of the suspension is greater than 1,000,000 dyn-cm due to the high specific surface or the high percentage of solids, the suspension is not syringeable. The relationship of structural breakdown to various specific surfaces and percentages of solids is shown in Figure 147. The line AB represents a maximum limit of 1,000,000 dyn-cm for easy

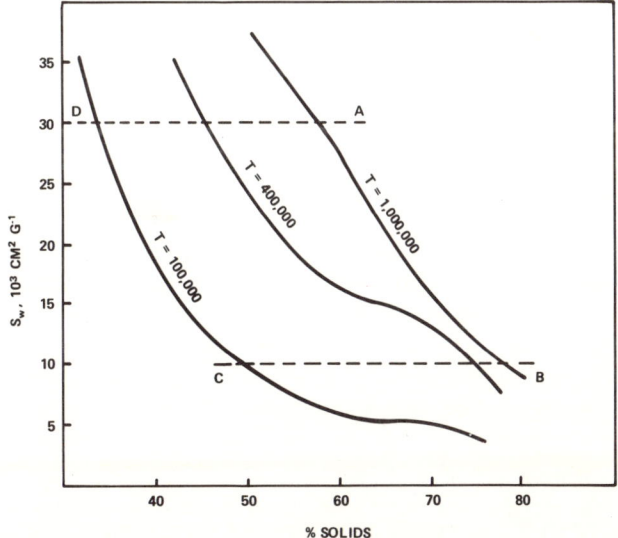

Figure 147. Locus of given suspension T values for various combinations of S_W and per cent solids for powders with a broad particle size distribution. [S.S. Ober, H.C. Vincent, D.E. Simon and K.J. Frederick, J. Am. Pharm. Assoc., Sci. Ed. 47, 673 (1958).]

injection. The line BC represents a minimum limit of 10,000 cm² g⁻¹ for injectability. The suspension has good syringeability, if the specific surface is greater than 10,000 cm² g⁻¹ and if the structural breakdown point is from 150,000 to 750,000 dyn-cm. The region of operation for powders of broad particle size distribution is enclosed by lines AB and BC. If the particle size distribution is narrow and clogging of the needle is to be avoided, a lower maximum structural breakdown and a higher minimum specific surface is required. This decreases the operational region of an acceptable suspension. Injection of the suspension forms a spherical depot in the muscle. If the injection flattened into a fan-shaped deposit, much of the repository effect is lost due to the increased surface from which the tissue fluid leaches the penicillin. Owing to the high degree of thixotropy and the high yield values, a 40 to 70 per cent procaine penicillin G suspension can pass through a hypodermic needle and yet provide a respository effect in the muscle by rapidly regaining its structure.

86. Procaine penicillin G, milled — 150,000 units
    Procaine penicillin G, micronized — 150,000 units
    Lecithin — 12.0 mg
    Sodium citrate — 5.7 mg
    Sodium carboxymethylcellulose, low viscosity — 5.0 mg
    Polyvinylpyrrolidone — 5.0 mg
    Methylparaben — 2.6 mg
    Water for injection, q.s. — 1.0 ml

    Sig.: Procaine penicillin G injection

Equal amounts of milled and micronized procaine penicillin G having a particle size from 40 to 60 μ and 2 to 10 μ, respectively, are used. The broad and controlled particle size distribution contributes to the flow of the suspension through the hypodermic needle without clogging and to the spherical shape of the depot in the muscle. Both milled and micronized procaine penicillin G are blended with the lecithin before being comminuted. The procaine penicillin G is then sterilized by treatment with ethylene oxide. The vehicle is prepared by dissolving the sodium citrate, sodium carboxymethylcellulose, and polyvinylpyrrolidone in sufficient water for injection. The vehicle is sterilized at 120° for 30 minutes. The methylparaben is sterilized by treatment with ethylene oxide. After the vehicle has cooled, the sterile methylparaben is added aseptically. The sterile milled and micronized procaine penicillin G is added aseptically to the vehicle. The sterile suspension is passed through a sterile colloid mill and filled aseptically into sterile containers. The methylparaben is a preservative. The sodium citrate is used to buffer the suspension at approximately a pH 6.8, at which a penicillin G solution has its maximum stability. The lecithin is a wetting agent that aids in the dispersion of the hydrophobic procaine penicillin G powder. The sodium carboxymethylcellulose is a suspending agent that retards sedimentation. The polyvinylpyrrolidone facilitates the clean drainage of the suspension from the container and the syringe.

Suspending Agents

A suspending agent is a substance that increases the viscosity of a suspension so that sedimentation is retarded. A suspending agent also slows the rate of creaming or rise of oil globules in an emulsion. Advantageous flow characteristics are conferred on a polyphasic system by the proper selection of a suspending agent. An ideal suspending agent should be therapeutically inert and chemically stable over a wide range of pH; in low concentrations it should provide adequate viscosity and physical stability for the polyphasic system.

The specific suspending agents discussed are prototypes of their class. All are widely used in pharmaceuticals and may be used internally. Although they are typical suspending agents, it should be recognized that due to similarities in structure to emulsifying agents, certain of the suspending agents may be used with proper technique to prepare emulsions.

Algin. The term "algin" or "alginate" is applied to derivatives of alginic acid obtained from kelp. Alginic acid has a molecular weight of approximately 14,000 g mole^{-1}. Alginic acid is a polyglycuronoside composed of anhydro β-D-mannuronic acid linked so that the carboxylic group is free and the aldehyde is linked as a glycoside and L-glucuronic acid. In pharmacy water-soluble salts of alginic acid are used; they are anionic and are stable at pH 5 and greater. At pH less than 4 the insoluble alginic acid is precipitated.

Sodium alginate dissolves in cold water after standing overnight. Dissolution is hastened by heat and gentle agitation. Prolonged heating at temperatures exceeding 50° causes hydrolysis and loss of viscosity. The viscosities produced by various types of commercial algins depends on the degree of hydrolysis that occurred during processing. The concentration of the algin influences the viscosity. An algin may form a solution with a viscosity of 1000 cp at 1 per cent concentration and a gel at 5 per cent concentration. Moderate concentrations of salts of alkali metals and alcohol only slightly decrease the viscosity; high concentrations dehydrate and precipitate the algin. Heavy metal ions precipitate the corresponding salt of alginic acid as a stringy precipitate. The careful addition of calcium ions to a solution of algin increases the viscosity. This is probably due to the linking of alginic acid moieties through the divalent calcium to produce a longer linear molecule, which offers an increased resistance to flow. At low concentrations of calcium some of the carboxylic groups have not reacted and in ionic form they maintain the algin in solution. A further addition of a low concentration of calcium produces a gel in which the long molecules of insoluble calcium alginate have trapped some of the dispersion medium.

Algin is typical of the hydrophilic colloids obtained from plants. These hydrophilic colloids, e.g., agar, chondrus, pectin, and tragacanth, are carbohydrate in nature. They have a high molecular weight, but they are water soluble and highly hydrated, owing to hydrogen bonding of their hydroxyl groups with water. They are generally linear polymers, which at random dispersion tend to intertwine and flow past one another with considerable resistance. In aqueous medium the strong hydration and the resistance of the linear macromolecules to flow produces a viscous solution. Although the viscosity is increased by the same mechanism, the degree of viscosity increase varies with the various hydrophilic colloids; and often it varies for a given substance, owing to differences in processing and standardization. There is batch variation of these plant hydrophilic colloids as a result of the variation of growing environment, and the content of extraneous matter depends on the method of collection and processing. Synthetic agents are more uniform and provide reproducible properties with less batch variations.

The plant hydrophilic colloids are anionic and acidic. The exception is guar gum, which is nonionic. In general, the hydrophilic colloids are available as water-soluble salts from which the acid form is precipitated at values less than pH 4. High concentrations of electrolytes and alcohol dehydrate the hydrophilic colloids; fortunately sufficiently high concentrations are seldom encountered in pharmaceuticals. The viscosity of hydrophilic plant sols decreases with an increase in temperature. Excessive heat and excessive shear in high-shear mixing equipment can depolymerize a hydrophilic colloid with the accompanying loss of viscosity.

When water is initially added to a hydrophilic colloid, it swells and absorbs water with the formation of a very viscid layer surrounding each particle. The particles tend to stick together in lumps, which are difficult to break up, because they are coated by a slippery layer that hinder exposure to high shear. The slow diffusion of water through the extremely viscid layer greatly retards dissolution of the entire particle. Usually the powdered suspending agent is slowly sprinkled on water with mechanical agitation. Even with mechanical blending complete hydration may not occur for days. Consequently, the rheological properties at the time of production are not necessarily those of the marketed product. Hydration may be facilitated by the addition of alcohol, glycerin, or a suitable wetting agent a short time before the addition of water.

350 • fluid suspensions and emulsions

87. Camphor spirit   100 ml
    Alcohol   100 ml
    Tragacanth   15 g
    Precipitated sulfur   60 g
    Purified water, q.s.   1000 ml

Sig.: Kummerfeld's lotion

The tragacanth is sprinkled on 500 ml of water and allowed to stand. The sulfur is added to the tragacanth mucilage. The alcohol and camphor spirit are added, and the lotion is adjusted to final volume with water. Tragacanth has a molecular weight of 840,000 g mole^{-1} and hydrates very slowly. Even after homogenized it is probably not completely hydrated for several days. For a given concentration of plant hydrophilic colloid, tragacanth yields the highest viscosity.

Gelatin. Gelatin is obtained by the partial hydrolysis of collagen derived from skin, connective tissue, and bones of animals. Gelatin consists of polypeptide chains of various length. Some of the amino acids in the gelatin are diaminomonocarboxylic acids and others are discarboxylic monoamino acids. Since the peptide linkage involves one amino and one carboxylic acid group, gelatin is amphoteric, owing to the presence of free amino and carboxylic groups. Thus, the charge of gelatin depends on the pH. Gelatin is available in two types, as shown in Figure 148. Type A is prepared by acid hydrolysis and is highly hydrated and positively charged at pH 4 to 4.5. The isoelectric point of type A is pH 7 to 9, at which the gelatin has no net charge and exists as a zwitterion. At the isoelectric point the ζ potential is zero, and the gelatin sol is the least hydrated and has its lowest viscosity.

Although gelatin does not significantly lower interfacial tension, an oil-in-water emulsion may be formed with gelatin if the system is homogenized or passed through a colloid mill. If sufficient energy is expended to disperse the oil globules, the gelatin will form a tenacious film with an intense charge about the globules.

88. Mineral oil   500.0 ml
    Gelatin, type A   8.0 g
    Tartaric acid   0.6 g
    Alcohol   60.0 ml
    Purified water, q.s.   1000   ml

Sig.: Mineral oil emulsion

The tartaric acid and the gelatin are added to 300 ml of water. After a few minutes they are heated until the gelatin dissolves. A gelatin sol undergoes hydrolysis and loss of viscosity during storage; however, if the gelatin sol is heated at 98° for 20 minutes, there is a minimum of loss of viscosity during storage. The solution is cooled to 50°, and the alcohol and sufficient water are added to make 500 ml. The mineral oil is added with agitation, and the formulation is processed by a homogenizer or a colloid mill until an emulsion is formed. An emulsion cannot be prepared by trituration in a mortar. If the concentration of oil is 50 per cent or more, the viscosity contribution of the dispersed phase permits the formation of a stable emulsion. Dilute emulsions are very difficult to form unless the viscosity is increased by the addition of a suspending agent. Type A gelatin is cationic, owing to the acid pH produced by the tartaric acid; it cannot be used with negatively charged hyrophilic colloids, e.g., acacia and tragacanth, as coacervation occurs.

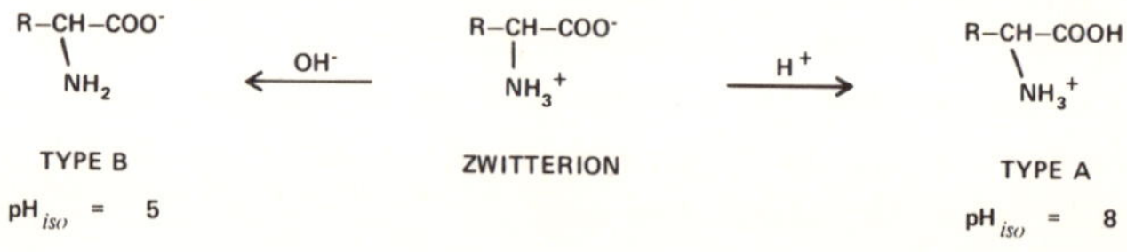

Figure 148. Type structures illustrating the amphoteric species of gelatin.

$$\underset{\substack{\text{TYPE B}\\ \text{pH}_{iso} = 5}}{\text{R–CH–COO}^-\!\!\!\diagdown\!\text{NH}_2} \quad \underset{\text{OH}^-}{\longleftarrow} \quad \underset{\substack{\text{ZWITTERION}}}{\text{R–CH–COO}^-\!\!\!\diagdown\!\text{NH}_3^+} \quad \underset{\text{H}^+}{\longrightarrow} \quad \underset{\substack{\text{TYPE A}\\ \text{pH}_{iso} = 8}}{\text{R–CH–COOH}\!\!\!\diagdown\!\text{NH}_3^+}$$

Type B gelatin is prepared from alkali-treated precursors and is used at a pH of about 8. The alkaline medium may be maintained by the addition of sodium bicarbonate. Since type B is anionic, it may be used with negatively charged hydrophilic colloids.

Methycellulose. Cellulose is composed of long chains of anhydroglucose units in a β-glucosidic linkage. The cellulose derivatives used in pharmacy as suspending agents are long-chain polymers in which R groups have been etherified at the hydroxyl groups, as shown in Figure 149. Since each anhydroglucose unit in the cellulose structure contains three reactive hydroxyl groups, the extent of reaction is often expressed in terms of degree of substitution. If all three hydroxyl groups are reacted, the degree of substitution is three. If chemical analysis shows an R content corresponding to etherification with 1.3 of the three hydroxyl groups, the degree of substitution is 1.3. In general the degree of substitution controls the solubility of the derivative. The degree of polymerization or length of the chain controls the viscosity characteristics of the derivative. Thus, for a given degree of substitution there are several viscosity types, depending upon the length of the molecule.

Cellulose, which has been etherified to contain 1.3 to 2.6 methoxyl groups per anhydroglucose unit, is water soluble. The methycellulose used in pharmacy has a degree of substitution from 1.64 to 1.94, which is equivalent to a methoxyl content of 27.5 to 31.5 per cent. Methylcellulose has a molecular weight ranging from 30,000 to 150,000 g mole^{-1}. The resulting viscosity types are usually designated in terms of the viscosity produced by a 2 per cent solution at 20°. For example, a 2 per cent aqueous solution of methylcellulose, 1500 cp will have a viscosity of 1500 cp at 20°. The types of premium-grade methylcellulose available to the pharmacist are 15, 25, 100, 400, 1500, and 4000 cp. The affect of concentration on viscosity is shown in Figure 150. The viscosity is an exponential function of concentration, c, and for many cellulose derivatives it may be expressed by the equation

$$\frac{2.3 \log \eta_{rel}}{c} = k + \frac{75k^2}{1 + 1.5kc}$$

where k is a constant for a specific cellulose derivative.

Cellulose is insoluble in water because of intermolecular hydrogen bonding, which ties up the hydroxyl groups so that they are unavailable for association with water. When cellulose is partially methylated, association between the cellulose molecules is hindered, and the free hydroxyl groups may more readily associate with the water. The preferred method of preparing methylcellulose solutions is to use hot water. The powdered methylcellulose is blended with one-fourth to one-half of the required volume of water at 90°. After the methylcellulose is thoroughly wetted, the remainder of the water is added as ice or cold water. For maximum clarity the solution of methylcellulose should be cooled in a refrigerator. If cold water is first added to the powdered methylcellulose, a viscid film is formed on the surface of each particle, which causes lumping and slows diffusion of the water into the interior of the particles.

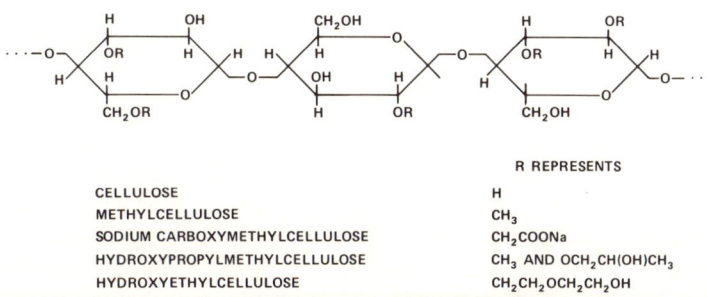

Figure 149. Structure of various cellulose derivatives.

352 • fluid suspensions and emulsions

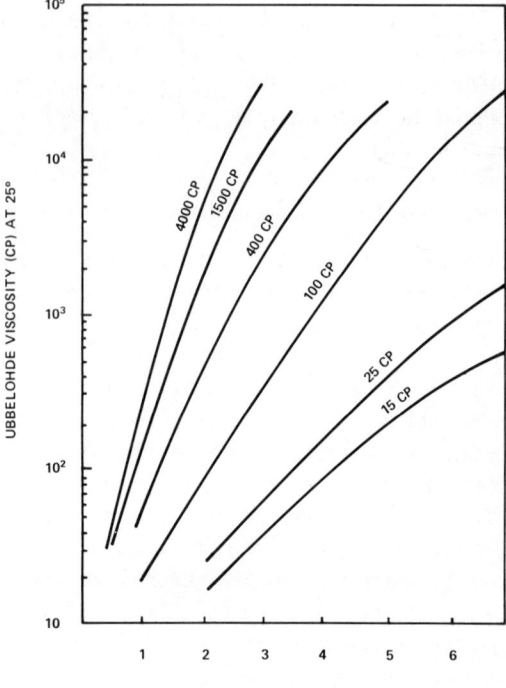

Figure 150. Relation of viscosity to concentration for six types of methylcellulose.

A solution of methylcellulose may also be made by making a slurry of the powder with 5 parts of alcohol, glycerin, or propylene glycol. If less of the polyol is used, the mixture is too viscid and forms lumps. Water is then added gradually with stirring to the slurry. A wetting agent may be used in a manner similar to the polyols; however, certain wetting agents affect the viscosity. At 1 per cent solution of dioctyl sodium sulfosuccinate increases the viscosity of methylcellulose 65 HG 4000 cp by 48 per cent; a 1 per cent solution of sodium stearate increases the viscosity of a 2 per cent methylcellulose 100 cp by 540 per cent.

As a solution of methylcellulose is heated, its viscosity initially decreases until a temperature is reached at which gelation occurs. As the temperature is raised, the energy of the water molecules is increased, and the hydrogen bond to the methylcellulose is ruptured. With the rupture of the hydrogen bonds the methylcellulose is no longer hydrated, and its linear molecules intertwine and precipitate as a gel at approximately 45 to 55°. In general, the addition of salts and additives lowers the gel temperature. Methylcellulose in which 7 to 16 per cent of the substitution is hydroxypropyl groups, gels at a higher temperature and is known in pharmacy as hydroxypropyl cellulose. The high-gel methylcelluloses are designated by HG, which is preceded by a number indicating the gel temperature. Thus, methylcellulose 65 HG is a mixed methyl and hydroxypropyl ether of methylcellulose and its 2 per cent aqueous solution gels at 65°.

Methylcellulose moderately lowers interfacial tension. At viscosities less than 500 cp the surface tension of methylcellulose is approximately 50 dyn cm^{-1} at 25°. Although primarily a suspending agent, methylcellulose can be used as a protective colloid, and it forms oil-in-water emulsions. At 25° the interfacial tension between mineral oil and methylcellulose solution is approximately 20 dyn cm^{-1}. In general, the low-viscosity types possess greater surface activity than the high-viscosity types. The high-viscosity types possess more film-forming properties than the low-viscosity types. The low-viscosity types had been used as a wetting and dispersing agent in intramuscular parenteral suspension for reconstitution. As methylcellulose is not metabolized, its use in parenterals is not recommended.

Methylcellulose is nonionic and neutral. It is stable from pH 3 to 11. Methylcellulose can be salted out of solution by high concentrations of additives. This is caused by a competition of the additive for water and the dehydration of the methylcellulose that precipitates. Eight grams of anhydrous magnesium chloride, 4 g of anhydrous sodium sulfate, or 65 g of sucrose is the maximum amount that can be added to 100 ml of a 2 per cent solution of methylcellulose, 4000 cp. A 2 per cent solution of methylcellulose may be prepared with up to 40 per cent alcohol in water. Methylcellulose 65 HG and 60 HG will tolerate a maximum of 60 and 80 per cent alcohol, respectively.

Sodium Carboxymethylcellulose. The water-soluble sodium carboxymethylcellulose used in pharmacy is a substituted cellulose containing from 0.65 to 0.85 sodium carboxymethyl groups per anhydroglucose unit. Like methylcellulose, the degree of substitution controls the solubility, and the length of the linear molecule controls the viscosity for each degree of substitution. The viscosity types of premium sodium carboxymethylcellulose are designed as low, medium, and high. In the designation sodium carboxylmethylcellulose-P-75-L, the letter P indicates that it has been refined to a premium grade, the number refers to the degree of substitution of 0.75, and the letter L indicates it is a low-viscosity type. The viscosity of sodium carboxymethylcellulose decreases with an increase in temperature. The relationship of concentration to apparent viscosity is shown in Figure 151. It should be recalled that solutions of cellulose derivatives have a pseudoplastic flow.

Sodium carboxymethylcellulose dissolves in cold or hot water. Solutions can be most rapidly prepared when the water is heated, a high-shear mixing is used, and the powder is added properly. The powder is added to the vigorously agitated water at a rate slow enough so that the particles remain separate and are individually wetted without clumping but not so slow that the solution becomes viscid before all the powder is added.

Sodium carboxymethylcellulose is anionic and is soluble in water by ion-dipole and dipole-dipole interactions. Solutions of sodium carboxymethylcellulose are slightly alkaline and are stable from pH 6 to 10. As the pH is decreased the solution loses viscosity, and at pH 2 the free acid is precipitated.

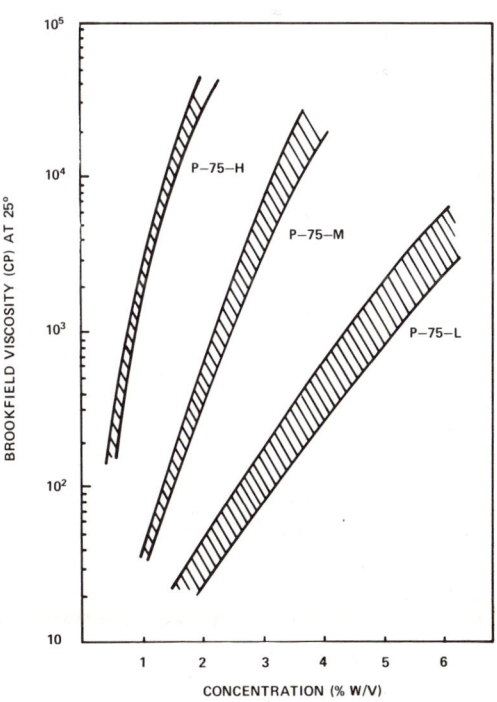

Figure 151. Relation of viscosity to concentration for three types of sodium carboxymethylcellulose.

In general, the compatibility of sodium carboxymethylcellulose with salts depends on whether or not the cation of the added salt forms a soluble salt of carboxymethylcellulose. Moderate concentrations of potassium chloride have little effect; however, if zirconium sulfate is added, the insoluble zirconium carboxymethylcellulose is precipitated. Usually monovalent cations form soluble salts, and polyvalent cations form insoluble salts.

Microcrystalline cellulose in combination with sodium carboxymethylcellulose or methylcellulose may be used as a suspending agent. The commercially available microcrystalline cellulose, Avicel®, is a water-dispersible colloid, which contains 8 per cent sodium carboxymethylcellulose to aid in its dispersion. When stirred in water it forms a sol. At concentrations exceeding 1 per cent the elongated cellulose particles interact to form an opaque, thixotropic gel. A microcrystalline cellulose sol is flocculated by small amounts of electrolytes and cationic polymers and surface-active agents. The flocculated system settles to a large sedimentation volume and retards caking. When methylcellulose or sodium carboxymethylcellulose are added to a microcrystalline cellulose dispersion, the polymers act as a protective colloid and are adsorbed on the cellulose particles. A network is formed of the solid particles linked by the polymer chains to produce a thixotropic system. This pseudoplastic and thixotropic system is an excellent vehicle for a suspension, because the dispersed phase is held in the thixotropic structure during storage, and the suspension provides a pourable consistency when in use.

89.	Aluminum hydroxide	52 g
	Magnesium trisilicate	100 g
	Avicel	11 g
	Sodium carboxymethylcellulose-70-M	9 g
	Purified water	828 ml

Sig.: Antacid suspension

The microcrystalline cellulose is dispersed in the water by means of a high-shear mixer. The sodium carboxymethylcellulose is added and dissolved by means of high-shear mixer. The aluminum hydroxide and magnesium trisilicate are added and mixed. The suspension is homogenized.

Montomorillonite Clay. The clays used as suspending agents in pharmacy have primarily a montomorillonite structure, as shown in Figure 152. Their plate-like crystals probably consist of alternate layers of alumina and silica bonded by various bridges. The units of the montmorillonite clays are loosely held together by weak O-O associations. In the presence of water, these weak O-O associations are broken to an extent, and the clay imbibes water. With the sorption of water into its structure, the clay swells and effectively the particles spread and interfere with the movement of other particles. The amount of free water is reduced as the dipole is oriented in some manner with the swollen particle and is not free to move at random. These effects produce an increase in viscosity. Montmorillonite clays are usually anionic, owing to the lattice arrangement. In an aqueous medium the unbalanced charge in the lattice usually results in a negative charge on the particle. Thus, cations are attracted toward the particle, and a diffuse double layer with a ζ potential is formed. The flow characteristics of aqueous dispersion of montmorillonite clays are altered by electrolytes, which change the ζ potential.

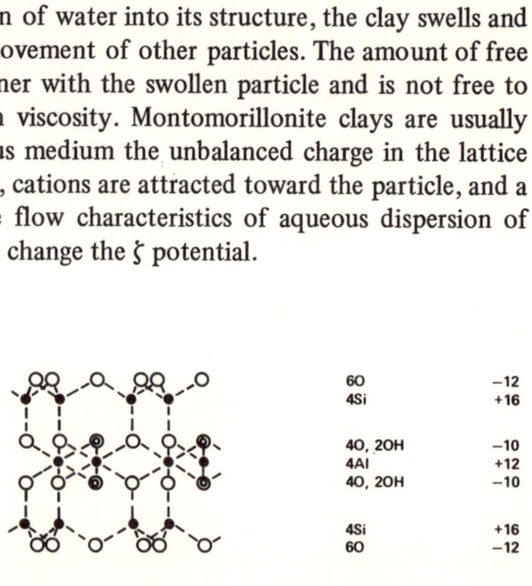

Figure 152. Planar representation of the unit cell of an ideal montmorillonite clay. The number and type of atom or group in every lattice plane are given in the left column. The necessary or available electrons in each sheet are given in the right column; if the (+) and (-) are not equal, the lattice has a charge.

6O	−12
4Si	+16
4O, 2OH	−10
4Al	+12
4O, 2OH	−10
4Si	+16
6O	−12

Different montomorillonite clays vary in metallic component. Bentonite is colloidal hydrated aluminum silicate. It exhibits plastic flow and is thixotropic at concentrations exceeding 4.3 per cent. Veegum® is a purified mixture of magnesium and aluminum silicates. It is lighter in color, odorless, and tasteless in comparison to bentonite. Veegum may adsorb bitter-tasting drugs and improve the palatability of a liquid medication; however, clinical tests should demonstrate that the drug is not so strongly adsorbed that its biological availability is significantly lessened.

The plastic and thixotropic behavior is due to the interparticular interaction, which is influenced by electrolytes and pH. Bentonite is anionic and exhibits maximum viscosity in the alkaline range. It is not suitable for use at pH less than 6 and is coagulated by strong acids. The viscosity and yield value of bentonite suspensions are relatively unaffected by a change in temperature.

To prepare an aqueous dispersion the bentonite or Veegum is slowly added to the water with continuous agitation. More complete hydration is obtained by dispersing the clay before adding any electrolyte. Hydration is slow and the maximum viscosity may not be attained in a single day. The most significant factor in reducing the time required for hydration is the use of high-shear mixers. The use of hot water accelerates hydration and is recommended if low-shear mixers are used. To further shorten the time required, it is suggested that a 4 or 5 per cent dispersion be initially prepared and diluted to the required concentration after hydration.

Although bentonite is a suspending agent, it can be used to form emulsions because of its adsorption at the oil-water interface to form a protective film about the dispersed globules.

90. Calamine   6.0 g
    Zinc oxide   6.0 g
    Olive oil   40.0 ml
    Bentonite 6% in lime water, q.s. 100 ml

    Sig.: Calamine emulsion with bentonite

It is interesting to note that the order of mixing determines the type of emulsion formed in this formulation. If the olive oil is blended with the dry powders in a high-shear mixer and the bentonite in lime water is added last, a water-in-oil type of emulsion is formed. One might anticipate this type of emulsion due to the presence of calcium oleate formed by the reaction between the oleic acid in the olive oil and the calcium hydroxide solution. An oil-in-water emulsion may be formed by adding the calamine and zinc oxide to the bentonite in lime water in a high-shear mixer and last adding the olive oil.

EMULSIONS

Emulsification involves high-shear mixing. Emulsion formation is facilitated by the emulsifying agent, which reduces interfacial tension and allows the formation of a greatly enlarged interfacial area with a reduced energy input. The viscosity, phase volume ratio, densities, and interfacial tension contribute to one phase being dispersed in globules while the other phase reforms the dispersion medium. For example, in using acacia as an emulsifying agent the 4:2:1 ratio of oil to water to acacia has been found to be optimum for the formation of an oil-in-water emulsion, which is diluted to the desired volume after the primary emulsion is formed. Different ratios are required by other emulsifying agents.

Coalescence and Creaming

An emulsion is energetically unstable, and even in the presence of an emulsifying agent the globules cannot be subdivided and stabilized in the colloidal state. Any globules of colloidal size undergo Brownian movement and upon colliding coalesce with a reduction in free surface energy. In the presence of an emulsifying agent this continues until the globules no longer undergo Brownian movement. Thus, an emulsion seldom has globules less than 0.5 μ even if it is homogenized. An emulsion prepared manually in a mortar with a pestle probably has particles as large as 25 μ. It is the strength of the film of adsorbed emulsifying agent that slows coalescence to the extent that a practical emulsion is formed.

Creaming is the displacement of the less dense oil globules in an oil-in-water emulsion toward the surface. If a proper emulsifying agent is present, coalescence will be prevented by the film of adsorbed emulsifying agent, and the emulsion can be redispersed by shaking. Although phase separation does not occur in a creamed emulsion, the emulsion has a poor appearance and lacks uniformity. The Stokes equation indicates the influence of particle size, viscosity, and difference in densities upon the rate of creaming. Since particle size is the most important factor in slowing creaming, most emulsions are routinely homogenized.

Mathematically, when a given number of uniform spheres are packed as closely as possible, they occupy 74 per cent of the total volume. In actual emulsions the globules have a size distribution, and the smaller globules fit within the spaces between the larger globules. In real emulsions as the dispersed phase is progressively increased beyond 50 per cent, the viscosity increases from that of a fluid to a paste. As the phase volume of the dispersed phase is progressively increased, the particles become more and more distorted, with very close packing. This large surface offers resistance to flow of the particles, and the viscosity is increased.

The rate of creaming is inversely proportional to the viscosity of the emulsion. In most pharmaceutical emulsions the emulsifying agent is in excess of that necessary to form a monomolecular layer about the globules. The excess emulsifying agent forms micelles, which may solubilize some of the oil or oil-soluble medicinal compounds. The viscosity is increased by the excess emulsifying agent. The viscosity of an emulsion may be increased by (1) increasing the phase volume ratio of the dispersed phase, (2) reducing the particle size of the dispersed phase, (3) increasing the amount of emulsifying agent, and (4) adding a suspending agent.

Emulsions exhibit non-Newtonian flow. Concentrated emulsions show pseudoplastic flow, i.e., a high viscosity at rest and a low viscosity at high shear. The emulsifying agent and any added suspending agent influence the flow properties.

The emulsifying agent contributes to the stability by the tenacity of its film, its relative partial solubility in the two phases, and its formation of an electric double layer at the interface. The addition of polar solvents to an emulsion reduces the stability because the emulsifying agent is extracted from the interface by the polar solvent.

In some emulsions the type of emulsion is determined by the phase volume ratio. A sodium soap is generally thought to produce an oil-in-water emulsion. For a given concentration of soap, if the oil phase volume ratio exceeds a critical ratio, a water-in-oil emulsion is formed. The addition of sodium salts to an oil-in-water emulsion may salt out the soap with the formation of a water-in-oil emulsion. Phase inversion may also occur as the result of chemical reaction. An oil-in-water emulsion that is emulsified by a monovalent soap can be inverted by the addition of a polyvalent cation. Initially the polyvalent cation reduces the ζ potential; and as it enters the electrostatic field of the fatty acid anion it forms an insoluble soap, which favors the formation of a water-in-oil emulsion.

Uses of Emulsions

Oral Emulsions. The purpose of emulsification is to administer a uniform blend of immiscible liquids in a single preparation. An emulsifying agent is required to prepare a stable emulsion; it must be nontoxic and nonirritating for cosmetic and pharmaceutical use. Oral emulsions are the oil-in-water type. The emulsifying agent surrounds the oil so that the oily feel and taste are minimized. Flavoring agents are added to improve the palatability. The flavoring agent may partition between the two phases. This is desirable, as an emulsion in which both phases are flavored has a better initial and aftertaste than an emulsion, in which only the external phase is flavored. In selecting the concentration of a flavor to be used, consideration must be made for its partition ratio so that an adequate concentration remains at equilibrium in the external phase. A similar consideration must be given to the partitioning of preservatives in order that a concentration sufficient to prevent microorganic growth remains in the aqueous phase.

Emulsification may increase the intestinal absorption of fats. An emulsion homogenized to dispersed oil globules of less than 1 μ is rapidly assimilated. An antioxidant may be added to the oil to prevent rancidity. Propyl gallate, nordihydroquaiaretic acid, β-tocopherol, and tert-butyl hydroxyanisole are recognized antioxidants.

91.	Mineral oil	50.0 ml
	Agar	1.0 g
	Acacia	4.0 g
	Phenolphthalein	0.4 g
	Alcohol	6.0 ml
	Vanillin	5.0 mg
	Saccharin	5.0 mg
	Purified water, q.s.	100 ml

Sig.: Phenolphthalein in liquid petrolatum emulsion

The agar is boiled with 35 ml of water until dissolved. The agar solution is cooled to 45°. Sixteen milliters of the mineral oil is emulsified with the acacia and 8 ml of water. The remainder or the mineral oil is gradually added to the primary emulsion. The agar solution is added as required to maintain a suitable consistency. The vanillin, saccharin, and phenolphthalein are dissolved in the alcohol and gradually added to the emulsion. The emulsion is adjusted to final volume and is homogenized. The viscosity of the emulsion required that it be dispensed in a wide-mouthed bottle.

Topical Emulsion. By proper formulation a topical emulsion may be prepared with the fluidity of a lotion or the firmness of an ointment. Liniments are applied with massage; the consistency and slippery feel of these topical emulsions facilitates the rubbing involved in their application. Emulsification generally decreases the rate and extent of absorption of a drug by the skin; however, at times the presence of an emulsifying agent increases the rate of percutaneous absorption, i.e., absorption into and through the skin. Emulsions appeal to the patient, as they are easily washed from the surface, do not stain clothing, and do not feel greasy.

92.	Chlorophenothane	1.0 g
	Benzyl benzoate	11.5 ml
	Polysorbate 80	2.0 g
	Purified water, q.s.	100 ml

Sig.: Benzyl bensoate chlorophenothane lotion

The chlorophenothane, benzyl benzoate, and benzocaine are mixed with the polysorbate 80. The water is gradually added to form an oil-in-water emulsion. Purified water is added to final volume.

Intravenous Emulsion. A few parenteral emulsions have been used successfully in the administration of phytonadione and in the intravenous feeding of fats. Unwanted physiological effects, e.g., febrile reaction, and hemolysis, have limited the use of intravenous emulsions. Only a few emulsifying agents, e.g., lecithin, gelatin, Pluronic® F-68, serum albumin, and polysorbate 80, have been utilized. The intravenous emulsions are prepared by standard procedures and are then homogenized to a size less than 1 μ. The emulsion is then sealed in its container and sterilized in an autoclave.

93. Cottonseed oil   15.0 ml
    Dextrose   4.0 g
    Lecithin   1.2 g
    Pluronic®F-68   0.3 g
    Water for injection, q.s. 100 ml

Sig.: Fat emulsion for intravenous feeding

The lecithin is mixed with the cottonseed oil and is heated to 70°. The dextrose and Pluronic® F-68 are dissolved in water at 90°. The lecithin in cottonseed oil is added with agitation to the aqueous phase. The oil-in-water emulsion is homogenized until most of the particles are less than 1 μ in diameter and none are larger than 5 μ. The emulsion is filled into its final container and is autoclaved at 15 psi for 20 minutes.

Emulsifying Agents

An emulsifying agent is a surface-active agent that markedly lowers interfacial tension and concomitantly forms a tenacious film about the dispersed globules. Emulsifying agents may be classified as natural agents derived from animal, mineral, and vegetable sources, and as synthetic emulsifying agents. The synthetic agents are conveniently categorized as anionic, cationic, and nonionic agents. As cationic surface-active agents are not used as emulsifying agents, they are not discussed in this section.

Natural Emulsifying Agent. *Acacia.* Acacia is the dried gummy exudation of *Acacia senegal* and other species of acacia trees. It is one of the oldest emulsifying agents suitable for extemporaneous compounding of emulsions for oral administration. Acacia is typical of a natural vegetable product in that its properties vary with growing conditions, and it may contain extraneous matter acquired during collection. Acacia is a carbohydrate with a molecular weight of approximately 270,000 g mole^{-1}. As commercially available it is a mixture of calcium, magnesium, and potassium salt of arabic acid. Analysis of arabic acid indicates that it is composed of 30.3 per cent L-arabfuranose, 11.4 per cent L-rhamnopyranose, 36.9 per cent D-galactopyranose, and 13.8 per cent D-glucuronic acid. The chain consists of a 1,3 linkage of β-D-galactopyranose units. In the postulated structure given in Figure 153 arabinose and rhamnose, which are easily hydrolyzed from the arabic acid, are represented as R. The structure is branched with the D-glucuronic acid, being linked to the main chain through at least one D-galactose unit. Acacia is anionic and acidic, owing to the glucuronic acid in its structure; it will form a coacervate with positively charged macromolecules.

Acacia lowers interfacial tension and forms an oil-in-water emulsion. A 3.5 per cent acacia mucilage has a viscosity of approximately 135 cp. Since the viscosity is low, a suspending agent is often added to an acacia emulsion to retard creaming. Acacia mucilage retains its viscosity from pH 4 to 10. The acidic groups react with heavy metal ions to form a stringy precipitate. Any ingredients that have a strong affinity for water tend to dehydrate acacia; however, acacia mucilage can be prepared in 40 per cent alcohol. An enzyme in acacia promotes the oxidation of phenolic compounds, but it may be inactivated by heat.

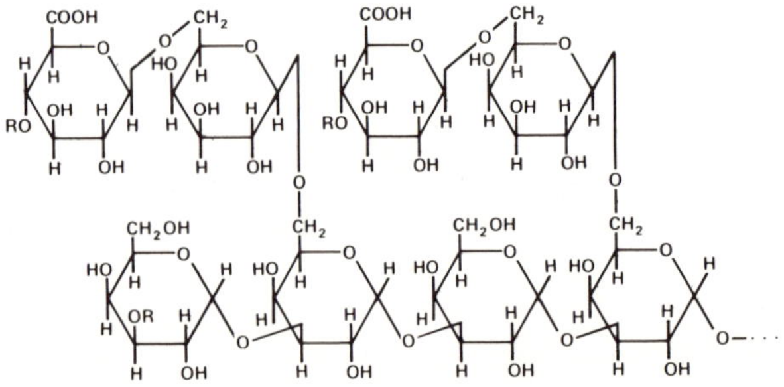

Figure 153. Postulated structure for arabic acid, with R representing L-arabofuranose and L-rhamnopyranose.

Lecithin. The term "lecithin" applies to a group of compounds that are glyceryl esters of two fatty acid molecules and esterified at the third carbon atom with phosphoric acid, which has an ester linkage to choline:

$$\begin{array}{c} \quad\quad\quad\quad\quad O \\ \quad\quad O\ \ CH_2\text{-}O\text{-}\overset{\|}{C}\text{-}R \\ R'\text{-}\overset{\|}{C}\text{-}O\text{-}CH \\ \quad\quad | \quad\ O \\ \quad\quad CH_2\text{-}O\overset{\|}{P}\text{-}OCH_2CH_2\overset{+}{N}(CH_3)_3 \\ \quad\quad\quad\ \ \overset{|}{O_-} \end{array}$$

Lecithin is present in animal and vegetable materials. Much of the lecithin used in pharmacy is obtained from soybean. In the natural lecithins the phosphoryl choline group is attached to the α-carbon atom. Although the β-carbon is asymmetric, the L isomers are found in nature. The lecithins differ in their fatty acids. In general the saturated stearic and palmitic acid are attached to the α-carbon; the unsaturated oleic, linoleic, linolenic, and arachidonic acid are attached to the β-carbon.

Purified lecithin is a waxy, colorless solid. It is readily oxidized and turns yellow on exposure to air and light. It is insoluble in water, but it is hygroscopic and forms a colloidal sol with water. Lecithin is decomposed by alkali.

Lecithin greatly reduced interfacial tension and forms oil-in-water emulsions. It has been used successfully in intramuscular parenteral suspensions and intravenous parenteral emulsions as a wetting and emulsifying agent.

Cholesterol. Lanolin is a purified, fat-like substance from the wool of sheep. It contains cholesterol and its esters, which impart a water-absorbing ability, owing to the formation of a water-in-oil emulsion. Cholesterol has the structure

Cholesterol is nonionic and is unaffected by moderate changes in pH. Pure cholesterol is not as effective an emulsifying agent as its mixture with the esters. Modifications of lanolin prepared by physical and chemical treatment are commercially available for use as emulsifying agents in cosmetic and dermatological preparations.

Synthetic Anionic Agents. *Soap.* The term "soap" refers to the salt of a long-chain fatty acid and an alkaline substance. A general formula is R—COOM. Soaps prepared from C_{12} to C_{18} fatty acids produce a marked lowering of interfacial tension. The monovalent alkali soaps, e.g., ammonium, potassium, or sodium salts of aluric, myristic, oleic, palmitic, or stearic acid form oil-in-water emulsions. A potassium soap is known as a soft soap; a sodium soap is know as hard soap. A low concentration of soap dissolves in water and alcohol. As the concentration exceeds the CMC, a colloidal sol is formed. If the concentration is further increased, the soap will form a gel. Aqueous soap dispersions are strongly alkaline; they are not used for internal preparations because of their acrid taste and purgative action. Soaps find their widest use as detergents. Soaps may be used to form solubilized liquids and emulsions for external use.

In an acidic medium the emulsifying characteristics of soap are destroyed as the insoluble free fatty acid is formed. In the presence of excessive polyvalent cations, the water-insoluble polyvalent or metallic soap is precipitated. Calcium soap is the only metallic soap used in pharmacy as an emulsifying agent. It is used to form water-in-oil dermatological emulsions. It is usually prepared by mixing calcium hydroxide solution with olive oil, which contains oleic acid. If an oil, e.g., cottonseed oil or linseed oil, with a low acid value is used, oleic acid may be added to produce sufficient emulsifying agent.

94. Phenol   1 g
     Calamine   8 g
     Zinc oxide   8 g
     Olive oil   50 ml
     Calcium hydroxide solution, q.s.   100 ml

Sig.: Calamine emulsion

The calamine, phenol, and zinc oxide are mixed with the olive oil. The calcium hydroxide solution is gradually added to the olive oil with agitation to make 100 ml. The calcium hydroxide reacts with the free acid in olive oil to yield calcium oleate:

$$2CH_3(CH_2)_7 CH=CH (CH_2)_7 COOH + Ca(OH)_2 \rightarrow$$

$$[CH_3(CH_2)_7 CH=CH (CH_2)_7 COO]_2 Ca + 2H_2O$$

The calcium oleate forms a water-in-oil emulsion.

The reaction of an organic amine with a fatty acid produces an organic soap. The organic soap formed by the reaction of triethanolamine with oleic or stearic acid is widely used to form oil-in-water emulsions for topical application.

Sodium Lauryl Sulfate. A sulfated surface-active agent is an alkaline or amine salt of a sulfated long-chain alcohol. Sodium lauryl sulfate has the formula

$$CH_3(CH_2)_{10} - CH_2O\overset{O}{\underset{O}{-\overset{\uparrow}{\underset{\downarrow}{S}}-}}ONa$$

It forms oil-in-water emulsions. As its calcium salt is water soluble, it finds use in dental and topical preparations. It is not precipitated by an acidic medium because the acid form is readily soluble in water.

Glyceryl monostearate is a waxy, nonionic solid that is insoluble in water. Although two hydroxyl groups and a long alkyl chain confer some degree of surface activity, pure glyceryl monostearate is too hydrophobic to be an effective emulsifying agent. A mixture of glyceryl monostearate and sodium lauryl sulfate or a monovalent soap is water dispersible and is known as glyceryl monostearate, self-emulsifying. Glyceryl monostearate, self-emulsifying, is effective in forming oil-in-water emulsions. The surface-active agent added to the glyceryl monostearate determines the suitability for internal use.

Dioctyl Sodium Sulfosuccinate. Dioctyl sodium sulfosuccinate is a waxy solid that is soluble in water and most nonpolar organic solvents. It has the formula

$$\begin{array}{c} \quad\quad\quad\quad\quad\quad C_2H_5 \\ \quad\quad\quad\quad\quad\quad | \\ CH_3(CH_2)_3 - CHCH_2\text{-OOC-CH}_2 \\ \quad\quad\quad\quad\quad\quad\quad\quad\quad\quad | \quad\; O \\ \quad\quad\quad\quad\quad\quad\quad\quad\quad\quad\quad\;\; \uparrow \\ CH_3(CH_3)_3 - CHCH_2\text{-OOC-CH-}\overset{}{\underset{\downarrow}{S}}\text{-ONa} \\ \quad\quad\quad\quad\quad\quad | \quad\quad\quad\quad\; O \\ \quad\quad\quad\quad\quad\quad C_2H_5 \end{array}$$

It is a strong wetting agent. A 0.1 per cent solution lowers the surface tension of water to 28.7 dyn cm^{-1}. Its calcium salt is soluble as a result of high polarity of the sulfonate group. It will form oil-in-water emulsions; however, the emulsion is improved by incorporation of a hydrophilic colloid.

Synthetic Nonionic Agents. Most of the nonionic emulsifying agents used in pharmacy are complex esters and/or ethers of alcohols. They possess the advantages of being stable over a wide pH range and of not reacting with ions. In general, they are prepared from a hydrophobic compound, possessing a polar group having a free hydrogen atom, by reaction with ethylene oxide. As the length of the polyoxyethylene chain is increased, the substance becomes more water soluble. A wide range of emulsifying ability is obtained by varying the length of the polyoxyethylene chain so that the HLB of the molecules is controlled. The large number of emulsifying agents and their complex structure make it necessary to utilize the HLB system to determine the type of emulsion formed and the proper blend of emulsifying agents to be used.

Polyoxyl 40 Stearate. The polyol esters are formed by the reaction of a polyhydric alcohol, e.g., glycerin, propylene glycol, and polyethylene glycol, with a fatty acid. Many of the glycol esters, e.g., glyceryl monostearate, are poor emulsifying agents unless they are blended with an anionic surface-active agent.

Polyoxyl 40 stearate is an effective emulsifying agent for forming oil-in-water emulsions. It is polyoxyethylene 40 monostearate with a general formula

$$C_{17}H_{35}COO(CH_2CH_2O)_{40}H$$

Polyoxyl 40 stearate or Myrj® 52 is a waxy solid that is water soluble and has an HLB value 16.9. It is especially useful in preparing topical emulsions that contain astringent electrolytes.

Polysorbate 80. Arlacels® are partial esters of sorbitan and fatty acids, e.g., lauric, oleic, palmitic, and stearic acid. Arlacels® are oil dispersible or oil soluble and have a HLB value less than 8.6. Tweens® are prepared by reacting the nonesterified hydroxyl groups of Arlacels with ethylene oxide. The polyoxyethylene chain confers water dispersibility or solubility upon the Tween®. The length of the polyoxyethylene chain determines the solubility and HLB of the emulsifying agent. Tweens® have an HLB value greater than 9.6. The chemical relationship between an Arlacel® and a Tween® of like number is shown in Figure 154. A blend of an Arlacel® and a Tween® is routinely used to obtain the proper HLB value to form a stable emulsion.

Polysorbate 80 is an oleate ester of sorbitol and its anhydrides condensed with approximately 20 oxyethylene units. It is a liquid with a density of 1.1 g cc^{-1} and a viscosity of 350 to 550 cp at 25°. Polysorbate 80 is soluble in water and forms oil-in-water emulsions. As a surface-active agent that may be used internally, it is widely used in pharmacy in the role of an emulsifying agent, a solubilizing agent, and a dispersing agent.

Preservatives

The preservation of pharmaceuticals against microorganic growth is a complex problem that must be experimentally evaluated for each product. The effectiveness of a preservative depends on the constituents of the product, the variety of microorganisms present, pH, and type of container. Sterility is obligatory for all ophthalmic and parenteral products; sterility is recommended for nasal and otic products. If these products are sterilized and packaged in a single-dose container, a preservative is not required. If the sterile product is packaged in a multiple-dose container, a bacteriostatic agent is added to prevent microorganic growth if the product is contaminated during withdrawal of a portion of the contents. The use of bacteriostatic agents is limited to injections with a dose not exceeding 5 ml.

In oral and topical products sterility is not necessary; however, good manufacturing practice requires careful procedures to prevent contamination. Products that are not hermetically sealed and that would support microorganic growth under normal shelf life should contain chemical preservatives. The active growth of microorganisms in an emulsion results in an unaesthetic appearance and spoilage; it also changes the rheological properties and may break the emulsion. Although any constituent used in preparing the product may have been contaminated, the microorganisms grow in the aqueous phase, in which the nutrient constituents provide a favorable environment for growth. Thus, to be effective an adequate concentration of the preservative must be dissolved in the aqueous phase.

Pharmaceutical polyphasic systems are good media for molds and yeasts, because they have a high water content and may contain carbohydrates and/or proteins. In an emulsion the partition ratio of the preservative between the oil and aqueous phases influences the concentration of the preservative to which the microorganisms are exposed. A preservative with a high oil solubility and relatively low water solubility is less effective and requires a higher concentration in an emulsion than in an aqueous solution. The effective concentration of a preservative in a polyphasic system is affected by any interactions, micellular solubilization, or complexation between the preservative and other ingredients, e.g., methylparaben and polysorbate 80, and phenol and soap.

The ideal preservative should be (1) effective against all microorganisms, (2) effective in low concentrations, (3) nontoxic, (4) compatible, and (5) tasteless and odorless. Some preservatives that have been used in pharmaceuticals are given in Table LXVIII.

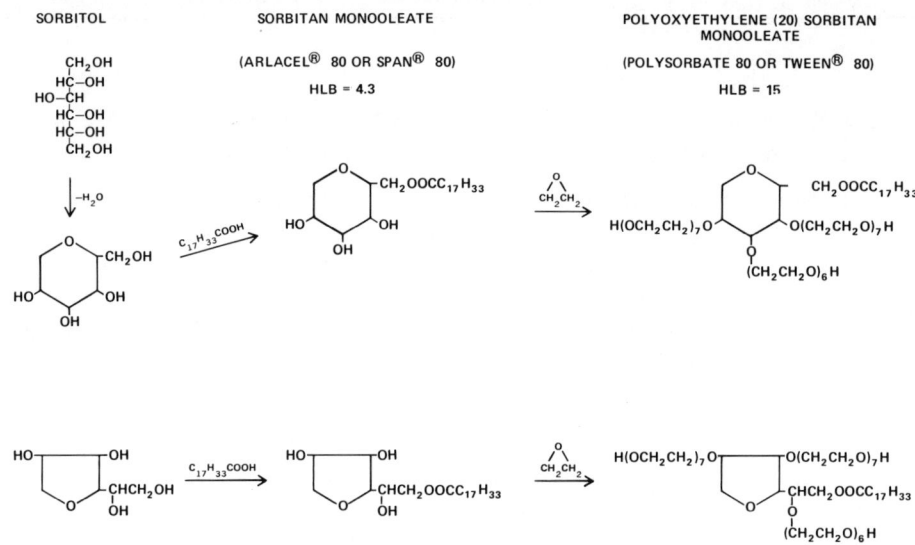

Figure 154. Formulas for a typical Arlacel®, which is formed by anhydrization of sorbitol to hexitans and their esterification, and a typical Tween®, which is formed by the addition of polyoxyethylene chains to the nonesterified hydroxyls of the Arlacel®.

Table LXVIII Preservatives Frequently Used in Pharmaceuticals

Preservative	Concentration (%)	Ineffective in	General Uses
Alcohol	15		Oral, topical
Benzalkonium chloride	0.002-0.01		Ophthalmic, oral, topical
Benzoic acid	0.1-0.2	Alkaline media	Oral, topical
Chlorobutanol	0.5	Alkaline media	Ophthalmic, parenteral
p-Chloro-*m*-cresol	0.1-0.2		Parenteral, topical
Cresol	0.4		Biological, parenteral
Methylparaben	0.2		Oral, ophthalmic, parenteral, topical
Phenol	0.5		Biological, parenteral
Phenylmercuric nitrate	0.004-0.01		Oral, ophthalmic, parenteral, topical
Sorbic acid	0.2	Alkaline media	Oral
Thimerosal	0.01	Acidic media	Parenterals

14 | PLASTIC PHARMACEUTICAL SUSPENSIONS AND EMULSIONS

A substance is said to be deformed when the application of an appropriate stress or force per unit area changes the shape or size of the material. A substance is said to flow if its degree of deformation changes continually with time. If a substance is an elastic solid, the application of a nonhomogeneous stress, i.e., different stress at different positions, causes deformation or strain but not flow. Upon the release of the stress, the elastic solid returns to its original state.

In the fluid polyphasic systems discussed in Chapter 13, the application of any anisotropic stress, i.e., different stress in different directions, and nonhomogeneous stress, however small, results in flow. This pseudoplastic flow is exhibited by most of the hydrophilic colloidal sols utilized in pharmacy.

A plastic substance flows at a rate that is a function of the applied stress if the stress exceeds the yield value. The yield value represents the shearing stress required to break the interactions between the constituent particles either in selective planes of deformation or in all directions with deflocculation and an increase in particulate movement. If a shearing stress less than the yield value is applied to a plastic substance, it is deformed. Upon the release of the shearing stress, the plastic substance does not return to its original state but remains in a deformed state. Dispersions of carboxyvinyl polymer and homogenized tragacanth exhibit plastic characteristics.

Creams, jellies, ointments, pastes, and suppositories are polyphasic systems that possess plastic properties; they deform under applied stress, but they retain their shape after the stress is removed. When an ointment or jelly flows from the orifice of a tube, it flows with a viscosity that is a function of the applied shearing stress. No flow occurs unless the applied stress exceeds the yield value. When a plastic material flows through a cylinder such as the nozzle of an ointment tube, the shear stress is a minimum at the center of the cylinder and a maximum at the wall. Under certain conditions, the stress near the wall exceeds the yield value at the same time that the stress near the center of the cylinder is less than the yield value. The plastic substance then flows along the cylinder as a solid plug surrounded by liquid.

Petrolatum is a gel consisting of liquid hydrocarbons held in a matrix of microcrystalline solid hydrocarbons. Petrolatum has a yield value and exhibits plastic flow. The hysteresis loop shown in Figure 155 demonstrates that petrolatum is thixotropic. The thixotropic breakdown of petrolatum is slower then the gel-sol transformation of more fluid thixotropic substances. Under the range of rates of shear to which petrolatum is exposed in normal use, its yield value ranges from 1000 to 10,000 dyn cm^{-2} and its plastic viscosity is from 5 to 50 cp. At low rates of shear the rheogram of petrolatum has a spur or bulge on the initial upcurve. This bulge may be explained by considering the composition of petrolatum. Petrolatum varies according to its source and the methods of processing and refining. It is composed of a mixture of n-, iso- and cyclic-paraffins. The rheological properties of a given petrolatum depend on the ratio of these constituents. The best pharmaceutical grade has a low content of n-paraffins. Under mechanical stress the structural collapse of the finer gel of the iso-paraffins is less than that of the n-paraffins. At rest petrolatum is a three-dimensional gel composed of the various paraffins associated by random entwinement and physical interaction. As the rate of shear is increased, the

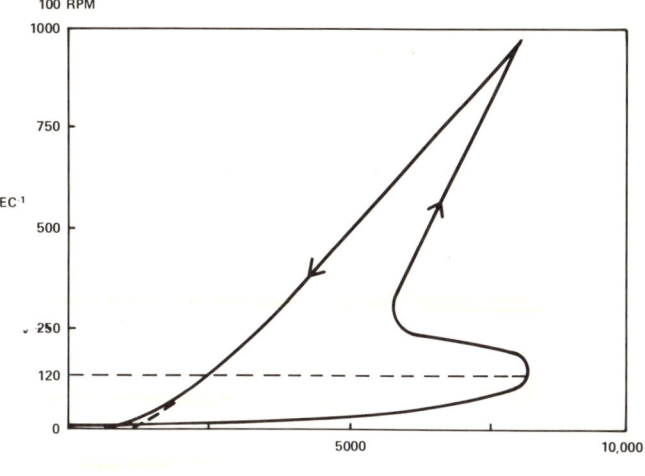

Figure 155. Rheogram of petrolatum exhibiting thixotropy and a yield value. [J.C. Boylan, *J. Pharm. Sci. 55*, 710 (1966).]

n-paraffins tend to align in the direction shear, but the cyclic- and iso-paraffins do not align as readily and retain some of the three-dimensional gel structure. As the rate of shear is further increased, the paraffins become further aligned, with the separation of some of the entwined paraffin chains. With this separation and breakdown of the gel the bulge in the rheogram disappears and the difference between the upcurve and the downcurve becomes minimal. This pheonomenon is desirable in an ointment. When petrolatum is applied to the skin, the initial few seconds of shearing stress destroys much of the gel structure making it easy to spread.

OINTMENTS

Ointments are plastic preparations intended for external application to the body. The plastic viscosity of most ointments is lowered by the stress of application, so they are easily spread; the plastic viscosity is controlled by modification of the formulation. Ointments may be used topically as emollients, which make the skin more pliable, and as protective barriers, which prevent harmful substances from coming in contact with the skin. A therapeutic ointment is used for systemic effect; the therapeutic ointment base acts as a vehicle for a medicinal compound that is intended to undergo percutaneous absorption, i.e., absorption through the skin into the deep tissue and blood vessels.

Ointments should be chemically and physically stable. The medicinal compound must be uniformly distributed. As ointments are applied to sensitive, diseased, or denuded skin, any insoluble substances must be reduced to a size small enough to avoid a gritty sensation or irritation. The viscosity of the ointment should permit it to be easily extruded from the tube and easily applied while it still adheres to the skin. If ointments are stored in an environment warm enough to soften the ointment, insoluble powders may settle from suspension-type ointments and the dispersed phases may separate in emulsion-type ointments.

Ointments are packaged in tubes or jars. When an ointment is packed in a jar, manual pressure is applied with a spatula to eliminate air spaces. The surface is smoothed by passing a flexible spatula over the surface of the packed ointment. Ointments prepared by fusion are packaged while they are still fluid enough to be poured. Ointment tubes are available in various sizes with plain tips or nasal, ophthalmic, rectal, and vaginal tips. Ointments packaged in tubes are less messy and the amount removed is better controlled than those packaged in jars. A tube is more sanitary than a jar because it minimizes contamination. Loss of moisture and uptake of oxygen is reduced because of the small area that is briefly exposed to the atmosphere by ointments in tubes.

The community pharmacist can easily dispense extemporaneous ointments in collapsible tubes. The tube is cleaned by flushing it with water and then rinsing it in alcohol. The ointment is placed in the center of a square piece of paper at least as long as the tube to be filled, and it is rolled tightly in the paper to form a narrow cone. The cone is inserted as far as possible into the uncapped, empty tube. With the tube on a flat surface the ointment is gradually pushed toward the apex of the cone by a broad spatula. The spatula is advanced along the paper and along the tube flattening it until the ointment extrudes from the tip. The spatula is pressed firmly on the flattened lower portion of the tube, and the paper is rapidly withdrawn from the tube. The cap is replaced, and the lower end is trimmed, if necessary, and is folded over at least once and crimped firmly in position.

A paste is a thick, stiff ointment that does not soften at body temperature. The high solid content and the adhesion between the solid particles account for the stiffness of a paste. The high per cent of powder absorbs serous secretions from acute lesions that tend toward crusting, oozing and vesiculation. Pastes are difficult to remove from the skin and are unsuitable for application to hairy regions.

Suspension-Type Ointments

Ointments in which a finely divided medicinal solid is uniformly dispersed are plastic suspensions. The medicinal compound is the dispersed phase, and the base is the dispersion medium. The consistency of the dispersion medium is such that sedimentation does not normally occur; however, if the ointment is exposed to heat, it may soften or liquefy so that sedimentation can occur.

Bases. The oleaginous bases consist mainly of hydrocarbons. The hydrocarbons have the advantage of being physiologically inert, chemically stable and unreactive with medicinal compounds.

Petrolatum is a mixture of liquid hydrocarbons held in a gel matrix of microcrystalline solid hydrocarbons. Petrolatum has a melting range from 38 to 60°. It is available as yellow petrolatum and decolorized white petrolatum. Mineral oil may be added to decrease the viscosity of petrolatum. Nonpolar stiffening agents, e.g., ceresin (61 to 78°), paraffin (50 to 57°), or spermaceti (42 to 50°), may be added to increase the consistency of petrolatum. White ointment and yellow ointment are white and yellow petrolatum in which 5 per cent white and yellow wax, respectively, has been incorporated. These bases are prepared by the fusion method.

    95. White wax   50 g
          White petrolatum   950 g

          Sig.: White ointment

The white wax is melted on a water bath to avoid charring, and the white petrolatum is added and warmed until liquefied. The mixture is stirred until congealed. The addition of wax or an insoluble powder to a petrolatum base increases its thixotropy, yield value, and plastic viscosity. The effect on the concentration of wax on the plastic viscosity and on the yield value and the thixotropy are shown in Figures 156 and 157.

Plastibase® is a gel prepared by shock cooling of liquid petrolatum and 5 per cent polyethylene with an approximate molecular weight of 1300 g mole^{-1}. The mobility of the liquid petrolatum permits the drug to diffuse readily from the base. Plastibase melts around 90°, and its consistency changes only slightly over the temperature range 15 to 60°. Drugs that dissolve in Plastibase® tend to lower its viscosity. Plastibase® should not be melted, as it congeals to a smooth base only if flash cooled.

The oleaginous bases are occulsive, i.e., prevent passage of moisture and heat, and are objectionable if the physician desires the escape of heat and the evaporation of serous discharges from inflamed areas. They are used as emollients and as inert bases for readily hydrolyzable drugs. Their stability, which permits heat sterilization, make the oleaginous bases a widely used vehicle for ophthalmic ointments. Oleaginous bases do not conveniently take up aqueous solutions. Cosmetically, they are greasy and difficult to wash from the skin and clothing.

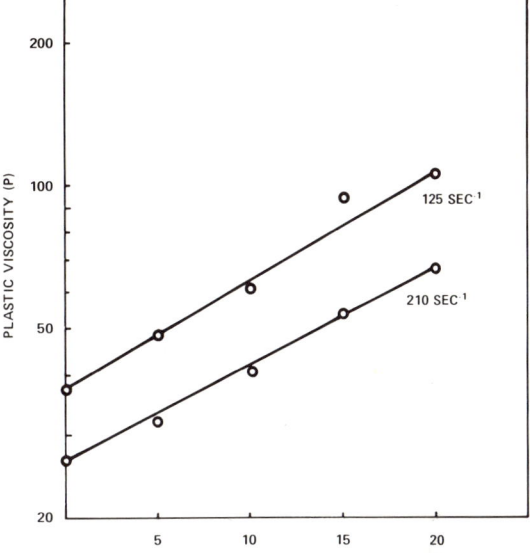

Figure 156. Influence of concentration of white wax on viscosity of petrolatum. [H.B. Kostenbauder and A.N. Martin, *J. Am. Pharm. Assoc., Sci. Ed.* **43,** 401 (1954).]

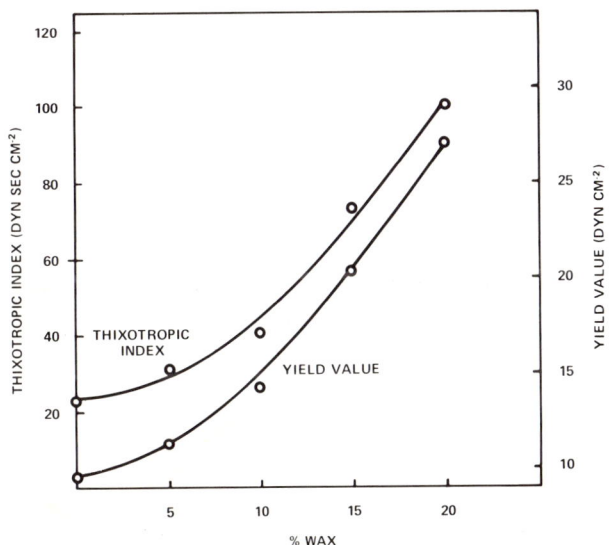

Figure 157. Influence of concentration of white wax on thixotropy and yield value of petrolatum. [H.B. Kostenbauder and A.N. Martin, *J. Am. Pharm. Assoc., Sci. Ed.* **43,** 401 (1954).]

Ointment bases that readily take up water are known as absorption bases. Absorption bases are often anhydrous but upon being mixed with water form emulsions.

Wool fat is the refined fat-like material obtained from the wool of sheep. It melts from 36 to 42°. Wool fat absorbs large amounts of water, owing to the presence of cholesterols and their esters, which produce a water-in-oil emulsion. Wool fat forms an occlusive layer that softens and makes the skin more pliable. Wool fat is seldom used alone, as it is tacky and not cosmetically acceptable. Lanolin is wool fat that contains 25 to 30 per cent water.

Hydrophilic petrolatum absorbs up to 30 per cent water with the formation of a water-in-oil emulsion. As the amount of water incorporates is increased, the yield value is decreased and the plastic viscosity and thixotropy are increased. Hydrophilic petrolatum is superior to wool fat because it is not tacky and is practically ordorless. Although it will take up aqueous solutions, hydrophilic petrolatum is not easy to wash from the skin.

96.	Cholesterol	30 g
	Stearyl alcohol	30 g
	White wax	80 g
	White petrolatum	860 g

Sig.: Hydrophilic petrolatum

The stearyl alcohol, white wax, and white petrolatum are melted on a steam bath. The cholesterol is dissolved in the molten mixture. The mixture is removed from the bath and stirred until it congeals.

A water-soluble base is one that dissolves in water. The only available water-soluble base is composed of polyethylene glycols, which have the general structure

$$H(OCH_2CH_2)_xOH$$

The consistency of the polyethylene glycol depends on its molecular weight. Polyethylene glycol 400 is a liquid with $x = 8$ or 9 and a molecular weight of approximately 400 g mole^{-1}; polyethylene glycol 4000 is a solid with $x = 68$ to 84 and a molecular weight of approximately 4000 g mole^{-1}. The various polyethylene glycols can be blended to obtain a wide range of consistency.

97.	Undecylenic acid	50 g
	Zinc undecylenate	200 g
	Polyethylene glycol 4000	300 g
	Polyethylene glycol 400	450 g

Sig.: Compound undecylenic acid ointment

The polyethylene glycol is melted on a water bath at 65°. The undecylenic acid and the zinc undecylenate are added. The ointment is removed from the water bath and is stirred until congealed. Polyethylene glycol ointments are anhydrous and can be easily washed from the skin. They may be somewhat irritating to inflamed tissue. There is little percutaneous absorption from polyethylene glycols, as they are nonocclusive and the moisture loss lessens the hydration of the skin.

In the mechanical incorporation method of preparing suspension-type ointments the drug is reduced to a powder before it is incorporated into the ointment base. Manually an ointment slab and spatula or a mortar and pestle may be used. The community pharmacist levigates or triturates the drug with a small portion of the base or with a levigating agent, e.g., mineral oil, to ensure that there has been adequate reduction of particle size. Then it is blended geometrically with the remainder of the base. An ointment slab is a porcelain plate or heavy glass that is ground on one side to aid in reducing particle size. A broad flexible spatula is used to rub the ointment on the slab. A mortar and pestle are suggested if appreciable amounts of a liquid are to be incorporated. If a further reduction of particle size of the commercially available medicinal compound is not required, it is convenient to mix the ointment base and the drug on a sheet of disposable parchment paper. This eliminates the need to clean a slab or mortar.

98.	Ammoniated mercury, very fine	50 g
	Mineral oil	30 g
	White ointment	920 g

Sig.: Ammoniated mercury ointment

The ammoniated mercury is levigated on an ointment slab with the levigating agent, mineral oil, to form a smooth paste. The white ointment is then geometrically added and levigated until uniform.

99. Coal tar   10.00 g
    Polysorbate 80   5.00 g
    Zinc oxide   246.25 g
    Starch   246.25 g
    White petrolatum   492.50 g

Sig.: Coal tar ointment

The zinc oxide, starch, and white petrolatum are mixed to form zinc oxide paste. The polysorbate 80 is mixed with the coal tar, and the mixture is geometrically mixed with the zinc oxide paste. The polysorbate 80 lowers interfacial tension and facilitates the uniform dispersion of the coal tar in the paste; it also acts as a detergent to aid the removal of the ointment from the skin.

Water-soluble solids may be dissolved in a small volume of water to facilitate uniform incorporation into the base. Volatile solvents are not recommended, as they evaporate rapidly and may leave large crystals.

100. Epinephrine bitartrate   1.0 g
     Purified water   10.0 ml
     Hydrophilic petrolatum, q.s.   100 g

Sig.: Epinephrine bitartrate ophthalmic ointment

The epinephrine bitartrate is dissolved in the water. The solution is gradually incorporated into the hydrophilic petrolatum.

Ophthalmic ointments require that the drug be micronized or in solution. It is good manufacturing practice to manufacture sterile ophthalmic ointments. In general, the sterile drug is added aseptically to the sterile base. After uniform incorporation the ointment is filled aseptically into sterile tubes. Petrolatum is most frequently used in ophthalmic ointments because it is stable and may be sterilized by 2 hours of exposure to 170°. A soft ophthalmic ointment may be produced by adding mineral oil to the petrolatum. As it is anhydrous, petrolatum may be used as a base for water-sensitive drugs, e.g., chlortetracycline, nystatin, and isoflurophate. Petrolatum is bland and is preferred to emulsion-type ointments that contain a potentially irritating surface-active agent.

In the industrial preparation of suspension-type ointments the solid drug, prior to incorporation, may be reduced to a fine particle size by milling in a ball mill or micronizer; this is obligatory for ophthalmic ointments. The micronized drug may be sprinkled into the base or molten base and distributed by a mechanical mixer. Mixers for ointments and pastes operate by direct action on the material adjacent to the mixing elements. They do not set up flow currents because of the high viscosity. The agitator or blades move throughout the material or the material is brought to the agitator. The mixers used in pharmacy for the preparation of ointments are chiefly the planetary mixer and the roll mill. The previously described colloid mill, hammer mill, or homogenizer may be used for the finishing operation to ensure the proper reduction of particle size and homogeneity of the ointment.

A planetary mixer utilizes mixing arms rotating about their own axis and also about a common axis, which is usually the center of the mixing vessel. This increases the mixing action, which is important for materials that are not fluid. Planetary mixers are known as change-can mixers because the mixing vessel or can is conveniently separated from the mixing element for batch production. In the pony-mixer design of a planetary mixer, the agitator consists of several vertical blades held on a rotating head and positioned near the wall of the can. The blades are slightly twisted. The agitator is mounted eccentrically with respect to the axis of the can. The can rests on a turntable driven in a direction opposite to that of the agitator, so that during the operation the entire contents of the can are brought to the blades to be mixed. When mixing is completed, the agitator head is raised to lift the blades out of the ointment; the blades are cleaned; and the can is replaced with another containing a new batch.

In the beater version of the planetary mixer as shown in Figure 158, the can is stationary. The agitator has a planetary motion; as it rotates, it precesses, so that it repeatedly mixes all parts of the can. The blades may overlap with a clearance as low as 0.04 in. The blades also have a close clearance with the walls of the can. Thus, the blades and can provide a kneading action and shear.

Ointments and pastes may be subjected to intense shear by passing them between smooth metal rollers revolving at different speeds. By repeated passes between mixing rollers as shown in Figure 26, solid drugs can be comminuted and throughly dispersed. In pharmacy, roller mills are not generally used for initial mixing, but they are used to grind and complete the homogeneity of the ointment. The roller mills are generally the three-roller type with adjustable clearances. The differential speed and the narrow clearance between the rollers develop high shear over small volumes of material.

Fusion is required when an ointment contains waxy materials. In general, the ingredient with the highest melting point is melted and the other ingredients are then added. It is desirable to use a steam kettle with sweeper blades to melt the material and avoid charring. If the medicinal compound is thermostable and soluble, it is added to the molten base and stirred until dissolved. If the medicinal compound is insoluble, the powder is sifted into the molten base and stirred until congealed. Obviously, volatile ingredients should not be added to the ointment until it has cooled. The ointment is then milled to complete its preparation.

Emulsion-Type Ointments

The emulsion-type ointments may be oil-in-water or water-in-oil emulsions. Anionic and nonionic surface-active agents are used as emulsifying agents. The nonionic emulsifying agents are usually nonirritating, tolerant to hard water, and compatible with acidic substances. As emulsion-type ointments contain considerable water, they must contain a preservative to protect them from microorganic growth. In the selection of a preservative consideration must be given to the possibility of its interaction with nonionic emulsifying agents.

After the application of most emulsion-type ointments the water evaporates, leaving an oily layer on the skin. This oily film is responsible for their emollient action. Emulsion-type ointments are cosmetically acceptable to the user as they do not feel greasy, they provide a cooling effect as the water evaporates, and they are readily washed from the skin and clothing.

Bases. Cold cream is a classical example of a water-in-oil type of ointment. Its name relates to the cooling effect caused by the slow evaporation of water. The remaining layer of oil acts as an emollient. Cold cream consists of 40 to 70 per cent oil, 5 to 15 per cent wax or spermaceti, and 20 to 35 per cent water. The borax reacts with the free fatty acids in the wax to form a sodium soap of a high molecular weight acid, e.g., cerotic acid. The HLB of the emulsifying agent is such that the phase volume ratio determines the type of emulsion formed. If the aqueous phase is less than 45 per cent, a water-in-oil emulsion is formed. Strong acids destroy the emulsion by forming the free acid from the soap.

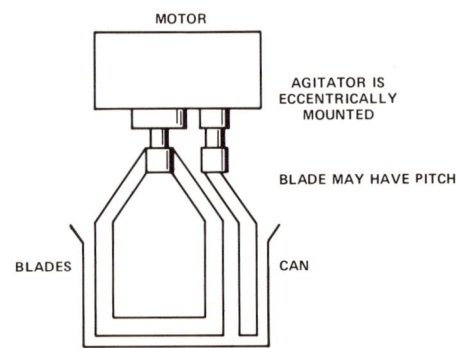

Figure 158. Planetary mixer with stationary can. Clearance between blades and can may be only 1/32 in.

101.
Spermaceti	125 g
White wax	120 g
Mineral oil	560 g
Sodium borate	5 g
Purified water	190 g

Sig.: Cold cream

The spermaceti and white wax are comminuted to small pieces. They are melted with the mineral oil on a steam bath at 70°. The sodium borate is dissolved in water and heated to 70°. The warm aqueous solution is gradually added to the oily phase with agitation and stirred until the cream congeals. Emulsion-type ointments are soft if stirred until congealed, but they frequently become hard and unacceptable if not stirred during cooling. Some cosmetic cold creams do not contain soaps, but they are emulsified by nonionic emulsifying agents.

Washable ointments are emulsion-type ointments that can be easily washed from the skin with water. Hydrophilic ointment is an oil-in-water emulsion that is easily cleansed from the skin and clothing. Its initial yield value is high, but it softens when rubbed and is easily spread.

102.
Methylparaben	0.25 g
Propylparaben	0.15 g
Sodium lauryl sulfate	10.00 g
Propylene glycol	120.00 g
Stearyl alcohol	250.00 g
White petrolatum	250.00 g
Purified water	370.00 g

Sig.: Hydrophilic ointment

The stearyl alcohol and the white petrolatum are melted on a steam bath at 75°. The remaining ingredients are dissolved in water and warmed to 75°. The aqueous solution is added to the oily phase with agitation, and the emulsion is stirred until the ointment congeals. The sodium lauryl sulfate is the emulsifying agent that forms an oil-in-water emulsion. The stearyl alcohol and petrolatum contribute to the viscosity of the ointment. The stearyl alcohol is oriented with the sodium lauryl sulfate to form a more tenacious layer about the emulsified oily phase. The propylene glycol is a humectant which, owing to its hygroscopic nature, retards loss of water by evaporation.

Vanishing creams are oil-in-water emulsions that contain 60 to 80 per cent water and 10 to 25 per cent stearic acid. From 15 to 25 per cent of the stearic acid is reacted with alkali, e.g., potassium hydroxide or triethanolamine, to form a soap. The unreacted stearic acid forms the oily dispersed phase, which is left as a film on the skin after the water evaporates. Fatty alcohols, e.g., cetyl and stearyl, may be included in the formula to increase the viscosity and to impart a pleasing feel during application. Approximately 5 per cent glycerin, sorbitol, or propylene glycol may be added as a humectant.

103.
Stearic acid	18.00 g
Potassium hydroxide	0.80 g
Glycerin	5.00 g
Methylparaben	0.02 g
Propylparaben	0.01 g
Purified water	76.20 g

Sig.: Vanishing cream

The stearic acid is melted on a steam bath at 75°. The remaining ingredients are dissolved in the water at 75°. The aqueous solution is added to the oily phase with agitation. The potassium hydroxide reacts with a portion of the stearic acid to form potassium stearate, which emulsifies the unreacted

plastic suspensions and emulsions

stearic acid as the dispersed phase. Excessive agitation should be avoided so that air is not entrapped within the vanishing cream. In cosmetic vanishing creams the perfume is added after the cream has cooled, and the product is then milled.

Percutaneous Absorption

A prime requirement for a therapeutic ointment is that the medicinal compound incorporated reach the skin surface at an adequate rate and in an adequate amount. The ointment base does not appreciably penetrate the skin or function as a carrier in transporting the drug through the skin barrier; however, the ointment base affects the release of the drug. The choice of an ointment base depends on the condition of the skin and the physical properties of the drug in the ointment.

Percutaneous absorption is the penetration of a medicinal compound from the surface of the skin into and through the skin to the bloodstream. Anatomically the drug must pass consecutively through a surface film of the emulsified lipids, the stratum corneum, the skin barrier, the stratum germinativum, and the dermis and blood vessels as shown in Figure 159. The film on the surface of the skin is discontinuous and is composed of sebum, sweat, and desquamated horny cells. It is generally believed that this film does not significantly affect penetration. The horny layer or stratum corneum is 20 to 40 μ thick and is largely composed of proteinaceous keratin, which may absorb large amounts of water. The surface lipids may spread between the cell walls and dissolve lipid-soluble materials. The barrier layer is in intimate contact with the stratum corneum, and it is an electronegative barrier that repels anions and holds cations so that ions do not penetrate. The barrier layer is 10 μ thick and prevents the penetration of molecules with molecular weights exceeding approximately 300 g mole^{-1}; however, the diameter of pores in the material and the intercellular spaces in the barrier are greater than the largest penetrating molecule. The fact that drugs with a partition ratio approaching 1 penetrate most easily suggest that the skin barrier has polar and nonpolar characteristics. The un-ionized molecules that penetrate the barrier layer pass readily through the living epidermis or stratum germinativum and dermis and are carried away by the lymphatic or blood vessels. In general, lipid-soluble drugs penetrate the skin more readily than highly water soluble drugs; however, some water solubility is necessary for absorption.

Hair follicles and sweat glands open onto the surface of the skin. In the upper part of the follicular canal the hair shaft does not adhere to the wall, and the space is filled with air and horny scale.

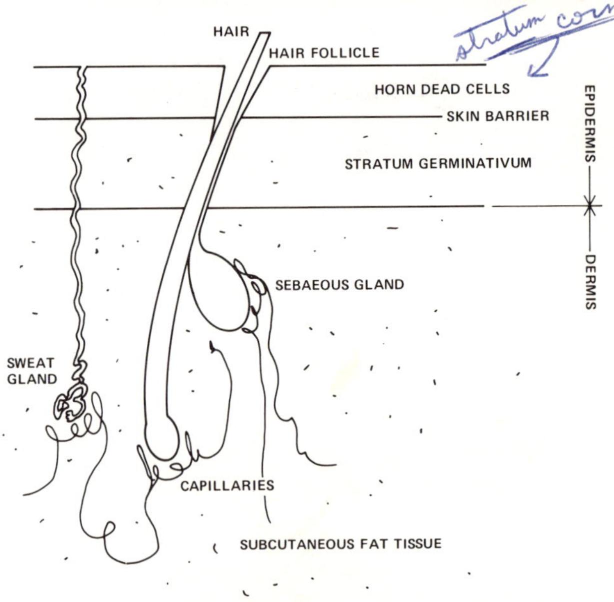

Figure 159. Diagrammatic representation of intact human skin and routes of penetration.

This space is continuous with the duct of the sebaceous gland from which sebum flows. Any drug that is soluble in sebum reaches this space and the inside of the sebaceous gland, whose membrane is more permeable than the skin barrier. Likewise, the wall of the follicular sheath is more readily penetrated than the skin barrier. In transfollicular penetration the drug need not penetrate the skin barrier.

The fundamentals of percutaneous absorption are incompletely understood. It may be that both transfollicular and transepidermal penetration are involved.

From the physiological viewpoint the factors influencing the rate and extent of percutaneous absorption are (1) condition of the skin, (2) area of application, and (3) frequency of application. With diseased or abraded skin there is frequently a large increase in rate and extent of absorption. When the skin barrier has been destroyed, the affect of the ointment on absorption is minimized. Penetration is slow in areas having a thick callus, e.g., palm and heel, and rapid in regions of thin keratic layer, e.g., the face. Absorption is directly proportional to the area covered and inversely proportional to the thickness of the skin barrier. A more frequent application with inunction provides a greater total amount of drug absorbed.

Moisture. Although the skin is intuitively thought of as being waterproof, clinical experience has shown that a watertight covering over the skin influences absorption. The hydration of the stratum corneum favors the rate of penetration of all materials that penetrate into the skin. Water is sorbed by the proteinaceous material of the skin and may increase the size of the pores. At high relative humidities the increased activity of the water changes the diffusion coefficient and activity of the drug. As shown in Figure 160, the absorption of methyl salicylate is enhanced by an increase in moisture. The effect of moisture on absorption rates is proportional to the partition coefficient and the water solubility of the drug. The greater increase in penetration enhanced by hydration occurs with a drug that has the greater water solubility and a smaller partition coefficient. This is illustrated in Figure 160 for methyl salicylate, which has a solubility in water of 0.08 per cent and a partition coefficient of 7.7. The glycol salicylate is more water soluble and has a lower partition coefficient than methyl salicylate; its ratio of rate of absorption in hydrous to anhydrous system is three times as great as the ratio for methyl salicylate.

Hydration of the stratum corneum arises from water diffusing from the stratum mucosum, from the atmosphere, or from perspiration that accumulates after the application of an occlusive ointment. It is the water content of the stratum corneum that determines the softness and flexibility of the skin. Oleaginous ointments are the most occlusive bases and induce increased hydration through the

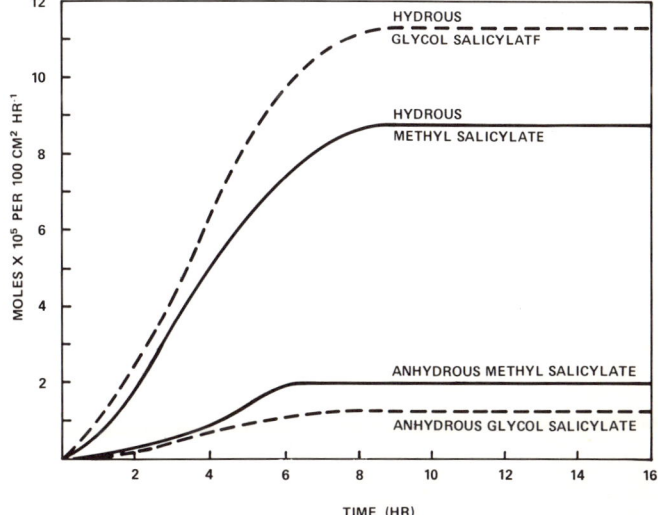

Figure 160. Urinary excretion data showing influence of moisture on percutaneous absorption of methyl salicylate (solid line) and glycol salicylate (dashed line). [D.E. Wurster and S.F. Kramer, *J. Pharm. Sci. 50*, 288 (1961).]

accumulation of perspiration at the skin-ointment boundary. Oleaginous ointments act as emollients by retarding moisture loss from the stratum corneum and by lubricating the outer surface. Water-in-oil emulsions are slightly less occlusive, but they are good emollients. Oil-in-water emulsions tend to invert as the water evaporates and leave a continuous oil film containing the drug. Humectants tend to decrease hydration by preventing the formation of a continuous oil film and may abstract moisture from the skin. Water-soluble ointments offer the least change in hydration, and they do not have an emollient action. Hydrophilic powders decrease hydration by increasing the surface area and rate of evaporation of water; all powders interfere with the continuity of the oil film and probably decrease the occlusive effect. A bandage covering an ointment tends to retain perspiration and increase hydration.

The dermatologist expresses percutaneous absorption in terms of the rate of absorption into and through the skin; since the pharmacist is concerned with the formulation and development of an ointment he is apt to express the same process in terms of the rate of release of the drug from the ointment.

In therapeutic ointments the maximum extent and rate of drug absorption is generally desired. The drug is transported from the ointment to the skin by diffusion. The pharmaceutical scientist assumes that the diffusion process is passive; i.e., it is not energetically associated with a biological transport process. From the physicochemical viewpoint the factors affecting the rate and extent of percutaneous absorption are (1) the activity of the water in the ointment, (2) the activity of the drug in the ointment and the skin barrier, and (3) the diffusion coefficient of the drug in the ointment and the skin barrier. The release from the ointment can be described by simple models for conditions in which the rate-controlling steps in transport are in the skin barrier and the rate-controlling steps in transport are in the ointment.

Rate-Controlling Steps Are in Transport through the Skin Barrier. Assuming that the ointment base does not affect the skin, the relationship between the steady-state rate of penetration, dq/dt, for the simple model shown in Figure 161, and several properties of a water-soluble drug is

$$\frac{dq}{dt} = \frac{KCDA}{h}$$

where K is the partition coefficient of the drug between the base and the skin barrier, C the concentration of the drug in the base, D the effective average diffusion coefficient of the drug in the barrier phase, A the effective cross-sectional area, and h the effective thickness of the barrier phase.

The important properties of the drug that determine its rate of penetration through the skin are its partition coefficient and its diffusion coefficient in the barrier phase. The product of the partition coefficient and the diffusion coefficient is known as the permeability coefficient. According to the Stokes-Einstein equation, the diffusion coefficient varies approximately as the cube root of the molecular weight; therefore, the diffusion coefficients of substances of a similar molecular weight and

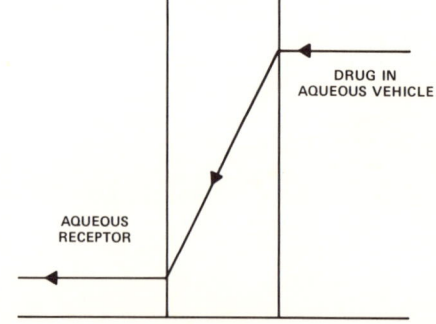

Figure 161. Diagrammatic representation of simple steady-state diffusion across a barrier layer of thickness h. [T. Higuchi, *J. Soc. Cosmetic Chemists* **11**, 85 (1960).]

shape are only slightly different. The partition coefficient varies greatly with the molecular weight and structure; therefore, the partition coefficient is an important factor in the permeability coefficient.

The complex structure of skin has polar and nonpolar regions. A drug at the ointment-skin boundary may easily penetrate a membrane if it has a high partition coefficient, i.e., ratio of concentration in membrane to concentration in base. If the partition coefficient between the membrane and the tissue fluid is high, the drug cannot easily leave the membrane. Thus, to achieve a satisfactory rate of penetration through all regions of the skin and base, a drug should have a partition coefficient of approximately unity.

The driving force behind drug diffusion is the activity gradient between the ointment and the deep tissue. Obviously, the activity of the drug decreases with the depth of penetration, and diffusion is always in the direction of lower activity.

In this simple model only the concentration or activity of the drug in the vehicle appears; therefore, the properties of the vehicle do not affect absorption. When the rate-determining step in absorption is the passage of the barrier phase, the rates of absorption from different ointments are the same if the activity of the drug in the base is maintained constant. All ointments containing finely milled particles of water-soluble drugs in suspension provide the same rate of absorption.

To obtain a fast rate of absorption the drug should be used under conditions whereby it has a high activity. Since activity is important, for a given concentration of a drug, a base that has a low affinity for the drug increases its activity and consequently produces faster absorption. Drugs firmly held by the base have low activities and slow rates of absorption. Polyethylene glycols complex salicylic acid and reduce its activity; thus a given concentration of salicylic acid in a polyethylene glycol base has a slower release than from a petrolatum base.

For sparingly water soluble drugs the rate-controlling step in transport does not involve transport through the skin barrier but transfer from the barrier to the tissue fluid. Examination of the multilayer model in Figure 162 shows that the decrease in activity of the drug occurs largely below the barrier layer. The partition coefficient is unfavorable for the transport of the water-insoluble drug to the aqueous tissue fluids, and consequently the rate of absorption is very slow.

The multilayer model consists of a lipidal and a hydrous barrier. The rate of diffusion, dq/dt, through a double-layer model is

$$\frac{dq}{dt} = \frac{aA}{\frac{h_1}{P_1} + \frac{h_2}{P_2}}$$

where a is the activity of the drug in its vehicle; A is area; h_1 and h_2 are the thickness of barrier layers 1 and 2, respectively; and P_1 and P_2 are defined for their respective barrier layer as $P = D/\gamma$, where γ is the

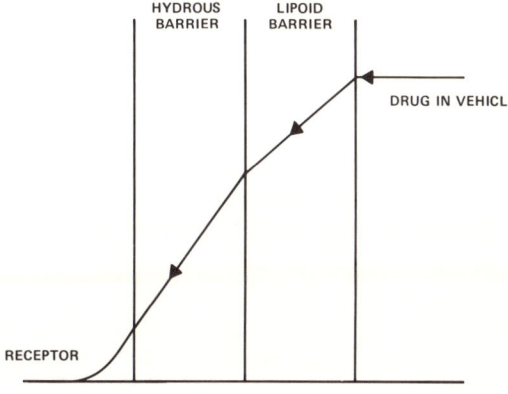

Figure 162. Diagrammatic representation of diffusion across a double barrier layer. [T. Higuchi, *J. Soc. Cosmetic Chemists 11,* 85 (1960).]

activity coefficient of the drug in the barrier. If it is assumed that the diffusion coefficients in the layers are approximately equal,

$$\frac{dq}{dt} = \frac{aAD}{h_1\gamma_1 + h_2\gamma_2}$$

where D is the mean diffusion coefficient and γ_1 and γ_2 are the activity coefficients of the drug in the respective layers. A drug that minimizes the summation in the denominator will penetrate the fastest. Hence, a compound with a balance of hydrophilic and hydrophobic groups more readily penetrates a multilayer system.

If the activity coefficients, except for the activity coefficient in hydrous layer, are very small, the rate of absorption of the drug would be greatly influenced by the rate of capillary blood flow. The rate of absorption of hydrophobic compounds is influenced by the capillary flow; the rate of absorption of hydrophilic compounds is little affected by capillary flow.

Rate-Controlling Steps Are in Transport in the Applied Ointment. In systems in which the rate-controlling steps of penetration are in the skin barrier, it is assumed that the activity of the drug is uniform throughout the ointment, and if the concentration of the drug did change in the ointment, there is only a negligible and uniform concentration gradient developed in the direction normal to the skin surface. There must be some gradient for diffusion to occur; however, the very small gradient can be ignored because of the resistance of the intact skin to penetration.

With highly insoluble, suspension-type ointments or injured skin, large concentration gradients may develop in the ointment. In these systems in which the rate-controlling steps are in the applied ointment and the skin has no role, it is assumed that the concentration of the drug in the skin is essentially zero because the diffusing drug is rapidly removed to the deeper tissue. Thus, all concentration gradients occur in the ointment.

Absorption from Emulsion-Type Ointments. When the rate of absorption is limited by drug transport below the skin barrier or by passage through the barrier, the absorption of salicylic and benzoic acid from aqueous buffered solutions as found in emulsion-type ointments through intact skin can be expressed as

$$\frac{dC}{dt} = -\frac{AC}{RV} = -\frac{A(1-\alpha)}{RV}$$

Integration yields

$$C = C_0 \exp(-A(1-\alpha)/RV)$$

where C_0 is the initial concentration of the drug in the ointment, C the concentration in the ointment at time t, R the resistance of the skin barrier, V the volume of the ointment, A the area of application, and α the degree of dissociation of the weak acid. The above expression can be expanded to

$$t = \left(\ln \frac{C_0}{C_0 - C}\right) \frac{RV}{A(1-\alpha)}$$

Inspection of the above equation shows that the time necessary to reduce the concentration of drug from C_0 to C is inversely related to the fraction of the undissociated molecules, i.e., $(1-\alpha)$.

The simplest model consists of an ointment in which the drug is initially dissolved. It is assumed that the diffusion coefficient of the drug is constant in the ointment and that components other than the drug do not diffuse out of the ointment. According to the Fick law of diffusion, q, the amount of drug released at the skin-ointment boundary per unit area of application, is

$$q = hC_0 \left\{ 1 - \frac{8}{\pi^2} \sum_{m=0}^{\infty} \frac{1}{(2m+1)^2} \exp[-D(2m-1)^2 \pi^2 t/4h^2] \right\}$$

where h is the thickness of the applied layer, C_0 the initial concentration of the drug in the ointment, D the diffusion coefficient of the drug in the ointment, and t the time after application; m is an integer.

The application of this equation can be illustrated by the release of radioiodide from an emulsion-type ointment. Thirty grams of isotopically labeled ointment was prepared by mixing 0.3 ml of $Na^{131}I$ solution with 29.7 g of the following base.

104.
Sipon® ES (sodium lauryl ether sulfate)	2.000 g
Stearyl alcohol	24.500 g
White petrolatum	24.500 g
Purified water	37.000 ml
Propylene glycol	12.000 ml
Methylparaben	0.025 g
Propylparaben	0.015 g

The dispersed phase is impermeable to sodium iodide, and the sodium iodide diffused only in the aqueous phase. In Figure 163 the fraction released is plotted as a function of time. The circles represent experimental data, and the smooth curve represents values calculated using the above equation with $D = 2.0 \times 10^{-6}$ cm^2 sec^{-1}.

In terms of f, fraction of the drug released, the above equation may be written

$$f = \frac{q}{hC_0} = \left\{ 1 - \frac{8}{\pi^2} \sum_{m=0}^{\infty} \frac{1}{(2m-1)^2} \exp\left[-D(2m-1)^2 \pi^2 t/4h^2\right] \right\}$$

If f does not exceed 0.3, the above equations are approximately

$$q = 2C_0 \sqrt{\frac{Dt}{\pi}}$$

and

$$\frac{dq}{dt} = 2\sqrt{\frac{Dt}{\pi h^2}}$$

The distribution of the drug in the ointment is shown in Figure 164. Initially, at time t_0 the concentration is uniform through the ointment from $x = 0$, which is the ointment-skin boundary, to $x = h$, which is the ointment-air boundary. At a later time the distribution in the ointment is shown by t_1 after the drug near the skin-ointment boundary has been taken up by the skin. The curve continues to fall toward the abscissa as time elapses and more drug is removed.

Examination of the simplified equation above shows that the rate and amount released can be

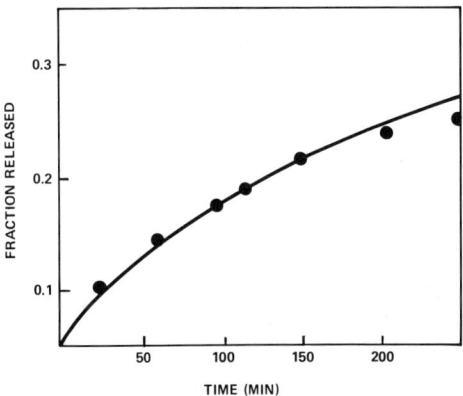

Figure 163. Comparison of experimental release of $Na^{131}I$ represented by circles with calculated release represented by smooth curve from an emulsion-type ointment. [W.I. Higuchi, *J. Pharm. Sci.* 51, 802 (1962).]

378 • plastic suspensions and emulsions

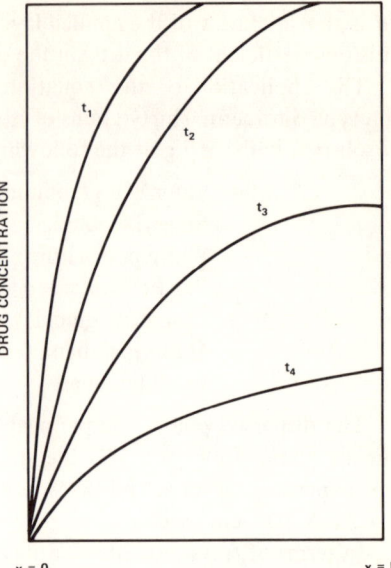

Figure 164. Concentration profiles in an ointment when the Fick law is obeyed and diffusion is into a perfect absorber at $x = 0$. (W.I. Higuchi, A.A.C.P. *Proceedings Teachers' Seminar on Pharmacy,* Madison, Wis., 1961, p. 162).

altered by the concentration of the drug in the ointment and its diffusion coefficient. The amount and rate of release is directly proportional to the initial concentration.

If an ointment is a solution composed of molecules of a size comparable to or smaller than the drug molecule, the diffusion coefficient is inversely proportional to the viscosity as approximated by the Stokes-Einstein equation,

$$D = \frac{kT}{6\pi\eta a}$$

where k is the Boltzmann constant, T the absolute temperature, a the molecular radius of the drug, and η the viscosity of the ointment. In general, the radius of the drug molecule is roughly proportional to the cube root of the molecular weight of the drug, so that values of the diffusion coefficient are of the magnitude 10^{-5} cm^2 sec^{-1}. Thus, in several minutes an appreciable fraction of the drug is released from the ointment and absorbed.

In the heterogenous system of an emulsion-type or a suspension-type ointment the estimation of the diffusion coefficient is not simple. In these polyphasic ointments relationships are available that relate the effective drug diffusion coefficient to the volume fractions of the phases and to the diffusion coefficients and partition coefficients of the drug in each of the phases. Assuming that the Fick law of diffusion applies and that the volume fraction of the dispersed sphere does not exceed 0.1, the effective diffusion coefficient D_e of the system is given by

$$D_e = \frac{D_1}{V_1 + KV_2}\left(1 + 3V_2 \frac{KD_2 - D_1}{KD_2 + 2D_1}\right)$$

where D_1 is the diffusion coefficient in the dispersion medium, D_2 the diffusion coefficient in the dispersed phase, V_1 the volume fraction of the dispersion medium, V_2 the volume fraction of the dispersed phase, and K the equilibrium partition coefficient, i.e., ratio of concentration of drug in dispersed phase to the concentration in the dispersion medium. For larger volume fractions of the dispersed phase and for highly irregular particles, this expression is only qualitative.

Inspection of the above equation indicates that if the partition coefficient is small, i.e., drug preferentially partitions into the dispersion medium, and the diffusion coefficients in both phases are approximately equal, the dispersed phase acts as a mechanical barrier within the ointment. This situation does not make the effective diffusion coefficient in the ointment much smaller than about ½ D_1 for most values of the volume fraction of dispersed phase. Thus, the dispersed phase of an emulsion does not appreciably alter drug release.

If the partition coefficient is large, i.e., drug favors partition into the dispersed phase, the effective diffusion coefficient can be smaller than the diffusion coefficient in the dispersion medium by a magnitude of $\frac{1}{KV_2}$. Consequently, for a given initial concentration, the release to a good absorber may be slowed by a factor of the magnitude of KV_2 if an emulsion-type ointment with a large K is used instead of an ointment of only the dispersion medium.

While the preceding model involves the partitioning of the drug into the dispersed phase, the equation may be used to calculate the effective diffusion coefficient for other situations. It may be used if most of the drug is initially adsorbed onto the particles of the dispersed phase and if the adsorption is proportional to the concentration in the dispersion medium and if

$$K = \frac{M_2}{C_1}$$

where M_2 is the weight of drug adsorbed per unit volume of adsorbent and C_1 is the weight of drug per unit volume of the dispersion medium. The Langmuir adsorption isotherm is a good approximation when the solute is adsorbed on a solid from solution. It may be expressed as

$$m = \frac{M_2}{\rho} = \frac{k_1 k_2 C_1}{1 + k_1 C_1}$$

where m is the amount of adsorbed drug per unit weight of adsorbent, ρ is the density of the adsorbent, and k_1 and k_2 are constants. When $k_1 C_1 \ll 1$, this expression may be approximated by a linear isotherm,

$$M_2 \cong \rho k_1 k_2 C_1$$

Thus, the equations expressing D_e and K can be used to predict the rate of release with $D_2 = 0$ for most situations in which no more than a monolayer of drug is initially adsorbed. The release from an ointment in which the adsorbent has a large K value is slowed by a factor of KV_2.

The equation for calculating the effective diffusion coefficient can be applied to an ointment in which an immobile complexing agent binds most of the drug according to a linear binding law. Then

$$K = \frac{M_2}{C_1} = \frac{kC_1}{C_1} = k$$

where k is the complexing constant.

In a gel, e.g., mineral oil gelled with polyethylene, the polymeric chains offer little mechanical resistance to diffusion of the drug molecule. Thus, in general

$$D_e \cong D_1 \cong D_2$$

Although the gross viscosity of the ointment is high, the environmental viscosity of the drug is that of the liquid constituent of the gel. Hence, the effective diffusion coefficient is given by the Stokes-Einstein equation, with η being the viscosity of the liquid constituent.

Absorption from Suspension-Type Ointments. The amount q released at time t per unit area of application of a finely divided solid drug from a homogeneous base, e.g., penicillin in petrolatum or tetracaine in petrolaturm, does not follow the Fick law of diffusion and may be expressed as

$$q = (2C - C_S) \sqrt{\frac{Dt}{1 + 2(C - C_S)/C_S}}$$

where C is the concentration of the drug, C_S the solubility of the drug in the ointment, and D the diffusion coefficient of the drug molecule in the dispersion phase. Differentiating with respect to time gives the rate of absorption,

$$\frac{dq}{dt} = \frac{1}{2}(2C - C_S)\sqrt{\frac{Dt}{1 + 2(C - C_S)/C_S}}$$

Generally, there is considerably more drug present than required to saturate the dispersion medium, i.e., $C \gg C_S$, and the relationship simplifies to

$$q = \sqrt{2CDC_S t}$$

and

$$\frac{dq}{dt} = \sqrt{\frac{CDC_S}{2t}}$$

The fraction of the drug released is expressed as

$$f = \frac{q}{hC} = 0.01\sqrt{\frac{h^2 C^2}{C_S(2C - C_S)}Dt}$$

The drug distribution during release from a suspension-type ointment is shown in Figure 165. The boundary recedes only as fast as the free drug molecules can diffuse out. At time t the solid line represents the concentration gradient in the layer of ointment. The total drug concentration shows a sharp discontinuity at the distance h from the ointment-skin boundary if none of the suspended phase dissolves until the environmental concentration drops below C_S. From the distance h above the ointment-skin boundary the concentration gradient is essentially constant. Over the distance h the linearity of the concentration gradient obeys the Fick law. The change in the concentration profile after the elapse of additional time is shown by the dashed line corresponding to the extension of the zone of partial depletion by distance Δh. At that time the amount of drug absorbed from the ointment is represented by the shaded area.

The amount of drug released from a suspension-type ointment to a perfect absorber is proportional to the square roots of the amount of drug per unit volume, the diffusion coefficient, the drug solubility, and time. In formulating ointments the rate of release can be controlled by regulating these factors. Obviously, the concentration of the drug can be easily varied. The diffusion coefficient is inversely proportional to the viscosity of the vehicle and may be altered by a change of vehicle. Different salts and derivatives of a drug may have different diffusion coefficients. The diffusion coefficient of sodium salicylate in oleaginous bases, e.g., petrolatum and hydrophilic petrolatum, is probably less than that of salicylic acid. The solubility can be altered by the addition of a complexing agent, e.g.,

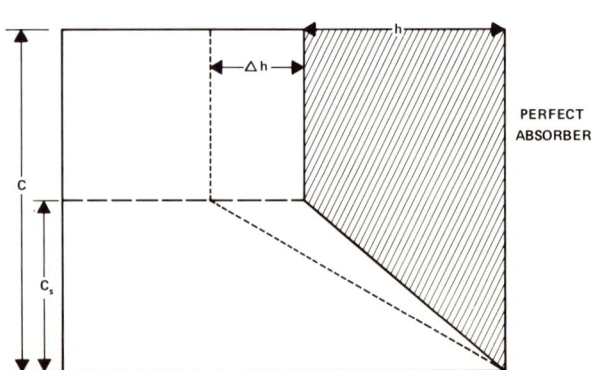

Figure 165. Concentration profiles in a suspension-type ointment in contact with a perfect absorber. [T. Higuchi, *J. Pharm. Sci.* **50**, 874 (1961).]

polyvinylpyrrolidone and iodine. The solubility may be altered by a change of ointment base. In emulsion-type ointments, e.g., hydrophilic ointment, the activity of salicylic acid is fairly high and the rate of release is rapid. In a suspension-type ointment, e.g., salicylic acid in polyethylene glycol, in which complexation occurs, the activity and rate of release of the salicylic acid is low. The activity and release of salicylic acid in an anhydrous base, e.g., hydrophilic petrolatum, is intermediate between those in emulsion-type and suspension-type ointments.

If a partially aqueous ointment is used, the solubility of slightly soluble weakly acidic and basic drugs can be altered by changing the pH. The concentration or activity of the molecular form of a weakly acidic drug changes rapidly with a change in pH for values greater than pK_a of the drug. The dissociation of a weakly acidic drug

$$HA \rightleftharpoons H^+ + A^-$$

is quantitatively expressed by its dissociation constant,

$$K_a = \frac{a_{A^-} a_{H^+}}{a_{HA}}$$

where a represents the activity or effective concentration of each species (see page 187).

By rearrangement and substitution of the relationship $a_{H^+} = 10^{-pH}$, the expression relating the activities of each species of the drug to the pH is

$$a_{HA} = \frac{a_{A^-} a_{H^+}}{K_a} = \frac{a_{A^-} \cdot 10^{-pH}}{K_a} = \frac{a_{A^-}}{K_a 10^{pH}}$$

As the pH of the ointment is increased, the activity of the undissociated species is rapidly decreased in the region where $pH > pK_a$. Within this region a change of 1 pH unit in the ointment causes a tenfold change in the activity of the undissociated species. Since the rate of release is increased by an increase in the activity of the undissociated species, a decrease in pH increases the rate of absorption of a weakly acidic drug.

A similar argument for a weakly basic drug shows that

$$a_B = \frac{a_{BH^+} 10^{pH}}{K_b 10^{pK_w}}$$

As the pH of the ointment is increased, the activity of the undissociated molecular species of the basic drug is rapidly increased in the region where $pH > pK_b$ or $pH > pK_w - pK_a$. Within this region an increase in pH of 1 unit causes a tenfold increase in the ratio of the undissociated form of an alkaloidal drug to the ionized form and an increase in rate of release by a factor of $\sqrt{10}$.

For both systems of ointments, i.e., drug in solution or drug in suspension, the release is a function of the square root of time. If $C >> C_s$ and if the diffusion coefficients are approximately the same, the rates of release in the two systems will differ by a factor $\sqrt{\frac{2C_s}{C}}$. This applies when the skin is a perfect absorber and the rate-limiting step in absorption is the release of the drug from the ointment. If the rate-limiting step is the penetration of the skin, there may be no difference or the suspension-type ointment may provide faster release than the emulsion-type ointment because the activity of the drug then becomes the important factor. If the skin is impermeable to a drug, the ointment is useless. When the skin is readily penetrated by a drug, there is opportunity to vary the rate of release by formulation. In diseased and abraded skin the skin barrier is destroyed and the drug penetrates freely into the dermis.

382 • plastic suspensions and emulsions

SUPPOSITORIES

Suppositories are a unit dosage form intended for insertion into the rectum, vagina, or urethra. Suppositories melt, soften, or dissolve in the body cavity. Some vaginal suppositories or inserts are ovoid, compressed tablets which disintegrate in the vaginal fluid. Inserts are dipped in warm water immediately before use to facilitate insertion. Although the insertion of a suppository is not esthetically appealing, the suppository is useful for local effect and for systemic effect. Nauseating drugs and products for infants and debilitated persons are often conveniently administered in a suppository.

Rectal suppositories are conical or cylindrical and tapered. A rectal suppository weighs approximately 2 g and is approximately 30 mm long and 10 mm in diameter. One design is tapered at both ends with the maximum diameter approximately one-fourth the distance from the tip; this suppository is moved inward by any contractions of the rectum and is not readily expelled. Infant suppositories weigh approximately 1 g. Suppositories are used locally to treat hemorrhoids, pruritis ani, and infections. To provide a proper local effect a prolonged, intimate contact is desired. Rectal leakage of suppository melts having a low viscosity is undesirable. Tenesmus is produced by a solid in the rectum, and unless the suppository dissolves or melts quickly after insertion explusion may occur. Glycerin suppositories are used to produce a quick fecal discharge in constipation; in addition to stimulating the defecation reflex, they act through irritation produced by the sodium stearate and the osmotic effect of the glycerin.

Vaginal suppositories vary in weight, from 3 to 5 g, and in design, but many are globular or ovoid. They are usually used for local effect in the treatment of trichomonal, bacterial, and monilial infections.

The community pharmacist usually dispensed suppositories in cardboard boxes with dividers. Industrially prepared suppositories are frequently individually wrapped in foil or waxed paper. There are individual plastic molds that serve as containers. The molten suppositories are poured into the plastic mold, and the mold is capped. The mass congeals in the plastic mold.

The combination mold and package is opened by placing a knife in a longitudinal slot and applying a twist to split the mold lengthwise. Suppositories containing glycerin are packaged in a wide-mouthed, well-closed containers, as they are hygroscopic. It is good practice to store all suppositories in a cool place.

Suspension-Type Suppositories

A suppository base should be nonirritating, chemically and physiologically inert, and easily formed into a suppository. A suppository must melt or dissolve rapidly so that it releases its medication, but it must be firm enough so that it can be inserted and will retain its shape during storage.

A rectal suppository should not be deformed by a 500-g weight applied to its base. This corresponds to a yield value in the order of 625,000 dyn cm^{-2}. Unfortunately, rheological investigations of suppositories are practically nonexistent, and the melting point is used to characterize the suppository. Frequently the melting point is determined on only a small sample of the base in a capillary tube. This is not satisfactory, because the presence of medicinal compounds and the method of manipulating the capillary tube influence the melting point. The apparatus shown in Figure 166 is used to determine characteristics of the entire suppository.

The apparatus consists of a glass tube with an internal diameter 1 to 3 mm larger than the diameter of the suppository to be tested. The tube is constricted to 3 mm to support the suppository. The temperature of the water circulating in the jacket about the tube is controlled and can be raised at the rate of 0.1° min^{-1}. After the suppository is placed in the tube, a glass rod is placed on it. A rubber tube is fitted over the rod so that when the rod rests on the suppository there is a distance of 14 mm between the lower end of the rubber tube and the upper end of the glass tube. The weight of the rod and rubber tubing is adjusted by a lead cylinder to 500 g. When the suppository deforms, the lead cylinder

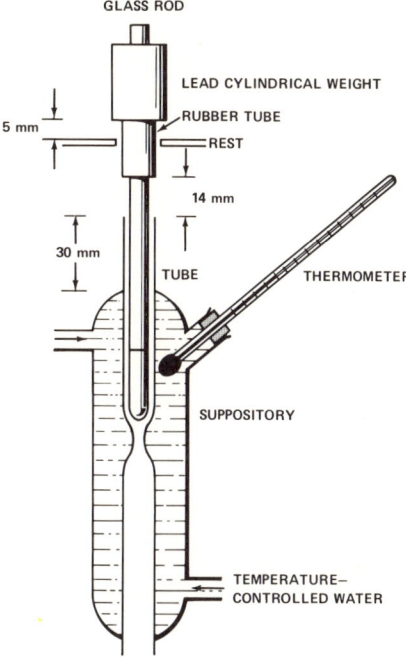

Figure 166. Apparatus for determining the softening and liquefaction temperature of a suppository. [Modified from I. Setnikar and S. Fantelli, *J. Pharm. Sci.* **52**, 38 (1963).]

drops 5 mm and is supported by a rest so that only the weight of the glass rod remains on the suppository. The temperature at which deformation occurs is the softening temperature. The softening temperature is indicative of the ease of insertion and physical stability during handling of the suppository.

The hardness of a suppository may also be determined in this apparatus. Weights are added to the glass rod until the suppository collapses; at 25° the weights required to collapse a suppository of theobroma oil, polyethylene glycol 4000, and glycerinated gelatin are 3.4, > 5, and 0.5 kg, respectively.

At the softening temperature the suppository supports only the glass rod. As the temperature rises, the suppository liquefies and the glass rod drops 9 mm, until it is supported by the glass tube. The temperature at which this occurs is the liquefaction temperature. Most liquefied suppositories flow through the constriction in the glass tube. The temperature at which this flow occurs is the flow temperature; it is the same as the liquefaction temperature except for very viscous liquids.

Bases. Theobroma oil or cocoa butter is a widely used oleaginous base because it is easily molded and it retains its shape at room temperature but melts at body temperature. Theobroma oil is the fat obtained from the roasted seed of *Theobroma Cacao*; it softens at 30° and melts at 34°. Theobroma oil is a mixture of liquid triglycerides trapped in a network of crystalline, solid triglycerides (see page 130). Approximately half of the triglycerides contain two saturated fatty acids, e.g., palmitic acid and stearic acid, and one unsaturated fatty acid, e.g., oleic acid.

Triglycerides exhibit polymorphism and commonly exist in four forms: vitreous, α, β' (crystalline, montropic), and β (crystalline, stable), in order of ascending melting point. Table LXIX shows the melting point of polymorphs of oleodipalmitin and oleodistearin. The vitreous form is obtained by rapid cooling of the completely melted solid. The lower-melting-point polymorphs are metastable, and transition to a higher-melting-point form takes place in the solid state. The transition is slow with unsymmetrical, mixed triglycerides. The formation of the higher-melting-point polymorph from the molten triglycerides is hastened by the presence of seed crystal of that form. The formation of the β polymorph is facilitated by slow cooling.

If in the fusion method of preparing suppositories the theobroma oil is melted at excessive heat and poured into a chilled mold, the theobroma oil does not congeal until the temperature is below 15°, and it crystallizes in a polymorphic form that melts from 23 to 24°. The resulting suppository melts at room temperature and is impossible to insert. Upon standing there is transition to the stable β form; however, the length of time required for this transition is considerable as illustrated in Table LXX.

Table LXIX Melting Points of Various Polymorphs (°C)

	Vitreous	a	β''	β'	β
Oleodipalmitin	12	21.5	29.0	35.0	37.5
Oleodistearin	23	29.5	37.0	41.5	43.5

Table LXX Comparison of Physical Properties of Theobroma Oil Suppositories Prepared by Proper Fusion Technique and by Excessive Heat *

Time (days)	Heated at 35°			Heated at 55°		
	CMT† (°C)	LT‡ (°C)	ST§ (°C)	CMT (°C)	LT (°C)	ST (°C)
0.1	32.2			25.1		
1	31.6	34	30	27.5	29	24
10	33.6	34	30	27.7	29	24
20	34.3	34	30	28.0	29	24
30	34.9	34	30	32.8	30	24
60	35.0	35	32	32.4	34	24
120	34.6	35	32	32.0	34	30

* I. Setnikar and S. Fantelli, *J. Pharm. Sci.* 52, 38 (1963).
† CMT, capillary melting temperature. ‡ LT, liquefaction temperature. § ST, softening temperature.

The proper technique for the preparation of theobroma oil suppositories by fusion requires the use of a warm-water bath to prevent the temperature from exceeding 35°. The theobroma oil is just melted so that it is opaque and fluid. Then some β nuclei remain to initiate crystallization as the β polymorph when the mass cools. The mold should not be chilled because the formation of the stable β polymorph is favored by slow cooling. From the mechanical viewpoint the mold should not be chilled before the melt is poured because the rapid solidification may cause cracks in the center of the suppository and breakage upon removal from the mold.

Substances, e.g., chloral, menthol, and phenol, that dissolve in theobroma oil depress its melting point. The depression of the melting point may occur to the extent that the suppository is too soft for insertion or liquefies at room temperature. Assuming that the molal freezing-point depression constant for theobroma oil is 10°, the melting point of the following suppository can be calculated.

      105. Chloral hydrate   0.5 g
             Theobroma oil   2.0 g

             Sig.: Chloral hydrate suppository

The molality of the chloral hydrate is the number of moles of chloral hydrate dissolved in 1000 g of theobroma oil,

$$\frac{0.5/165}{2} = \frac{x}{1000}$$

$$x = 1.5 \, m$$

The depression of freezing point is

$$\Delta T_f = K_f m = 10 \times 1.5 = 15°$$

Thus, the suppository melts at 35 - 15 = 20° and is too soft for use.

The addition of white beeswax has been suggested to raise the melting point. The addition of wax up to 3 per cent lowers the melting point of theobroma oil. The addition of wax beyond 6 per cent raises the melting point of theobroma oil-wax mixture above that of the body temperature. The presence of soluble drugs further alters the melting point. From 18 to 20 per cent spermaceti has also been used to raise the melting point of theobroma oil.

The effect of a soluble drug and a stiffening agent on the properties of a suppository can be illustrated by

106. Chloral hydrate   0.5 g
     Beeswax   0.5 g
     Theobroma oil   1.0 g

Sig.: Chloral hydrate suppository

The wax is melted on a water bath. The chloral hydrate is dissolved in the melted wax. The solution is removed from the heat and the theobroma oil is added. The melt is stirred and poured into the mold. After the suppository has congealed, it is placed in the refrigerator. After storage for 1 day in the refrigerator the suppository at room temperature is too soft to be inserted, and it is deformed by a 50-g weight applied to its base. This is anticipated, as the beeswax melts at a temperature approximately 30° higher than the melting point of theobroma oil; thus, the melting temperature differential is great enough to completely melt and eliminate all crystalline structure from the theobroma oil, when it is mixed with the melted wax. The suppository then congeals in a metastable form. The combined effect of depression of melting point due to the chloral hydrate solute and the metastable theobroma polymorph produces an unsatisfactory suppository. Upon storage the metastable polymorphs of the theobroma oil will undergo transition to the β polymorph and the melting point will be raised. This transition required approximately a month. After the transition to the β polymorph the final melting point will exceed the body temperature, owing to the high wax content. Unfortunately for the community pharmacist the length of time for the transition to the stable polymorph and the melting point of the suppository after the transition is unknown. Obviously it is not practical for the community pharmacist to evaluate these factors for a single prescription, although they could be determined; thus, the fusion method should be avoided. The community pharmacist may prepare the chloral hydrate suppositories by a manual or compression technique.

The two most common water soluble bases are glycerinated gelatin and polyethylene glycol. A glycerinated gelatin suppository is preferred to a theobroma oil suppository for vaginal use, as it does not leak. Glycerinated gelatin suppositories are hygroscopic and are packaged in well-closed containers. If the suppositories are to be stored, methylparaben may be added as a preservative. To facilitate insertion, the suppository is dipped into water. Glycerinated gelatin suppositories are not recommended for rectal use, as the swelling of the protein and the water attracted by the osmostic effect of the glycerin initiate the defecation reflex.

107. Medicinal compound and purified water   10 g
     Gelatin, granular   25 g
     Glycerin   65 g

Sig.: Glycerinated gelatin

The medicinal compound is dissolved or dispersed in sufficient water to weigh 10 g. The glycerin and the gelatin are added, and the mixture is heated. A water bath should be used to avoid charring. The mixture is stirred gently until the gelatin is dissolved. Entrapment of air is to be avoided. The mixture is poured into molds and allowed to gel. Type A or B gelatin may be used unless there is a specific reaction between the medicinal compound and the gelatin, e.g., mild silver protein and type A, or boric acid and type B.

The water-soluble polyethylene glycols are nonirritating and can be blended to produce suppositories with a wide range of hardness and melting point. As polyethylene glycol suppositories do not melt at body temperature, the release of the drug depends on the dissolution of the suppository. This has the advantage of ease of storage and no leakage from the body orifice. The small volume of fluid in the rectum is insufficient to rapidly dissolve the suppository. This may result in a slow release of the medication or loss of the medication if the individual cannot suppress the defecation reflex. Drugs that dissolve in polyethylene glycol lower the melting point of the suppository; however, this may be offset by use of a higher-molecular-weight polyethylene glycol. Drugs that complex with polyethylene glycol may be more or less readily released from the suppository, depending on the solubility of the complex. A high content of insoluble powder in polyethylene glycol tends to produce a brittle suppository.

In the clinical use of water-soluble suppository bases it should be realized that they dissolve by dehydration of the rectal mucosa and that the dehydration is physiologically abnormal and may be irritating.

Preparation. Suppositories are prepared by a manual compression and fusion method. Small numbers of extemporaneous suppositories are usually shaped by hand using theobroma oil. This is a simple operation that does not require elaborate apparatus or an accurate determination of the amount of base displaced by the drug; however, it is not a satisfactory method in hot weather and it requires practice to make a well-shaped suppository. The community pharmacist usually grates the theobroma oil in advance and stores it in the refrigerator. To compound a prescription the pharmacist pulverizes the medicinal compound and geometrically blends it in a mortar into the grated theobroma oil. When the drug is uniformly incorporated, the mass is taken into the hands and kneaded until it is pliable. The pliable mass is shaped into a cylinder having the same diameter as the suppository to be formed. The cylinder is cut into the required number of segments of equal length. Each segment is shaped with the hands to a pointed cylinder. To avoid contact with the hands some pharmacists suggest kneading and shaping the suppository through a piece of filter paper. Starch may be used as a dusting powder to reduce the stickiness. Aqueous solutions may be emulsified into a small quantity of wool fat, which is then uniformly incorporated into the theobroma oil base.

In the compression method suppositories are molded by forcing the mixture into molds by pressure. One end of the cylinder of the suppository machine is threaded so that various molds may be screwed onto the cylinder. Brass molds are available for making three 1- or 2-g rectal suppositories, a single 5-g vaginal suppository, or a length of urethral suppository that is cut to the desired length. The drug and the base are mixed thoroughly, and the mass is transferred to the cylinder of the suppository machine. As shown in Figure 167, pressure is applied by a piston as the wheel of the suppository machine is tightened to force the material into the cavity of the mold.

The mass enters the mold through a small opening at the apex of each cavity. A movable plate or gate closes the opposite end of the cavity and forms the base of the suppository. When the cavities are filled, the pressure is released, the end plate is removed, and the wheel is turned to eject the

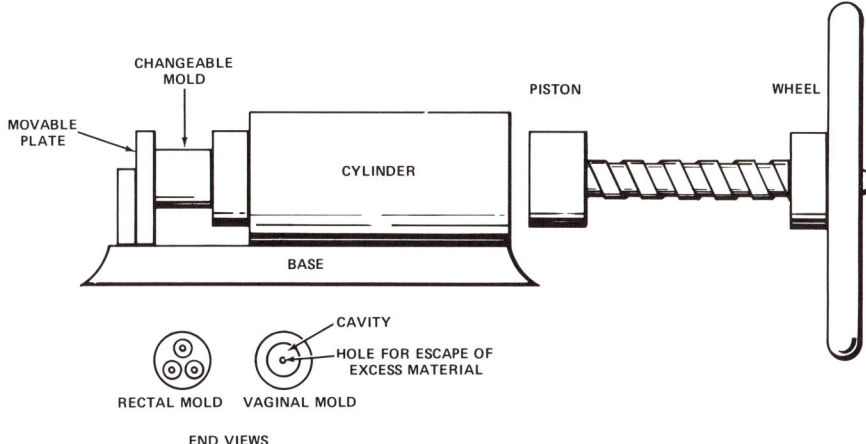

Figure 167. Basic suppository machine with changeable molds for the compression method.

suppositories from the mold. The end plate is replaced and the procedure is repeated. It is good practice to use enough material for several extra suppositories to accommodate for any loss in production. It is advantageous to chill the cylinder containing the formulation prior to compression. Industrial equipment is fundamentally the same; however, it is motor driven, has larger capacities, and may be jacketed for circulating cold water about the cylinder.

If the drug has a different density than that of the base, the volume of the base that the drug displaces must be considered in both the compression and fusion method.

> **108.** Tannic acid   0.2 g
> Theobroma oil, q.s.
> Sig.: 200-mg rectal tannic acid suppository

From previous work the pharmacist knows that the average weight of a rectal theobroma oil suppository made in his mold is 2.0 g. As there are three cavities in the mold, 6.0 g of theobroma oil is required to make three pure theobroma oil suppositories. Tannic acid has a density of 1.4 g cc^{-1}; it is, therefore, 1.4/0.86, or 1.6, times as dense as theobroma oil, which has a density of 0.86 g cc^{-1}. The amount of theobroma oil displaced by the tannic acid required for three suppositories is

$$\frac{0.2 \times 3}{1.6} = 0.38 \text{ g}$$

Three suppositories will require 6.00 - 0.38 = 5.62 g of theobroma oil and 0.6 g of tannic acid.

Frequently the values of the densities are not available and the correct amount of base must be determined experimentally. The mold may be calibrated by mixing the amount of tannic acid for three suppositories with insufficient theobroma oil to fill the cavities. This is then placed in the suppository machine and compressed into the cavities of the mold. The cylinder is then removed and theobroma oil is added. The machine is assembled and three complete suppositories are compressed. The suppositories are removed and weighed. The difference between the total weight and the weight of drug equals the amount of theobroma oil. The ingredients are then weighed out, mixed uniformly, and compressed into the desired suppositories.

In the fusion method the drug is added to the melted base and the mixture is allowed to cool after pouring into a mold. In the community pharmacy fusion is best carried out in a glass beaker immersed in hot water. With theobroma oil it is important that the temperature does not exceed 35° if any crystal nuclei of the stable β polymorph are to be maintained. The pulverized drug is mixed with the melted base. It is then removed from the source of heat and stirred until just pourable. The melt is poured in a steady stream along one side of the mold so that air is not entrapped. With insoluble drugs the melt should be stirred while pouring so that a homogenous suspension is obtained. If the melt is not poured in a steady stream into a mold, transverse ridges appear in the suppository wherever the stream was interrupted. The cavities of the mold are filled to excess so that there will not be a depression in the base of the suppository after the melt has cooled and contracted. A chilled mold may cause supercooling and cracking of the suppository. With theobroma oil a slow rate of cooling favors the crystallization of the stable β polymorph. After congealing the excess above, the mold is removed and opened. The finished suppositories are then stored in a cool place.

The mold does not require lubrication with theobroma oil and polyethylene glycol suppositories because upon cooling they contract away from the wall of the cavity. As shown in Figure 168, molds are divided longitudinally so they may be opened to remove the suppositories. They are made of brass, aluminum, stainless steel, and plastic. The plastic molds are not satisfactory, as they lose their polish and are poor conductors of heat. After use the mold should be cleaned. A clean and polished mold does not require a lubricant. Suppositories may stick to a scratched mold. A light coating of mineral oil for water-soluble bases or water for oleaginous bases facilitates removal from damaged molds.

109. Aminophylline   0.25 g
     Polyethylene glycol 1540   0.80 g
     Polyethylene glycol 6000   1.10 g
     Polyethylene glycol 400   0.50 g

     Sig.: 250-mg aminophylline suppository

100. Hydrocortisone acetate   15 mg
     Glyceryl laurate   10%
     Polyethylene sorbitan monstearate   90% q.s.

     Sig.: 15-mg hydrocortisone acetate suppository

Melt the glyceryl laurate and the polyethylene sorbitan monstearate on a water bath. Add the powdered hydrocortisone acetate and stir until homogeneous. Pour with stirring into mold and allow to congeal.

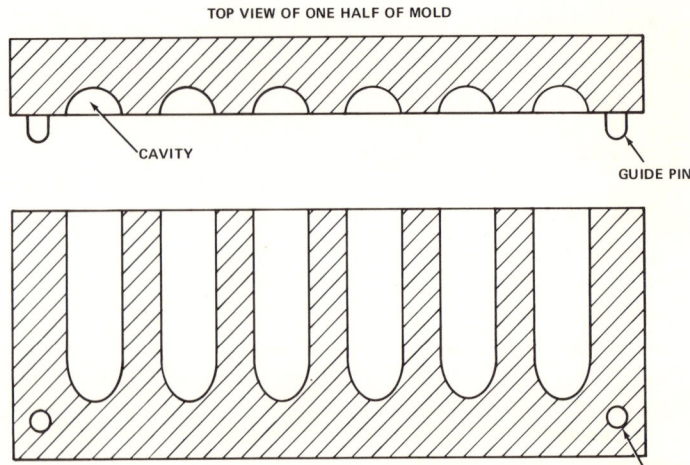

Figure 168. Basic suppository mold used in the fusion method.

111. Glycerin   91 g
     Sodium stearate   9 g
     Purified water   5 g

     Sig.: Glycerin suppositories

The sodium stearate is dissolved in the glycerin heated at 120°. Water is added to the solution and the mixture is immediately poured into a warm metal mold. The glycerin acts osmotically, so water diffuses into the rectum. One purpose of the sodium stearate is to form a gel, which allows convenient insertion of the glycerin. The sodium stearate also acts to produce fecal discharge by its local irritation of the mucous membrane of the rectum.

Emulsion-Type Suppositories

A phase volume ratio that favors an oil-in-water emulsion produces an emulsion that is too fluid to make a physically acceptable suppository. If a firm suppository could be formed, it would be unstable, as the external aqueous phase would tend to evaporate. A limited number of suppositories are water-in-oil emulsions. In theobroma oil 10 per cent wool fat or 2 per cent cholesterol are used to incorporate up to 15 per cent aqueous solutions.

Rectal Absorption

Two-thirds of the rectum follows the curvature of the lower spine. At the height of the coccyx, the rectum assumes a more horizontal position and turns downward just above the anal sphincter. The rectum is approximately 15 cm long with a maximum diameter of 6 cm. The normal rectum has a temperature of 37°, exerts a pressure from 0 to 6 g cm^{-2}, and exhibits practically no peristaltic movement. It may contain feces. Water is not present in the liquid state, but it composes about 80 per cent of the feces. Normally the rectum contains only about 2 ml of mucus, which has a pH 7.4. This small volume of mucus has little buffer capacity, and consequently the pH of the rectal cavity is determined by the medicinal compound present.

Passive absorption or diffusion occurs through the mucosa. The submucosal region has an abundance of lymphatic and blood vessels. The inferior hemorrhoidal vein near the anal sphincter and the middle hemorrhoidal vein drain into the inferior vena cava and do not drain directly into the general circulation. The superior hemorrhoidal vein near the upper rectum joins the inferior mesenteric vein, which empties into the portal vein. This has suggested that drugs may be absorbed rectally and bypass modification and detoxification in the liver. If this effect in initial circulation exists, it has little significance in the administration of most drugs. In addition, the anastomoses between the venous branches of the rectal circulation do not afford a distinct separation to the two circulatory routes. Usually a suppository comes to rest approximately 5 cm above the anal sphincter, and a rapid-melting suppository would favor absorption by the blood vessels connected to the vena cava. After a suppository has melted, there appears to be an upward displacement of a few centimeters. The time required for liquefaction of a rectal suppository is from 3 to 7 minutes for theobroma oil, 30 to 40 minutes for glycerinated gelatin, and 30 to 50 minutes for polyethylene glycol. Owing to its rapid liquefaction, theobroma oil is a good base for local soothing action and for the rapid release of water-soluble drugs.

Rectal absorption involves (1) the release or dissolution of the drug from the suppository and (2) the absorption of the dissolved drug through the mucosa. Either of these steps may be the rate-limiting step in rectal absorption. In general, it is assumed that absorption is a faster process than the diffusion of the drug from the suppository to the rectal fluid. It is the release which the pharmacist may control by various formulations of suppository bases.

The release of a drug is influenced by its partition coefficient. Diethylstilbesterol is practically insoluble in water and in glycerinated gelatin; it is soluble in theobroma oil. Although diethylstilbesterol has limited water solubility, it is dissolved and absorbed faster from a glycerinated gelatin suppository than from a theobroma oil suppository. Its partition coefficient so strongly favors the theobroma oil, that it is only very slowly released. Theobroma oil melts quickly, but it is immiscible with rectal mucus and generally releases oil-soluble drugs less readily than glycerinated gelatin and polyethylene glycol.

With drugs that are only slightly soluble in both the aqueous and the oily medium, the absorption of the drug is only slightly influenced by the suppository base. In Figure 169 it can be seen that aspirin is absorbed at approximately the same rate from a theobroma oil and a polyethylene glycol suppository. Even with its limited solubility, the absorption of aspirin from a rectal suppository is comparable to its gastrointestinal absorption from a compressed tablet.

As a general practice, faster and more complete rectal absorption is obtained by the selection of a water-soluble salt, e.g., sodium hexobarbital, sodium salicylate, or sodium tolbutamide, than the corresponding water-insoluble parent compound. For oleaginous suppository bases this may be rationalized on the basis of the partition coefficient of the drug. In each of the three suppository bases shown in Figure 170 the water-soluble sodium salt of sulfisomidine is absorbed more rapidly than the poorly soluble free acid. In Figure 171 the absorption of sulfisomidine from polyethylene glycol and theobroma oil suppositories is approximately the same for the first 12-hour period, after which there is a greater release from the polyethylene glycol base. The gastrointestinal absorption following oral administration is much greater than rectal absorption. The large difference between the oral and rectal absorption may be partially due to the very small volume of rectal fluid available for dissolving the drug. Since the initial absorption from theobroma oil and polyethylene glycol is nearly the same, it is conceivable that the apparently better absorption from polyethylene glycol at a later time reflects the leakage and loss of drug from the rectum with the fluid theobroma oil.

For suppository bases that do not melt at body temperature the drug is available for absorption as the suppository dissolves. Dissolution of a suppository is a slow process, owing to the small volume of mucus and the small surface area of the suppository. In such formulations the transport from the base to the mucus is the rate-limiting step in rectal absorption. The onset of therapeutic action will be slow and the effect may be of prolonged duration from drugs that are dissolved or suspended in polyethylene glycol.

A model may be proposed for the dissolution of a water-soluble suppository containing a drug that does not react with the base. The rectal fluid dissolves the drug and the base at rates proportional to their solubilities and diffusion coefficients. At some time one of the components becomes depleted at the solid-liquid interface region. As a result, a surface layer is formed that is composed of only one

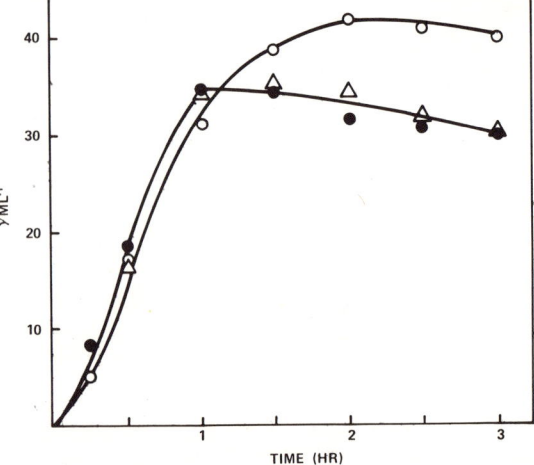

Figure 169. Mean plasma concentration of salicylic acid after administration to humans of 0.75 g of aspirin as oral tablet (open circles), theobroma oil suppository (solid circles), and polyethylene glycol suppository (open triangles). [Modified from U. Samelius and A. Astrom, *Acta Pharmacol. Toxicol.* **14**, 240 (1958).]

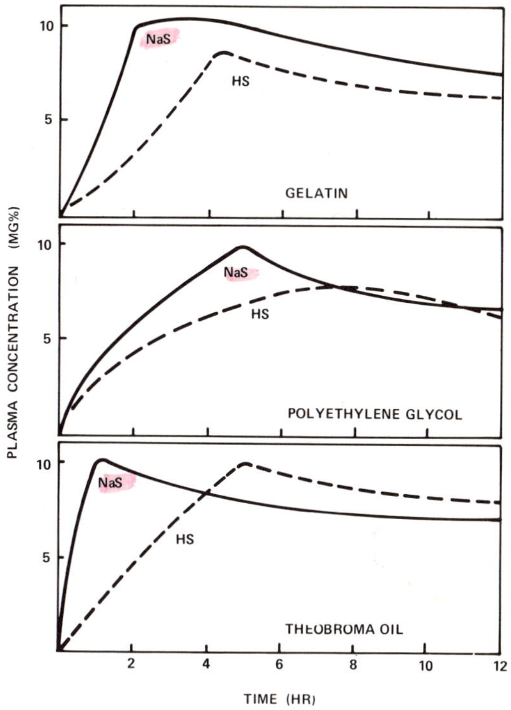

Figure 170. Mean plasma concentration of sulfisomidine after administration to rabbits of free acid (HS) and salt (NaS) in gelatin, polyethylene glycol, and theobroma oil suppositories. [Modified from L. Pennati and K. Steiger Trippi, *Pharm. Acta Helv. 33,* 663 (1958).]

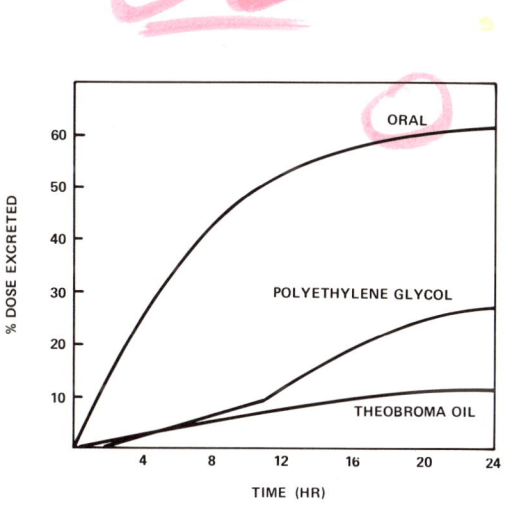

Figure 171. Cumulative urinary excretion from humans of sulfisomidine after the oral and rectal administration of sulfisomidine sodium. [Modified from T.W. Schwarz and K. Bichsel, *Pharm. Acta Helv. 38,* 861 (1963).]

component. After an elapse of time three situations may exist for the single-dimensional, two-component model assuming there is no build up of the components.

In case I, drug A dissolves fast enough to leave a layer of pure suppository base, B. Under these conditions

$$\frac{N_A}{N_B} < \frac{D_A C_A^0}{D_B C_B^0}$$

where N_A and N_B are the initial amounts of A and B in the suppository, D_A and D_B the respective diffusion coefficients, and C_A^0 and C_B^0 the respective solubilities. The dissolution rates, R, are

$$R_B = \frac{D_B C_B^0}{h}$$

and

$$R_A = \frac{N_A}{N_B} R_B$$

where h is the effective diffusion layer thickness. The influence of the ratio of the amount of drug to the amount of base on dissolution is shown in Figure 172. The rate of dissolution as represented by the slope of the line is increased as the amount of drug per unit volume of suppository is increased.

In case II, the suppository base, B, dissolves fast enough to leave a layer of pure drug A. Under these conditions

$$\frac{N_A}{N_B} > \frac{D_A C_A^0}{D_B C_B^0}$$

and the rates of dissolution are

$$R_A = \frac{D_A C_A^0}{h}$$

and

$$R_B = \frac{N_B}{N_A} R_A$$

In case III, the dissolution rates of A and B are proportional to their relative amounts in the suppository. Under these conditions

$$\frac{N_A}{N_B} = \frac{D_A C_A^0}{D_B C_B^0}$$

and the dissolution rates are

$$R_A = \frac{D_A C_A^0}{h}$$

and

$$R_B = \frac{D_B C_B^0}{h}$$

These equations apply only to the steady state, which requires that the solubilities of A and B do not greatly differ. If one of the components is very much less soluble than the other, the model reduces to solute release from an inert matrix. This has been previously considered in the release of drugs from ointments.

For suspension-type suppositories with a base that melts at body temperature, the availability of the drug for absorption depends on the melting characteristics. Although the partition coefficient of a water-soluble drug favors the partition from the theobroma oil into the rectal fluid, a water-soluble medicinal compound suspended in theobroma oil is not readily released from the intact suppository. This is the result of the slow rate of diffusion in the intact suppository and the small surface area of the suppository. When the suppository is melted, there is a greater area of theobroma oil-mucus interface

plastic suspensions and emulsions • 393

than with an intact suppository. The melted theobroma oil has a lower viscosity than the intact suppository, and diffusion is more rapid in the liquefied theobroma oil. The greater area from which the partition occurs and the faster diffusion rate facilitate rectal absorption.

A medicinal compound, e.g., aminopyrine, with a partition coefficient that does not strongly favor either phase will dissolve in the theobroma oil. The solute molecules partition from the intact suppository to a greater extent than the larger particles of a water-soluble drug suspended in a suppository. Upon melting of the suppository the rate of diffusion is increased only slightly. Thus, the availability and absorption of a drug dissolved in the base is not increased by the melting of the suppository to as great an extent as that of a drug suspended in the base.

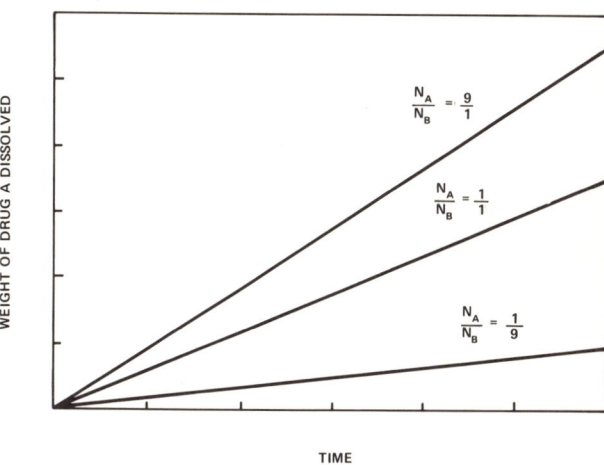

Figure 172. Influence of the ratio of drug to base, N_A/N_B, on dissolution rate of water-soluble drug from a water-soluble suppository base.

APPENDIX

ALGEBRA

Quadratic Equation

The solution of a quadratic equation $ax^2 + bx + c = 0$ is

$$x = \frac{-b \pm \sqrt{b^2 - 4ac}}{2a}$$

If $b^2 - 4ac$ is positive, the roots are real and unequal, but for a real problem usually only one root is physically possible. If $b^2 - 4ac$ is zero, the roots are real and equal. If $b^2 - 4ac$ is negative, the roots are imaginary and unequal.

$$x^2 + 1.8 \times 10^{-5} x - 2.52 \times 10^{-6} = 0$$

$$x = \frac{-1.8 \times 10^{-5} \pm \sqrt{(1.8 \times 10^{-5} \times -(-2.52 \times 10^{-6} \times 4)}}{2}$$

$$= \frac{-1.8 \times 10^{-5} \pm \sqrt{3.24 \times 10^{-10} + 10.08 \times 10^{-6}}}{2}$$

$$= 1.58 \times 10^{-3}$$

Exponents

Small numbers are conveniently manipulated by expressing the numbers as powers of 10. For example, 0.00015 may be expressed as 1.5×10^{-4}. The first part is the coefficient and the second is the exponential factor of 10.

An exponent is a symbol written above and to the right of another symbol, denoting how many times the latter is repeated as a factor.

The properties of exponents are as follows:

1. In the process of multiplication, exponents are added and the coefficients are multiplied.

$$a^x a^y = a^{x+y}$$

$$1.5 \times 10^{-4} \times 5 \times 10^2 = 7.5 \times 10^{-2}$$

2. A product raised to a power is equal to the product of each factor raised to the given power.

$$(ab)^x = a^x b^x$$

$$(1.5 \times 6)^2 = (1.5^2)(6^2) = 81$$

3. When an exponent is raised to a power, the exponent and the power are multiplied.

$$(a^x)^y = a^{xy}$$
$$(\pi^2)^{4/3} = \pi^{8/3}$$

4. If $a \neq 0$, the negative exponent of a number is equal to the reciprocal of that number raised to the positive exponent.

$$a^{-x} = \frac{1}{a^x}$$

$$125^{-1/2} = \frac{1}{125^{1/2}} = 0.089$$

5. In the process of division, exponents are subtracted and coefficients are divided.

$$\frac{a^x}{a^y} = a^{x-y}$$

$$\frac{28 \times 10^6}{6 \times 10^{23}} = 4.67 \times 10^{-17}$$

Logarithms

The logarithm of a positive number, N, to a given positive base, b, other than 1, is the exponent of the power, x, to which the base must be raised to equal the number.

$$N = b^x \quad \text{or} \quad \log_b N = x$$

Thus, in the exponential form, $100 = 10^2$, and in the logarithmic form, $2 = \log_{10} 100$.

Although any positive number, except 1, may be chosen as a base of a system of logarithms, two bases are most commonly used. The common logarithms use the base 10 and are designated as log. The natural logarithms use as a base the irrational number e (2.71828) and are designated as ln. Mutliplying the common logarithm by 2.303 converts it to the natural logarithm,

$$2.303 \log N = \ln N$$

A logarithm consists of an integer known as the characteristic, and a decimal known as the mantissa. The characteristic determines the position of the decimal point in the number; the mantissa determines the actual digits and is independent of the decimal point.

The characteristic of a number may be found using the following rules:

1. The characteristic of any number greater than 1 is one less than the number of digits before the decimal point.

2. The characteristic of any number less than 1 is negative and is found by subtracting from 9 the number of ciphers between the decimal point and the first significant digit, and writing -10 after the result.

The common logarithms of the same sequence of digits have the same mantissa. To find the mantissa in a four-place logarithm table, look in the column marked N for the first two digits and pick the column headed by the third digit — the mantissa is the number appearing at the intersection of this row and column.

For example, to find log 229 using a four-place logarithm table, first determine the characteristic which is 1 less than the number of digits before the decimal, or 2. The mantissa is found by following the row after the number 22 until it intersects with the column under 9, or 0.3598. The log of 229 = 2.3598.

When the characteristic is negative, it is often more convenient to use an equivalent form, writing the characteristic as the difference of two positive numbers of which the second is a multiple of 10. Thus, -1 is equivalent to 9 - 10, and -12 is equivalent to a 8 - 20.

For example, to find the log 0.0229, first determine the characteristic, which is found by subtracting 1 from 9 and writing -10 after the result. The mantissa is found exactly as shown in the previous example. The logarithm may be expressed as

$$\log 0.0229 = 8.3598 - 10 = -2 + 0.3598 = -1.6402$$

To find the number corresponding to a given logarithm, the process is reversed. The number found is known as the antilogarithm. The sequence of digits of the given mantissa is found in the table, and the proper position for the decimal point in this sequence of digits is determined by the given characteristic.

For example, if $\log N = 0.6990$, examination of the logarithm tables shows the antilogarithm to be 500. The characteristic shows that there is one digit before the decimal. Thus, the number is 5.

The logarithm of the reciprocal of a number is equivalent to the negative logarithm of the number,

$$\log \frac{1}{N} = \log 1 - \log N = -\log N$$

The negative logarithm of a number can be found by subtracting the logarithm of the number from 10.0000 - 10.

For example, to determine $-\log(5 \times 10^{-5})$, first find the logarithm and subtract from 10.0000 - 10,

$$\log(5 \times 10^{-5}) = \log 5 + \log 10^{-5} = 0.6990 + (5.0000 - 10) = 5.6990 - 10$$

$$\begin{array}{r} 10.0000 - 10 \\ 5.6990 - 10 \\ \hline 4.3010 \end{array}$$

Thus, $-\log(5 \times 10^{-5}) - = 4.3010$.

If the negative logarithm is known, reversal of the previous operation will provide the number. For example, if $-\log N = 6.8$, multiply by -1 to obtain $\log N = -6.8$; then convert this logarithm to one with a positive mantissa by adding to 10.0000 - 10, and find the antilogarithm.

$$\begin{array}{r} 10.0000 - 10 \\ -6.8 \\ \hline 3.2000 - 10 \end{array}$$

$\log N = 3.2000 - 10$

$N = 0.000000158$, or 1.58×10^{-7}

Calculations are often simplified by using the properties of logarithms. Three properties of logarithms taken to the same base are as follows:

1. The logarithm of a product is equal to the sum of the logarithms of its factors.

$$\log AB = \log A + \log B$$

$$\log(525 \times 27) = \log 525 + \log 27 = 2.7202 + 1.4314 = 4.1516$$

Using four-place logarithm tables the antilogarithm of 0.1516 is 142 and from the characteristic the number corresponding to this multiplication is 1.42×10^4.

2. The logarithm of a quotient is equal to the logarithm of the dividend minus the logarithm of the divisor.

$$\log \frac{A}{B} = \log A - \log B$$

$$\log \frac{4.7 \times 10^{-5}}{1.9 \times 10^{-3}} = \log(4.7 \times 10^{-5}) - \log(1.9 \times 10^{-3})$$

$$\begin{array}{rl} \log 4.7 = & 0.6721 \\ \log 10^{-5} = & -5 \\ \hline & -4.3279 \\ \log 1.9 = & 0.2788 \\ \log 10^{-5} = & -3 \\ \hline & 2.7212 \end{array}$$

$$\log \frac{4.7 \times 10^{-5}}{1.0 \times 10^{-3}} = -4.3279 - (-2.7212) = -1.6067$$

$$\begin{array}{r} 10.0000 - 10 \\ -1.6067 \\ \hline 8.3933 - 10 \end{array}$$

Antilog 0.3933 = 247, and with a characteristic of -2 the number is 0.0247.

3. The logarithm of a power of a number is equal to the exponent times the logarithm of the number.

$$\log A_P = p \log A$$
$$\log 2.7^{0.3} = 0.3 \log 2.7 = 0.3 \times 0.4314 = 0.1294$$

Antilog 0.1294 = 135, and with a characteristic of 0 the number is 1.35.

Trigonometric Terms

The following definitions are based on the right-angle triangle ABC in Figure 173:

$$\text{sine } \alpha = \frac{\text{opposite side}}{\text{hypotenuse}} = \frac{a}{c}$$

$$\text{cosine } \alpha = \frac{\text{adjacent side}}{\text{hypotenuse}} = \frac{b}{c}$$

$$\text{tangent } \alpha = \frac{\text{opposite side}}{\text{adjacent side}} = \frac{a}{b}$$

$$\text{cotangent } \alpha = \frac{\text{adjacent side}}{\text{hypotenuse}} = \frac{b}{a}$$

$$\text{secant } \alpha = \frac{\text{hypotenuse}}{\text{adjacent side}} = \frac{c}{b}$$

$$\text{cosecant } \alpha = \frac{\text{hypotenuse}}{\text{opposite side}} = \frac{c}{a}$$

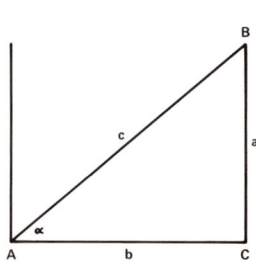

Figure 173.

ANALYTIC GEOMETRY

The equation for a straight line is

$$y = mx + b$$

where m is the slope when y is plotted against x and b is the intercept on the y axis where $x = 0$. The slope may be calculated from any two points $(x_1, y_1$ and $x_2, y_2)$ on the line.

$$m = \frac{y_2 - y_1}{x_2 - x_1}$$

In Figure 174 the line is extrapolated to intersect the y axis at $b = 0.114$. The slope is calculated by values at 2 and 10 hours:

$$m = \frac{\log C_2 - \log C_1}{t_2 - t_1}$$

$$= \frac{\log 0.8 - \log 0.13}{2 - 10}$$

$$= \frac{-(0.0969) - (0.8861)}{-8}$$

$$= -0.1$$

The equation of the line is

$$\log C = -0.1t + 0.114$$

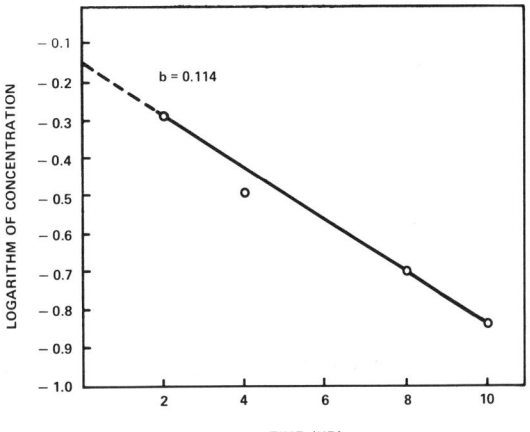

Figure 174.

DIFFERENTIAL CALCULUS

Definitions. A variable is a quantity that may have different values. A constant is a quantity that retains the same value throughout any given system.

A variable, y, is said to be a function of another variable, x, if for every one of some set of values of x there corresponds a value of y. Mathematically, the statement "y is a function of x" is written $y = f(x)$, which is read "y is the f of x."

Limit of a Variable and of a Function. The concept of a limit is essential to understanding the differential. Consider a bead with a hole strung on a wire so that the bead is movable. Let a black spot on the wire represent a fixed point whose abscissa is a. The statement "the variable x approaches the constant a" is analogous to the bead moving along the wire. Permit the bead to come closer to the spot than 0.1 mm. Then mark off on each side of the spot 0.1-mm intervals. Move the bead until it gets between the marks and never let it out again. It may now be said that the bead comes and remains closer than 0.1 mm to the spot.

The intervals or increments can be made as small as one desires, and the bead enters and remains inside this interval. At no time is there any consideration that the bead will actually coincide with the black spot — nothing has been said to imply that x is eventually equal to a. There is no interest in having $x = a$; it is what is going on close to a that is of interest.

To expand further on the concept of a limit, consider the equation

$$x_n = \frac{n}{n+1}$$

where $x_1 = 1/2$, $x_2 = 2/3$, $x_3 = 3/4$, ... If these points are plotted along the x axis, it appears that x is approaching 1. If this is a fact, one must be able to surround 1 by an interval as small as desired, so that eventually all the remaining plotted points will fall inside the interval.

Choose an interval of width 2/100 of which 1 is the middle point. Now, one expects the differences

$$1 - \frac{1}{2},\ 1 - \frac{2}{3},\ 1 - \frac{3}{4},\ \ldots,\ 1 - \frac{n}{n+1}$$

will become and remain less than 1/100. To see whether or not they will, consider

$$1 - \frac{n}{n+1} = \frac{n+1-n}{n+1} = \frac{1}{n+1}$$

Evidently, $\frac{1}{n+1} < \frac{1}{100}$ if $n + 1 > 100$, i.e., if $n > 99$. It can be said with certainty that $1 - x_n$ will be numerically less than 1/100 provided that n is greater than 99. Thus, the difference in question eventually become and remain numerically less than 1/100. Symbolically, this may be stated using vertical bars to mean abstract values:

$$[1 - x_n] < 1/100 \quad \text{for all } n > 99$$

This does not mean that x is approaching 1; it says that x eventually differs from 1 by less than 1/100 and that x might eventually reach 999/1000 and still satisfy this equation.

It must be assured that the difference between 1 and x will become and remain less than any arbitrarily small positive number. Determine if $[1 - x_n]$ will be less than some arbitrarily small number, $e = 1/N$.

Now

$$[1 - x_n] = 1 - \frac{n}{n+1} = \frac{1}{n+1}$$

will be less than $e = 1/N$ if $n + 1 > N = 1/e$. For brevity, using symbols,

$$|1 - x_n| < e = 1/n \quad \text{for all } n > \frac{1}{e} - 1 = N - 1$$

Now it is certain that x approaches 1 (written $x \to 1$), because no matter how small an interval (of width $2e$) is chosen to surround 1, all values, after a certain one, assumed by x fall inside this interval. This certain value of x depends only on the size of the interval chosen. This discussion should clarify what is meant by the statement "that x is approaching a value," so that the limit of a function may now be discussed.

Consider y as a function of x defined by the equation

$$y = \frac{2x^2 - 2x}{x - 1}$$

The interest lies in what happens to y as x approaches 1. If $x = 1$ is substituted in the equation, it takes the meaningless form 0/0, which is not defined. Examine the values of x tabulated and note that it appears that y is approaching 2.

x	1.1	1.01	1.001	1.0001	1.00001
y	2.2	2.02	2.002	2.0002	2.00002

To test this observation, note that

$$y = \frac{2x(x-1)}{x-1} = 2x$$

for every value of x except $x = 1$. Thus

$$|y - 2| = |2x - 2| = 2|x - 1|$$

can be arbitrarily small by taking x close to 1.

This is interpreted graphically in Figure 175. When drawn, the equation is that of a straight line with a single point omitted. The omitted point has an abscissa of 1 for which y is not defined.

Draw a horizontal strip of width $2e$. All points in this strip have ordinates that differ from 2 by less than e. From where these horizontal lines intersect the curve, draw vertical lines to intersect the x axis.

When the value of any point between 1 and the intersections on the x axis is substituted for x in the equation, the resulting value of y will differ from 2 by less than e. It is then said that the limit of y is 2 as x approaches 1. This illustrates that the function y may be a limit as x approaches some particular value, although the function may be undefined for the value of x in question.

If $y = f(x)$ is a function of x and if y approaches b as x approaches a, the limit of y is b as x approaches a and is written

$$\lim_{x \to a} y = b \quad \text{or} \quad \lim_{x \to a} f(x) = b.$$

The limit of a function may now be defined. If $y = f(x)$ is a function of x, then y is said to have a limit b as x approaches a, provided that the numerical value of the difference between y and b becomes and remains less than any arbitrarily assigned small positive number for all values of x close enough, but not equal, to a.

Expressed symbolically, the limit of $f(x)$ is said to be b as x approaches a if for any preassigned number $e > 0$ there exist a number $\delta > 0$ such that for $0 < [x - a] < \delta$ so that $[f(x) - b] < e$.

It must be emphasized that this definition and the idea of a limit has nothing to do with the value of the function y for $x = a$. It must be recognized that x may approach a in any manner.

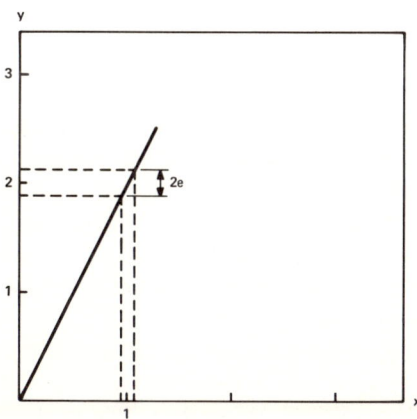

Figure 175.

Variables Becoming Infinite. A variable is said to become infinite if it becomes and remains larger than any arbitrarily given number. Consider the function plotted in Figure 176,

$$y = \frac{2}{x}$$

When x approaches 0, the function $y = 2/x$ has no limit but may be numerically as large as desired by making x close enough to 0. It is said that "y becomes infinite as x approaches 0," and it is symbolically written

$$y \to \infty \quad \text{as} \quad x \to 0$$

This says that y is a variable that becomes and remains numerically greater than any number we care to assign, or "y increases numerically without limit." It is not to be erroneously thought that ∞ represents a very large, although unknown, number.

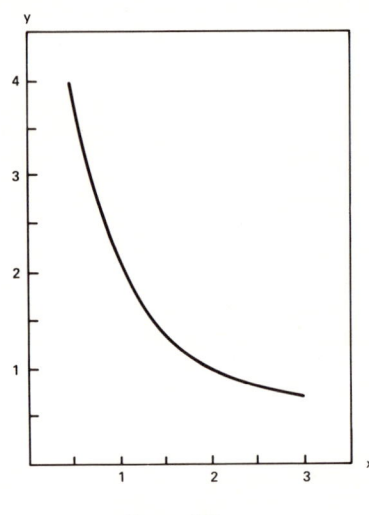

Figure 176.

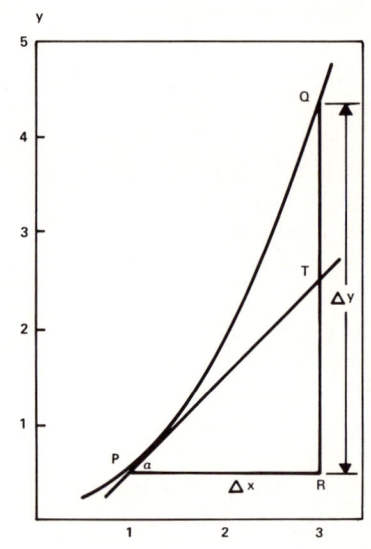

Figure 177.

Derivative. An understanding of the derivative is essential to the discussion and comprehension of the rates of change in many pharmaceutical functions. Perhaps the simplest way to investigate the properties of any function is to consider its curve. For example, the curve $y = \frac{1}{2}x^2$ is a continuous curve for all values of x. It can be shown that the curve has a tangent for every point on the curve.

In Figure 177 the tangent to the curve at point P $(1, \frac{1}{2})$ is defined as follows: Let P be a fixed point on the curve and Q any other point on the curve. The tangent at P is the limiting position PT of the secant PQ as Q approaches P along the curve from either side of P. Draw PR parallel to the x axis and RQ parallel to the y axis.

This definition is equivalent to saying that the limit of the variable angle RPQ is a fixed angle α as Q approaches P along the curve; and if $\alpha \neq 90°$ this is equivalent to saying that the limit of $RQ/PR = \tan RPQ$ as Q approaches P along the curve.

Returning to point P $(1, \frac{1}{2})$ of the curve $y = \frac{1}{2}x^2$, designate the distance PR by Δx (read delta x and to be considered as a single symbol, not as a product) and the distance RQ by Δy. Then Q has the coordinates $(1 + \Delta x, \frac{1}{2} + \Delta y)$, and $\tan RPQ = \Delta y/\Delta x$. Note that as Q is to the right and above P, RQ and RP are positive, but if Q is to the left and below P, then RQ and PR are negative; however, in both cases $RQ/PR = \Delta y/\Delta x$ is positive.

If Q approaches P from either side of the curve, Δx approaches 0. So, if $\Delta y/\Delta x$ has a limit as Δx approaches 0, this limit must be $\tan \alpha$. Suppose Q is the point (2, 2). Then, the value $\Delta y/\Delta x$ may be determined,

$$\Delta x = \text{abscissa of } Q \text{ minus abscissa of } P = 2 - 1 = 1$$
$$\Delta y = \text{ordinate of } Q \text{ minus ordinate of } P = 2 - \tfrac{1}{2} = 3/2$$

and

$$\frac{\Delta y}{\Delta x} = \frac{3}{2} \div 1 = \frac{3}{2}$$

Other values of $\Delta y/\Delta x$ are:

Abscissa of P	Abscissa of Q	Δx	Ordinate of P	Ordinate of Q	Δy	$\dfrac{\Delta y}{\Delta x}$
1	2	1.0	0.5	2.0	1.5	1.5
1	1.5	0.5	0.5	1.125	0.625	1.25
1	1.1	0.1	0.5	0.605	0.105	1.05
1	1.01	0.01	0.5	0.51005	0.01005	1.005
1	1.001	0.001	0.5	0.5010005	0.0010005	1.0005

It appears that $\Delta y/\Delta x$ is approaching 1. To find the ordinate of Q we need only to replace x by $1 + \Delta x$ in the equation $y = \tfrac{1}{2}x^2$,

$$\text{ordinate of } Q = \tfrac{1}{2}(1 + \Delta x)^2 = \tfrac{1}{2}(1 + 2\Delta x + \Delta x^2)$$
$$= \tfrac{1}{2} + \Delta x \cdot \tfrac{1}{2} + \Delta x^2$$

To find Δy we subtract from this ordinate of Q the ordinate of P or $\tfrac{1}{2}$:

$$\Delta y = \Delta x + \tfrac{1}{2}\Delta x^2$$

Thus

$$\frac{\Delta y}{\Delta x} = 1 + \tfrac{1}{2} \Delta x$$

and

$$\lim_{\Delta x \to 0} \frac{\Delta y}{\Delta x} = \lim_{\Delta x \to 0} (1 + \tfrac{1}{2} \Delta x) = 1$$

It is now certain that the curve has a tangent at P and the direction, since its slope is 1, is an angle of $45°$ with the horizontal.

Other points P may be investigated. Suppose P has the coordinates (x, y). For any point Q on the curve, the coordinates are $(x + \Delta x, y + \Delta y)$. Again $\tan RPQ = \Delta y/\Delta x$ and it can be determined if $\Delta y/\Delta x$ has a limit as Δx approaches 0.

Placing the coordinates of Q in the equation as before one obtains

$$y + \Delta y = \tfrac{1}{2}(x + \Delta x)^2 = \tfrac{1}{2}x^2 + x\Delta x + \tfrac{1}{2}\Delta x^2$$

To find Δy subtract the ordinates of P from the ordinate of Q giving

$$\Delta y = x\Delta x + \tfrac{1}{2} \Delta x^2$$

so that

$$\frac{\Delta y}{\Delta x} = x + \tfrac{1}{2} \Delta x$$

and therefore

$$\lim_{\Delta x \to 0} \frac{\Delta y}{\Delta x} = \lim_{\Delta x \to 0} (x + \tfrac{1}{2} \Delta x) = x$$

Since it is known that $\lim_{\Delta x \to 0} \dfrac{\Delta y}{\Delta x}$ is $\tan \alpha$, at any given point on the curve $\tan \alpha$ is equal to the abscissa of that point.

The remarks made may be generalized. Given a function $y = f(x)$ that is continuous and single-valued throughout an interval, say $a \leq x \leq b$, the slope of the tangent may be found for any point. Let a point be $P(x, y)$ and let Q be another point on the curve. The coordinates of Q are $(x + \Delta x, y + \Delta y)$. To calculate the ordinate of Q, replace x by $x + \Delta x$, obtaining

$$y + \Delta y = f(x + \Delta x)$$

To find Δy subtract the ordinate of P from this ordinate:

$$\Delta y = f(x + \Delta x) - f(x)$$

Hence

$$\frac{\Delta y}{\Delta x} = \frac{f(x + \Delta x) - f(x)}{\Delta x}$$

and therefore

$$\lim_{\Delta x \to 0} \frac{\Delta y}{\Delta x} = \lim_{\Delta x \to 0} \frac{f(x + \Delta x) - f(x)}{\Delta x}$$

Rate of Change of a Function. The function $y = \tfrac{1}{2}x^2$ may be regarded from a different viewpoint by a chemist or a pharmacist. Instead of a graphical interpretation, they would be interested in how fast y increases with an increasing x. Examination of Figure 177 shows that near $x = 0$, the curve rises slowly and y changes slowly with increasing x, whereas for large values of x the curve rises rapidly and y changes rapidly with increasing x. The rate of change of the function y is not a constant but varies with x.

To find the average rate of change of y between $x = 1$ and $x = 2$, compute the number of units change in y and divide by the number of units change in x. When $x = 1$ and $y = \tfrac{1}{2}$, and when $x = 2$ and $y = 2$ the change in y is $\Delta y = 2 - \tfrac{1}{2} = 3/2$. The change in x is $\Delta x = 1$. The average rate of change of y between the two values of x is

$$\frac{\Delta y}{\Delta x} = \frac{3}{2} \div 1 = \frac{3}{2}$$

Then $\dfrac{\Delta y}{\Delta x}$ is the average rate of change of y between the original and new values of x. This average rate of change of y approaches 1 as a limit as the interval Δx is made to approach 0. This limit is called the instantaneous rate of change of y at the point where $x = 1$ or at the point $(1, \tfrac{1}{2})$.

The rate of change of y at any other point (x,y) of the function $y = \frac{1}{2} x^2$ may be found. The original value of x is x and the original value of y is $y = \frac{1}{2} x^2$. The new value of x is $x + \Delta x$ and the new value of y is

$$y + \Delta y = \frac{1}{2}(x + \Delta x)^2$$

The change in y is

$$\Delta y = x \Delta x + \frac{1}{2} \Delta x^2$$

and

$$\frac{\Delta y}{\Delta x} = x + \frac{1}{2} \Delta x$$

Therefore the rate of change of y at the point (x, y) is

$$\lim_{\Delta x \to 0} \frac{\Delta y}{\Delta x} = x$$

In general, the average rate of change of the function $y = f(x)$ between two values of x is simply the new value of y minus the original value of y divided by the new value of x minus the original value of x,

$$\frac{\Delta y}{\Delta x} = \frac{f(x + \Delta x) - f(x)}{\Delta x}$$

and the rate of change of y at the point (x, y) is

$$\lim_{\Delta x \to 0} \frac{\Delta y}{\Delta x} = \lim_{\Delta x \to 0} \frac{f(x + \Delta x) - f(x)}{\Delta x}$$

The result is expressed in number of units change in y per unit change in x.

Derivation of a Function. The calculations involved in find the slope of the tangent line to a curve and in calculating the rate of change of a function are exactly the same. The difference is in terminology and viewpoint. These two examples have been given to introduce a concept. A general process and definition entirely independent of these examples may now be introduced.

Let $y = f(x)$ be a function that is single-valued and continuous in the interval $a \leq x \leq b$. Let (x, y) be any particular pair of numbers satisfying the equation $y = f(x)$ and having x in the specified interval. Then

1. Let x receive an increment Δx. Replace x by $x + \Delta x$, obtaining a new value of y,

$$y + \Delta y = f(x + \Delta x)$$

2. Subtract the original value of y from the new value of y to obtain Δy,

$$\Delta y = f(x + \Delta x) - f(x)$$

3. Form the quotient

$$\frac{\Delta y}{\Delta x} = \frac{f(x + \Delta x) - f(x)}{\Delta x}$$

4. Take the limit of this quotient as x approaches 0. The result is denoted by $\frac{dy}{dx}$ and is called the derivative of y with respect to x at the point (x,y):

$$\frac{dy}{dx} = \lim_{\Delta x \to 0} \frac{\Delta y}{\Delta x} = \lim_{\Delta x \to 0} \frac{f(x + \Delta x) - f(x)}{\Delta x}$$

The process of finding a derivative is called differentiation. The symbol $\frac{dy}{dx}$ is only to be regarded as a single symbol and is on no account to be thought of as a quotient of two numbers dy and dx. It is important to note that $\frac{dy}{dx}$ means the derivative at the particular point whose coordinates are (x, y). The derivative is independent of geometric considerations.

If the derivative of a function is positive at a given point, the function is increasing in the neighborhood of this point; if the derivative is negative, the function is decreasing in the neighborhood.

General rules for differentiation of algebraic functions are:

1. If $y = x^n$, then $\frac{dy}{dx} = nx^{n-1}$.

   If $y = x^3$ then $\frac{dy}{dx} = 3x^2$.

2. The derivative of any constant is zero:

   $$\frac{dc}{cx} = 0$$

3. The derivative of the sum of any finite number of functions is the sum of the derivatives of the separate functions. Thus,

   $$\frac{d(a+b)}{dx} = \frac{da}{dx} + \frac{db}{dx}$$

   $$y = x^2 + x^{-1/3} \quad \text{then} \quad \frac{dy}{dx} = 2x - 1/3x^{-4/3}$$

4. The derivative of the product of two functions is the first times the derivative of the second plus the second times the derivative of the first. Thus,

   $$\frac{d(ab)}{dx} = a\frac{db}{dx} + b\frac{da}{dx}$$

   $$y = x^2(x^3 + x + 5)$$

   $$\frac{dy}{dx} = x^2(3x^2 + 1) + 2x(x^3 + x + 5) = 5x^4 + 3x^2 + 10x$$

5. The derivative of a constant times a function is that constant times the derivative of the function. Thus,

   $$\frac{d(cu)}{dx} = c\frac{du}{dx}$$

6. The derivative of the quotient of two functions is the denominator times the derivative of the numerator minus the numerator times the derivative of the denominator, all divided by the square of the denominator:

   $$\frac{d}{dx}\left(\frac{u}{v}\right) = \frac{v\frac{du}{dx} - u\frac{dv}{dx}}{v^2}$$

$$y = \frac{x^2 + 5}{x + 1}$$

$$\frac{dy}{dx} = \frac{(x+1)2x - (x^2+5)(1)}{(x+1)^2} = \frac{x^2 + 2x - 5}{x^2 + 2x + 1}$$

7. The derivative of a function may be expressed as

$$\frac{dy}{dx} = \frac{dy}{du}\frac{du}{dx}$$

$$y = (x^2 - 3)^{2/3}$$

Let $y = u^{2/3}$:

$$\frac{dy}{du} = \frac{2}{3}u^{-1/3} \quad \text{and} \quad \frac{du}{dx} = 2x$$

$$\frac{dy}{dx} = \frac{dy}{du}\frac{du}{dx} = \frac{2}{3}u^{-1/3}\,2x = \frac{2}{3}(x^2-3)\,2x = \frac{4x}{3}(x^2-3)$$

8. The derivative with respect to x of the nth power of a function of x is n times the function to the $(n-1)$ power times the derivative of the function with respect to x:

$$\frac{d}{dx}(u^n) = nu^{n-1}\frac{du}{dx}$$

$$y = (x^2 + 6)^{3/2}$$

$$\frac{dy}{dx} = \frac{3}{2}(x^2+6)^{1/2}\,2x = 3x(x^2+6)^{1/2}$$

Partial Derivatives. Corresponding to the concept of the derivative of a function of one variable, the concept of partial derivatives of a function of several variables may be defined.

If $u = f(x, y)$, and if y is kept fixed, then u becomes a function of x only; its derivative with respect to x is called the partial derivative of u with respect to x and is denoted symbolically as

$$\left(\frac{\delta u}{\delta x}\right)_y$$

In the function $u = x^2 + xy + y^2$ the partial derivative with respect to x when y is constant is

$$\left(\frac{\delta u}{\delta x}\right)_y = 2x + y$$

and the partial derivative with respect to y when x is constant is

$$\left(\frac{\delta u}{\delta y}\right)_x = x + 2y$$

INDEX

Abbreviations, vii
Absorption, percutaneous, 372
    rectal, 389
Acacia, 318, 358
    as emulsifying agent, 339, 358
    mucilage, 318
    structure of, 358
N-acetyl-p-aminophenol, 258
    hydrolysis of, 258
    influence of temperature on, 259
    pH profile, 260
Acid-base catalysis, 258
Acid-base equilibria, 209
Activity, 187
    coefficient, 188
    of solute, 188
    of solvent, 187
    of strong electrolyte, 189
Adsorption, 20
    at liquid interface, 20, 307
    at solid interface, 21, 130
    Langmuir isotherm, 23
    of ions, 296
    physical, 21
Aerosol, 295, 322, 323
    classification of, 295, 324
    cold fill, 329
    compressed gases, 326
    container and valve, 328
    liquefied gases, 326
    operation, 323
    pressure fill, 329
    propellants, 326, 327
    spray pattern, 325
Algins, 349
Aliquot method, 60
Amine soaps, 360
Amphoretic nature of gelatin, 360
Ampul, 287
Andreasen pipet, 14
Antioxidants, 357
Arlacels, 361
Aromatic waters, 170
Arrhenius, dissociation, 209
    equation, 256, 270
Aspirin, hydrolysis of, 251
    first-order, 251
    influence of temperature on, 256
    pH profile, 258
    zero order, 254
Atkins and Pantin buffer, 234
Atomizers, 322
Autoclave, 274
Autoxidation, 266

Balance, Class A, 59
Bases, 209
    salts and, 225
    weak, 211
Bentonite, 355
Benzocaine, hydrolysis of, 265
    retarded by complexation, 265
    retarded by solubilization, 265
Biological half-life, 93
Blenders, 334
    for dispersing liquid in a solid, 55
    for preparing solutions, 162
    immiscible liquids, 340
    solid-solid, 51
    suspensions, 331
Blood level, after repeated administration, 96
    first-order elimination from, 92
    minimum effective, 94
Boiling-point elevation, 191
    constant, 191
Bonding forces in solids, 107, 113
    covalent, 112
    dipole-dipole, 107
    induced dipole-induced dipole, 111
    ionic, 111
    metallic, 112
Brønsted-Lowry theory, 209
Brownian movement, 296
Brunauer, Emmett, and Teller (BET) equation, 24
Buccal tablet, 74, 83
Buffer, 224
    capacity, 227
    equation, 225
    solutions, 231, 263
Bulk powders, 61
Bulkiness, 18

Caking, 28, 128, 132, 341
Calibration of suppository mold, 387
Calibration of T.T. mold, 70
Capsules, 66
    capacities, 67
    elastic, 69
    filling, 67
Catalysis, acid-base, 258
Cellulose, 351, 354
Cellulose acetate phthalate, 88
Chartulae, 63
Chlorpromazine, zero-order photolysis of, 269
Cholesterol, 359
Clark and Lubs buffer, 232
Clausius-Clapeyron equation, 122
Coacervation, 316
Coating, 86
    air suspension, 90
    enteric, 88
    evaluation of, 91
    film, 89
    press, 89
    sugar, 86
Colligative properties, 190
    of colloids, 299
    of concentrated solutions, 196
    of electrolytic solutions, 195
    of nonelectrolytic solutions, 190
Colloids, definition, 295
    gel, 320
    hydrophilic, 296, 298, 318, 349
    hydrophobic, 296, 317
    preparation, 317, 318
    properties, 296
    protective, 315
    purification, 318
    sol, 295
    stability of, 315
Collyria, 290

Color, 179
   stability of, 272
Comminution, 37
Complex formation, 176, 264, 375
Compressed tablets, 73
Concentration expressions, 139
Conductance, equivalent, 185
   specific, 185
Conjugate pair, 209
Continental method for preparing emulsions, 339
Coulomb principle, 144
Creaming, 337, 355
Critical micelle concentration, 264, 314
Crystal hydrate, 133
Crystal systems, 113

Dalton's law of partial pressures, 153
Debye-Hückel theory, 189
Deflocculation, 298
Deformation, 364
Degradation, by hydrolysis, 251, 257
   by oxidation, 266
   by photolysis, 269, 272
Degree of dissociation, 186, 212
Deliquescence, 135
Density, apparent, 17, 80
   true, 17
Detergent, 313
Dialysis, 318
Diameter, average, 4
   definition of, 1, 10
   geometric mean, 8
   median, 5
   statistical, 1, 2, 10
Dielectric constant, 145
Diffusion, 299
   constant, 159, 299
   Fick's law of, 159, 299
   from ointment, 374
   from suppository, 389
Dilatant flow, 306
Dioctyl sodium sulfosuccinate, 360
Dipole, 107, 143
Dipole moment, 108
Disintegration of tablets, 82
Dissociation constants, 210
   of acids, 210, 215
   of bases, 211, 219
   of water, 214
Dissolution, 27, 84, 158
   apparatus, 85, 162
   factors affecting, 160
   forces involved, 147
   in reactive medium, 165, 166
   in nonreactive medium, 160
   rate, 28, 159
Distribution coefficient, 247
Divided powders, 63
Donnan membrane equilibrium, 300
Double layer, 297
Dry-heat sterilization, 276
Dundon and Mack equation, 27
Dusting powders, 61

Effervescent granulation, 64
Efflorescence, 135

Einstein equation, 303
Elastic material, 364
Electrokinetic potential, 297
Electrolytes, 195
   classification of, 188
   colligative properties of, 195
   conductance of, 185
   dissociation of, 209
   strong, 189
   weak, 209
Electromeric effect, 109
Elixirs, 238
Emulsification, 337, 339
Emulsifying agents, 313, 335, 358
   acacia, 358
   calcium oleate, 360
   cholesterol, 359
   dioctyl sodium sulfosuccinate, 360
   lecithin, 359
   polyoxyl 40 stearate, 361
   polysorbate 80, 361, 362
   sodium lauryl sulfate, 360
Emulsions, 334, 355
   coalescence of, 355
   creaming of, 356
   intravenous, 357
   ointments, 370
   oral, 356
   phase volume ratio, 336
   stability of, 337
   types of, 335
Emulsion-type ointment, 370
Emulsoid, 316
Enantiotripic polymorph, 126
Energy of activation, 256
English method of preparing emulsions, 339
Enteric coat, 88
Eutectic point, 118
Extraction, 30, 241
   liquid-liquid, 247
   processes of, 242, 245
Extracts, 246

Feldman buffer, 235
Fick's law of diffusion, 159,
Film balance, 309
Filters, 277
   asbestos, 278
   membrane, 278
   porcelain, 277
   siliceous earth, 278
   sintered-glass, 278
Filtration, bacterial, 277
   pressure, 280
   vacuum, 280
First-order reaction, 250, 258, 261, 265, 268
Flavor, 177
Flocculation, 307, 320, 343
Flow, dilatant, 306
   Newtonian, 302
   plastic, 305, 364
   pseudoplastic, 305
Fluidextracts, 245
Folding of divided powders, 63
Force, compressional, on tablets, 80
   affect on apparent density, 80

affect on disintegration, 83
affect on hardness, 82
affect on porosity, 81
affect on surface area, 80
Free energy, 154
Freezing-point depression, 192
    constant, 193
Freundlich adsorption isotherm, 22
Fumagillin, second-order oxidation of, 268
Fusion, in preparing ointments, 370, 371
    in preparing suppositories, 384

Gas, constant, 154
    ideal and real, 153
Gastric fluid, simulated, 83
Gel, 320
    structure, 320
Gelatin, 298, 320, 350
Geometric dilution, 38
Gibbs equation, 309
Gifford's buffer solution, 235
Glycerin suppositories, 389
Glycerinated gelatin, 385
Gold number, 316
Granulation, effervescent, 65
    of tablets, 75
Granules, 64

Half-life, 251
Hardness, 82
Hatch-Choate equations, 9, 13
Heat of solution, 147
Hemolysis, 196
Henderson-Hasselbalch equation, 225
Henry's law, 155
Hofmeister series, 315
Homatropine methyl bromide, second-order hydrolysis of, 255
Homogenizer, 333
Humectant, 371
Hydrates, 133, 152
Hydration of colloids, 349
    of ions, 151
    of skin, 373
Hydrogen bonding, 109, 144
    affect on physical constants, 121, 145, 147
    intermolecular, 145
    intramolecular, 121
Hydrogen ion concentration, 213
    and pH, 213
Hydrolysis, 257
    degree of, 224
    protection from, 262
    rate of, 257
Hydrophile-lipophile balance (HLB), 310, 338
    tables,
Hygroscopicity, 130

i factor, 195
Ideal gas law, 154
Imbibition, 131, 320
Implant, 34, 74
Induced dipole, 111
Inductive effect, 107, 143
Inhalers, 323
Injections, 283
    emulsion, 357

preparation, 285
solution, 283
suspension, 347
types, 283
Insufflations, 62, 323
Insulin activity vs. size, 32
Interionic attractive forces, 111
Intermolecular force, 113
    attraction, 107
    dipole-dipole, 107, 143
    induced dipole-dipole, 148
    induced dipole-induced dipole, 111, 142
    ion-dipole, 133
    ion-induced dipole, 111
    van der Waals, 111, 142
Intestinal fluid, simulated, 83
Invert sugar, 173
Ionic, equilibria, 209
    mobility, 183
    strength, 189
Ionization, 209
    constants, 210, 215
    of water, 214
    of weak acids, 210
    of weak bases, 211
Isoelectric point, 350
Isotonic solutions, 196
    tables, 198, 200, 208

Kinetics, 250
Kohlrausch law, 186

L values, 198
$L_{iso'}$, 197
Lacrimal fluid, 233
Langmuir adsorption isotherm, 23
Lecithin, 359
Levigation, 37
Lewis electronic theory, 209
Light, affect on stability, 269
Liniment, 357
Liquefaction of solid mixtures, 117
Logarithm, 396, back cover
Lozenges, 72
Lubricants, 68, 76
Lyophilization, 48, 123

Maceration, 242
Magmas, 321
Marc, 241
Mass-action law, 210
Mathematics, review of, 395
Mean, arithmetic, 4
    geometirc, 8
Melting point, 116
    and intermolecular forces, 111
    of binary systems, 118
Mestatable form, 126
Methylcellulose, 318, 351
Micelle, 314, 319
    critical concentration, 314
    solubilization by, 314
Milliequivalents, 140
Mills, 38
    ball, 41
    colloid, 44, 332

fluid-energy, 45
hammer, 42
micronizer, 45
roll, 42
table of, 46
Mixers, 54, 162
blade and paddle, 164
change can, 369
colloid mill, 44, 332
homogenizer, 333
planetary, 369
tumbler, 54
turbine, 163, 331
V blender, 54, 57
Mixing, by geometric dilution, 38
liquid-liquid, 340
liquid-solid, 55, 331
solid-solid, 51
Mobility, ionic, 183
Moist-heat sterilization, 274
Moisture, atmospheric, 130
Molality, 140
Molded solids, 70
Mole fraction, 140
Molecule, affect of structure on physical properties, 142
cross-sectional area of, 309
length of, 309
water, 133
Moment, dipole, 108
Monotropic polymorph, 126
Montomorillonite clays, 354
Morphine oxidative degradation of, 266
Mucilages, 318

Nernst equation, 247
Neutralization curve, 226
Newtonian flow, 302
Non-Newtonian flow, 304
Nonpolar solvents, 146, 238
Normal distribution, 4
Normality, 139
Noyes-Whitney equation, 28, 158
Number of degrees of freedom, 118

Ointments 365
emulsion type, 370
oleaginous, 366
ophthalmic, 369
preparation by fusion, 366, 371
preparation by incorporation, 368
release from, 374
rheology of, 364, 367
suspension type, 366
washable, 371
water soluble, 368
Oleoresins, 246
Ophthalmic ointments, 369
Order of reactions, 250
first, 250, 259, 261, 265
higher, 254
second, 255, 269
zero, 254, 272
Osmosis, 194
Osmotic pressure, 194
of electrolytes, 195
van't Hoff equation, 195

Ostwald viscometer, 303
Oxidation, 266

Packaging, 64, 124, 131, 133, 171, 265, 266, 365
Packing, close st, 15
open, 16
Palitzsch buffer, 236
Parenteral injections, 283
emulsions, 357
solutions, 283
suspensions, 347
sterility of, 289
types, 283
Partial vapor pressure, 155,
Particle, 1
affect of size on therapeutic action, 30, 103
diameters, 1, 4, 5, 8, 10
influence of size on properties of, 19, 27, 30, 39, 52
reduction of, 37
shape, 1, 51
size frequency distribution, 3, 5, 8
Particle size measurement, 11
Andreasen pipet, 14
microscope, 11
sieves, 11
Partition coefficient, 247, 357, 362, 372, 389
Pastes, 366
Pencillin G procaine, blood level and particle size, 33, 34
hydrolysis of, 264
parenteral suspension of, 348
rheology of suspension of, 348
solubility and stability of, 264
suspension of, 344
Percentages, 139
Percolation, 173, 242
Percutaneous absorption,
Petrolatum, 364, 366
hydrophilic, 371
pH, 213
affect on stability, 258, 260, 262
affect on tissue, 233, 234
and solubility, 228
conversion to hydrogen ion concentration, 213
determination of, 231
equation for indicator solution, 231
equation for solution of salts, 221
equation for solution of weak acid, 210
equation for solution of weak base, 211
Phase diagram, 117, 126
Phase inversion, 340
Phase rule, 117
Phase volume ratio, 370
Phenethicillin, base catalysis of, 263
pH profile, 262
Photolysis, 269
Pills, 71
pK_a, 215
pK_b, 215
pK_w, 215
Planetary mixer, 369
Plastic flow, 305, 364
Plastic viscosity, 305
Poise, 301
Poiseuille's equation, 302
Polar, groups, 149
solvents, 146, 238

Polarity, 146
Polarizability, 143
Polyethylene glycols, 368, 386
Polymorphism, 124, 384
    cortisone acetate, 125
    enantiotropic, 126
    monotropic, 126
    theobroma oil, 129, 384
    transition, 125
Polyoxyl 40 stearate, 361
Polysorbate 80, 361
Porosity, 17, 80
Potential, electrokinetic, 297
    zeta, 297
Powder, 1
    bulkiness of, 18
    density of, 17
    fineness of, 30
    flammability of, 39
    flow properties of, 18
    packing of, 15
    particle size measurement, 11
    porosity of, 17
    repose angle of, 18
Powders, bulk, 60
    divided, 63
    dusting, 61
    effervescent, 65
    hygroscopic drugs, 131
    insufflation, 62
    liquefaction of, 116
    mixing of, 51
    water of crystallizing in,
Prescription balance, 59
Preservatives, 288, 292, 319, 362, 363
Preserving quality of sucrose, 174
Propellants, 326
Protective colloids, 315
Pseudoplastic flow, 305
Pulverization, factors affecting, 38
    abrasion, 38
    composition, 41
    flammability, 39
    temperature, 40
    toxicity, 41
    size, 39
Pyrogens, 170, 290

Raoult law, 155
Rate constants, 250, 254
Rate equations, 250, 254
Reactions, 250
    bimolecular, 250, 268
    factors influencing, 257
    half-life of, 251
    orders of, 250, 254, 168
    photochemical, 269
    unimolecular, 250
Rectal absorption, 389
Reference state, 187
Relative humidity, 135
Repose angle, 18
Resins, 246
Resistance, specific, 185
Rheology, 301
    of ointments, 364, 367
    of solutions, 301
    of suspensions, 347
    significance of, 343, 365

Salting out, 171
Salts, of strong acids and weak bases, 223
    of weak acids and strong bases, 222
    of weak acids and weak bases, 223
    pH of solutions of, 221
    solubility of, 151
Saturated solutions, 140
Schulze-Hardy rule, 298
Second-order reaction, 255, 268
Sedimentation, 306
    and Brownian movement, 306
    and caking, 341
    rate, 306, 342
    ratio, 307
Selective adsorption of ions, 297
Sensitivity requirement, 59
Sieve, analysis, 11
    Tyler series, 12
    U.S. Standard, 12
Size frequency distribution, 3, 5, 8, 13
Skin, 372
Slugging, 79
Soaps, 359
Sodium carboxymehoylcellulose, 353
Sodium chloride equivalent, 199
    derivation of, 199
    tables, 200
Sodium chloride lattice, 115
Sodium lauryl sulfate, 360
Solubility, 140
    descriptive terms, 141
    expressions of, 140
    factors affecting,
    pH and, 166, 228
    product, 141
    structure and, 143, 152
    temperature and, 161
    total, 166, 229
Solubilization, 264, 314, 319
Solute-solvent interactions, 147
    dipole-dipole, 148
    induced dipole-dipole, 148
    induced dipole-induced dipole, 147
    ion-dipole, 151
Solution, 139, 174
    adjusted, 196
    aqueous, 174
    buffered, 231
    colligative properties of, 190
    ideal and real, 153, 154, 155
    isotonic, 196
    mechanism of, 142
    nonaqueous, 238
    ophthalmic, 237, 290
    parenteral, 283
    preparation of, 162
    rate of, 159
    stability of, 250
Solvents, nonpolar, 146
    polar, 146, 284
Sorensen modified phosphate buffer, 236
Specific conductance, 185

Specific resistance, 185
Specific surface, 2
Spirits, 240
Spray drying, 50
Sprays, 322
Stability of drugs, 250
    accelerated analysis of, 270
    enhancement of,
    prediction of, 269
    to hydrolysis, 257
    to oxidation, 266
    to photolysis, 269, 272
Standard deviation, 5
Steric hinderance and solubility, 147
Sterilization, 274, 286
    autoclave, 274
    bacterial filtration, 277
    dry heat, 276
    gaseous, 280
    radiation, 281
Stokes equation, 306, 342
    and creaming, 337
    and sedimentation, 306, 342
    and size determination, 14
Sublimation, 122
Sugar coating, 86
Sulfa drugs, 31, 93
Suppositories, 382
    bases, 383
    preparation, 384, 386
    shape and size, 382
Surface, specific, 2
    tension, 20, 308
Surface-active agents, 308, 335
    anionic, 359
    as emulsifying agents, 358
    characteristics of, 334, 337, 356
    classification of, 358
    in ointments, 370
    hydrophilic-lipophilic balance of, 311
    nonionic, 361
Suspending agents, 348
    algins, 349
    bentonite, 355
    gelatin, 350
    methylcellulose, 351
    microcrystalline cellulose, 354
    sodium carboxymethylcellulose, 353
    Veegum, 365
Suspensions, 330, 341
    caking of, 28, 128, 341
    deflocculated and flocculated,
    oral, 344
    parenteral, 346
    preparation of, 330
    rheology of, 343
    sedimentation of, 342
    topical, 345
Suspension-type ointments, 366
Suspensoid, 316
Sustained release, 92
    evaluation of, 103
    types of, 100
Sutherland-Einstein equation, 300
Symbols, v
Syneresis, 320
Syringeability, 346
Syrups, 171

Table of, aerosol propellants, 327
    Atkins and Pantin buffer, 234
    boiling-point constant, 192
    Clark and Lubs buffer, 232
    colloidal properties, 316
    colloidal systems, 295
    common dyes, 181
    composition of theobroma oil, 130
    cortisone acetate polymorphs, 125
    descriptive solubility, 141
    dielectric constants, 146
    dipole moments, 108
    dissociation constants, acid, 215
    dissociation constants, base, 219
    effect of intramolecular hydrogen bonding, 121
    effect of ionic distance, 122
    effect of types of bonding, 113, 123
    electrostatic field and solubility, 152
    Feldman buffer, 235
    fineness of powders, 30
    freezing-point constant, 193
    freezing point of 1 per cent solutions, 208
    Gifford buffer, 235
    granulating agents, 75
    HLB values, 311
    heat of solution, 150
    hydrogen bonding, 110, 145, 147
    ion product of water, 214
    ionic mobility, 184
    L values, 198
    L_{iso} values, 200
    mills for fine grinding, 46
    mixers, comparison of, 334
    molecular structure on physical properties, 144
    ophthalmic preservatives, 292
    Palitzsch buffer, 236
    preservatives, 363
    sodium chloride equivalents, 200
    Sorensen modified buffer, 236
    sterilization methods, 286
    transference numbers, 184
    U.S. Standard sieves, 12
    viscometer range, 303
    viscosity, definitions of, 304
    volume of injection, 287
    weight variation, 80
Tablet, 73
    buccal, 74, 83
    coated, 86
    disintegration of, 76
    hardness of, 82
    hypodermic, 71
    lubricant for, 76
    molded, 70
    precompression preparation of, 79
    preparation of, 74, 79
    slugging preparation of, 79
    sublingual, 74
    testing of, 70
    triturate, 80
    weight variation of, 80
    wet granulation of, 74
Tablet machine, 77

Tastes, 177
Temperature, affect on reaction rate, 256
    affect on vapor pressure, 155
    affect on viscosity, 304
Tension, interfacial, 308
Tetracycline, 31
Thiamine, stability of,
Thixotropy, 305, 365
Tinctures, 243
Transference numbers, 183
Triethanolamine soaps,
Triple point, 124
Trituration, 37
Troches, 72
Tube, collapsible, ointment, 365
Tyndall effect, 296

Ultraviolet light, 281

Vaginal insert, 74, 382
Van der Waals equation, 154
Van der Waals force, 111, 142
Van't Hoff equation, 195
Van't Hoff *i* factor, 195
Vanishing cream, 371
Vapor pressure, 155
    lowering of, 190
    partial, 155
Vials, 287
Viscosity, 301
    definitions, 304
    affect of temperature, 304
Void, 17
Volatility of solids, 122
    affect of type of bonding on, 123

Washable ointments, 371
Water, 170
    aromatic, 170
    in crystals, 133
    ion product of, 214
    structure of, 133
    types of water, 170
Weight-variation test, 80
Wet granulation, 75
Wetting agents, 313
Work of emulsification, 335
Wurster apparatus, 90

Yield value, 305, 364

Zero-order reaction, 254, 269
Zeta potential, 297
Zwitterion, 298